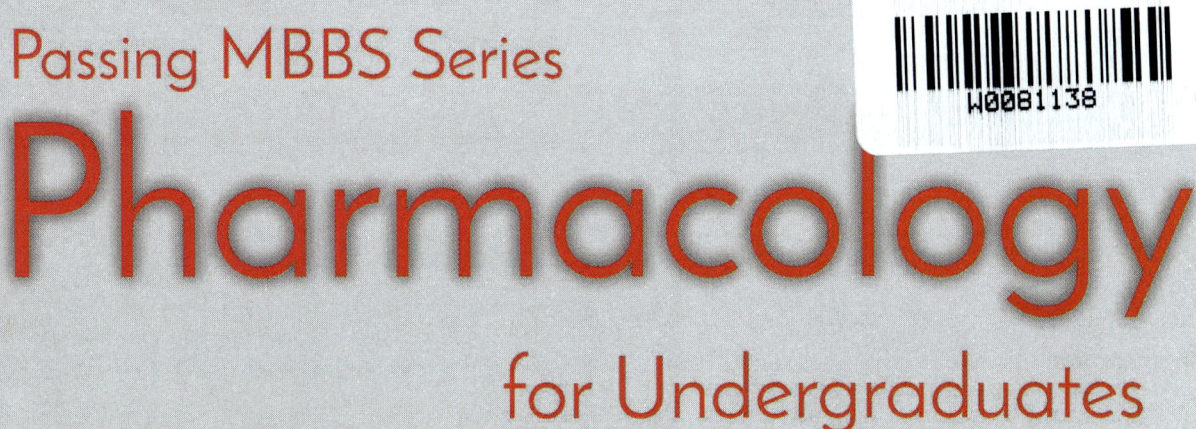

Passing MBBS Series

Pharmacology

for Undergraduates

Yogesh Gulati MBBS, MD

MBBS (King George Medical College, Lucknow)
MD (Pharmacology, King George Medical College, Lucknow)

Sumit Verma MBBS, MD, DNB

MBBS (Maulana Azad Medical College, New Delhi)
MD (Anaesthesia, Vardhman Mahavir Medical College & Safdarjang Hospital, New Delhi)
DNB (Anaesthesiology, National Board of Examinations, New Delhi)

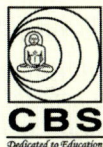

CBS
Dedicated to Education

CBS Publishers & Distributors Pvt Ltd

• New Delhi • Bengaluru • Chennai • Kochi • Mumbai
• Hyderabad • Kolkata • Nagpur • Patna • Vijayawada

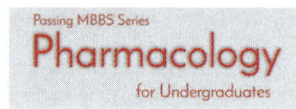

ISBN: 978-93-88108-85-0

Copyright © Publishers

First Edition: 2019

All rights reserved. No part of this book may be reproduced or transmitted in any form or by any means, electronic or mechanical, including photocopying, recording, or any information storage and retrieval system without permission, in writing, from the publishers.

Published by **Satish Kumar Jain** and produced by **Varun Jain** for
CBS Publishers & Distributors Pvt Ltd

4819/XI Prahlad Street, 24 Ansari Road, Daryaganj, New Delhi 110 002, India.
Ph: +91-11-23289259, 23266861, 23266867   Website: www.cbspd.com
Fax: 011-23243014
e-mail: delhi@cbspd.com; cbspubs@airtelmail.in.

Corporate Office: 204 FIE, Industrial Area, Patparganj, Delhi 110 092
Ph: +91-11-4934 4934   Fax: 4934 4935
e-mail: feedback@cbspd.com; bhupesharora@cbspd.com

Branches

- **Bengaluru:** Seema House 2975, 17th Cross, K.R. Road,
  Banasankari 2nd Stage, Bengaluru 560 070, Karnataka
  Ph: +91-80-26771678/79   Fax: +91-80-26771680   e-mail: bangalore@cbspd.com

- **Chennai:** 7, Subbaraya Street, Shenoy Nagar, Chennai 600 030,
  Tamil Nadu
  Ph: +91-44-26680620, 26681266   Fax: +91-44-42032115   e-mail: chennai@cbspd.com

- **Kochi:** Ashana House, No. 39/1904, AM Thomas Road, Valanjambalam, Ernakulam 682 018, Kochi, Kerala
  Ph: +91-484-4059061-65   Fax: +91-484-4059065   e-mail: kochi@cbspd.com

- **Kolkata:** 6/B, Ground Floor, Rameswar Shaw Road, Kolkata-700 014, West Bengal
  Ph: +91-33-22891126, 22891127, 22891128   e-mail: kolkata@cbspd.com

- **Mumbai:** 83-C, Dr E Moses Road, Worli, Mumbai-400018, Maharashtra
  Ph: +91-22-24902340/41   Fax: +91-22-24902342   e-mail: mumbai@cbspd.com

Representatives

•	**Hyderabad**	+91-9885175004	•	**Nagpur**	+91-9021734563	•	**Patna**	+91-9334159340
•	**Pune**	+91-9623451994	•	**Vijayawada**	+91-9000660880			

Printed at:

Dedication

Disclaimer

From Publisher's Desk

Dear Readers

I extend my heartfelt welcome to you to the fifth successful year of CBS Exam Books. It has been an amazing journey so far and I am highly grateful for your support and cooperation to help us achieve various milestones in this whole span of time. The mission with which we started in 2015 was to bring nothing but the best of everything to our target audience and today I am proud to say that we have maintained that standard and aspire to continue the same in future as well.

Every single title under the banner of CBS Exam Books has been developed and nurtured like an infant. The authors and our complete team work day and night to bring you the best in everything. Be it content, presentation, social media contests and offers, we strive to meet your expectations with every passing year and your trust has motivated us to maintain and upgrade ourselves all this time. I am extremely grateful to all our authors who are the real pillars of our complete series of CBS Exam Books. Their contribution is the foundation stone of CBS Exam Books.

I am reminded of these lines by Drake,

"Sometimes it's the journey that teaches you a lot about your destination".

We have grown and changed with the passage of every single year to upgrade our ways of providing our readers with maximum benefits and help them effectively manage their time and efforts. 2018 was a year of great achievements. Let me walk you through our successful journey of last year.

○ Most of the titles of CBS Exam Books received wide acceptance and recognition in being the best by the readers. To mention a few, SARP Anatomy, CRISP, Surgery Sixer, Complete Review of Pathology, Conceptual Review of Pharmacology, SOCH, Forensic Medicine, Complete Review of Medicine, Conceptual Review of PSM, MICRONS, My PGMEE Notes, AIIMS Med Easy and PRIMEs. With your constant support and our consistent efforts, I am sure that we will together witness an exponential acceptance of all CBS Exam Books in 2019.

○ The social presence of CBS Exam Books has broadened in 2018 through Facebook. We received great appreciation for our regular Facebook activities and contests like Free Complimentary copies of our books, Bid 2 Win, Fastest Finger First, Book Fair and Social Community Awards. To make 2019 more exciting and engaging for you all, we are expanding ourselves through a YouTube channel, Instagram and Telegram along with Facebook. Join us on all these platforms and enjoy our exciting offers and benefits.

Every book is incomplete if it does not have the right readers. We value you and your feedbacks. Please share your feedbacks and suggestions directly with me at bhupesharora@cbspd.com. We promise to deliver in our books, what you desire to see. I would like to sum up with these lines of Robert Frost:

Woods are lovely dark and deep,
But I have promises to keep.
And miles to go before I sleep,
And miles to go before I sleep!

Wishing you success in all your endeavors!

Bhupesh Arora
Vice President – Publishing & Marketing
(PGMEE Division)
Email: bhupesharora@cbspd.com
Mobile: (+91) 9555590180

Preface

Pharmacology is a complex subject with many important aspects related to the drugs such as their uses, mechanisms of action, classifications, adverse effects, interactions, etc. This makes the subject difficult to understand, comprehend and most importantly, difficult to remember.

During interactions with the students (both undergraduate and postgraduate), their problems and challenges were predominantly identified and were found to be related to the vastness and complexity of this subject. Such challenges often increase manifold prior to the examinations, when it is nearly impossible to remember all the drug names and their associated pharmacological features.

This motivated us to author **Pharmacology for Undergraduates** under Passing MBBS Series that summarizes and presents this challenging subject into basic elements while keeping intact all the important topics that are needed by the undergraduate students.

The current book is designed with a vision of being an examination-oriented preparatory manual. The content is presented in a concise, clear, point-wise and clutter-free manner.

Huge number of tables, figures and flowcharts have been incorporated to facilitate easy understanding, fast review and quick revision immediately before the examinations.

We would like to thank **Mr Satish Kumar Jain** (Chairman) and **Mr Varun Jain** (Managing Director), M/s CBS Publishers and Distributors Pvt Ltd for providing me the platform in bringing out the book. We have no words to describe the role, efforts, inputs and initiatives undertaken by **Mr Bhupesh Arora,** (Vice President- Publishing and Marketing, PGMEE and Nursing Division) for helping and motivating us.

We sincerely thank the entire CBS team for the creative fully colored presentation. We thank Dr Mrinalini Bakshi (Editorial Head and Content Strategist) for her editorial support and Ms Nitasha Arora (Production Head & Content Strategist), Dr Anju Dhir (Senior Scientific Coordinator/Editor), Mr Nitish Dubey (Senior Editor) and all the production team members Mr Ashutosh Pathak, Mr Prakash Gaur, Mr Phool Kumar, Mr Bunty Kashyap, Mr Chaman Lal, Ms Tahira Parveen, Ms Babita Verma, Mr Chander, Mr Raju Sharma, Mr Manoj Chaudhary, Mr Vikram Chaudhary, Mr Manoj Malakar and Ms Manorama for devoting laborious hours in designing and typesetting of the book.

We are also grateful to all the individuals who have directly or indirectly contributed towards the authoring and publication of this book.

We would love to hear from the students regarding their feedback and suggestions for improvement, so that it may benefit numerous students over the years to come.

Yogesh Gulati
Sumit Verma

Contents

SECTION C   **DRUGS ACTING ON THE CARDIOVASCULAR SYSTEM**

SECTION D — DRUGS ACTING ON THE CENTRAL NERVOUS SYSTEM

SECTION E   DRUGS USED FOR ANESTHESIA

SECTION G — DRUGS ACTING ON THE RESPIRATORY SYSTEM

SECTION H — DRUGS ACTING ON THE ENDOCRINE PHYSIOLOGY

SECTION K   **DRUGS ACTING ON THE GASTROINTESTINAL SYSTEM**

SECTION L   ANTIMICROBIALS

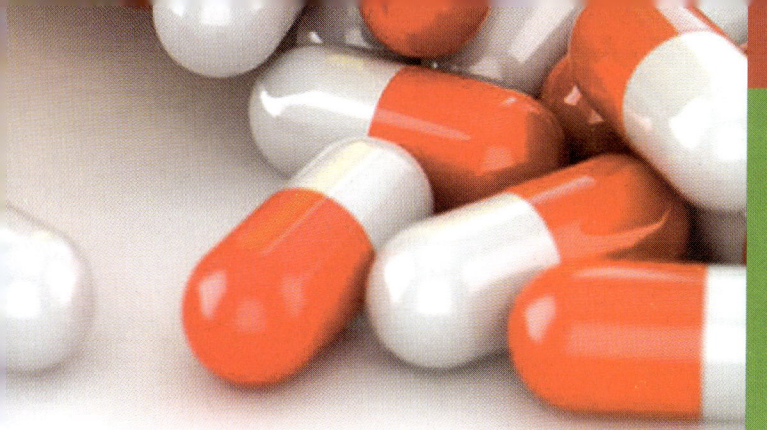

General Pharmacology

SECTION OUTLINE

1 Introduction and General Principles

INTRODUCTION

Pharmacology is the branch of science that deals with the effects of drugs on living beings and the effects of living beings on the drugs. The two key subdivisions of pharmacology are pharmacokinetics and pharmacodynamics (Figure 1).

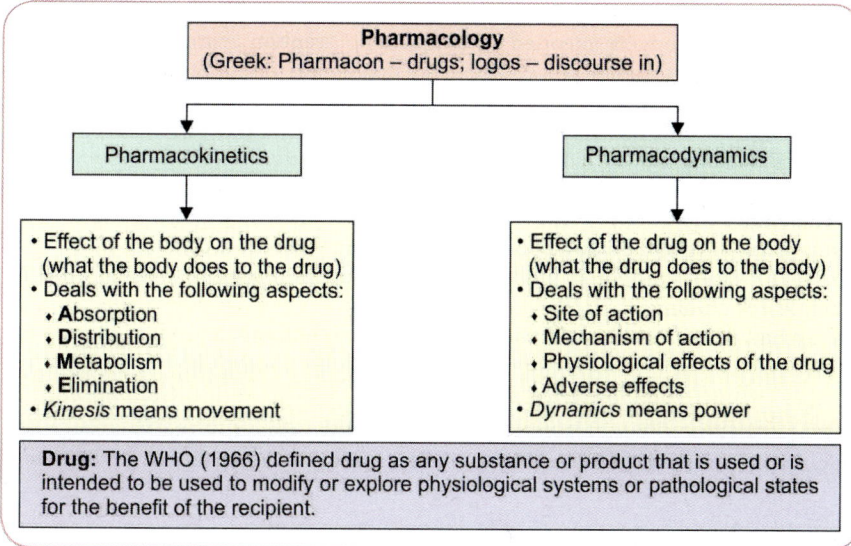

Figure 1: Pharmacology

Clinical Pharmacology

It deals with the study of drugs in human beings. Some of the key factors in clinical pharmacology include:

- Clinical evaluation of new drug in patients and in healthy volunteers
- Assessment of the clinical efficacy and safety of a drug in comparative clinical trials
- Postmarketing safety surveillance
- Patterns of drug use.

Chemotherapy

It is the treatment of systemic infections/malignancies with drugs that demonstrate selective toxicity towards the offending organism/malignant cells with limited or minimal toxicity to the host cell.

Essential Medicines

The WHO defines essential medicines as those that satisfy the priority health care needs of the population. The following factors are considered for selection of essential medicines:

- Prevalence of disease
- Relevance to public health

- Cost effectiveness and comparative costs
- Adequate evidence of safety and efficacy

The essential medicines should be available all the time in the required quantities, having assured quality, in appropriate dosage forms at a cost-effective price.

The list of essential medicines is available at the WHO website and contains medicines such as atropine, dexamethasone, phenytoin, epinephrine, amoxicillin, etc.

Prescription Drugs

These drugs can only be obtained by producing a prescription from a licensed medial practitioner. The examples include benzodiazepines (diazepam), antibiotics (azithromycin), etc.

Nonprescription Drugs (Over the Counter Drugs)

These drugs can be obtained by the patient directly without the need of a prescription from a licensed medial practitioner.

Orphan Drugs

Orphan drugs are medicinal products intended for diagnosis, prevention or treatment of rare diseases. A rare disease is any disease that affects a small percentage of the population (e.g. in Europe, a rare disease is a disease that affects less than 1 in 2,000 citizens).

Some regulatory agencies provide incentives to the drug manufacturers for developing therapies for rare diseases. Some of these benefits may include:

- Market exclusivity—meaning that other manufacturers cannot place similar products in the market for a specific time duration
- Assistance in protocol development to aid in clinical development of the drug
- Reduction in fees for various regulatory procedures such as authorizations
- Assistance in research funding

Examples of the orphan drugs include nelarabine for acute lymphoblastic leukemia, riluzole for amyotrophic lateral sclerosis etc.

Pharmacotherapeutics

It is the application of pharmacological information and disease information in diagnosis, treatment or prevention of a disease.

Pharmacy

It is a branch of science that deals with manufacture, preservation, compounding, dispensing, standardization, quality control and optimal utilization of drugs.

Pharmacovigilance

It is the science and activities relating to the detection, assessment, understanding and prevention of adverse effects or any other medicine-related problem. (The importance of pharmacovigilance: Safety monitoring of medicinal products. Genève: WHO; 2002)

In line with this general definition, the underlying objectives of pharmacovigilance in accordance with the applicable EU legislation are:

- Preventing harm from adverse reactions in humans arising from the use of authorized medicinal products within or outside the terms of marketing authorization or from occupational exposure; and
- Promoting the safe and effective use of medicinal products, in particular through providing timely information about the safety of medicinal products to patients, health care professionals and the public.

Pharmacovigilance is therefore an activity contributing to the protection of patients' and public health.

Toxicology

It is a science that deals with the biological effects of poisons along with the measures for prevention, detection and treatment of poisoning.

SOURCES OF DRUG INFORMATION

Pharmacopeia

It is a book which contains a list of officially approved drugs with their formulas, uses, preparation, dosages, tests for their strength, purity, and other related information, etc. Some of the pharmacopeias are Indian pharmacopeia (IP), British pharmacopoeia (BP), French Pharmacopoeia (Ph.Fr.), United States Pharmacopeia (USP) etc.

Formulary

A formulary is a list of medications that are approved to be prescribed in a particular health system or under a particular health insurance policy. The development of prescription formularies is based on evaluations of efficacy, safety, cost-effectiveness of drugs, side effects, contraindications and doses.

Other sources of drug information also include published literature, standard medical textbooks, Martindale, product monographs, prescribing information available from the drug manufacturers etc.

DRUG NOMENCLATURE

There are generally three types of drug names (Figure 2).

Drug nomenclature (Naming of drugs) There are generally three types of drug names		
Chemical name	**Generic or nonproprietary name**	**Brand or proprietary name**
• Chemical description of a substance • Usually follows the standards defined by IUPAC (International Union of Pure and Applied Chemistry) • Difficult to use in routine clinical practice as they are usually long and complex • Code names may be given by companies for drugs in the development phase	• Name assigned by a competent scientific body/council such as: ♦ United States Adopted Name (USAN) council ♦ British Approved Name (BAN) council • International nonproprietary name (INN) is a generic/official name that is given to a drug or active ingredient. The World Health Organization coordinates the granting of the INN • A nonproprietary name is also called an official name once it appears in a pharmacopeia • Advantages of use of generic name include standardization of drug name, ease of understanding etc.	• Name assigned to a drug by a pharmaceutical company • These names are a trademark or a property of the manufacturer • The brand names differ across manufacturers and may also differ across countries with same manufacturer • Usually are short and easy to remember
Drug nomenclature for paracetamol		
Chemical name	**Generic or nonproprietary name**	**Brand or proprietary name**
N-acetyl-p-aminophenol	Paracetamol (also known as acetaminophen)	Crocin® Calpol® Panadol®

Figure 2: Drug nomenclature

SOURCES OF DRUGS

The sources of drugs along with some examples are shown in Figure 3.

Sources of drugs	
Plants	• Alkaloids – names usually end with 'ne' ◆ Morphine from *Papaverum somniferum* ◆ Atropine from *Atropa belladonna* • Glycosides – sugar moiety and a nonsugar moiety are joined ◆ Digoxin from *Digitalis purpurea*
Minerals	• Ferrous sulfate for use in anemia • Magnesium sulfate for use as a purgative
Animals	• Hormones (insulin from pork pancreas) • Vitamins (B_{12} from liver)
Microorganisms	• Penicillin from *Penicillium notatum* • Griseofulvin from *Penicillium griseofulvum*
Semisynthetic	• Diamorphine • Buprenorphine
Synthetic	• Fentanyl, alfentanil • Paracetamol, phenytoin
Genetic engineering/ biotechnology	• Recombinant hepatitis B vaccine • Human erythropoietin • Human insulin

Many of the drugs available today are either from a semisynthetic or the synthetic source. The advantages include a better control on the quality and process of manufacturing. Also, appropriate modifications (as required) can be made in the structure to identify a more efficacious drug having a better safety profile

Figure 3: Sources of drugs

ROUTES OF DRUG ADMINISTRATION

A route of administration is the path by which a drug or other substance is taken into the body.

Most drugs can be administered by different routes. The following drug- and patient-related factors are considered while determining a particular route of administration (Figure 4).

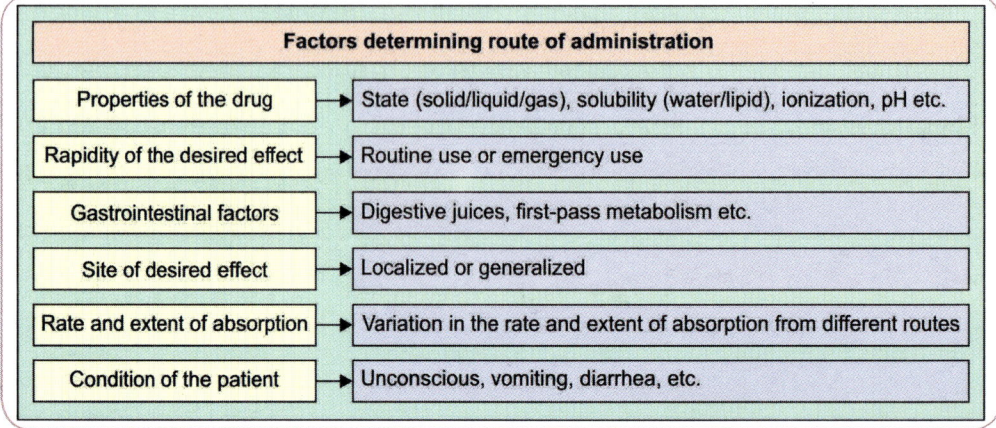

Factors determining route of administration	
Properties of the drug	State (solid/liquid/gas), solubility (water/lipid), ionization, pH etc.
Rapidity of the desired effect	Routine use or emergency use
Gastrointestinal factors	Digestive juices, first-pass metabolism etc.
Site of desired effect	Localized or generalized
Rate and extent of absorption	Variation in the rate and extent of absorption from different routes
Condition of the patient	Unconscious, vomiting, diarrhea, etc.

Figure 4: Factors determining route of administration

The major routes of administration can be classified as those for local action and those for systemic action (Figure 5).

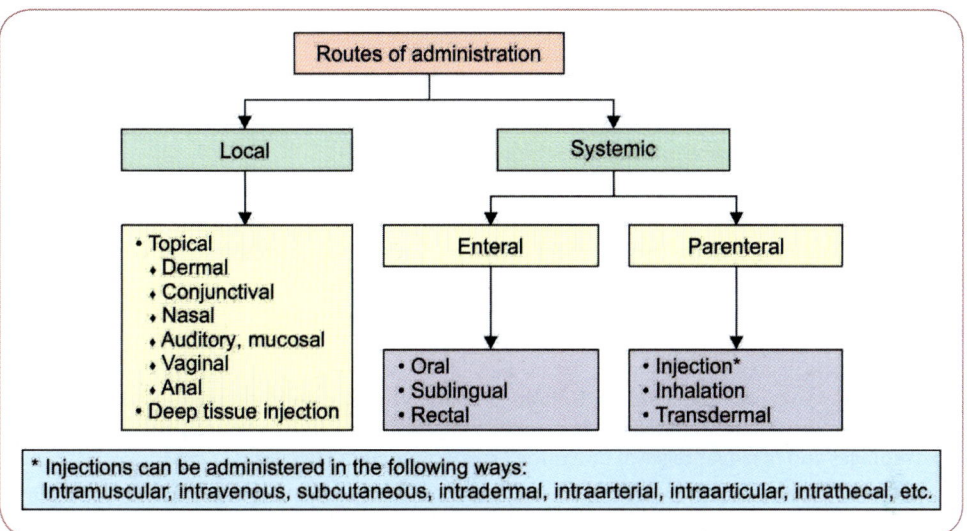

Figure 5: Routes of administration

Local Route

It is one of the simplest methods of drug administration. The drug is applied directly at the site where the effect is desired. The advantage of local application is that high concentration of the drug is attained at the desired site and systemic adverse effects are reduced.

The local routes are as follows:

Topical

The drug is applied to the surface (skin or mucous membrane) for localized action. It is often convenient for the patient.

The various type of topical applications commonly employed are mentioned in Table 1.

TABLE 1	Topical preparations
Location	**Preparations commonly used**
• Skin	As cream, ointment, lotion, powder (e.g. clotrimazole cream, powder)
• Mucous membranes	
▪ Eyes, ears, nose	As drops, ointment, spray (e.g. ciprofloxacin eye/ear drops)
▪ Mouth and pharynx	As paint, mouthwash, ointment, cream (e.g. lignocaine ointment, acyclovir cream)
▪ Gastrointestinal tract	As nonabsorbable drug (e.g. neomycin, sucralfate)
▪ Bronchi	As inhalational (e.g. salbutamol, cromolyn sodium)
▪ Urethra	As jelly (e.g. lignocaine jelly)
▪ Vagina	As pessary, cream, tablet, insert (e.g. gemeprost pessary, levonorgestrel insert)
▪ Anus	As ointment, suppository (e.g. bisacodyl suppository)

General Pharmacology ■ SECTION A

Deep Tissue Injection

The drugs are administered directly into the deeper issues by injection e.g. intra-articular steroid (triamcinolone) injection in the joint space.

Systemic Route

Drugs administered by this route enter blood and are distributed throughout the body, including the site of action. They are further subdivided into enteral and parenteral routes:

Enteral Routes

Enteral administration means that the drug is directly placed in any part of gastrointestinal tract. The enteral routes are further discussed below:

Oral Route

It is the most commonly used method.

The dosage forms may include solid and liquid preparations. The solid preparations may include tablet, capsule, powders etc. The liquid preparations may include syrups, emulsions, mixtures, etc.

Some advantages and disadvantages of oral route are mentioned in Figure 6.

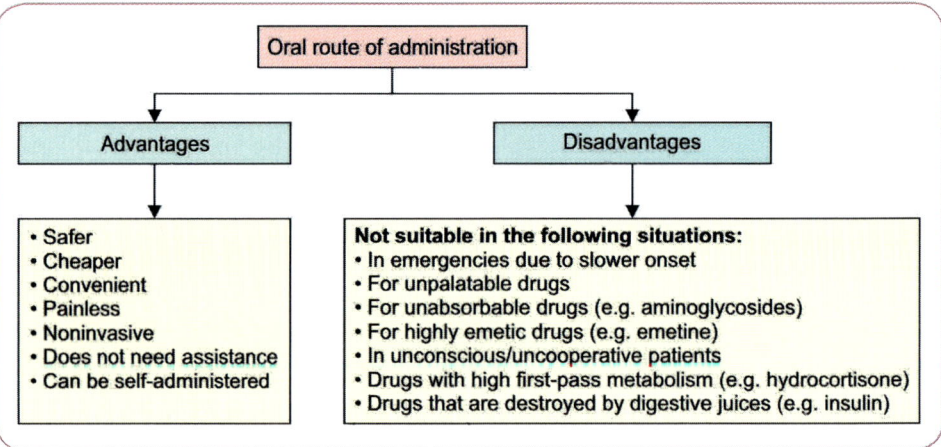

Figure 6: Oral route of administration

Sublingual Route

The tablet containing the drug is kept under the tongue. The drug diffuses into the capillary network and directly enters the systemic circulation (e.g. sublingual nitroglycerin for acute angina attack).

The buccal route (drug placed between the cheek and tongue) is equivalent to the sublingual route.

Some advantages and disadvantages of sublingual route are mentioned in Figure 7.

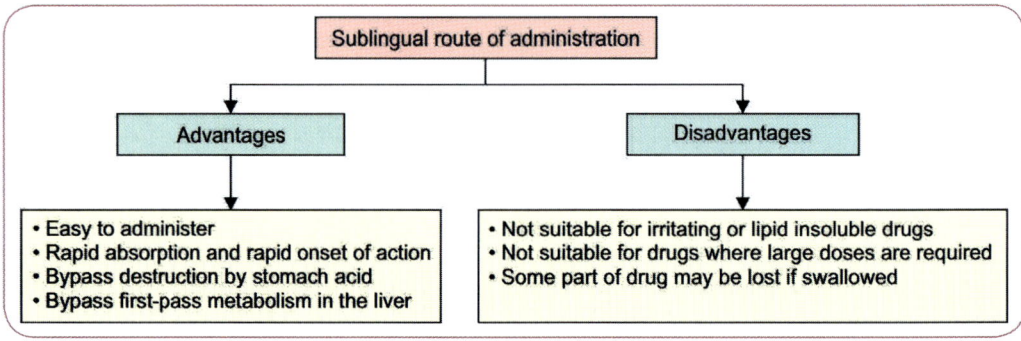

Figure 7: Sublingual route of administration

Rectal Route

Certain unpleasant drugs may be given by this route as suppositories or retention enemas for either local or systemic effect (Table 2).

TABLE 2	Rectal formulations
Local effect	• Bisacodyl and glycerin suppositories for bowel evacuation • Soap water enema for bowel evacuation • Methylprednisolone for ulcerative colitis
Systemic effect	• Indomethacin for rheumatoid arthritis • Diazepam for status epilepticus

The absorption occurs into internal and external hemorrhoidal veins. The drug absorbed into the external hemorrhoidal vein (around 50%) bypasses the liver and therefore, bypasses the first-pass metabolism.

Some advantages and disadvantages of rectal route are mentioned in Figure 8.

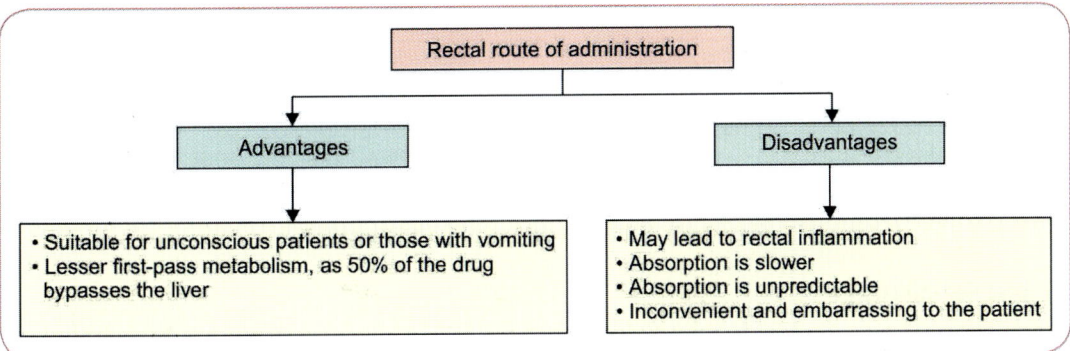

Figure 8: Rectal route of administration

Parenteral Routes

Parenteral administration means that the drug is introduced directly into the systemic circulation and does not reach the gastrointestinal tract.

Some advantages and disadvantages of parenteral route are mentioned in Figure 9.

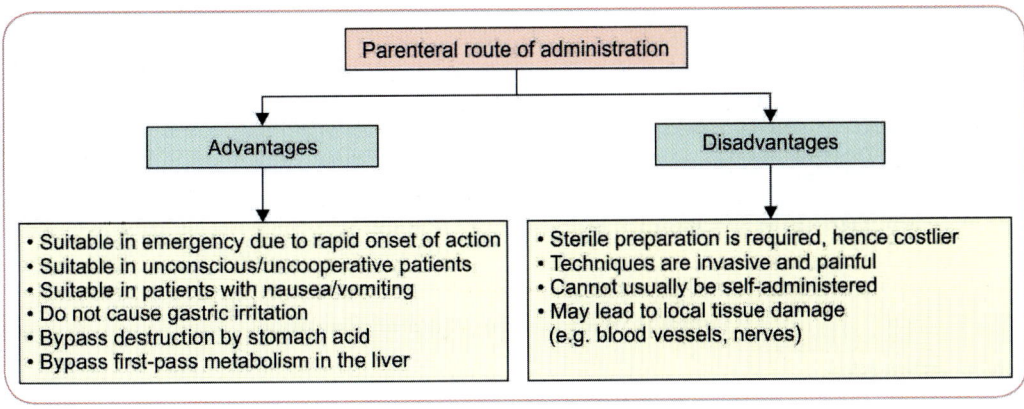

Figure 9: Parenteral route of administration

The parenteral routes are further discussed below:

Injections

Subcutaneous Injection

The drug is injected into the loose subcutaneous tissue beneath the skin. The subcutaneous tissue is richly innervated by nerves; hence, irritant drugs cannot be injected there. The drugs commonly given by this route include insulin and heparin.

Some advantages and disadvantages of subcutaneous route are mentioned in Figure 10.

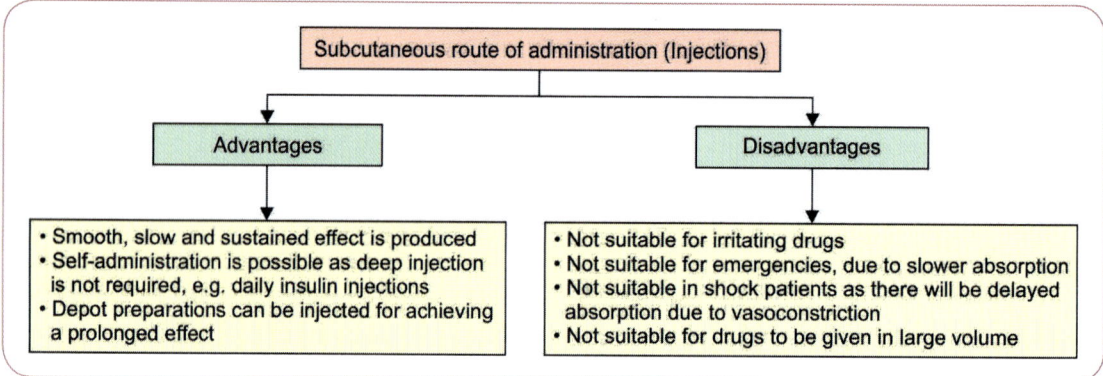

Figure 10: Subcutaneous route of administration

Intramuscular Injection

The drug is injected into one of the larger skeletal muscles, e.g. deltoid, gluteus maximus, etc. The muscles are less richly innervated by nerves; hence, some irritant drugs may be injected here.

The drugs commonly given by this route include antibiotics, neuroleptics, paracetamol, diclofenac, depot testosterone, etc.

Some advantages and disadvantages of intramuscular route are mentioned in Figure 11.

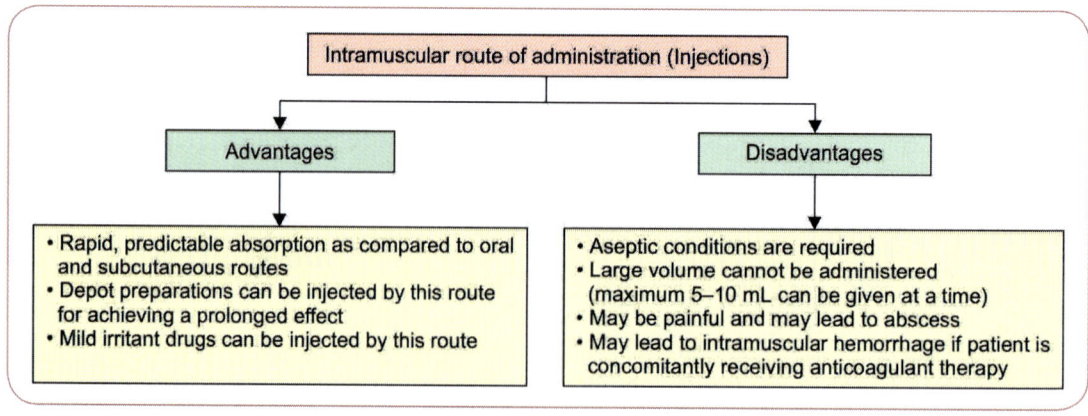

Figure 11: Intramuscular route of administration

Intravenous Injection

The drug is injected directly into one of the superficial veins as slow infusion or as bolus injection.

The drugs commonly administered by intravenous injection include antibiotics, diazepam, epinephrine, propofol, etc.

Some advantages and disadvantages of intravenous route are mentioned in Figure 12.

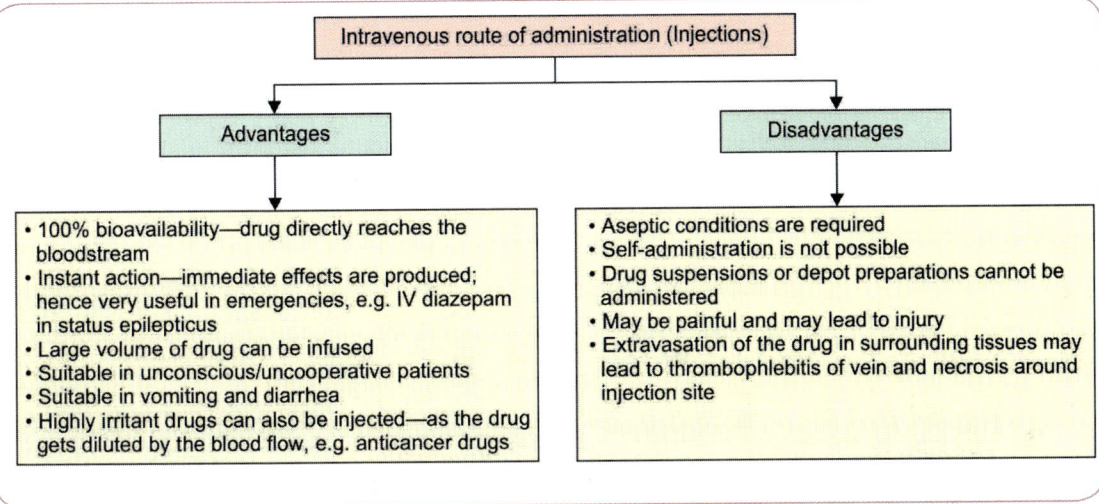

Figure 12: Intravenous route of administration

Inhalational Route of Administration

The drug is directly inhaled, and systemic action is achieved. The drugs commonly administered by inhalation include volatile gases and liquids.

Some advantages and disadvantages of inhalational route are mentioned in Figure 13.

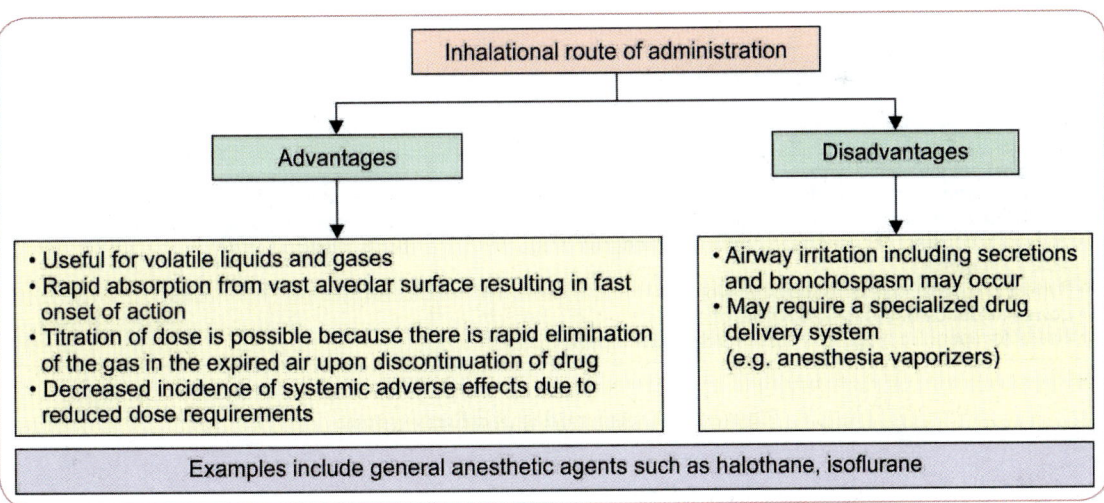

Figure 13: Inhalational route of administration

Transdermal Drug Delivery System

The transdermal drug delivery systems are designed to deliver a therapeutically effective amount of drug across the skin.

The delivery of the drug into the systemic circulation is at a constant rate and occurs via the stratum corneum.

The drug is absorbed percutaneously into the systemic circulation following diffusion at the skin surface. The various components of a transdermal drug delivery system are (Figure 14):

- Occlusive backing film
- Drug containing reservoir
- Rate controlling micropore membrane
- Adhesive layer that also contains the priming dose of the drug
- Layer that needs to be peeled off prior to application on the skin surface

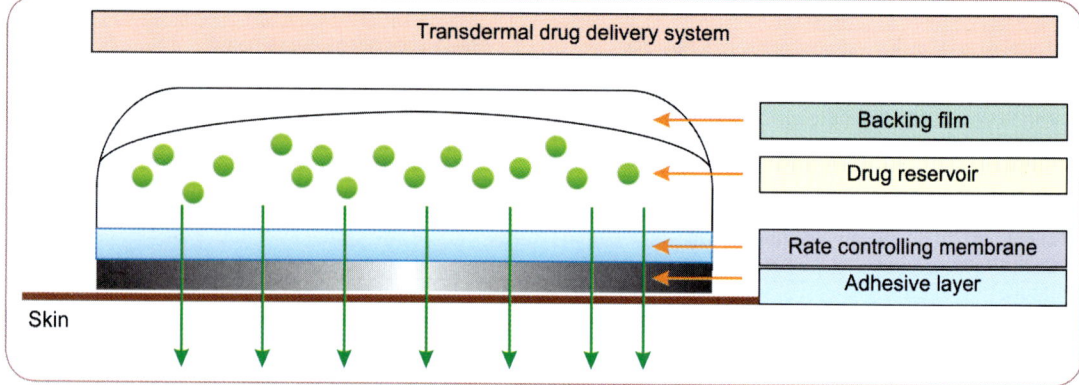

Figure 14: Transdermal drug delivery system

Some advantages and disadvantages of the transdermal drug delivery systems are mentioned in Figure 15.

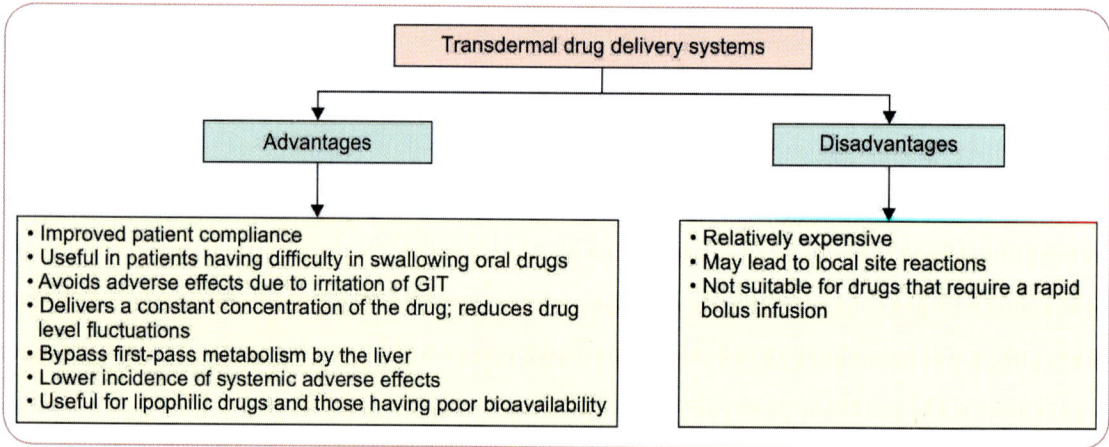

Figure 15: Transdermal drug delivery systems

SPECIAL DRUG DELIVERY SYSTEMS

The special drug delivery systems have been developed to enhance drug delivery at the target sites and to improve patient compliance (Table 3).

TABLE 3	Special drug delivery systems	
Type	**What is it?**	**Example(s)**
Progestasert	Intrauterine contraceptive device	Used for progesterone delivery

Contd...

Type	What is it?	Example(s)
Prodrug	Inactive form of the drug that gets converted to the active form in the body	Levodopa used for parkinsonism is a prodrug for dopamine—gets converted to dopamine; wherein dopamine cannot cross the blood brain barrier
Ocusert	Contains the drug in a reservoir from which the drug is released slowly	Pilocarpine ocusert—kept under the lower eyelid of glaucoma patients. It releases pilocarpine for 7 days.
Liposomes	Small vesicles made up of phospholipids that can be filled with drugs	Liposomal amphotericin B is used to treat systemic fungal infections. Liposomal preparation is less toxic and has a better adverse effect profile as compared to the conventional amphotericin B.
Monoclonal antibodies	Antibodies directed against a single antigenic determinant and produced by a single clone	• Palivizumab is used for respiratory syncytial virus infections; • Rituximab is used for non-Hodgkin's lymphoma, chronic lymphocytic leukemia
Computerized miniature pumps	Release drugs at a defined rate	Insulin pumps
Drug eluting stents	Stents that contain drugs which are released slowly (elute)	Sirolimus eluting stents

SECTION A ■ General Pharmacology

1. Name merits and demerits of rectal route of administration of drugs
2. Enumerate drugs given by intravenous route. Write advantages and disadvantage of intravenous route of administration.
3. Write advantages and disadvantages of transdermal route of administration.
4. Transdermal Drug Delivery System
5. What are advantages and disadvantages of subcutaneous route of drug administration
6. Mention different routes of drug administration with a few examples
7. Orphan drugs – define & give examples

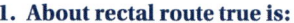

MULTIPLE CHOICE QUESTIONS

1. **About rectal route true is:**
   (Recent Question 2016)
   a. Used for irritant and unpleasant drugs
   b. Cannot be used in unconscious patient
   c. There is predictable absorption of drug
   d. Diazepam cannot be given via rectal route of administration

2. **Most variable absorption is seen with which route:** *(Recent Question 2016)*
   a. Oral
   b. Intramuscular
   c. Intravenous
   d. Per rectal

3. **True statement regarding the route of drug administration is:** *(PGI June 2004)*
   a. 80% bioavailability by IV injection
   b. IM administration needs sterile technique
   c. Intradermal injection produces local tissue necrosis and irritation
   d. Inhalational route produces delayed onset of action

4. **True about orphan drug is:** *(AIIMS May 2013)*
   a. Developed for orphans
   b. Drugs used very rarely
   c. Drugs used for rare diseases
   d. Rare drug for common diseases

5. **Essential medicines are those medicines:** *(Recent Question 2016)*
   a. That are required to manage emergency conditions
   b. That satisfy the priority healthcare needs of the population
   c. That are needed to manage serious diseases
   d. That are introduced recently into the market

Ans.

1. (a)	2. (a)	3. (b)	4. (c)	5. (b)

2 Pharmacokinetics

Pharmacokinetics is the study of drug absorption, distribution, metabolism and excretion in the body. In other words, it determines the fate of the administered drug, i.e. it is the study of how the body affects a drug. Pharmacokinetics can be depicted in Figure 1.

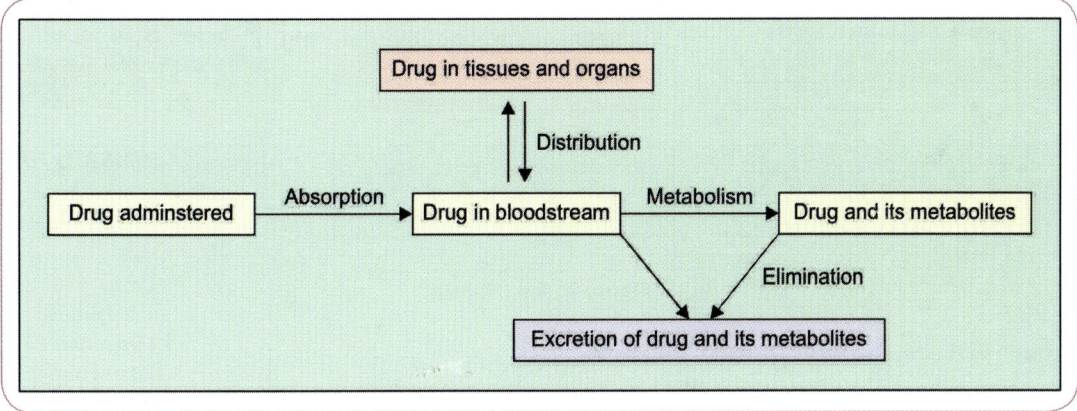

Figure 1: Pharmacokinetics

DRUG TRANSPORT ACROSS BIOLOGICAL MEMBRANES

The drug transport across various biological membranes in the body can occur through the following mechanisms:

Passive Diffusion

It is a process in which the drug molecules move across the membrane from a region of higher concentration to lower concentration (i.e. along the concentration gradient) till an equilibrium is attained.

The driving force in passive diffusion is the concentration gradient across the membrane (i.e. difference in drug concentration on either side of the membrane). The rate of diffusion is directly proportional to the degree of concentration gradient across the membrane.

The movement of the drug is passive, i.e. there is no requirement of energy. It is the most important mechanism for a majority of drugs.

The following situations require to be further mentioned:

Lipid Soluble Drugs

- Lipid soluble drugs diffuse rapidly by dissolving in the membrane lipid bilayers. The rate of diffusion depends upon the lipid solubility as well as concentration gradient across the membrane.
- The lipid soluble nonelectrolytes such as ethyl alcohol and diethyl ether rapidly cross the membranes.

Effect of pH of Surrounding Medium

- Most drugs are weak electrolytes (i.e. they are partly ionized drugs and their ionization is pH dependent). Hence, they exist as either weak acids or weak bases.
- Acidic drugs are unionized in the acidic medium and basic drugs are unionized in the basic medium. Hence, acidic drugs are better absorbed from the acidic medium and basic drugs are better absorbed from the basic medium (intestine).

The key implications of the degree of ionization and the surrounding pH are mentioned below:

Ion Trapping

Ion trapping is a phenomenon wherein a weak electrolyte on crossing a membrane encounters a particular pH, by the effect of which it gets ionized inside the cell and therefore, gets trapped in the cell. A specific example of ion trapping is mentioned in Figure 2.

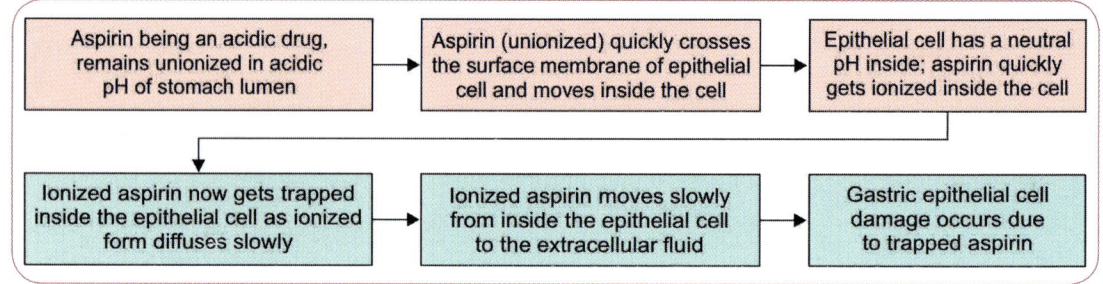

Figure 2: Ion trapping

Excretion of Acidic and Basic Drugs in the Urine

The kidney tubular membrane is a biological membrane. A lipid soluble unionized drug can be rapidly reabsorbed by passive diffusion.

Hence, by altering the pH of the urine and making the drug ionized, the reabsorption can be decreased, and the excretion can be promoted.

Thus, elevating the urine pH (i.e. making it alkaline) will fasten the excretion of acidic drugs (such as aspirin, uric acid etc.) and vice versa.

Filtration

It is the passage of drug molecules through pores in the membrane or through paracellular spaces. This passage can occur if the size of drug molecules is smaller than the size of the pores or spaces between the cells.

Specialized Transport

The specialized transport can occur by carrier mediated transport or can occur by endocytosis/exocytosis.

Carrier Mediated Transport

The transmembrane proteins function as carriers for transporting substrates (e.g. nutrients, transmitters, drugs) across the membrane.

The carrier attaches with the substrate, undergoes a conformational change and carries the substrate to the other side of the membrane.

Carrier mediated transport can be either by facilitated diffusion or by active transport (Figure 3).

Carrier mediated transport

Facilitated diffusion
- Does not require energy
- Carrier moves substrate along its electrochemical gradient
- Carrier moves substrate from higher to lower concentration
- Results in equilibrium, i.e. equal amount of substrate on both sides of the membrane
- Is saturable
- Can be inhibited competitively
- Example: Glucose transport into cells by GLUT4

Active transport
- Requires energy
- Carrier moves substrate against its electrochemical gradient
- Carrier moves substrate from lower to higher concentration
- Results in accumulation of substrate on one side of the membrane
- Is saturable
- Can be inhibited competitively
- Example: Levodopa transport (absorption) from the intestine

Active transport can be further divided into:
- **Primary active transport**—energy is obtained directly by ATP hydrolysis
- **Secondary active transport**—energy for movement of one substrate is obtained by simultaneous movement of other substrate (along its electrochemical gradient). If both move in same direction, it is called symport; if both move in opposite direction, it is called antiport.

Figure 3: Carrier mediated transport

Endocytosis/Exocytosis

This process is used to transport substrates of extremely large size across the membrane.

In this process, the substrate is engulfed (as a whole) by the cell membrane and carried inside the cell by pinching off the drug filled vesicle from the membrane. Exocytosis is the reverse process of endocytosis where substances are secreted out of the cell.

Common examples are:
- Transport of vitamin B_{12} (complexed with intrinsic factor) across the intestinal wall into the blood
- Transport of iron (in association with transferrin) into the red blood cells for hemoglobin synthesis.

ABSORPTION

Absorption is the movement of a drug from the site of its administration into the bloodstream.

The drugs given orally in solid dosage forms (tablets, capsules, etc.) should first dissolve in the aqueous phase, before they can be absorbed through a biological membrane. Hence, dissolution of the drug is a critical step in their absorption.

The drugs injected intravenously do not involve absorption as they are not required to cross any biological membrane. They directly reach the bloodstream; hence, the bioavailability is 100%.

Factors Influencing Drug Absorption

Physicochemical Properties of the Drug

Physical Form

The liquid forms (e.g. syrup/suspension) of the drug are better absorbed than solid forms (e.g. tablet/capsule).

This is because the solid forms must first dissolve before absorption can occur; hence, the rate of dissolution determines the availability of drug for absorption.

Ionization and Lipid Solubility

The unionized lipid-soluble form of the drug is better absorbed than the ionized water-soluble form.

This is because drug absorption mostly occurs by passive diffusion across the gastrointestinal (GI) membrane which is lipoidal in nature.

Particle Size

Drugs with smaller particle size have a shorter dissolution time (dissolve quickly in solution); hence, have a better rate of absorption.

In other words, smaller the particle size, faster will be the diffusion and absorption, and vice versa.

pH and Ionization

The basic concept is that the biological membranes exist in the form of a lipid bilayer.
○ The drug passes through the GI membrane more readily if it is uncharged (i.e. unionized).
○ The acidic drugs remain unionized in acidic medium and get ionized in alkaline medium.
○ The basic drugs remain unionized in alkaline (basic) medium and get ionized in acidic medium.

Hence, acidic drugs are better absorbed in acidic medium and basic drugs are better absorbed in alkaline medium.

The effect of pH and ionization on acidic and basic drugs is mentioned in Figures 4 and 5.

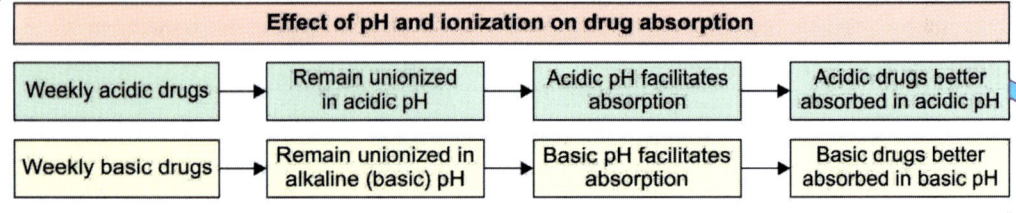

Effect of pH and ionization on drug absorption

| Weekly acidic drugs | → | Remain unionized in acidic pH | → | Acidic pH facilitates absorption | → | Acidic drugs better absorbed in acidic pH |
| Weekly basic drugs | → | Remain unionized in alkaline (basic) pH | → | Basic pH facilitates absorption | → | Basic drugs better absorbed in basic pH |

• Most drugs are either weak acids or weak bases
• A drug passes through membranes (lipid bilayers) more readily if it is uncharged (i.e. unionized)
• Acidic drugs are unionized in the acidic medium and basic drugs are unionized in the basic medium
  Hence, acidic drugs are better absorbed from the acidic medium and basic drugs are better absorbed from the basic medium (intestine)
Note: Although acidic drugs are expected to be better absorbed in the acidic medium (stomach); however, the rate of absorption for acidic drugs is higher in the intestine due to the following reasons:
  ♦ The stomach is lined with a thick mucus layer
  ♦ The stomach's surface area is small as compared to small intestine whose surface area is very large (~200 m²) due to multiple villi
• Hence, even for acidic drugs, the absorption from the stomach is slower
• The rate of absorption is therefore faster in the intestine for both acidic and basic drugs
• Therefore, any condition which increases gastric emptying increase the rate of absorption of the drugs

Figure 4: Effect of pH and ionization on drug absorption

Drug absorption scenarios

Scenario 1 Aspirin (acetylsalicylic acid) is primarily absorbed from the small intestine	Scenario 2 Lignocaine is not effective as a local anesthetic in pus/abscess

• Aspirin is an acidic drug
• It remains unionized in acidic medium (stomach) and gets ionized in alkaline medium (intestine)
• It is expected to be better absorbed from stomach; however, the reverse happens because:
  ♦ The stomach is lined with a thick mucus layer
  ♦ The stomach's surface area is small as compared to small intestine
• Hence, even for acidic drugs, the absorption is slower from the stomach
• The rate of absorption is therefore faster in the intestine for both acidic and basic drugs
	• Lignocaine is a basic drug
	• It remains unionized in alkaline medium and gets ionized in acidic medium
	• The active form of the drug is its unionized form because the unionized form can enter the cells and produce anesthetic effect
	• Pus/abscess is an acidic environment
	• If lignocaine is injected in pus/abscess, it gets ionized
	• The ionized form now cannot enter the cell membrane and cannot produce the desired anesthetic effect

Figure 5: Drug absorption scenarios

Gastric Emptying

Any factor that increases gastric emptying (lying on right side, recumbent position, increase in food temperature etc.) will likely lead to an increase in the drug absorption and vice versa.

Food

The presence of food in the stomach dilutes the drug and slows gastric emptying. Therefore, food usually decreases the absorption of many drugs.

Other Drugs

Certain drugs may affect absorption of other drugs when given together. The examples include:
- Antacids decrease the absorption of tetracyclines, iron, H_2-blockers, fluoroquinolones etc.
- Calcium decreases the absorption of tetracyclines by forming unabsorbable complexes

Total Surface Area Available for Absorption

The intestine has a much larger surface area compared to the stomach because of large number of microvilli; hence, drugs are more efficiently absorbed from the intestine.

Route of Administration

In the following situations, certain drugs cannot be given orally and must be given intravenously.
- Drugs that are highly ionized (e.g. gentamicin, neostigmine etc.) cannot be given orally as they are not absorbed from the GIT.
- Drugs that are degraded in the GIT (e.g. penicillin by acid and insulin by peptidases) cannot be given orally.

Expression of P-glycoprotein (P-Gp)

P-Gp is an efflux transporter protein that pumps certain drugs back into the intestinal lumen. This leads to low absorption of certain drugs from the GIT.

The examples include digoxin and cyclosporine which are substrates of P-Gp. Therefore, P-Gp inhibitors such as quinidine, erythromycin, verapamil, amiodarone etc. increase the bioavailability of digoxin and cyclosporine.

BIOAVAILABILITY

Bioavailability is the fraction of drug that reaches the systemic circulation in an unchanged form, following administration by any route.

For an intravenous dose, the bioavailability is 100% because all the drug directly reaches the bloodstream.

The bioavailability of an oral dose is <100% because of incomplete absorption across the intestinal wall and because of first-pass metabolism in the liver (Figure 6).

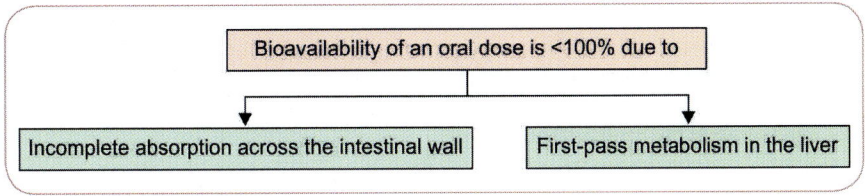

Figure 6: Bioavailability—oral dose

Factors Influencing Bioavailability of Drugs

The factors that influence drug absorption (mentioned in the preceding section) also influence the bioavailability of a drug. Apart from these, the following factors also influence the bioavailability of a drug:

SECTION A ■ General Pharmacology

First-pass Metabolism (First-pass Elimination)

The drugs when administered orally have to pass through the following sequence in the body (Figure 7).

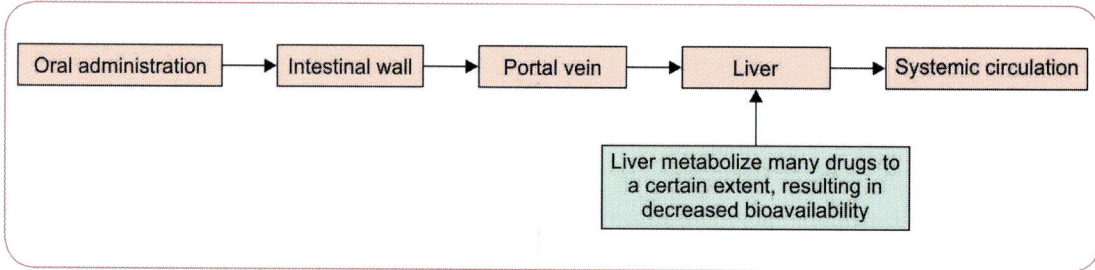

Figure 7: First-pass metabolism

During this passage, certain drugs are metabolized and inactivated in the liver (e.g. by the CYP3A4 system). Hence, a decreased concentration of the active drug reaches the systemic circulation. This results in decreased bioavailability of the drug and decreased therapeutic effect. This process is called first-pass metabolism.

Some examples of drugs with low and high oral bioavailability are mentioned in Figure 8.

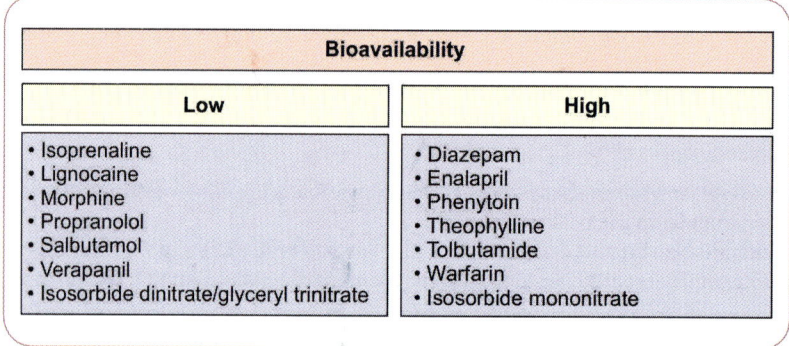

Figure 8: Bioavailability of some drugs

Features Regarding Drugs having High First-pass Metabolism

○ In drugs with high first-pass metabolism, the oral dose must be substantially higher than the parenteral dose e.g. nitroglycerine and morphine are given in high oral doses.
○ In drugs with extensive first-pass metabolism, the drugs must not to be administered orally. These drugs must be given by other routes (i.e. parenterally) e.g. lignocaine and isoprenaline are not given orally.
○ Oral bioavailability is increased if another drug which competes with the same metabolizing enzyme in the liver is given concomitantly. In this case, the oral dose should be decreased.

Enterohepatic Circulation (Enterohepatic Cycling)

It is a process where certain drugs (or their metabolites) are excreted through bile in the intestine but are subsequently reabsorbed back from the intestine into the bloodstream (e.g. digoxin, indomethacin).

In other situations, certain drug metabolites (mainly the glucuronide conjugates) are excreted through bile and delivered to the intestine. In the intestine, these conjugated metabolites are deconjugated or hydrolyzed by the intestinal bacteria releasing the parent active drug. The active drug then gets reabsorbed and reaches back to the liver (e.g. morphine, thyroxine, tetracyclines, chloramphenicol) (Figure 9).

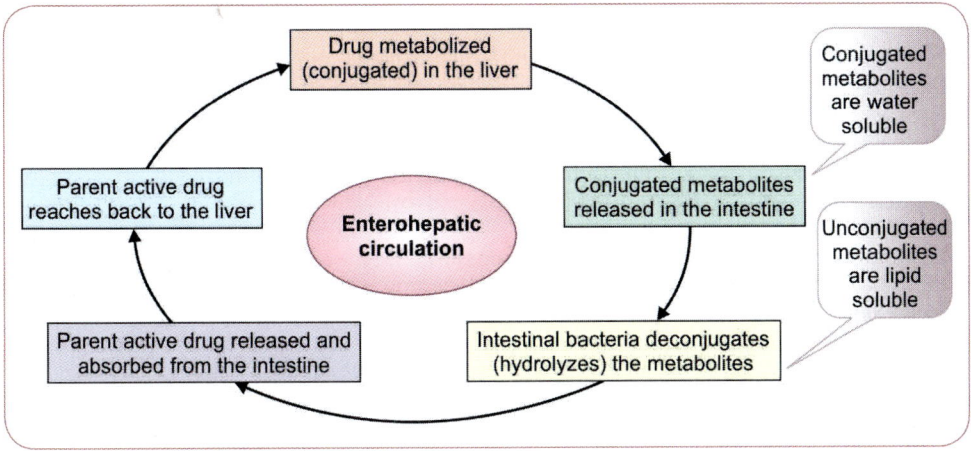

Figure 9: Enterohepatic circulation (Enterohepatic cycling)

Enterohepatic circulation functions as a small circulating reservoir; therefore, increases the bioavailability and prolong the actions of the above-mentioned drugs.

DISTRIBUTION

Drug distribution is defined as the process by which a drug reversibly leaves the blood and enters the extracellular fluid (interstitium) and other body tissues. It also refers to the transfer of drug from blood to the body tissues (Figure 10).

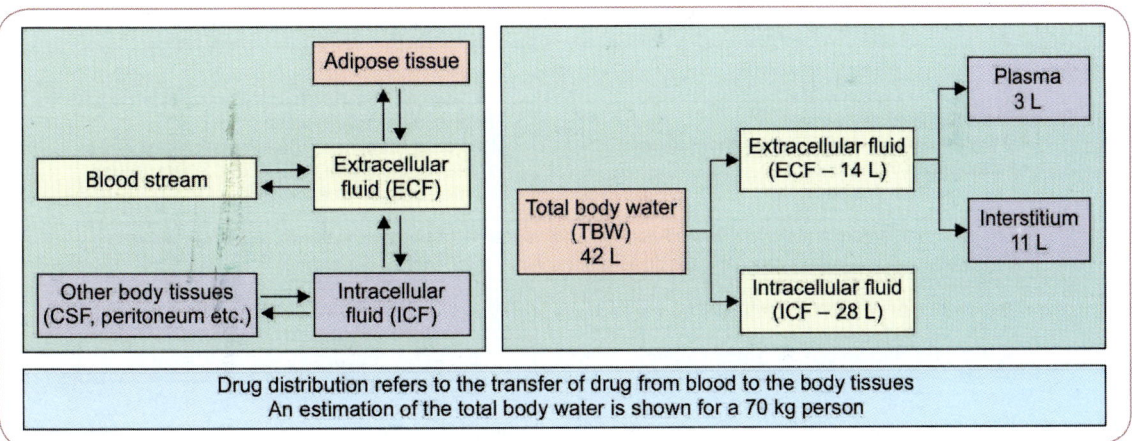

Figure 10: Drug distribution

Factors Affecting Drug Distribution

The factors affecting drug distribution include blood flow, capillary permeability, plasma protein and tissue binding, physical and chemical properties of the drug (such as lipophilicity) and volume of distribution.

Blood Flow

Rate of distribution is faster to organs with increased blood flow such as brain and liver, as compared to organs with decreased blood flow such as adipose tissue and muscles.

Capillary Permeability

It is determined by chemical properties of the drug and structure of the capillaries.

○ Liver and spleen have large slit junctions between endothelial cells with discontinuous capillaries that allows the drug to distribute from the blood to the liver and splenic cells

○ Blood brain barrier (BBB)

❑ It is a semipermeable membrane that separates the brain from the circulating blood

❑ It is formed by the endothelial tight junctions associated with astrocytes

❑ The functions of the BBB are as follows:

➢ Protection of the brain tissue from foreign/toxic substances

➢ Protection of the brain tissue from hormones and neurotransmitters

➢ Maintenance of a stable environment in the brain

❑ Lipid soluble (unionized) drugs such as morphine, barbiturates can cross the BBB

❑ Nonlipid soluble (ionized) drugs such as dopamine, neostigmine cannot cross the BBB

❑ Some drugs such as levodopa use a specific transporter to cross the BBB

❑ BBB can get disrupted in some inflammatory conditions such as meningitis; therefore, drugs such as penicillins can cross the BBB in such patients.

Plasma Protein and Tissue Binding

Plasma Protein Binding

Acidic drugs usually bind to albumin and basic drugs usually bind to α_1-acid glycoprotein (Figure 11).

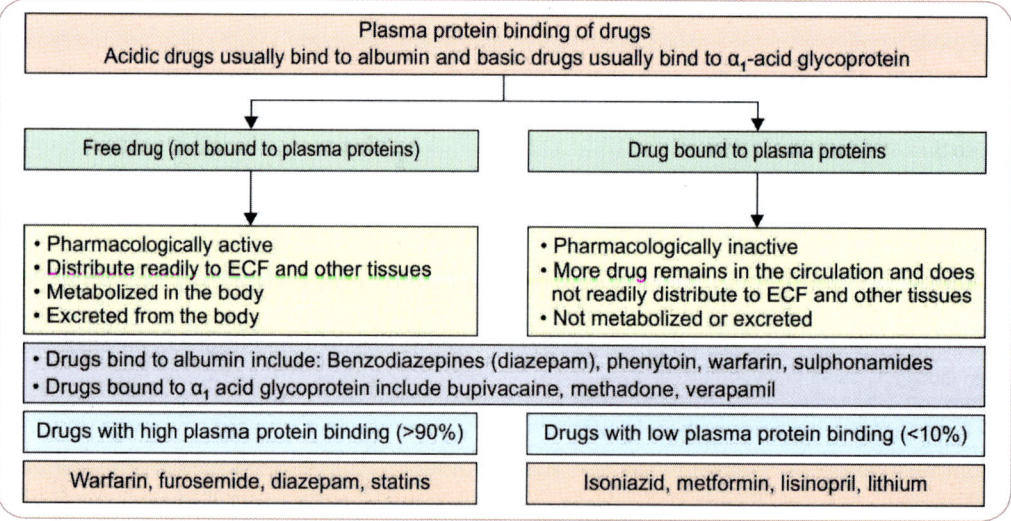

Figure 11: Plasma protein binding

The characteristics of drugs with high plasma protein binding are mentioned in Table 1.

TABLE 1	Drugs with high plasma protein binding
• More drug stays in the blood and does not distribute to the ECF and other tissues. Hence, the volume of distribution is low.	
• Bound drugs are not pharmacologically active and have a delayed metabolism and excretion.	
• Bound drugs have a longer duration of action because they are not available for metabolism and excretion.	
• Conditions such as renal failure, hepatic diseases and anemia have decreased albumin levels—hence, there is a reduction in plasma protein binding leading to an increase in the levels of free drug. This may result in drug toxicity.	

Contd...

- Hemodialysis does not cause removal of highly bound drugs in cases of poisoning.
- High plasma protein bound drugs can lead to displacement interactions due to competition for the protein binding sites. Some examples include:
  - Displacement of sulfonylurea by salicylates
  - Displacement of warfarin by phenytoin
  - Displacement of bilirubin by sulphonamides and vitamin K—may lead to kernicterus in neonates

Tissue Binding

There are many drugs that tend to accumulate in different body tissues (Table 2).

TABLE 2	Tissue binding of drugs
Body tissues	**Accumulation of drugs may lead to toxicities on chronic use**
Liver	Methotrexate, chloroquine
Lungs	Amiodarone
Bones and teeth	Tetracyclines
Adipose tissue	Thiopentone

Physical and Chemical Properties of the Drug (Such as Lipophilicity)

Lipophilic drugs can easily distribute across many biological membranes. Hydrophilic drugs cannot easily distribute across many biological membranes.

Apparent Volume of Distribution

It is a hypothetical volume of fluid that is needed to contain the entire drug in the body at a drug concentration that is equal to that in plasma (Figure 12).

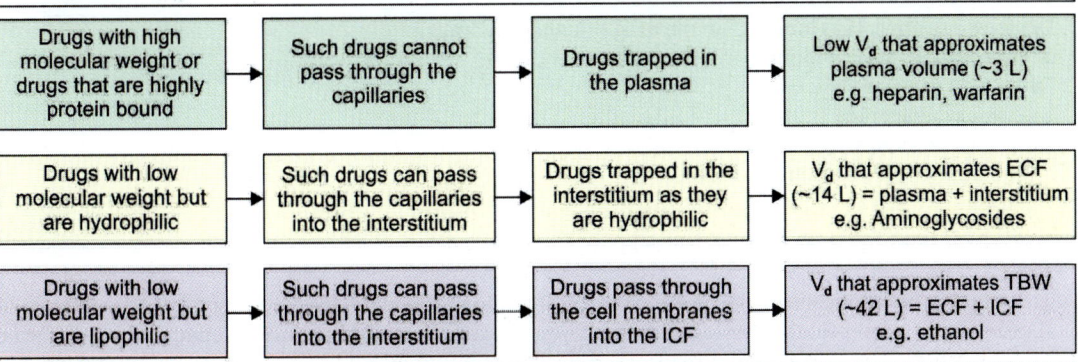

Figure 12: Apparent volume of distribution

Drug Redistribution

Drug redistribution is commonly seen with highly lipid soluble drugs that initially distribute to highly vascular organs (brain). Subsequently, these drugs are distributed into the less perfused organs such as adipose tissue or muscle (Figure 13).

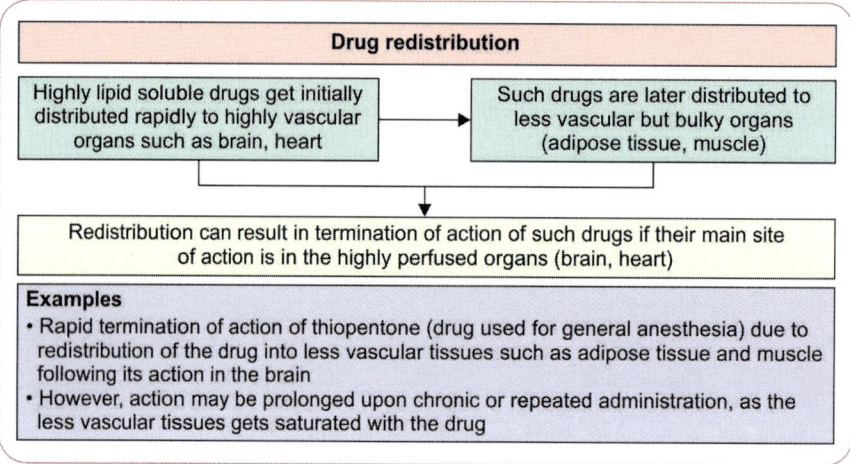

Figure 13: Drug redistribution

Therapeutic Drug Monitoring

It is the measurement of plasma drug concentration to monitor drug therapy in an individual patient. Therapeutic drug monitoring can be used in the following situations:
- Drugs having a narrow therapeutic index, e.g. digoxin, lithium, phenytoin
- Dugs having significant inter-individual variations in drug levels, e.g. antidepressants
- Unexplained lack of efficacy, e.g. antibiotics
- Use of potentially toxic drugs in patients with underlying renal failure, e.g. aminoglycosides
- To identify noncompliance of the patient with drug therapy

Therapeutic drug monitoring is not useful in the following situations:
- Drugs that produce a response which can be easily assessed:
  - Antihypertensives—measurement of blood pressure
  - Oral anticoagulants—measurement of coagulation parameters such as INR
  - Hypoglycemics—measurement of blood sugar levels
- Drugs whose effect lasts longer than the drug (hit and run drugs):
  - Omeprazole, MAO inhibitors
- Drugs with irreversible action:
  - Phenoxybenzamine
- Drugs that are activated in the body:
  - Levodopa used in Parkinson disease.

METABOLISM (BIOTRANSFORMATION)

Drug metabolism or biotransformation is the chemical alteration of the drug in a living organism. A drug is usually metabolized from a lipid-soluble (unionized) compound to a water-soluble (ionized) compound. Such water-soluble or ionized compounds are not reabsorbed in the renal tubules and hence, are excreted from the body (Figure 14).

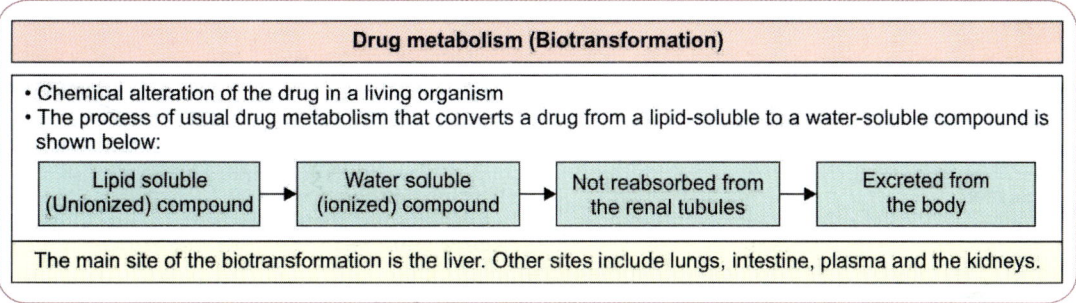

Figure 14: Drug metabolism (Biotransformation)

The metabolism can result in the following outcomes (Figure 15):

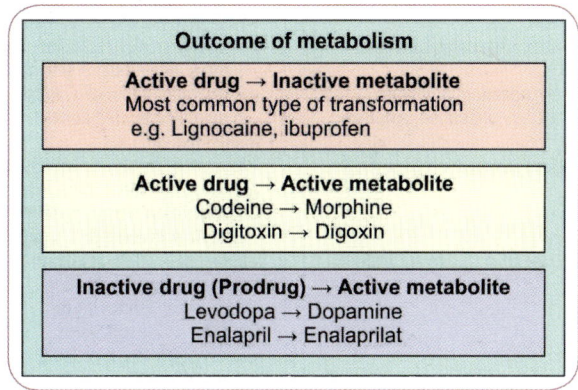

Figure 15: Outcome of metabolism

Prodrugs

Prodrugs are inactive compounds that get metabolized (biotransformed) in the body to an active compound (Inactive drug (Prodrug) → Active metabolite).
The advantages of administering a prodrug are:
○ Better bioavailability
○ Increased stability
○ Decreased toxicity
○ Selective delivery at the site of action
Some examples of prodrugs being converted to active drugs in the body are:
○ Levodopa → Dopamine for parkinsonism
○ Enalapril → Enalaprilat for hypertension
○ Bacampicillin → Ampicillin for infections
○ Prednisone → Prednisolone for rheumatoid arthritis
○ Sulfasalazine → 5-Aminosalicylic acid for ulcerative colitis
Other examples of prodrugs include sulindac, proguanil, cyclophosphamide, acyclovir, dipivefrin etc.

Classification of Biotransformation Reactions

The biotransformation reactions can be classified as follows (Figure 16)
○ Phase I reactions—also called nonsynthetic or functionalization reactions.
○ Phase II reactions—also called synthetic or conjugation reactions.

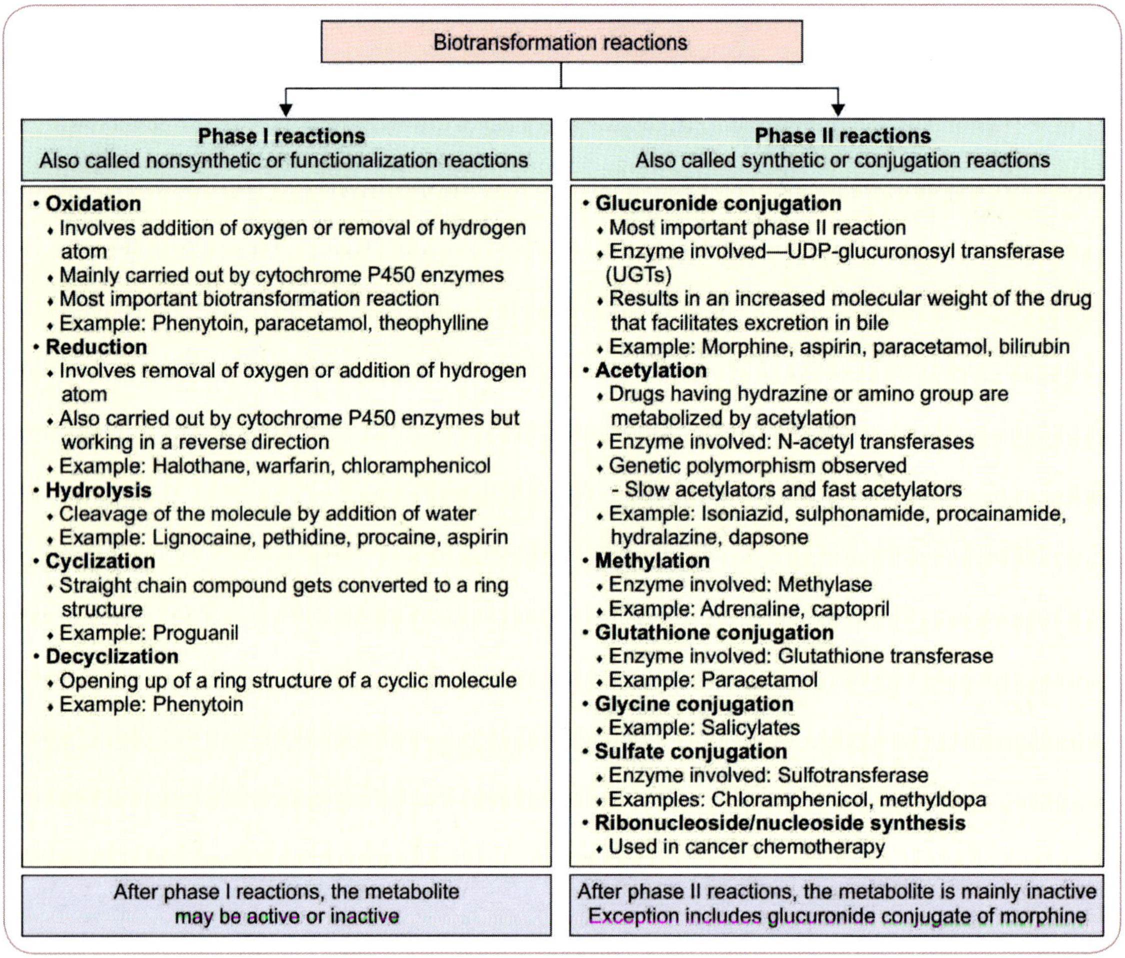

Biotransformation reactions	
Phase I reactions Also called nonsynthetic or functionalization reactions	**Phase II reactions** Also called synthetic or conjugation reactions
• **Oxidation** ♦ Involves addition of oxygen or removal of hydrogen atom ♦ Mainly carried out by cytochrome P450 enzymes ♦ Most important biotransformation reaction ♦ Example: Phenytoin, paracetamol, theophylline • **Reduction** ♦ Involves removal of oxygen or addition of hydrogen atom ♦ Also carried out by cytochrome P450 enzymes but working in a reverse direction ♦ Example: Halothane, warfarin, chloramphenicol • **Hydrolysis** ♦ Cleavage of the molecule by addition of water ♦ Example: Lignocaine, pethidine, procaine, aspirin • **Cyclization** ♦ Straight chain compound gets converted to a ring structure ♦ Example: Proguanil • **Decyclization** ♦ Opening up of a ring structure of a cyclic molecule ♦ Example: Phenytoin	• **Glucuronide conjugation** ♦ Most important phase II reaction ♦ Enzyme involved—UDP-glucuronosyl transferase (UGTs) ♦ Results in an increased molecular weight of the drug that facilitates excretion in bile ♦ Example: Morphine, aspirin, paracetamol, bilirubin • **Acetylation** ♦ Drugs having hydrazine or amino group are metabolized by acetylation ♦ Enzyme involved: N-acetyl transferases ♦ Genetic polymorphism observed - Slow acetylators and fast acetylators ♦ Example: Isoniazid, sulphonamide, procainamide, hydralazine, dapsone • **Methylation** ♦ Enzyme involved: Methylase ♦ Example: Adrenaline, captopril • **Glutathione conjugation** ♦ Enzyme involved: Glutathione transferase ♦ Example: Paracetamol • **Glycine conjugation** ♦ Example: Salicylates • **Sulfate conjugation** ♦ Enzyme involved: Sulfotransferase ♦ Examples: Chloramphenicol, methyldopa • **Ribonucleoside/nucleoside synthesis** ♦ Used in cancer chemotherapy
After phase I reactions, the metabolite may be active or inactive	After phase II reactions, the metabolite is mainly inactive Exception includes glucuronide conjugate of morphine

Figure 16: Biotransformation reactions

The drugs can be metabolized through metabolic phase reactions in the following ways:
- Drug → Phase 1 → Phase 2 → Excretion
- Drug → Phase 1 → Excretion
- Drug → Phase 2 → Excretion
- Unchanged Drug → Excreted

Drug Metabolizing Enzymes

There are two types of drug metabolizing enzymes: microsomal enzymes and nonmicrosomal enzymes (Table 3).

TABLE 3	Microsomal and nonmicrosomal enzymes	
Type	Microsomal enzymes	Nonmicrosomal enzymes
Location	Smooth endoplasmic reticulum (mainly in liver, kidneys, intestine and lungs)	Cytoplasm and mitochondria (mainly in liver cells and other tissues such as plasma)
Reactions catalyzed	Oxidation, hydrolysis, reduction, glucuronide conjugation	Many hydrolysis reactions, all conjugations except glucuronidation and some oxidations and reductions
Inducible	Inducible by various factors such as drugs	Not inducible, but some exhibit genetic polymorphisms
Example	Cytochrome P450 enzymes, glucuronyl transferase	Amidases, esterases

Cytochrome P450 Enzyme System

Cytochrome P450 enzyme system is involved in phase I biotransformation reactions. This enzyme system is also known as microsomal mixed function oxidases. It is also useful for the metabolism of endogenous compounds such as lipids, steroids etc. and exogenous compounds such as xenobiotics (Figures 17 and 18).

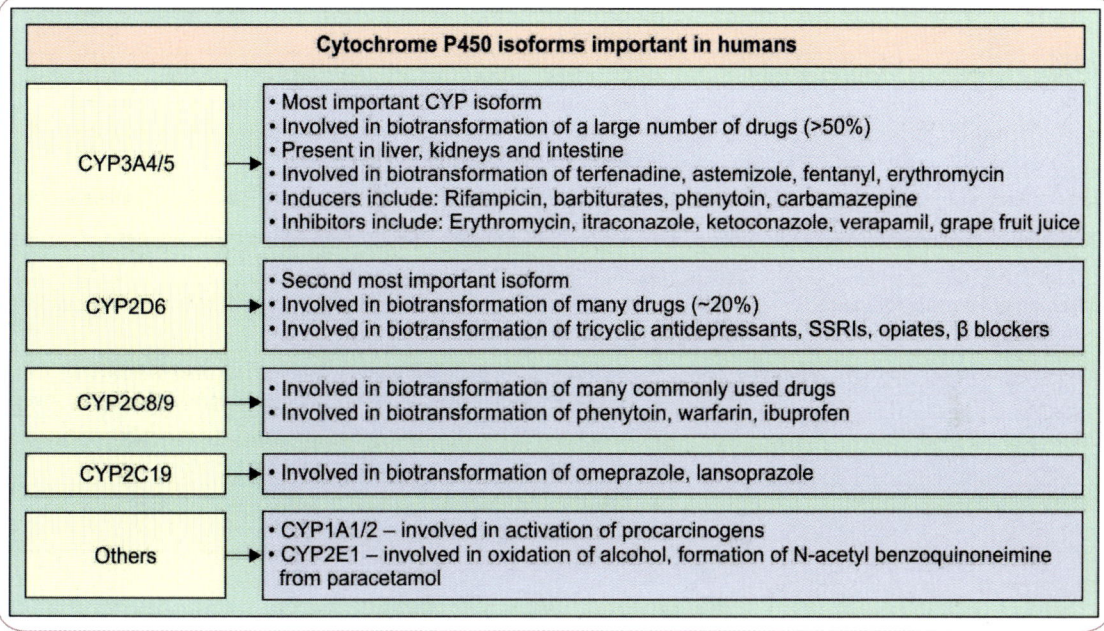

Figure 17: Cytochrome P450 isoforms

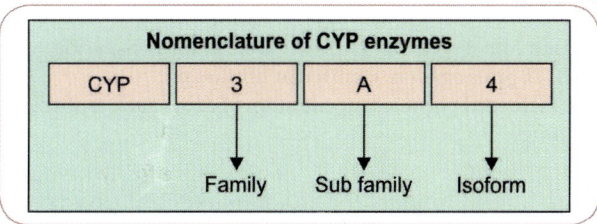

Figure 18: CYP enzymes—nomenclature

Some of the salient features regarding the significance of cytochrome P450 enzyme system are:
- Cytochrome P450 enzyme system is involved in the biotransformation of many drugs.
- Cytochrome P450 enzymes can be induced or inhibited by many drugs and compounds. This may result in various drug interactions that can lead to drug toxicity or result in altered efficacy of the drugs.
- Cytochrome P450 enzyme system demonstrate significant genetic variability across individuals/racial groups; hence, can lead to altered safety and efficacy profile of the drugs.
- Aging can have an effect on the drug metabolism due to reduced capacity of the CYP450 enzyme system in the liver. This may lead to altered safety and efficacy profile of the drug in the elderly.
- Many disease states can also lead to altered capacity of the CYP450 enzyme system.

Microsomal Enzyme Induction

Microsomal enzyme induction can occur due to many drugs, insecticides and carcinogens that can increase the activity of microsomal enzymes (such as CYP450 enzyme system and glucuronyl transferase). Some of the inducers and inhibitors of the CYP3A4/5 enzyme system are mentioned in Figure 17.

Microsomal enzyme induction can have multiple effects on the pharmacokinetics of drugs (Table 4).

TABLE 4	Significance of microsomal enzyme induction
Reduced intensity/duration of action of drugs	• Observed in drugs that are inactivated by metabolism → e.g. reduced efficacy of oral contraceptives resulting in contraceptive failure
Increased intensity of action of drugs	• Observed in drugs that are activated by metabolism → toxicity of paracetamol occurs because of one of its metabolites → in patients receiving microsomal enzyme inducers, toxicity occurs at lower paracetamol doses
Faster metabolism	• Observed in endogenous substances such as bilirubin and steroids
Precipitation of acute intermittent porphyria	• Microsomal enzyme induction can enhance the synthesis of porphyrin
Development of drug tolerance	• Observed when a drug induces its own metabolism (autoinduction) → carbamazepine
Use in congenial nonhemolytic jaundice	• Induction of hepatic bilirubin metabolism by phenobarbitone can increase bilirubin metabolism resulting in decreased bilirubin levels
Use in Cushing's syndrome	• Reduction of the clinical manifestation may be seen with phenytoin use, as it can increase adrenal steroid degradation
Use in chronic poisoning	• Induction of enzymes can lead to faster metabolism of toxic substances

Microsomal Enzyme Inhibition

Competitive inhibition of the metabolism of one drug by another drug is possible if the same enzymes or cofactors are utilized in the metabolism. Hence, the knowledge of various CYP isoforms along with their substrates, inducers and inhibitors is important to identify clinical effects on drug metabolism. Some drugs that can inhibit the enzymes involved in drug metabolism are:
- **Erythromycin:** Co-administration of erythromycin with drugs such as cisapride, astemizole and terfenadine can lead to arrhythmias such as QT prolongation, ventricular fibrillation.
- **Ciprofloxacin:** Can lead to increased plasma concentration of drugs such as theophylline and warfarin, that can result in toxicities of these drugs.

EXCRETION

Excretion is the process of elimination of drug(s) and their metabolite(s) from the body.

The polar (ionized) drugs are more efficiently eliminated from the body than high lipid-soluble (unionized) drugs.

The most important route of excretion is the kidney; the others include feces, lungs, saliva, sweat, milk, etc.

Kidney (Renal Excretion)

The kidney is the major organ for the excretion of drugs and their metabolites.

The excretion of drug by the kidneys involves 3 distinct processes: glomerular filtration, passive tubular reabsorption and active tubular secretion. The amount of drug finally excreted in the urine depends on these 3 processes as mentioned in Figure 19.

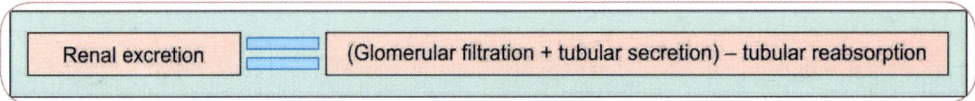

Figure 19: Renal excretion of drugs

Glomerular Filtration

The amount of drug entering the tubular lumen by glomerular filtration depends on the following factors (Table 5):

TABLE 5	Factors affecting glomerular filtration
Molecular size	• Drugs having smaller molecular size are more readily filtered at the glomerulus • Large molecules such as heparin or insulin cannot pass through the glomerulus
Plasma protein binding	• Only free drug (not bound to plasma proteins) can be filtered through the glomerulus
Glomerular filtration rate (GFR)	• Higher renal blood flow leads to a higher GFR, which leads to an increased glomerular filtration

Note: Lipid solubility and pH do not influence the passage of drugs through the glomerulus.

Passive Tubular Reabsorption

The reabsorption in the tubules occurs by passive diffusion. The key factors affecting the passive reabsorption are lipid solubility of the drug and the degree of ionization at a specific pH of surrounding medium (Figure 20).

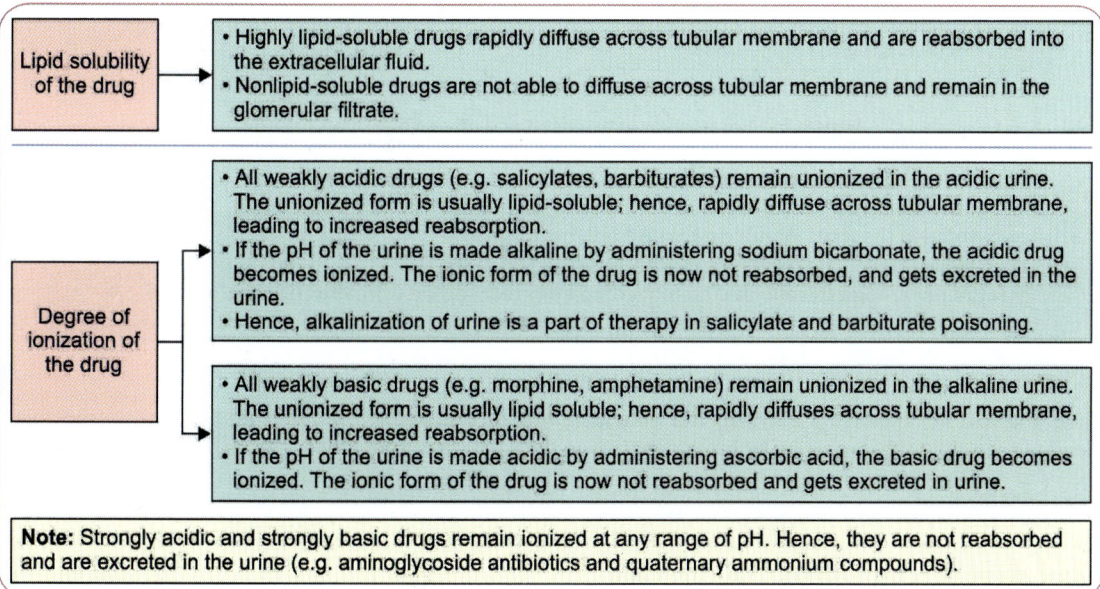

Figure 20: Factors affecting passive tubular reabsorption

Active Tubular Secretion

It is the carrier mediated active transport of drugs in the proximal tubule. It is an energy-requiring process.

The drugs which could not be filtered at the glomerulus moves on to the capillary network around proximal tubule, from where they are then secreted into the proximal tubule.

Tubular secretion is not affected by plasma protein binding (which was an obstacle during glomerular filtration) and changes in the pH of the surrounding medium.

Many acidic drugs (e.g. penicillin, probenecid, salicylates, indomethacin, barbiturates) and basic drugs (e.g. morphine, quinine, furosemide, procainamide) are actively secreted by employing separate transport carriers for acidic and basic drugs.

The transport carriers are relatively nonselective; therefore, drugs with similar physicochemical properties compete with each other for the same carrier system. For example, probenecid competes with penicillin and uric acid for the same carrier. This results in the outcomes mentioned in Figure 21.

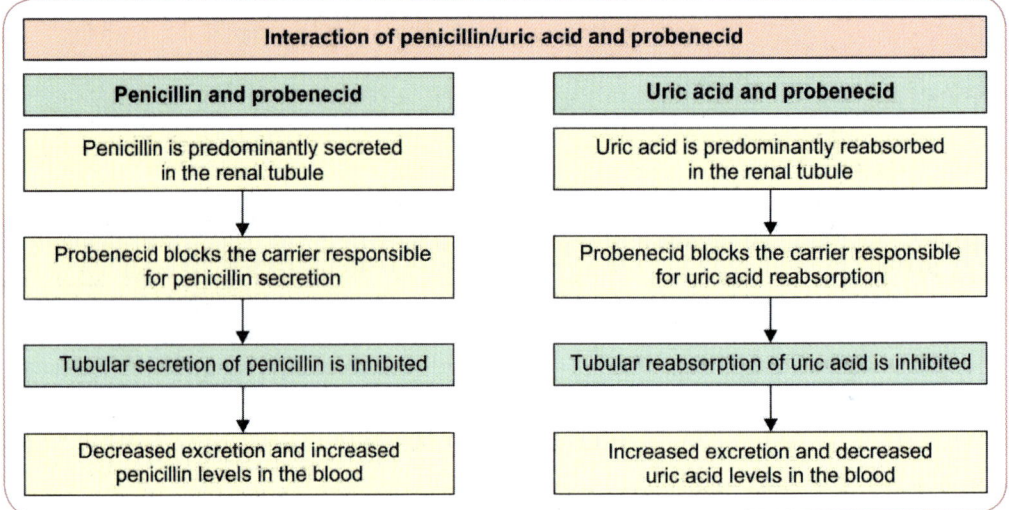

Figure 21: Interaction of penicillin and uric acid with probenecid

Feces

The drugs excreted in the feces mainly originate from the following:
- Orally ingested drugs that are not completely absorbed from the GIT
- Drugs secreted through the bile that are not completely reabsorbed from the GIT

Some drugs are directly secreted into the colon, e.g. anthracene purgatives.

Lungs

Gases and volatile liquids (e.g. ethyl alcohol, general anesthetics and ether) are excreted by lungs irrespective of their lipid solubility. The excretion by lungs depends on the partial pressure of these gases in the blood.

Breast Milk

The drugs consumed by the breastfeeding (lactating) mother may be excreted into the breast milk. This may lead to unwanted effects in the newborn suckling infant.

The pH of milk (7.0) is lower than plasma (7.4). Hence, basic drugs being mainly unionized in plasma diffuse into the breast milk. On reaching the breast milk (which has a lower pH), basic drugs get ionized; hence cannot diffuse back into the plasma.

Therefore, basic drugs (e.g. morphine, tetracycline, diazepam and estrogen/progesterone) are slightly more concentrated in the breast milk as compared to the acidic drugs.

Nonelectrolytes such as ethyl alcohol and urea rapidly enter the breast milk and reach the same concentration as that in plasma.

The administration of drugs to lactating women usually carries a caution that the suckling infant may be exposed to some amount of drug or its metabolites.

Sweat/Saliva/Hair

This is an unimportant route of excretion. Certain drugs like potassium iodide, lithium, phenytoin, rifampicin etc. are excreted through saliva. Certain heavy metals like arsenic, mercury etc. are excreted through hair follicles.

KINETICS OF ELIMINATION

The four key pharmacokinetic parameters include bioavailability, volume of distribution, plasma half-life and clearance.

The bioavailability and volume of distribution have been discussed in the preceding sections. The plasma half-life and clearance are discussed below:

Plasma Half-Life

It is the time taken for the plasma concentration of a drug to be reduced by 50% of its original value. The half-life is dependent upon 2 variables: volume of distribution (V) and clearance (CL) of the drug. The half-life is calculated by the following:

$$t1/2 = 0.693 \times \frac{V}{CL}$$

Assuming a simple case of a drug with one compartment distribution model and which follows a first order elimination, the following plasma concentration-time curve is usually obtained (Figure 22):

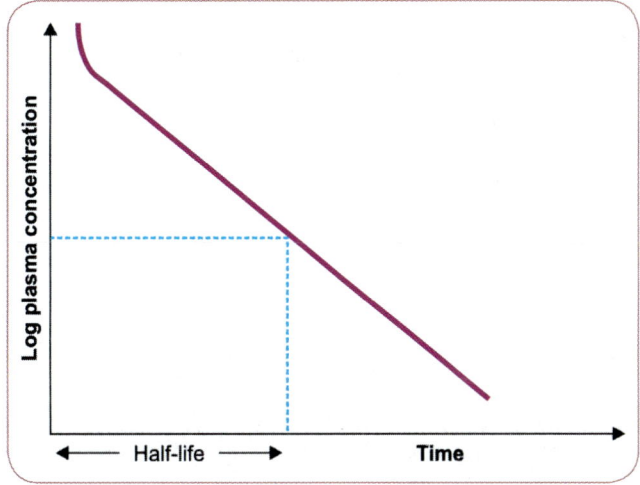

Figure 22: Log plasma concentration-time curve

It is a simple method of depicting drug elimination from the body in consecutive half-lives assuming first order elimination, where a constant fraction of the drug is excreted per unit time (Figure 23).

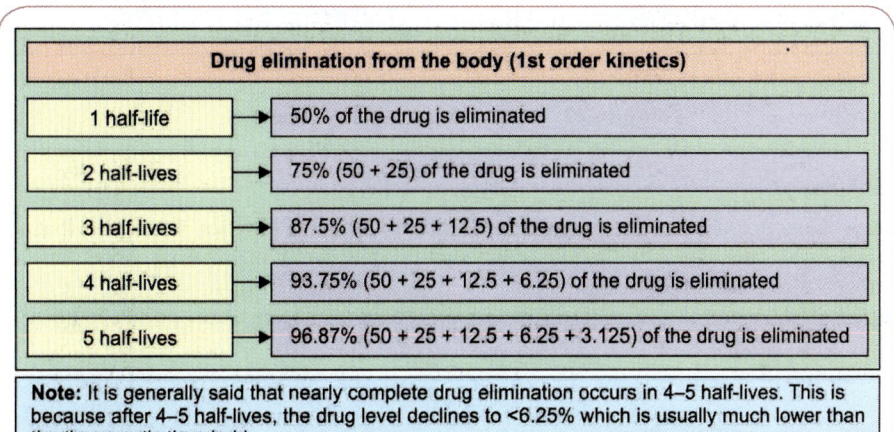

Drug elimination from the body (1st order kinetics)	
1 half-life	50% of the drug is eliminated
2 half-lives	75% (50 + 25) of the drug is eliminated
3 half-lives	87.5% (50 + 25 + 12.5) of the drug is eliminated
4 half-lives	93.75% (50 + 25 + 12.5 + 6.25) of the drug is eliminated
5 half-lives	96.87% (50 + 25 + 12.5 + 6.25 + 3.125) of the drug is eliminated

Note: It is generally said that nearly complete drug elimination occurs in 4–5 half-lives. This is because after 4–5 half-lives, the drug level declines to <6.25% which is usually much lower than the therapeutic threshold.

Figure 23: Drug elimination in successive half-lives

The plasma half-life has clinical significance because it helps in the following deductions:
○ Duration of action of a drug after a single dose
○ Dosing frequency
○ Time required to reach the steady state

Clearance

Clearance (CL) of a drug is the volume of plasma from which the drug is removed in unit time. In other words, it is the volume of plasma that is cleared of the drug in unit time. The usual units are mL/min.

$$CL = \frac{\text{Rate of elimination}}{\text{Plasma concentration}}$$

In majority of drugs, the processes involved in elimination are not saturated over the dose ranges used clinically. Hence, a constant fraction gets eliminated per unit time. This is the first-order kinetics.

For some of the drugs, the process involved in elimination gets saturated over the dose ranges used clinically. Hence, a constant amount gets eliminated per unit time. This is the zero-order kinetics.

The key differences between the first-order kinetics and the zero-order kinetics are mentioned in Figure 24.

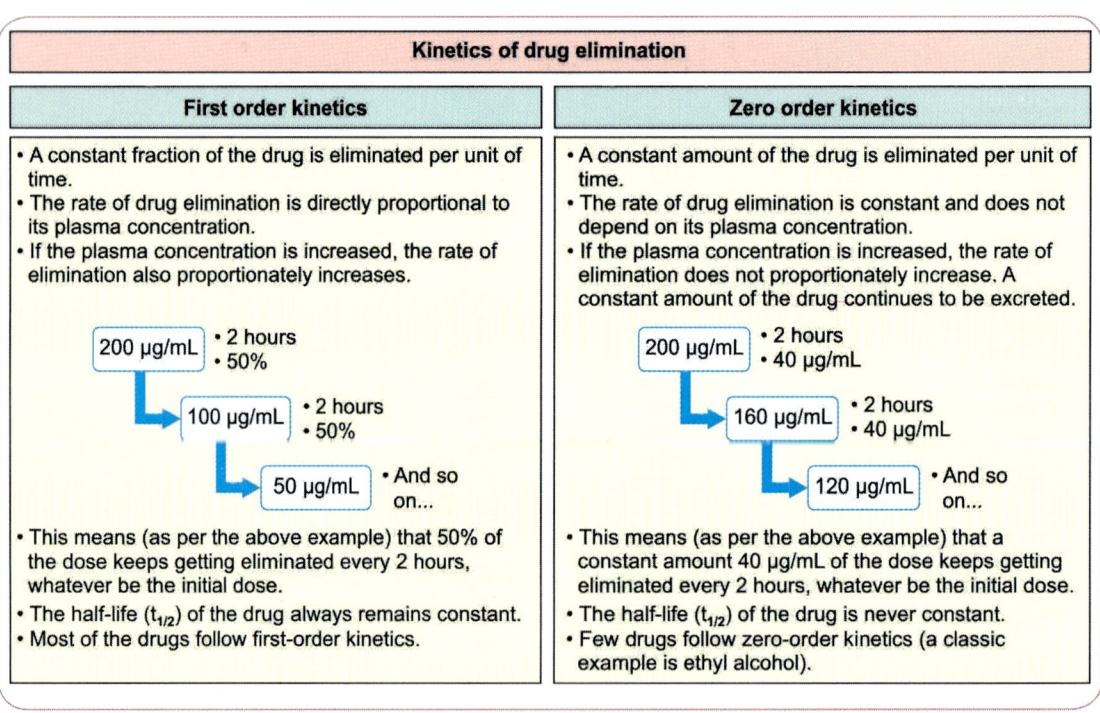

Figure 24: First order and zero order kinetics

Mixed Order Kinetics

There are certain drugs (e.g. aspirin, phenytoin) which follow mixed order kinetics. This means that at smaller drug concentration, the drugs are eliminated by first order kinetics. However, at higher drug concentration, the kinetics gradually changes to zero order (Figure 25).

This happens because the elimination processes (metabolizing enzymes, transporters, etc.) gets saturated at higher drug concentrations.

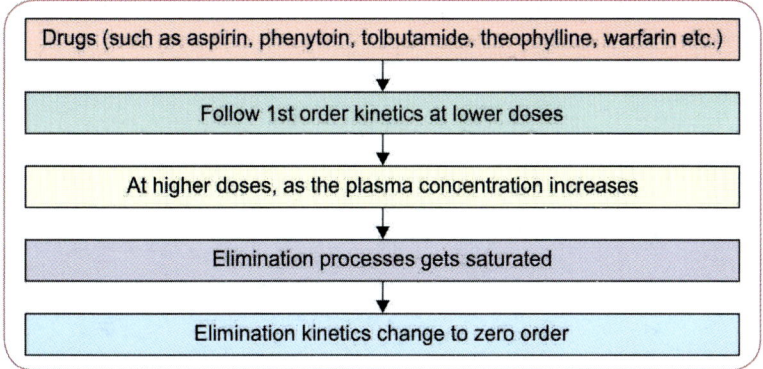

Figure 25: Mixed order kinetics

When the kinetics changes to zero order, a small increase in dose may result in a much higher increase in the plasma concentration, because the elimination process have become saturated. This may quickly lead to drug toxicity.

Therefore, appropriate therapeutic drug monitoring is required in such situations for proper monitoring of plasma concentrations.

Steady State

When a fixed dose of the drug is given repeatedly at regular intervals, the plasma concentration keeps on increasing until a steady state is reached.

This occurs because most drugs are repeated at intervals shorter than 4 half-lives. Hence, some drug from the 1st dose was still in the body when the 2nd dose was administered, some drug from the 2nd dose was still in the body when the 3rd dose was administered, and so on.

Therefore, the drug concentration keeps on increasing until within the dosing interval, the rate of drug elimination becomes equal to the rate of drug administration.

This is the point when the drug is said to have reached the plateau or the steady-state. Administration of the same doses thereafter, does not further lead to an increase in drug concentration.

The steady state is usually reached in 4–5 half-lives of the drug (Figure 26).

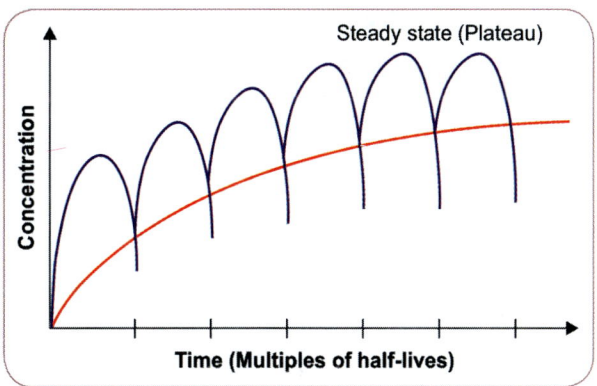

Figure 26: Steady state

Drug Dose Optimization and Target Level Strategy

The aim of drug therapy is to achieve and maintain plasma concentration within a therapeutic window while minimizing the adverse effects and/or toxicity (Therapeutic window means a concentration range that provides efficacy without causing adverse effects).

If the therapeutic window is narrow (digoxin, warfarin etc.), doses should be adjusted cautiously and monitoring of drug levels may be required.

Drug regimens are administered in the form of a maintenance dose, and if rapid effects are required, a loading dose also may be employed.

Loading Dose

A loading dose is a single dose or a series of doses, given at the beginning of therapy with the aim of quickly achieving the desired plasma concentration.

A loading dose is given when the time required to attain the steady state (4 half-lives) is long as compared to the patient's condition. It is generally used in clinical emergencies.

Example

The $t_{1/2}$ of lignocaine is 1–2 hours. Hence, it will take 4 half-lives i.e. 4–8 hours to attain the desired concentration (steady state). One cannot wait for 4–8 hours in a patient with life-threatening arrhythmias (for example, may be encountered after myocardial infarction) for attaining the therapeutic concentration of lignocaine. Hence, a loading dose of lignocaine is administered. Target concentration is quickly achieved. Then, the maintenance doses of lignocaine are continued to maintain the steady state.

Maintenance Dose

Maintenance dose is a dose which is repeated at fixed intervals of time (or given as a continuous infusion) to maintain the steady state once it has been attained.

It usually takes 4–5 half-lives of the drug to attain the steady state.

To maintain the steady state, the dose is adjusted such that the rate of drug administration is equal to the rate of drug elimination.

PROLONGATION OF DRUG ACTION

In certain situations, prolongation of drug action can be beneficial. The advantages of prolongation of drug action are:
- Frequency of drug administration is decreased
- Patient convenience and compliance is increased
- Fluctuations in plasma concentration is decreased

The drug action can be prolonged by the following methods:

Prolonging the Absorption from Administration Site

Oral

- The rate of absorption of solid oral dosage forms (e.g. tablets) is partly dependent on the rate of dissolution of the tablet in GI fluids.
- This is the basis for the development of prolonged action formulations (sustained release, extended release, prolonged release etc.).
- These preparations have special coatings or ingredients that release at different time points and therefore, control drug release.
- These preparations produce slow uniform absorption of the drug for 8 hours or more.
- The advantages are slower absorption, prolonged action, decreased dosing frequency, improved compliance, decreased adverse effects, and maintenance of therapeutic concentrations for longer periods (avoiding sudden peaks/troughs).
- It is valuable for drugs with short half-lives.

Parenteral

- By decreasing the vascularity of the absorbing medium e.g. adrenaline + lignocaine
  - Adding a vasoconstrictor (adrenaline) to a local anesthetic (lignocaine) produces the following beneficial action:

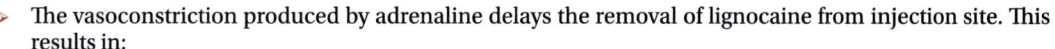

➤ The vasoconstriction produced by adrenaline delays the removal of lignocaine from injection site. This results in:
  • Prolongation of action of lignocaine
  • Decrease in toxicity of lignocaine (as systemic absorption of lignocaine is decreased)
  • Decrease in bleeding at the site of operation
○ By decreasing the solubility of the drug in subcutaneous or intramuscular injections, e.g. penicillin + procaine/benzathine
○ By injecting the drug as an oily solution, e.g. depot progestins
○ By esterification, e.g. esters of testosterone are slowly absorbed from injection site leading to prolongation of action
○ By pellet implantation.

Increasing the Plasma Protein Binding

The drug congeners having an increased plasma protein binding dissociate slowly form the proteins, leading to a prolonged duration of action.

Decreasing the Renal Excretion

The tubular secretion of certain drugs can be competitively inhibited by other drugs, e.g. probenecid competitively inhibits the tubular secretion of penicillin/ampicillin increasing their plasma levels and the duration of action.

Decreasing the Rate of Metabolism

The rate of metabolism of drugs can be decreased by either making a change in the molecular structure of the drugs or by inhibition of enzymes responsible for metabolism (degradation) of the drugs.
Examples include:
○ Adding ethynyl group to estradiol making the estrogen longer acting
○ Inhibition of dehydropeptidase 1 by cilastatin, thus protecting imipenem from hydrolysis and prolonging its action
○ Inhibition of dopa decarboxylase by carbidopa, thus protecting levodopa from metabolism and prolonging its action.

FIXED-DOSE COMBINATION (FIXED-DOSE RATIO COMBINATION [FDC])

Fixed-dose combination is the combination of 2 or more drugs in a fixed dose ratio in a single formulation. It means that a single tablet/capsule etc. contains both the drugs together.

It does not mean concomitant drug therapy wherein 2 or more drugs are separately consumed at the same time.

The advantages and disadvantages of fixed dose combinations are mentioned in Figure 27.

Fixed-dose combinations	
Advantages	**Disadvantages**
• Convenience (resulting in increased patient compliance) • Synergistic effect • Increased efficacy • Decreased adverse effects • Prevention of resistance	• Dose adjustment of a single drug is not possible • Pharmacokinetics incompatibility • Difficulty in identifying the drug causing adverse effect • Increased toxicity due to irrational combinations • Contraindication to one drug contraindicates the entire FDC
Examples of some of the FDCs: • Levodopa + carbidopa for parkinsonism • Estrogen + progesterone for oral contraception • Amoxicillin + clavulinic acid for infections • Sulfamethoxazole + trimethoprim for infections • Isoniazid + rifampicin + pyrazinamide for tuberculosis	

Figure 27: Fixed-dose combinations

ASSESS YOURSELF (Examination Questions of Various Universities)

1. What is biotransformation? Give an account of reactions involved with suitable examples. Enumerate factors affecting biotransformation
2. Define zero order kinetics with an example
3. First order kinetics in therapeutics
4. Define bioavailability of drug. Describe various factors affecting bioavailability
5. Microsomal enzyme induction
6. Entero-hepatic circulation of drugs
7. Apparent volume of distribution
8. Drug redistribution
9. Therapeutic drug monitoring
10. Cytochrome P450 enzyme system
11. Plasma half-life of drugs

MULTIPLE CHOICE QUESTIONS

1. Low volume of distribution indicates:
   (AIIMS Nov 2015)
   a. Low efficacy
   b. Decreased distribution in tissues and organ
   c. Short biological life
   d. Poor bioavailability

2. Which drug is not metabolized by acetylation?
   (AIIMS May 2008, Nov 2006, AIIMS May 2003)
   a. Isoniazid
   b. Dapsone
   c. Hydralazine
   d. Metoclopramide

3. Which of the following is a prodrug?
   (AIIMS May 2008, 2004, Nov 2006)
   a. Enalapril
   b. Clonidine
   c. Salmeterol
   d. Acetazolamide

4. Which of the following drugs is an inhibitor of cytochrome p450 enzymes? *(AIIMS May 2008)*
   a. Ketoconazole
   b. Rifampicin
   c. Phenytoin
   d. Phenobarbitone

5. Drug inhibiting the P-glycoprotein is:
   (Recent Question Dec 2016)
   a. Chloramphenicol
   b. Ketoconazole
   c. Tetracycline
   d. Erythromycin

6. Isoniazid is metabolized by:
   (Recent Question 2016)
   a. Acetylation
   b. Oxidation
   c. Reduction
   d. Hydrolysis

7. Plasma protein bound drug distributed in which compartment? *(Recent Question 2016)*
   a. Extracellular
   b. Intravascular
   c. Interstitial
   d. Extravascular

8. Alkaline dieresis is done for treatment of poisoning due to: *(Recent Question 2016)*
   a. Morphine
   b. Amphetamine
   c. Phenobarbitone
   d. Atropine

9. Urinary alkalinizing agents are administered in case of poisoning due to drugs which are:
   (Recent Question 2016)
   a. Weak bases
   b. Weak acids
   c. Strong bases
   d. Strong acids

10. Most common phase II drug metabolizing reaction: *(Recent Question 2016)*
    a. Glucuronidation
    b. Acetylation
    c. Oxidation
    d. Glutathione conjugation

11. Elimination after 4 half-life in first order kinetics: *(Recent Question 2016)*
    a. 84%
    b. 93%
    c. 80%
    d. 75%

Ans.											
1.	(b)	**2.**	(d)	**3.**	(a)	**4.**	(a)	**5.**	(d)	**6.**	(a)
7.	(b)	**8.**	(c)	**9.**	(b)	**10.**	(a)	**11.**	(b)		

12. **The elimination of alcohol follows:**
(Recent Question 2016)
   a. Zero order kinetics
   b. 1st order kinetics
   c. 2nd order kinetics
   d. 3rd order kinetics

13. **Which of the following is not a prodrug?**
(Recent Question 2016)
   a. Enalapril
   b. Imipramine
   c. Sulphasalazine
   d. Cyclophosphamide

14. **True about zero order kinetics:**
(Recent Question 2016)
   a. Constant fraction of the drug is eliminated per unit time
   b. Dependent on plasma concentration
   c. Constant amount of the drug is eliminated per unit time
   d. Half-life is constant

15. **Most common cytochrome associated with drug metabolism:** *(Recent Question 2016)*
   a. CYP3A
   b. CYP2C
   c. CYP2D6
   d. CYPA1E

16. **Which of the following is an effect of grapefruit juice on drug metabolism?**
(Recent Question 2016)
   a. Enzyme inducer
   b. Enzyme inhibitor
   c. Inhibits tubular secretion
   d. Inhibits tubular reabsorption

17. **Chemical modification of drug like oxidation by cytochrome P450 is called:** *(AP PG 2014)*
   a. First pass effect
   b. Presystemic extraction
   c. Phase I metabolism
   d. Phase II metabolism

18. **Bio-availability is defined:** *(TN PG 2005)*
   a. The volume of plasma completely cleared of a specific compound per unit time
   b. Percentage of drug that is detected in the systemic circulation after its administration
   c. Percentage of water solubility of the drugs
   d. Rate of elimination of drug

19. **Which of the following drug does not inhibit p-glycoprotein?** *(WB PG 2015)*
   a. Quinidine
   b. Verapamil
   c. Phenobarbitone
   d. Erythromycin

20. **From which of the following routes, bioavailability of the drug is likely to be 100 percent?** *(AIIMS May 2018)*
   a. Subcutaneous
   b. Intravenous
   c. Intramuscular
   d. Intradermal

21. **Hepatic first pass metabolism will be bypassed by the following routes of drug administration except?** *(AIIMS May 2018)*
   a. Oral
   b. Intravenous
   c. Sublingual
   d. Subcutaneous

Ans.

12.	(a)	13.	(b)	14.	(c)	15.	(a)	16.	(b)	17.	(c)
18.	(b)	19.	(c)	20.	(b)	21.	(a)				

3 Pharmacodynamics

Pharmacodynamics is one of the two subdivisions of pharmacology. It is the effect of the drug on the body and therefore is *what the drug does to the body*. Pharmacodynamics deals with the following aspects of drugs:

- Site of action
- Mechanism of action
- Physiological effects
- Adverse effects

TYPES OF DRUG ACTION

The main types of drug action can be classified as stimulation, irritation, depression, replacement and cytotoxicity (Table 1).

TABLE 1	Types of drug action			
Stimulation	**Irritation**	**Depression**	**Replacement**	**Cytotoxicity**
• Selective increase in the activity level of specialized cells • For example, stimulation of cardiac tissue by adrenaline	• Nonselective irritation of less specialized cells such as skin or epithelial cells • For example, increase of salivary secretion by bitters, relief of pain by counterirritants such as eucalyptus oil	• Selective decrease in the activity level of specialized cells • For example, depression of central nervous system by barbiturates	• Replacement of deficient endogenous substances • For example, hormone replacement (insulin in diabetes mellitus, thyroid hormone in hypothyroidism)	• Selective action against parasites, bacteria, viruses or cancer cells • For example, antibiotics, antiviral drugs, anticancer drugs etc.

MECHANISM OF DRUG ACTION

A majority of drugs act by targeting a discrete molecule, which is usually a protein molecule. The target proteins can be classified into 4 categories—enzymes, ion channels, transporters and receptors (Figure 1):

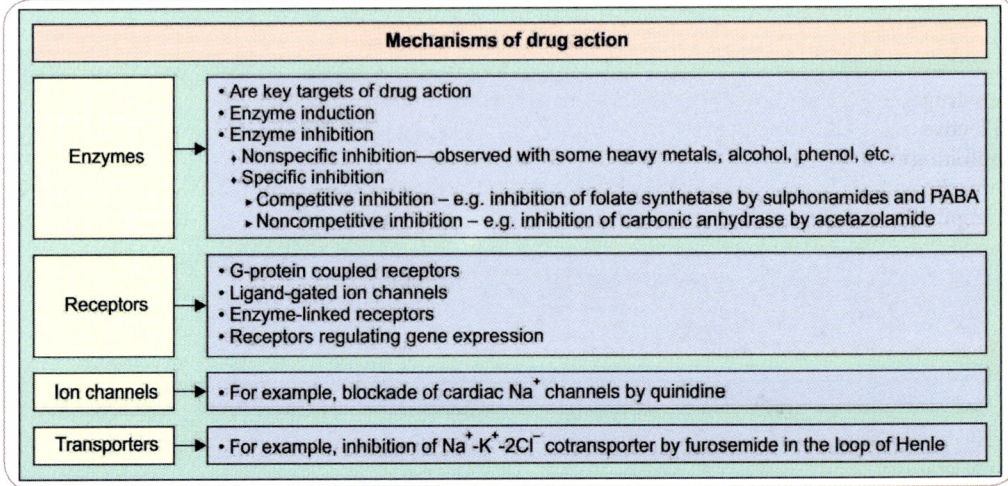

Figure 1: Mechanisms of drug action

Enzymes

Enzymes are involved in a majority of biological reactions. The drugs can act by causing either induction or inhibition of enzymes (Table 2).

TABLE 2	Enzyme induction and enzyme inhibition
Enzyme induction	
• Apparent increase of the enzyme activity • For example, induction of CYP3A4/5 enzymes by rifampicin, barbiturates	
Enzyme inhibition	
Nonspecific inhibition	• The structure of enzymes is altered by compounds such as heavy metals, strong acids, alcohols etc. • Inhibition is not limited to any specific enzyme, and affects any enzyme that comes in contact • Such compounds are generally too toxic for systemic use
Specific inhibition	• Only a particular enzyme is inhibited, other enzymes are not affected • Specific inhibition is of 2 types → Competitive and noncompetitive

Competitive inhibition (equilibrium type)	Noncompetitive inhibition
Drug competes with the substrate for binding to catalytic site of the enzyme	Drug binds to an adjacent site on the enzyme, instead of the catalytic site
This results in nonformation of a product or formation of a nonfunctional product	The enzyme is altered in such a way that the enzymatic catalytic activity is lost
For example, competition between sulfonamides and PABA for folate synthetase	For example, inhibition of carbonic anhydrase by acetazolamide

• **Nonequilibrium type of enzymatic inhibition:** Drug binds to the catalytic site of the enzyme; however, it binds either with a very high affinity or binds with strong covalent bonds. This results in an inability of the substrate to displace the drug from the enzyme.
• For example, higher affinity of methotrexate for dihydrofolate reductase

Ion Channels

Certain drugs bind to the ion channels and affect the flow of ions through these channels.

These drugs either bind to the ion channels directly (e.g. binding of local anesthetic to voltage gated Na^+ channels) or bind to the ion channels through specific receptors (e.g. ligand-gated ion channels, such as barbiturate binding to $GABA_A$ receptors).

Transporters

Certain drugs bind to the transporters in the membrane and produce their effects. The examples include:
- Selective serotonin reuptake inhibitors (SSRIs) such as fluoxetine bind to serotonin transporter, thereby inhibiting serotonin reuptake in the neurons
- Tricyclic antidepressants (TCAs) such as imipramine bind to norepinephrine transporter, thereby inhibiting norepinephrine reuptake in the neurons.

Receptors

The majority of drugs act by binding to receptors, which results in biological changes in the body.

The drug binds to the receptor leading to the formation of drug receptor complex. This results in the required effect of the drug (Figure 2).

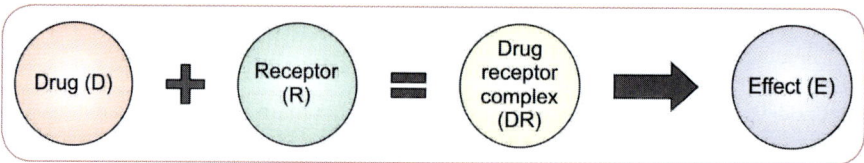

Figure 2: Drug receptor complex

The following terminology is important regarding the drug receptor complex:
○ **Affinity:** Ability of the drug to bind with the receptor
○ **Intrinsic activity (Efficacy):** Ability of the drug to produce a pharmacological effect after binding and inducing a functional change in the receptor.

The drug receptor interactions can be described as agonist, partial agonist, inverse agonist and antagonist (Figure 3).

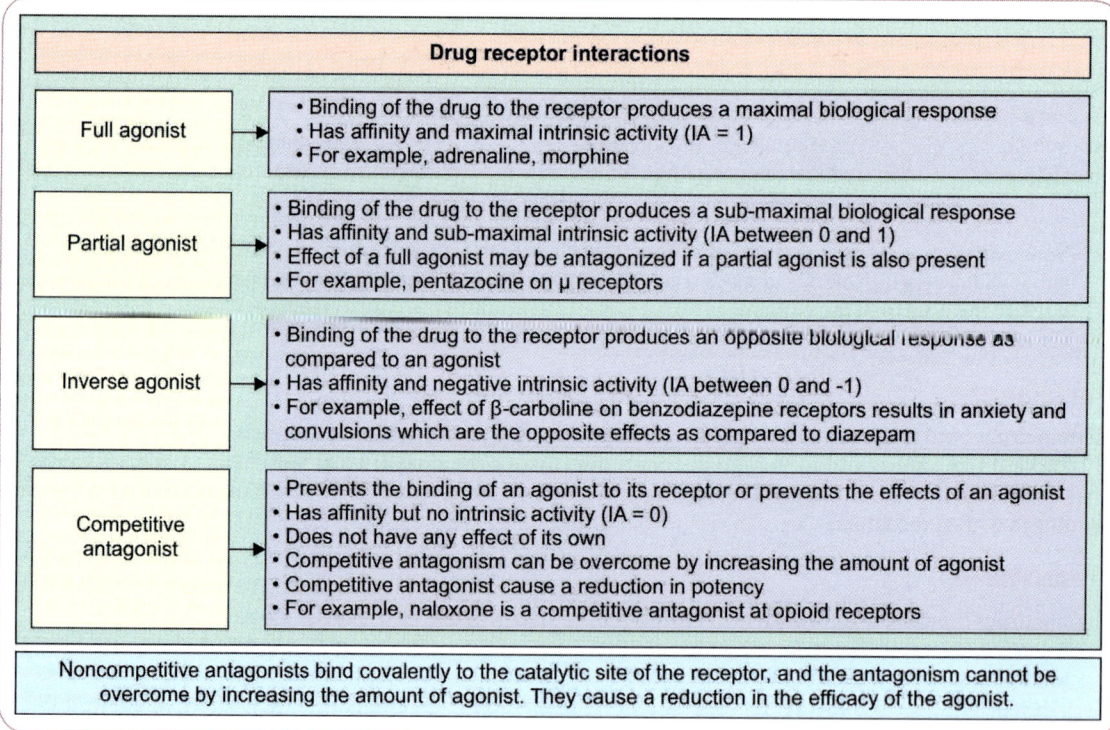

Figure 3: Drug receptor interactions

The drug receptor relationship is represented in Figure 4.

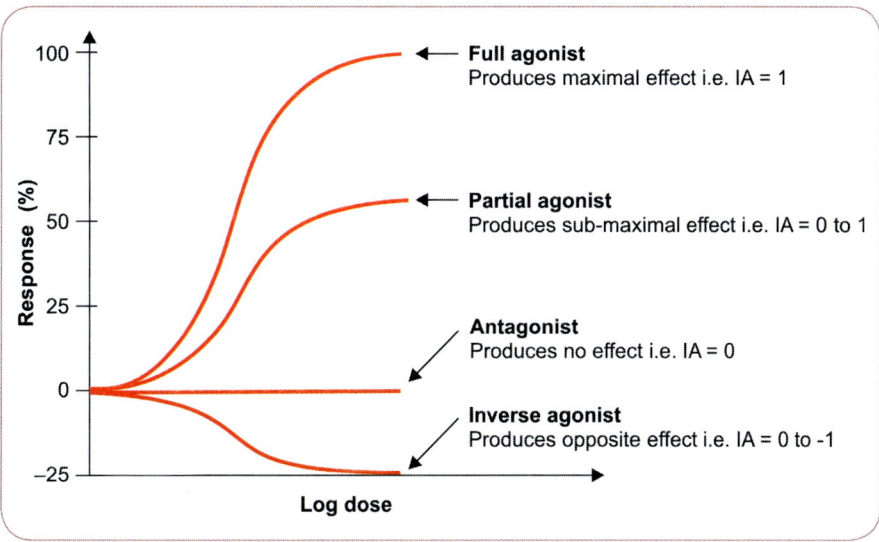

Figure 4: Drug receptor relationship

Types of Receptors

The receptors can be classified as cell surface receptors and intracellular receptors. Generally, the ligands for the intracellular receptors are smaller lipophilic molecules that can easily cross the plasma membrane to reach inside the cell (Figure 5).

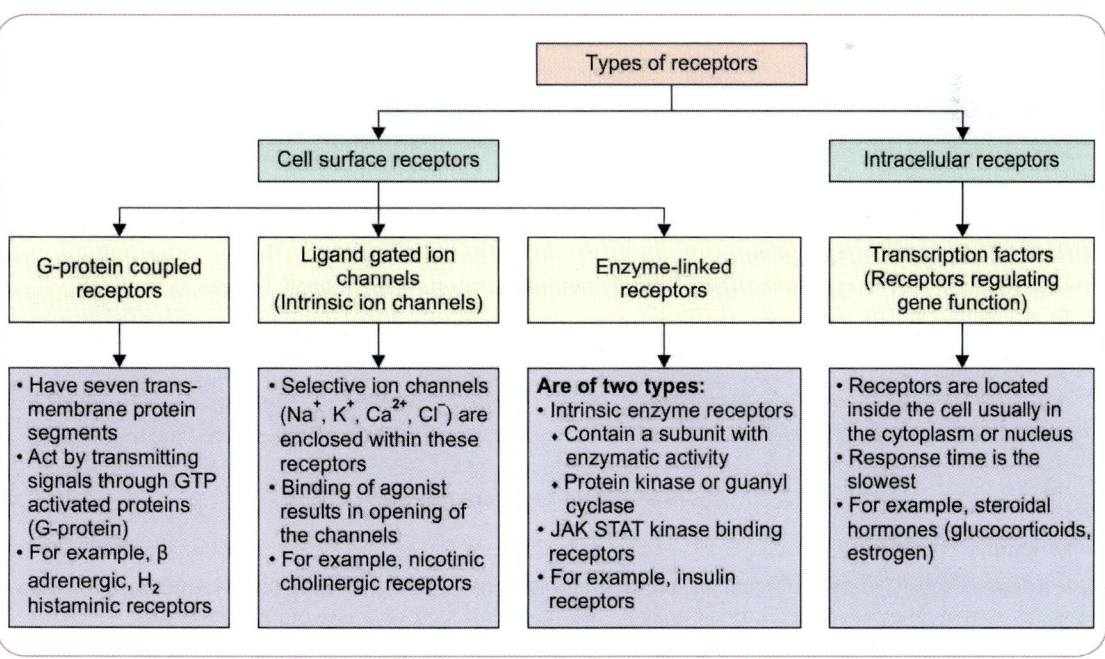

Figure 5: Type of receptors

G-protein Coupled Receptors

The G-protein coupled receptors (GPCR) are a large family of cell surface receptors that have seven transmembrane protein segments (Table 3).

TABLE 3	G-protein coupled receptors (GPCR)
Important type of G-proteins and their actions on the effector pathways	
• G_s: ↑ Adenylyl cyclase and ↑ Ca^{2+} channel • G_i: ↓ Adenylyl cyclase and ↑ K^+ channel • G_0: ↓ Ca^{2+} channel • G_q: ↑ Phospholipase C • G_{13}: ↑ Na^+/H^+ exchange	
Major effector pathways of G proteins	
Adenylyl cyclase → cAMP pathway (G_s)	• Stimulation of adenylyl cyclase → increase in cAMP levels → acts through protein kinase A (PK_A) → PK_A phosphorylates enzymes, transporters etc. → Pharmacological effects • Increased cAMP also opens calcium channels in heart, brain and kidneys • For example, β adrenergic, H_2 histaminic, D_1 dopaminergic
Adenyl cyclase → cAMP pathway (G_i)	• Inhibition of adenyl cyclase → decrease in cAMP levels → Pharmacological effects • For example, $α_2$ adrenergic, M_2 muscarinic, D_2 dopaminergic

Phospholipase C → IP_3-DAG pathway	• Phospholipase C activation → Second messenger generation, e.g. inositol triphosphate (IP_3) and diacylglycerol (DAG)
	  ▪ IP_3 mobilizes Ca^{2+} from intracellular stores
	  ▪ DAG increases protein kinase C activation by Ca^{2+}
	• This results in various pharmacological effects
	• For example, $α_1$ adrenergic, H_1 histaminic

Channel regulation	• Act through opening or closing of specific channels for Na^+, Ca^{2+}, K^+ • For example, $β_1$ adrenergic in heart

Ligand-gated ion Channels

These receptors enclose specific ion channels (e.g. Na^+, K^+, Ca^{2+}, Cl^-). The examples include nicotinic cholinergic, GABA, glycine and glutamate receptors.

The sequence of events following ligand binding to these receptors is mentioned in Figure 6.

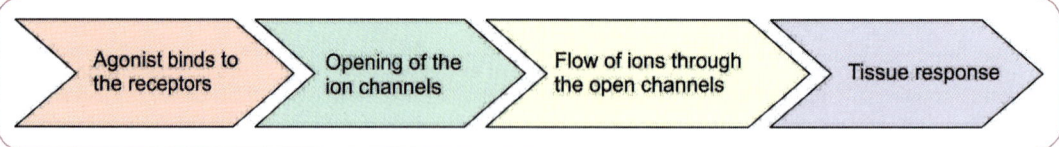

Figure 6: Ligand-gated ion channels

Enzyme-linked Receptors

These receptors consist of a protein that form dimers and undergo conformational changes resulting in increased enzymatic activity. They are either intrinsic enzyme receptors or JAK-STAT kinase binding receptors.

The examples include insulin and growth factor receptors.

The sequence of events following ligand binding to these receptors is mentioned in Figure 7.

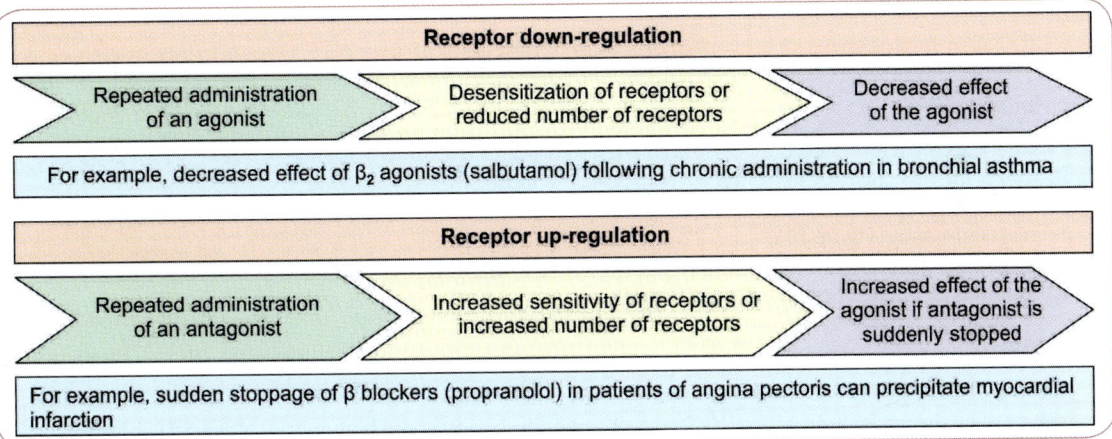

Figure 7: Enzyme-linked receptors

Regulation of Receptors

The receptors are regulated by many control mechanisms such as receptor activity, feedback regulation and other homeostatic processes.

The receptors can be down-regulated or up-regulated depending on the type of regulatory mechanisms (Figure 8).

Receptor down-regulation

| Repeated administration of an agonist | Desensitization of receptors or reduced number of receptors | Decreased effect of the agonist |

For example, decreased effect of β_2 agonists (salbutamol) following chronic administration in bronchial asthma

Receptor up-regulation

| Repeated administration of an antagonist | Increased sensitivity of receptors or increased number of receptors | Increased effect of the agonist if antagonist is suddenly stopped |

For example, sudden stoppage of β blockers (propranolol) in patients of angina pectoris can precipitate myocardial infarction

Figure 8: Receptor regulation

DOSE-RESPONSE RELATIONSHIP

Dose-response relationship is defined as a relationship between the concentration of drug at the receptors and the size of the response.

A dose-response relationship can be depicted by a dose-response curve. A dose-response curve shows the effects of an increasing dose of a drug and the resulting response.

A dose-response curve can be plotted using the normal doses or using the log doses on the X-axis (Figure 9).

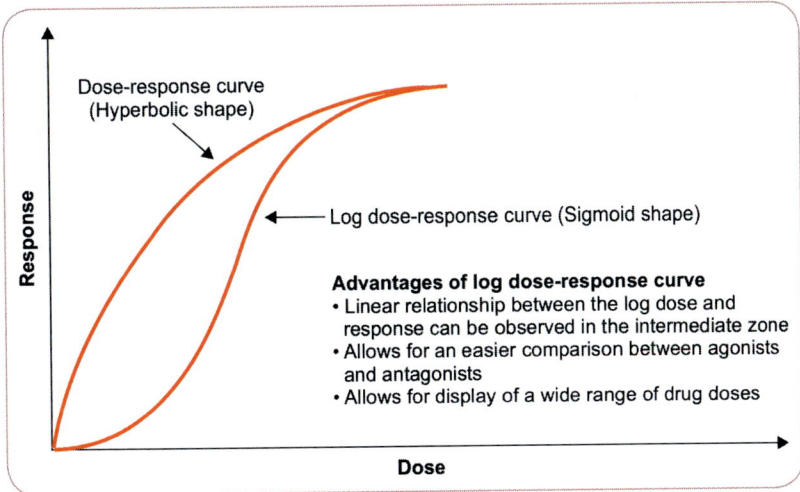

Dose-response curve (Hyperbolic shape)

Log dose-response curve (Sigmoid shape)

Advantages of log dose-response curve
• Linear relationship between the log dose and response can be observed in the intermediate zone
• Allows for an easier comparison between agonists and antagonists
• Allows for display of a wide range of drug doses

Response

Dose

Figure 9: Dose response curve and log dose-response curve

Types of Dose-Response Relationships

There are two types of dose-response relationships:
- Graded (Continuous)
  - Graph of a relationship between dose and response
  - Majority of drugs produce a graded response
  - Intensity of the response increases with the dose or concentration of the drug
  - Response can be measured on a continual basis
  - Easy to determine a linear relationship between drug concentration and response
- Quantal (All-or-none)
  - Some drugs produce a **quantal** or **all-or-none** response
  - The responses are not observed on a continual basis
  - Such drugs either produce a response or do not produce a response at all, i.e. all-or-none phenomenon
  - For example, ability of a sedative to induce sleep or not induce sleep.

Dose-Response Relationships—Potency, Efficacy and Slope

Drug Potency

- Potency is defined as the amount of dose needed to produce a desired response
- The lower the dose needed to produce a response, the more potent is the drug
- Indicated by the position of the dose response curve (DRC) on the X-axis (dose axis). Right shift indicates a decreased potency (Figure 10).
- For example, the analgesic dose of morphine is 10 mg while that of pethidine is 100 mg. This means that morphine is 10 times more potent than pethidine.

Drug Efficacy

- Efficacy is defined as the maximal response elicited by the drug
- Indicated by the upper limit of the DRC. Higher upper limit indicates a higher drug efficacy (Figure 10).

Slope of the DRC

- Steep slope indicates that the response will rapidly increase with moderate increase in dose—e.g. antihypertensive effect of hydralazine
- Flat slope indicates that response will gradually increase over a wide range of dose—e.g. antihypertensive effect of hydrochlorothiazide.

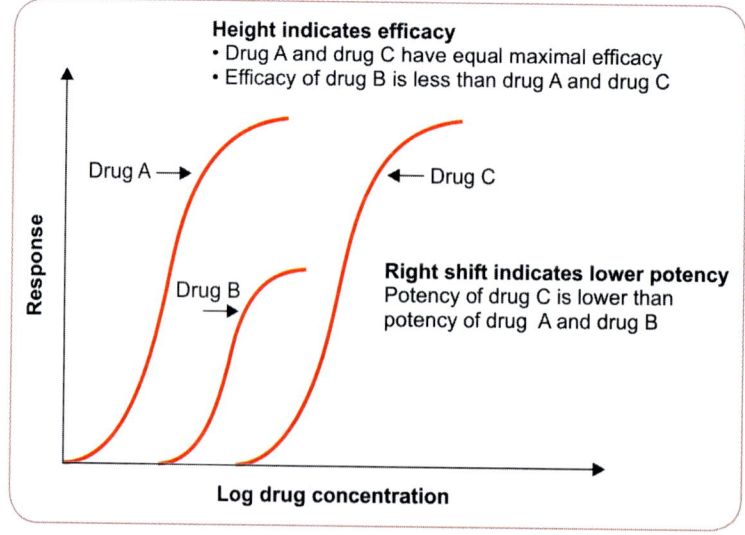

Figure 10: Dose-response relationship

Therapeutic Index and Therapeutic Window

Therapeutic index is an indicator of drug safety and is a ratio of median lethal dose and median effective dose of the drug. It is the distance between the therapeutic response DRC and the adverse effect DRC (Figure 11). In experimental animals, the following formula is used to calculate the therapeutic index:

$$\text{Therapeutic index} = \frac{\text{Median lethal dose (LD}_{50}\text{)}}{\text{Median effective dose (ED}_{50}\text{)}}$$

- LD_{50}: Amount of drug that is lethal in 50% of the population
- ED_{50}: Amount of drug that produces the desired response in 50% of the population

In humans, therapeutic index is very rarely known accurately and clinical drug trials along with clinical experience are used to identify a therapeutic window.

Warfarin, digoxin, lithium etc. have a small therapeutic window, while penicillin has a large therapeutic index.

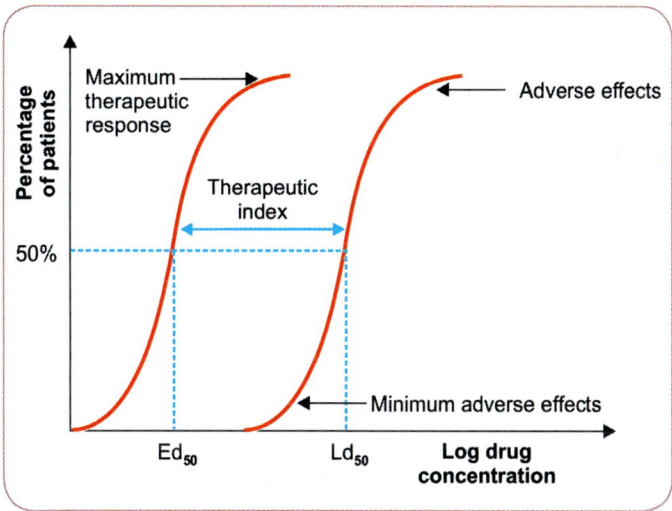

Figure 11: Therapeutic index

Therapeutic window is the range of drug doses which produces the desired response but with minimal toxic effects.

Drugs with a small therapeutic window must be carefully administered. There is a need for frequently measuring drug concentration in the blood.

▮ COMBINED EFFECT OF DRUGS

Administration of two or more drugs together or in rapid succession may lead to the following effects, based on the pharmacokinetic and pharmacodynamic properties (Figure 12).
- Additive effect (Summation)
- Synergism
- Antagonism
- Indifference—no effect on each other's pharmacologic properties

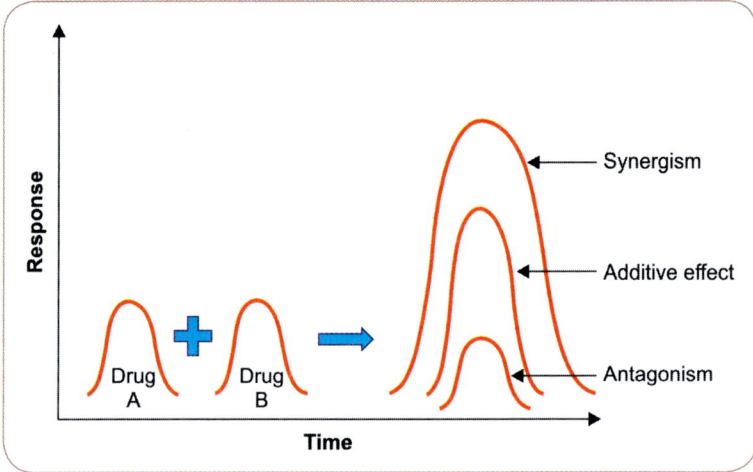

Figure 12: Combined effect of drugs

Additive Effect (Summation)

The combined effect of two or more drugs is equivalent to the sum of their individual pharmacological effect $(1 + 1 = 2)$.

Effect of drug $(X + Y)$ = Effect of drug X + Effect of drug Y

For example, paracetamol + aspirin → used as antipyretic/analgesic

Synergism

The combined effect of two or more drugs is more than the sum of their individual pharmacological effect $(1 + 1 = 3)$. This is usually a result of facilitation of the effect of one drug by another.

Effect of drug $(X + Y)$ >> Effect of drug X + Effect of drug Y

For example, levodopa + carbidopa → used in Parkinsonism

Antagonism

When one drug decreases or abolishes the effect of the other drug, they are said to be antagonistic.
The antagonism can be of following types (Figures 13 and 14):
- Physical antagonism
- Chemical antagonism
- Physiological/Functional antagonism
- Receptor antagonism
  - Competitive (equilibrium)
  - Noncompetitive
  - Competitive (nonequilibrium)

Types of antagonism		
	Competitive antagonism (equilibrium)	**Noncompetitive antagonism**
Receptor antagonism	Antagonist is structurally similar to the agonist and both bind to the same site of the receptor	Antagonist is not structurally similar to the agonist and bind to a different site of the receptor
	Prevents binding of agonist to the receptor or Prevents the effects of the agonist	Binding of antagonist to the receptor alters the receptor in such a way, that agonist is now no longer able to bind to the receptor
	Antagonism can be overcome by increasing the concentration of agonist	Antagonism cannot be overcome by increasing the concentration of agonist
	Reduction in potency of the agonist → right shift of the DRC with no reduction in efficacy	Reduction in efficacy of the agonist → flattening of the DRC
	For example, naloxone is a competitive antagonist at opioid receptors	For example, diazepam and bicuculline

Competitive (nonequilibrium)
- Antagonist binds covalently (i.e. strongly) to the same site of receptor, as that of the agonist
- Leads to flattening of the DRC
- For example, phenoxybenzamine is a nonequilibrium antagonist at α adrenergic receptors for adrenaline

Physiological antagonism
- Two drugs act on different receptors or by different mechanisms on the same physiological system, but have opposite physiological responses
- For example, insulin leads to hypoglycemia but glucagon leads to hyperglycemia; histamine causes bronchoconstriction but adrenaline causes bronchodilatation

Chemical antagonism
- The two drugs interact chemically and leads to the formation of inactive substance
- For example, oxidation of alkaloids by $KMnO_4$ used for gastric lavage, formation of complexes between chelating agents and heavy metals

Physical antagonism
- Antagonism of the two drugs is based upon their physical properties
- For example, adsorption of alkaloids by charcoal → used for alkaloid poisonings

Figure 13: Types of antagonism

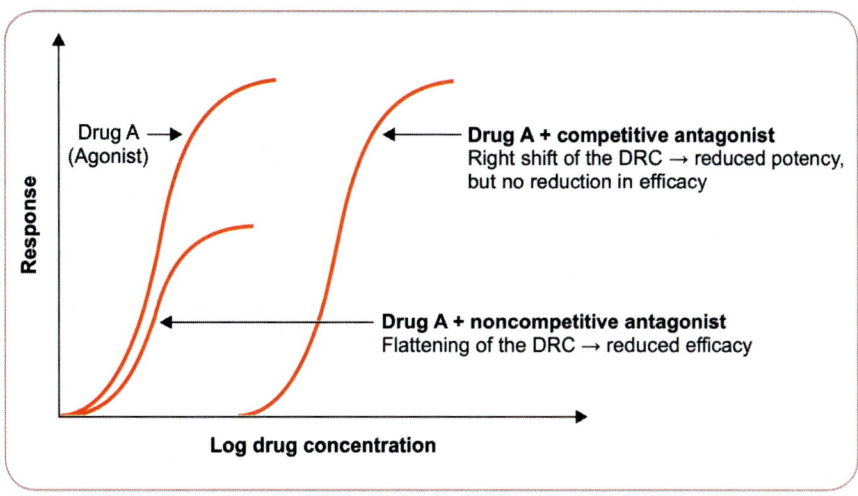

Figure 14: Competitive and noncompetitive antagonism

ASSESS YOURSELF (Examination Questions of Various Universities)

1. Therapeutic index
2. Therapeutic window
3. Competitive and noncompetitive antagonism
4. Inverse agonists
5. Dose-response curve

MULTIPLE CHOICE QUESTIONS

1. Which of the following statement is correct regarding the given DRCs? *(AIIMS Nov 2016)*

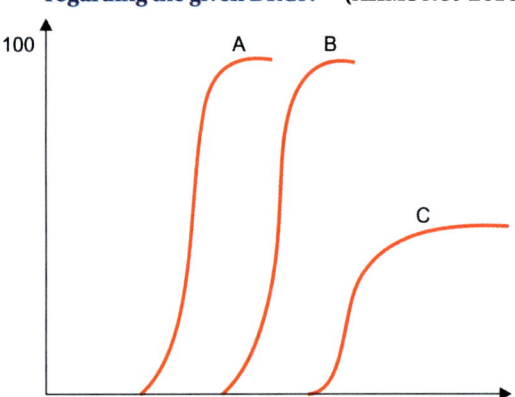

   a. A and B are full agonists
   b. C is noncompetitive antagonist
   c. B more potent than A
   d. A more efficacious than B

2. When two drugs acting on different receptors have opposite action, it is known as:
   (Recent Question Dec 2016)
   a. Physiological antagonism
   b. Competitive antagonism
   c. Noncompetitive antagonism
   d. Chemical antagonism

3. A partial agonist has: *(Recent Question 2016)*
   a. High affinity but low intrinsic activity
   b. High affinity but no intrinsic activity
   c. Low affinity but high intrinsic activity
   d. Low affinity but low intrinsic activity

4. Agonist is having: *(Recent Question 2016)*
   a. Affinity with intrinsic activity is 1
   b. Affinity with intrinsic activity is 0
   c. Affinity with intrinsic activity is -1
   d. None

5. Efficacy of a drug means:
   (Recent Question 2016)
   a. Maximum absorption of a drug
   b. Maximum metabolism of a drug
   c. Maximum response that can be elicited by the drug
   d. Maximum binding to its receptor

6. When a drug binds to the receptor and causes action opposite to that of agonist this is called as: *(Recent Question 2016)*
   a. Complete agonist
   b. Inverse agonist
   c. Partial agonist
   d. Neutral antagonist

7. When a drug binds to the receptor and causes action submaximal to that of agonist this is called as: *(Recent Question 2016)*
   a. Complete agonist
   b. Partial agonist
   c. Inverse agonist
   d. Neutral antagonist

8. Potency of a drug is a measure of its:
   a. Dose *(Recent Question 2016)*
   b. Efficacy
   c. Safety
   d. Therapeutic index

9. Which of the following act through G protein coupled receptors? *(AIIMS May 2018)*
   a. Ach muscarinic receptors
   b. Insulin receptors
   c. Ach Nicotinic receptors
   d. GABA-A receptors

10. Therapeutic index is a measure of:
    a. Potency *(AIIMS May 2018)*
    b. Efficacy
    c. Safety
    d. Potency + efficacy

Ans.

1.	(a)	2.	(a)	3.	(a)	4.	(a)	5.	(c)	6.	(b)
7.	(b)	8.	(a)	9.	(a)	10.	(c)				

4

Factors Modifying Drug Action

INTRODUCTION

Every individual responds differently to drugs. The way an individual respond to a drug is affected by many factors.

Individuals more commonly show quantitative differences in drug response (e.g. the plasma concentration or drug action increases or decreases) but sometimes show qualitative differences in drug response (type of response is different, e.g. drug allergy, idiosyncrasy).

The various factors modifying drug action are discussed below:

Age

Neonates

The excretory system of the kidney and the metabolizing system of the liver is immature and not fully developed in the neonates. This may lead to an increased half-life of drugs excreted by kidneys (e.g. gentamicin and penicillin), as well as gray baby syndrome with chloramphenicol (due to immature liver metabolizing enzymes).

Children

Children are growing and hence, are vulnerable to distinct adverse effects, e.g. steroids may lead to growth stunting, tetracyclines may lead to teeth staining, androgens may lead to premature epiphysis fusion, etc.

The dose of a drug in a child can be calculated by the following methods (Table 1):

TABLE 1	Dose calculation in children
Young's formula	**Dilling's formula**
Child dose = $\dfrac{\text{Age}}{\text{Age} + 12}$ × adult dose	Child dose = $\dfrac{\text{Age}}{20}$ × adult dose

Elderly

The kidney function and the liver metabolizing system gradually decline with progression of age in the elderly. The incidence of adverse effects is comparatively higher in the elderly as compared to adults; hence, the doses of the drug must be accordingly reduced, e.g. streptomycin dose reduction is required in the elderly.

The elderly populations are possibly taking multiple drugs due to concomitant diseases such as hypertension, diabetes, coronary syndrome, arthritis, etc.; hence, there are more chances of drug interactions.

Body Weight

The body weight (BW) impacts the drug concentration attained at the site of action. The adult dose refers to the dose required for an average sized adult. In cases of extremely obese or thin individuals and in children, the dosage can be calculated by the following:

$$\text{Dose} = \frac{\text{Body weight (kg)}}{70} \times \text{average adult dose}$$

A more accurate method of calculating the daily dose is by body surface area (BSA) instead of BW. However, since BSA calculation is difficult, BW is routinely used for dose calculations except in a few situations such as anticancer drugs.

Sex

Females have a smaller body size; therefore, they require smaller drug doses as compared to males.

Physiologic differences between males and females affect drug activity, including pharmacokinetics and pharmacodynamics.

Pharmacokinetic differences in females include slower GI motility, lesser intestinal enzymatic activity and slower glomerular filtration rate.

Pharmacodynamic differences in females include increased efficacy of drugs such as beta blockers, opioids, selective serotonin reuptake inhibitors and typical antipsychotics.

Additionally, females have a higher possibility of experiencing adverse drug reactions as compared to males. Examples include:

- Females are more susceptible to torsades de pointes; hence, medications known to prolong QT interval should be used with caution
- Females have higher mortality rates with the use of digoxin for heart failure

Further, menstruation, pregnancy and lactation must also be considered while prescribing drugs to females.

Environmental Factors

Cigarette smoking and consumption of charcoal broiled meat induce drug metabolizing enzymes, so the dose may need to be increased in smokers.

Food interferes with ampicillin absorption but a fatty meal increases the absorption of griseofulvin.

Genetic Factors (Pharmacogenetics)

The study of variability in drug response due to genetic factors is called pharmacogenetics.

Some specific genetic defects that lead to variation in drug response are mentioned in Table 2.

TABLE 2	Genetic defects and variation in drug response
G6PD deficiency and hemolytic anemia	• In G6PD deficiency, when oxidizing drugs (such as primaquine, quinine, sulfonamides, nitrofurantoin, etc.) are given, the reduction of glutathione and conversion of methemoglobin to hemoglobin cannot occur in the RBCs. This results in hemolysis.
Slow and rapid acetylators and peripheral neuritis	• Deficiency of the enzyme N-acetyl transferase results in slow acetylator status. • Isoniazid induced peripheral neuritis and hydralazine/procainamide induced lupus occurs mainly in slow acetylators.
Atypical pseudocholinesterase and apnea	• Succinylcholine which is a neuromuscular blocker is metabolized by plasma pseudocholinesterase enzyme within 5 minutes. • In some individuals, there is an atypical pseudocholinesterase which takes a long time to metabolize succinylcholine (1–2 hours). In such cases, therapeutic doses of succinylcholine lead to prolonged apnea due to paralysis of respiratory muscles.
UGT1A1*28 genotype and neutropenia	• Patients with UGT1A1*28 genotype of UDP-glucuronosyltransferase enzyme are more prone to development of irinotecan-induced neutropenia and diarrhea.
δ-aminolevulinic acid (ALA) synthetase enzyme and acute intermittent porphyria	• Barbiturates induce the enzyme involved in porphyrin synthesis, ALA synthetase, resulting in increased porphyrin synthesis. • Patients with a genetic defect in suppressing the enzyme ALA synthetase, may experience increased porphyrin synthesis (when barbiturates are given) leading to acute intermittent porphyria.

Psychosocial Factors

The nonpharmacological (psychosocial) factors can affect the patient's response to a drug. It is governed by patient's personality, beliefs and attitude.

Some patients respond to pharmacologically inert substances called the 'Placebo'.

Placebo

Placebo is a Latin word meaning 'I will please'. It is generally an inert substance like lactose tablet or distilled water injection. It does not have any pharmacological activity. The placebo works psychologically.

The response elicited in a patient is called placebo effect. The conditions where placebos may produce effects include pain, anxiety, etc.

Placebos are used in the following situations:
- As control (dummy) mediations in clinical trials
- As therapeutic agents that work psychologically for the relief of symptoms, e.g. pain, anxiety, insomnia, etc.

Pathological States

Gastrointestinal Disease

Achlorhydria (where acid secretion in the stomach is absent) decreases the absorption of weekly acidic drugs by favoring its ionization. Low acidity also decreases the absorption of iron from the stomach.

Liver Disease

The bioavailability of drugs having high first-pass metabolism (e.g. propranolol) is increased in chronic liver disease. This is because of limited capacity of liver for metabolizing drugs in liver disease.

The prodrugs which require hepatic metabolism for the release of active metabolites (levodopa, bacampicillin, etc.) are less effective.

Kidney Disease

The clearance of drugs that are excreted unchanged by the kidneys (aminoglycosides, digoxin, etc.) is decreased in kidney disease. This may lead to toxicity such as ototoxicity and nephrotoxicity with aminoglycosides.

Repeated doses of pethidine in kidney disease may lead to the accumulation of its metabolite norpethidine, which can cause convulsions.

Thyroid Disease

Hyperthyroid patients are very sensitive to sympathomimetics and are relatively resistant to morphine, digitalis or CNS depressants.

Tolerance

Tolerance refers to a decreased response to the drug, which occurs when the drug is repeatedly used and the body adapts to the continued presence of the drug.

In simple words, tolerance means a need for higher doses to produce a given response.

Examples include:
- Tolerance to antianginal effect of organic nitrates on long-term use
- Tolerance to alcohol, barbiturates, morphine, etc.

Types of Tolerance

The different types of tolerance are mentioned in Figure 1.

SECTION A ■ General Pharmacology

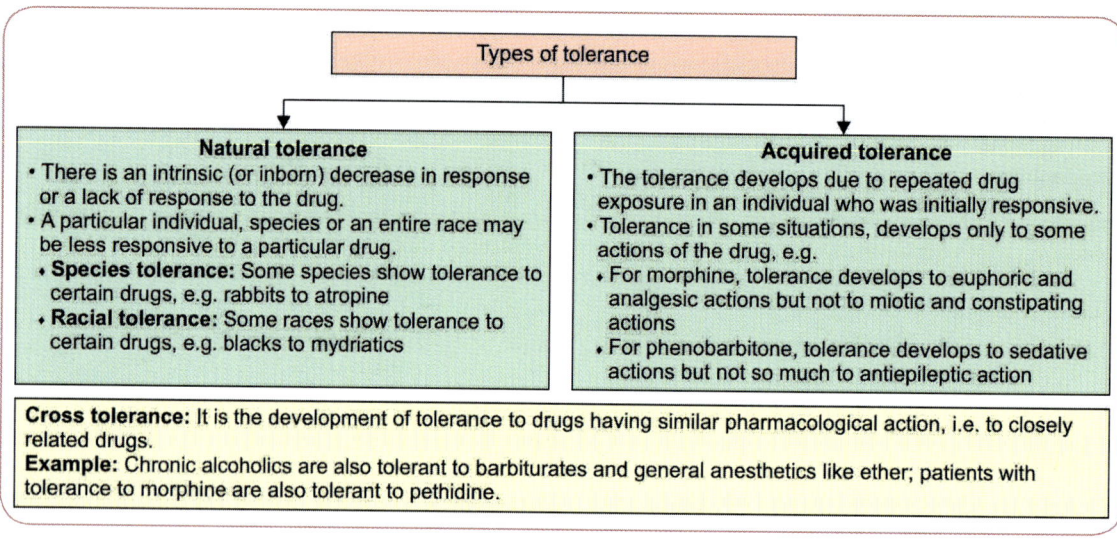

Figure 1: Types of tolerance

Tachyphylaxis (Greek: tachys – 'rapid', and phylaxis – 'protection')

It is the rapid decrease in response to certain drugs when they are administered repeatedly at very short intervals.

It is also known as acute tolerance.

It is mostly observed with indirectly acting drugs such as ephedrine, tyramine, amphetamine, etc.

These drugs act by rapidly releasing catecholamines (such as norepinephrine) from the storage sites, the synthesis of which is unable to match the release.

Other mechanism such as change in the sensitivity of the target tissues may also be responsible.

Drug Resistance

It refers to tolerance in microorganisms to the inhibitory action of antimicrobial drugs. Examples include staphylococcal resistance to penicillin, mycobacterial resistance to antitubercular drugs, etc.

Mechanisms of Development of Tolerance

The tolerance can be either pharmacokinetic (dispositional) or pharmacodynamic (functional) (Figure 2).

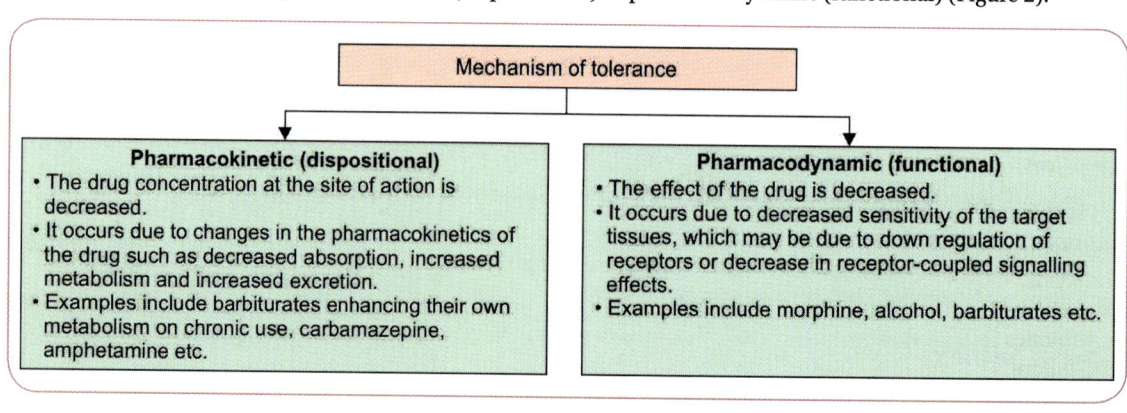

Figure 2: Mechanism of tolerance

DRUG INTERACTIONS

When two or more drugs are administered simultaneously or in quick succession, the effect of one drug can be modified or altered by another drug.

Drug interactions may lead to increased or decreased effects and may produce beneficial or harmful effects. The possibility of drug interactions increases with the number of drugs used.

Hence, a physician using multidrug therapy should be aware and cautious about the possibility of drug interactions.

The drug interactions can be classified as mentioned in Figure 3.

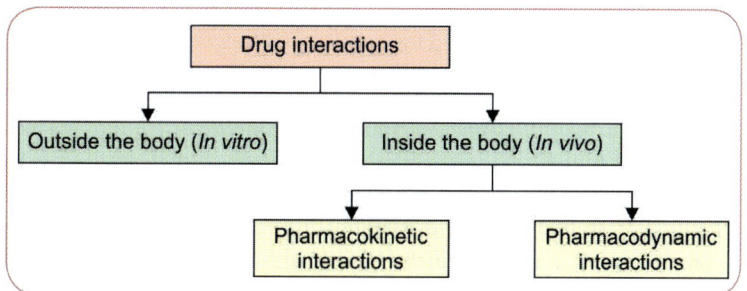

Figure 3: Types of drug interactions

Drug Interactions Occurring Outside the Body (*In vitro*)

This scenario is usually applicable when two or more drugs are mixed in an intravenous infusion or when they are mixed in the same syringe.

There may be inactivation or precipitation of one or more drugs due to physical or chemical incompatibilities.

Examples include the following:
- Penicillin/ampicillin should not be mixed with aminoglycosides in the same syringe because they interact chemically to form amides that are inactive. Hence, both penicillin and aminoglycosides are rendered ineffective.
- Phenytoin, barbiturates, methicillin should not be administered in highly acidic dextrose solution because these drugs get precipitated.

It is usually advised to avoid mixing two or more parenteral drugs before administration.

Drug Interactions Occurring Inside the Body (*In vivo*)

Pharmacokinetic Interaction

In this type of interaction, one drug affects the absorption, distribution, metabolism or excretion of the other drug. This results in an increase or decrease in concentration of the other drug at its site of action.

Absorption

The absorption of one drug is affected by the other concomitantly administered drug.

Examples include:
- Antacids, calcium, iron, etc. inhibits the absorption of tetracycline by forming an insoluble and poorly absorbed complex.
- Antibiotics such as tetracycline, ampicillin, etc. inhibit the absorption of oral contraceptives (OC) leading to OC failure.
  - Normally, the OC steroids are secreted in the bile as glucuronide conjugates. The intestinal bacteria deconjugate the steroids and release the steroids which are reabsorbed back from the intestine (enterohepatic circulation).
  - The antibiotics inhibit the intestinal bacteria and reduces the enterohepatic circulation. This leads to decreased OC levels in the blood resulting in OC failure.

Drugs inhibiting the gastrointestinal motility affects the absorption of other drugs, e.g. metoclopramide increases gastric emptying; hence, increases the absorption of other drugs.

Distribution

The interactions occurring due to distribution are those that involve plasma protein binding.

Multiple drugs can bind to the same site of plasma proteins. Hence, a drug with higher affinity for the plasma proteins will displace the other drug with lower affinity. This results in an increased concentration of the unbound (free) and pharmacologically active form of the drug that has been displaced.

Example include:
○ Salicylates (e.g. aspirin) displace warfarin and tolbutamide from protein binding sites leading to their increased blood levels that may result in hemorrhage and hypoglycemia respectively.

Metabolism

The metabolism of one drug is decreased (by enzyme inhibition) or increased (by enzyme induction) by the other drug.

Examples include:
○ Phenytoin, phenobarbitone, rifampicin, carbamazepine induces the metabolizing enzymes of antibiotics (e.g. metronidazole, tetracycline) and oral contraceptives resulting in failure of antibiotic therapy and OCs.
○ Erythromycin inhibits the metabolizing enzymes of carbamazepine, warfarin, theophylline and may lead to increase in their plasma levels and toxicity.

Excretion

The interaction during excretion mostly occurs at the level of tubular secretion.

Examples include:
○ Probenecid inhibits the tubular secretion of penicillins and cephalosporins, thereby increases their plasma levels and duration of action.
○ Aspirin inhibits the tubular secretion of methotrexate, thus increasing its toxicity.

The interaction during excretion may also occur by altering the pH of the urine. For example, excretion of weakly acidic drugs such as salicylates, barbiturates and sulfonamides can be increased by making the urine alkaline (i.e. by administering alkalization drugs). This method is mostly employed during treatment of drug poisonings.

Pharmacodynamic Interaction

In this type of interaction, the actions of one drug are modified at the target site by another drug. It does not lead to any change in concentration of the drugs.

The interaction mostly occurs at the level of receptors and may result in additive, synergistic or antagonistic effects.

Examples include:
○ Enhanced ototoxicity occurs when aminoglycosides are given with other ototoxic drugs, e.g. furosemide, ethacrynic acid.
○ Enhanced nephrotoxicity occurs when aminoglycosides are given with other nephrotoxic drugs, e.g. amphotericin B, cyclosporine.
○ Severe hyperkalemia occurs when ACE inhibitors are given with K^+-sparing diuretics.

▌ RATIONAL USE OF MEDICINES

As stated by the World Health Organisation (WHO) rational use of medicines requires that "the patients receive medication appropriate to their clinical needs in doses that meet their own individual requirements for an adequate period of time, and at the lowest cost to them and to their community".

It requires the administration of the right drug, in right dose, at right cost to the right patient.

Irrationalities in Prescribing

- Unjustified use of drugs, e.g. antibiotics for viral infections
- Use of drugs unrelated to the diagnosis, e.g. proton pump blockers for any abdominal pain
- Inappropriate use of drugs, i.e. incorrect drug, incorrect route, incorrect dose
- Unnecessary use of fixed drug combinations
- Unsafe use of drugs, e.g. using single antitubercular drug
- Use of drugs with doubtful efficacy, e.g. memory enhancers
- Polypharmacy without considering potential drug interactions

Dangers of Irrational use of Drugs

- Delay/failure in providing relief to the patient or treatment of the disease
- Increased chances of adverse drug reactions
- Increased chances of microbial resistance
- Increased cost of treatment
- Loss of patient's trust in the doctor
- Decreased health standards of the community.

Section A ■ General Pharmacology

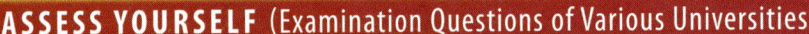

ASSESS YOURSELF (Examination Questions of Various Universities)

1. Describe drug tolerance. Give suitable examples
2. Tachyphylaxis
3. Drug interactions

MULTIPLE CHOICE QUESTIONS

1. Which of the following is most likely due to a pharmacogenetic condition?
   (Recent Question 2016)
   a. Hypoglycemia by insulin
   b. Tachycardia by albuterol
   c. Metoclopramide induced muscle dystonia
   d. Primaquine-induced hemolytic anemia

2. Idiosyncrasy is: *(Recent Question 2016)*
   a. Unpredictable reaction to a drug
   b. Predictable effect of a drug at normal concentration
   c. Predictable effect of a drug at high concentration
   d. Non of the above

3. True about Placebo: *(PGI May 2014)*
   a. It works only in psychiatric person
   b. Response is both objective & subjective
   c. Effect also seen in normal person
   d. It is an inert substance

Ans.

1. (d)   2. (a)   3. (b, c, d)

5 Drug Development, Pharmacovigilance and Adverse Drug Reactions

Medicines have been used by humans since ancient times. It is a known fact that medicines are not absolutely safe and do have the potential to cause harm.

In the year 1972, *Claude Bernard* stated that *"everything is poisonous, nothing is poisonous, it is all a matter of dose."*

Hence, medicines when used in large doses have the potential to cause harm (poison) and poison when used in small doses can have beneficial effect as medicines.

DRUG DEVELOPMENT

Drug development is the process of introducing a new medicinal product into the market following its discovery.

The approval to market a drug in a particular territory or country is given by a regulatory authority following review of data from various clinical studies conducted as a part of the drug development process.

Generally, the development process of a new drug goes through multiple phases as mentioned in Table 1.

TABLE 1	Drug development
Preclinical testing	• Animal studies including toxicology, carcinogenicity, teratogenicity
Phase I clinical trials (First in human)	• Objective is to identify the safe dosage range, observe adverse effects and understand the safety profile and tolerability of the drug • Phase I studies are conducted in a small number of subjects who are usually healthy volunteers
Phase II clinical trials (First in patient)	• Objective is to assess dosing recommendations, determination of efficacy and evaluation of safety • Phase II studies are generally conducted in a large number of volunteers who are usually patients
Phase III clinical trials (Multicenter trials)	• Objective is to confirm the efficacy of the new drug on the clinical course of the disease and to evaluate the risk-benefit profile • Phase III studies are generally conducted in a larger number of patients
Phase IV clinical trials (Postmarketing surveillance)	• Objective is to monitor and identify the safety concerns of a drug following its approval for marketing • Phase IV studies aim to provide further information about the safety and efficacy of a drug in a larger population

PHARMACOVIGILANCE

The World Health Organization (WHO) defines Pharmacovigilance (PV) as the science and activities relating to the detection, assessment, understanding and prevention of adverse effects or any other drug related problem.

The term pharmacovigilance originates from *pharmakon* (Greek) meaning "drug" and *vigilare* (Latin) meaning "to keep watch" (Figure 1).

Figure 1: Pharmacovigilance

Key Stakeholders in Pharmacovigilance

Pharmacovigilance is a collaborative engagement amongst the key stakeholders to ensure that the medicines have a positive benefit-risk balance.

The key stakeholders are as follows:

- Patient
- Physician or the healthcare professional (HCP)
- Marketing authorization holder (MAH)/Pharmaceutical company
- Regulatory agencies

■ ADVERSE DRUG REACTIONS

A key objective of pharmacovigilance is to ensure that the drug used in a patient has the maximum benefit with the lowest possibility of risk.

Collating information about adverse drug reactions (ADRs) is a critical part of pharmacovigilance and is required for monitoring the benefit-risk balance of a drug.

The ICH E2A guideline (*ICH Harmonized Tripartite Guideline: Clinical Safety Data Management: Definitions and Standards for Expedited Reporting - E2A*) mentions the following definitions:

Adverse event (AE): Any untoward medical occurrence in a patient or clinical investigation subject administered a pharmaceutical product and which does not necessarily have to have a causal relationship with this treatment.

An adverse event can therefore be any unfavorable and unintended sign (including an abnormal laboratory finding), symptom, or disease temporally associated with the use of a medicinal product, whether or not considered related to the medicinal product.

Adverse drug reaction (ADR): All noxious and unintended responses to a medicinal product related to any dose should be considered adverse drug reactions.

The phrase "responses to a medicinal product" means that a causal relationship between a medicinal product and an adverse event is at least a reasonable possibility, i.e. the relationship cannot be ruled out.

Types of Adverse Drug Reactions

The pharmacological classification of ADRs is mentioned in Table 2.

TABLE 2	Classification of ADRs
Type of ADRs	**Comments**
Type A (Augmented)	• Usually predictable and dose related • Due to augmentation of pharmacological effects of the drug • For example, respiratory depression in opioid overdose
Type B (Bizarre)	• Unpredictable and not related to dose • Unclear mechanism that may not be explained by the pharmacological effects of the drug • For example, hypersensitivity reactions
Type C (Chronic or continuing)	• Observed upon chronic exposure to a drug • For example, prednisolone induced adrenal suppression
Type D (Delayed)	• Observed sometime after exposure to drug • For example, teratogenicity, malignancy
Type E (End of use)	• These are reactions following drug withdrawal • For example, morphine withdrawal
Type F (Failure of therapy)	• Lack of efficacy following drug exposure • For example, resistance to antibiotics

ASSESS YOURSELF (Examination Questions of Various Universities)

1. Define the term pharmacovigilance. Discuss different type of adverse drug effects.

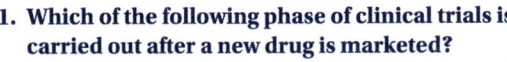

MULTIPLE CHOICE QUESTIONS

1. **Which of the following phase of clinical trials is carried out after a new drug is marketed?**
   (AIIMS May 2016)
   a. Phase 1
   b. Phase 2
   c. Phase 4
   d. Phase 0

2. **Pharmacovigilance means:** *(AIIMS May 2010)*
   a. Monitoring of drug safety
   b. Monitoring of unethical trade of drugs
   c. Monitoring pharma students
   d. Monitoring drug efficacy

3. **Pharmacovigilance is used:** *(AIIMS May 2009)*
   a. To monitor drug toxicity
   b. To monitor unauthorized drug manufacture
   c. For monitoring of students
   d. To check costs

4. **The aim of postmarketing studies is:**
   (Recent Question 2016)
   a. Efficacy of the drug
   b. Dosage of the drug
   c. Deals with alteration of the drug includes absorption, distribution, binding/storage
   d. Safety and comparisons with other medicines

5. **Stage IV clinical trial is also called as:**
   (Recent Question 2016)
   a. Human pharmacology and safety
   b. Postmarketing surveillance
   c. Therapeutic exploration and does ranging
   d. Therapeutic confirmation

6. **Phase I clinical trial involves:** *(TN PG 2011)*
   a. Large number of patients (2000–5000)
   b. Normal healthy individuals
   c. Small number of patients (300–500)
   d. Marketing surveillance

Ans.

| 1. | (c) | 2. | (a) | 3. | (a) | 4. | (d) | 5. | (b) | 6. | (b) |

NOTES

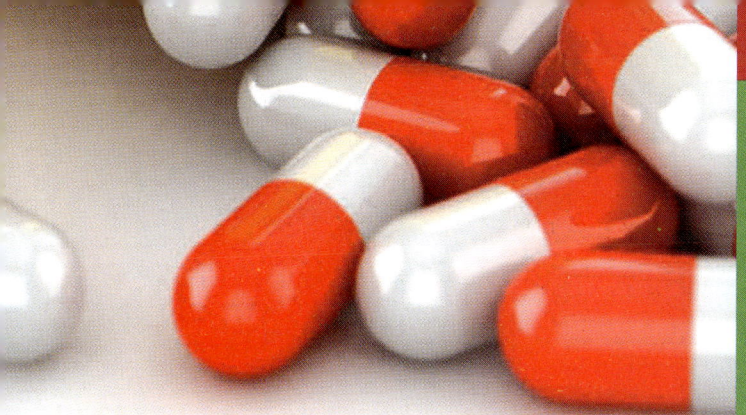

Drugs Acting on the Autonomic Nervous System

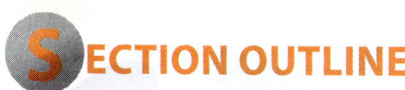 **SECTION OUTLINE**

Overview of the Autonomic Nervous System

The nervous system in the human body is divided into the central nervous system and the peripheral nervous system (Figure 1).

1. **Central Nervous System**
   - ❑ Consist of the brain and the spinal cord
2. **Peripheral Nervous System**
   - ❑ Consists of nerves derived from the brain and the spinal cord
   - ❑ It is subdivided into autonomic nervous system and the somatic nervous system

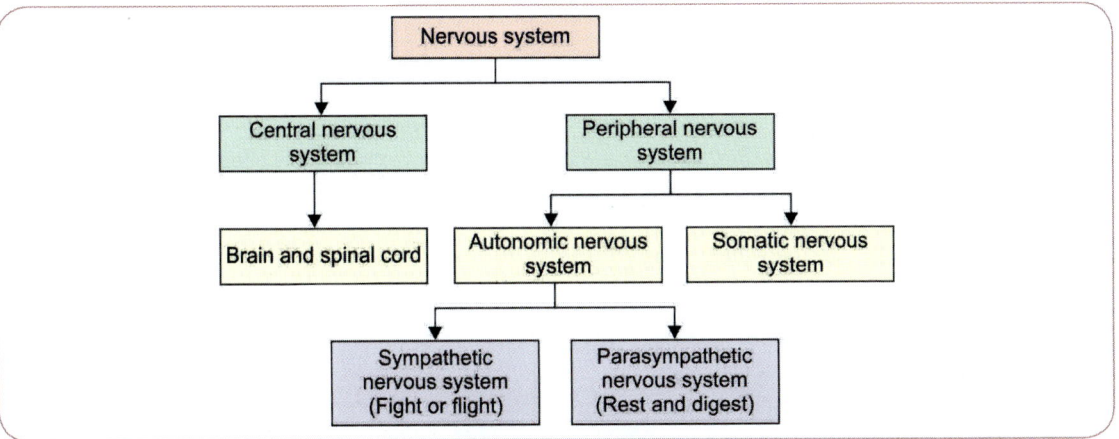

Figure 1: Nervous system

PERIPHERAL NERVOUS SYSTEM

The peripheral nervous system consists of the following (Figure 2):
- ○ Autonomic Nervous System
- ○ Somatic Nervous System

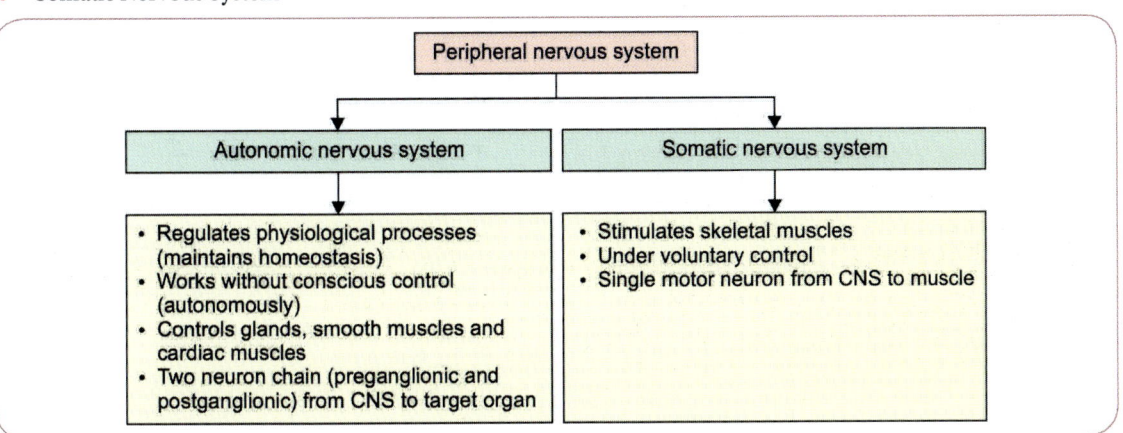

Figure 2: Peripheral nervous system

AUTONOMIC NERVOUS SYSTEM

The two major divisions of the autonomic nervous system (ANS) are as follows:
- Sympathetic Nervous System → Dominant system in fight or flight response
- Parasympathetic Nervous System → Dominant system in rest and digest activities

The parasympathetic nervous system originates from the craniosacral region; the Xth cranial nerve (vagus) contains most of the parasympathetic fibers.

The sympathetic nervous system originates from the thoracolumbar region (T1-L2).

Some of the key structural differences between the sympathetic and the parasympathetic system are mentioned in Table 1.

TABLE 1	Sympathetic versus parasympathetic system	
	Autonomic nervous system	
	Sympathetic	**Parasympathetic**
Predominant action(s)	• Stimulatory (except in GIT) • Dominant system in fight or flight response	• Inhibitory (except in GIT) • Dominant system in rest and digest activities
Origin of the fibers	• Thoracolumbar region of the spinal cord (T1 – T2)	• Cranial outflow along with III, VII, IX and X cranial nerves • Sacral outflow from S2–S4 nerve roots
Location of ganglia	• Close to the CNS, along the vertebral column	• In or close to the effector organ
Fiber length	• Preganglionic—short • Postganglionic—long	• Preganglionic—long • Postganglionic—short

The nerve fibers of the autonomic nervous system consist of two neurons that are arranged in series. Each fiber has two parts: the preganglionic and the postganglionic part.
- Preganglionic → before the ganglion
- Postganglionic → after the ganglion and goes to the effector organ

The length of the preganglionic and the postganglionic fiber varies in sympathetic and parasympathetic nervous system (Figure 3).

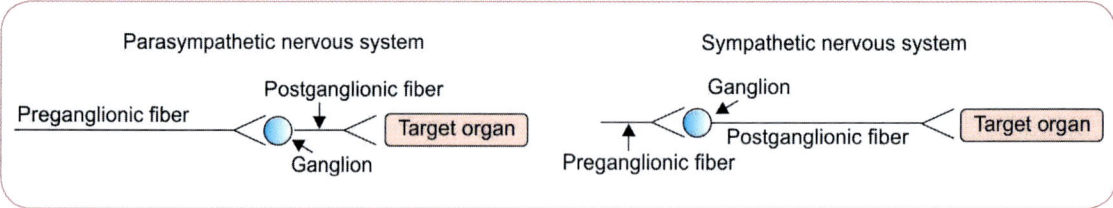

Figure 3: Pre and postganglionic fibers in the autonomic nervous system

Receptors and Neurotransmitters of the ANS

There are two types of receptors in the autonomic nervous system (Figure 4):
- Cholinergic receptors
- Adrenergic receptors

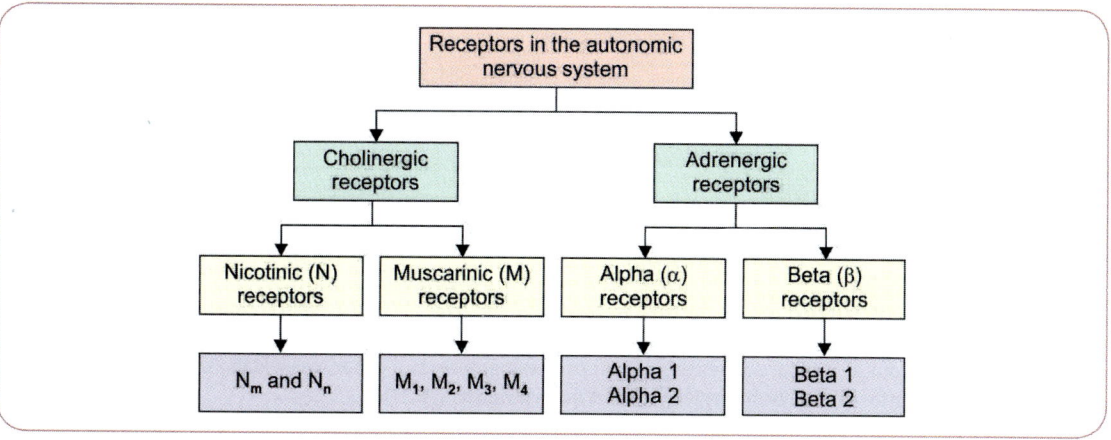

Figure 4: Receptors in the autonomic nervous system

Types of Fibers in the ANS

○ **Parasympathetic** → All pre and postganglionic fibers are cholinergic and they produce acetylcholine
○ **Sympathetic**
  ❑ Preganglionic → Cholinergic fibers and they produce acetylcholine
  ❑ Postganglionic → Most fibers are adrenergic and they produce norepinephrine (except sweat glands and blood vessels in skin)

Key Actions of the ANS

The autonomic nervous system plays a vital role in the internal homeostatic mechanism of the human body and has wide spread actions. Some of the key actions are mentioned in Table 2.

TABLE 2	Actions of ANS on some organ systems	
Organ system	**Sympathetic stimulation**	**Parasympathetic stimulation**
Eyes	• Pupillary dilatation (mydriasis)	• Pupillary constriction (miosis)
Salivary Glands	• ↓ Salivary production	• ↑ Salivary production
Cardiac	• ↑ Heart rate • ↑ Force of contraction	• ↓ Heart rate • ↓ Force of contraction
Lungs	• Bronchodilation	• Bronchoconstriction
GIT	• ↓ Motility	• ↑ Motility & ↑ Secretions
Adrenal medulla	• Secretion of norepinephrine and epinephrine	

7 Cholinergic System and Drugs

○ All pre- and postganglionic fibers in the parasympathetic nervous system are cholinergic.
○ Preganglionic fibers in the sympathetic nervous system are cholinergic. Most postganglionic fibers in the sympathetic nervous system are adrenergic (except sweat glands and blood vessels in skin).
○ The neurotransmitter in the cholinergic system is acetylcholine (ACh).

■ ACETYLCHOLINE—SYNTHESIS, STORAGE, RELEASE AND DESTRUCTION

Acetylcholine is synthesized locally in the nerve terminals. It is synthesized from acetyl CoA and choline and the reaction is catalyzed by the enzyme choline acetyltransferase (CAT).

Acetylcholine is stored in the synaptic vesicles. The release of acetylcholine occurs in response to the action potential that reaches the nerve terminals. Upon release, acetylcholine binds to the cholinergic receptors and causes their activation.

The binding of ACh to the cholinergic receptors is brief and upon dissociation, ACh is rapidly hydrolyzed to acetate and choline by the enzyme acetylcholinesterase (AChE).

The synthesis, storage and destruction of ACh is depicted in Figure 1.

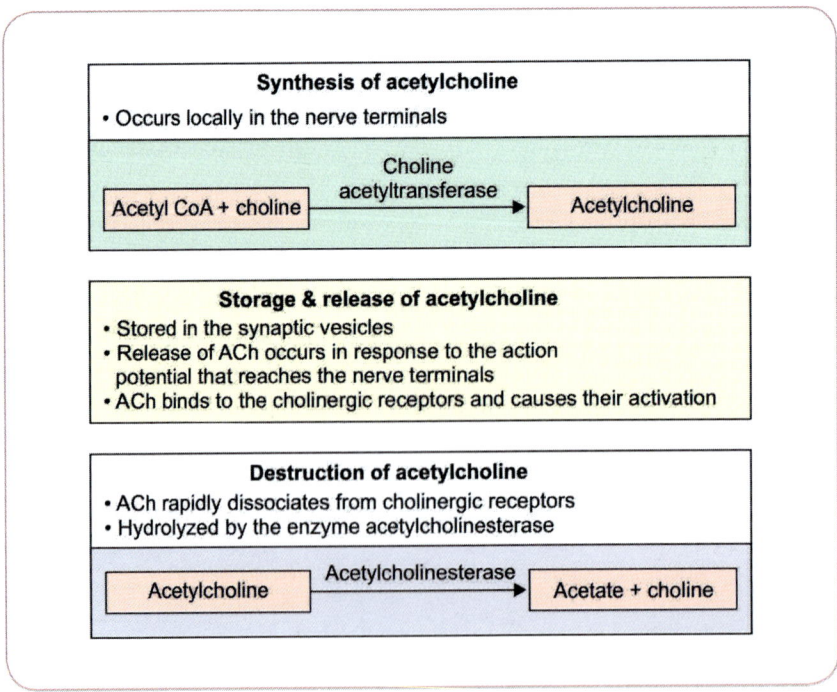

Figure 1: Acetylcholine synthesis, storage and destruction

Cholinesterase Enzyme

There are two types of cholinesterase enzymes present in the human body. Some of the salient differences amongst the two are mentioned in Table 1.

TABLE 1	Acetylcholinesterase (True) versus butyrylcholinesterase (Pseudo)	
	Acetylcholinesterase	**Butyrylcholinesterase**
Also known as	• True cholinesterase	• Pseudocholinesterase • Plasma cholinesterase
Distribution	• Neuromuscular junctions • Synapses • RBCs	• Plasma • Liver
ACh hydrolysis	• Fast	• Slow
Role (main)	• Hydrolysis of ACh	• Metabolism of ester anesthetics (procaine) • Metabolism of mivacurium, succinylcholine (muscle relaxant)

CHOLINERGIC RECEPTORS

Cholinergic receptors are of two types:
- Nicotinic receptors
- Muscarinic receptors

The types and subtypes of cholinergic receptors are mentioned in Figure 2.

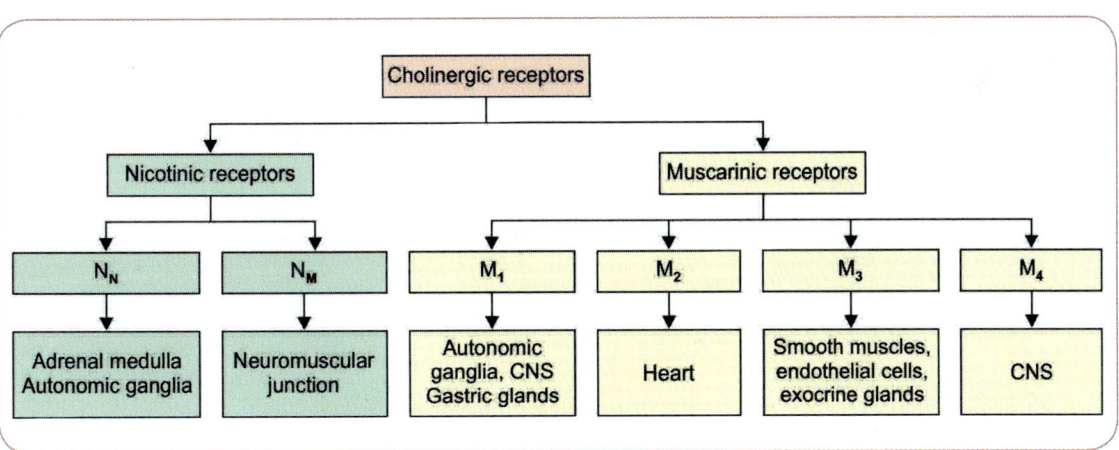

Figure 2: Cholinergic receptors

CHOLINERGIC DRUGS (CHOLINOMIMETICS, PARASYMPATHOMIMETICS)

Cholinergic drugs produce actions similar to those of acetylcholine (ACh).

These drugs produce actions either by directly acting on the cholinergic receptors or by indirectly acting to increase the availability of ACh (by inactivating the metabolizing enzyme cholinesterase). A classification of cholinergic agonists is mentioned in Figure 3.

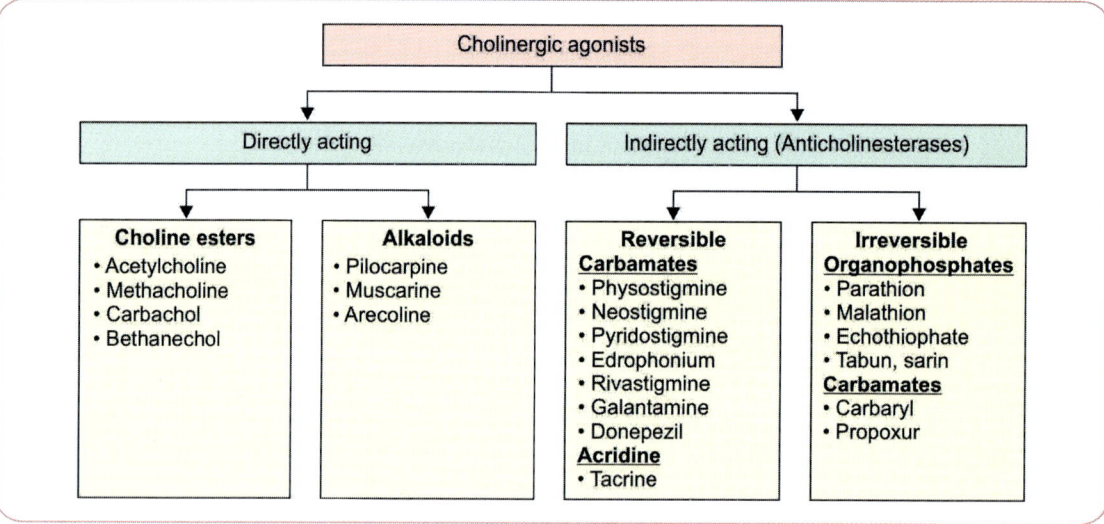

Figure 3: Classification of cholinergic agonists

DIRECTLY ACTING CHOLINERGIC AGONISTS

CHOLINE ESTERS

Acetylcholine is considered as the prototype. The other choline esters include carbachol and bethanechol. Some of the pharmacological properties of ACh and other choline esters is mentioned in Table 2.

TABLE 2	Pharmacological properties and clinical uses of choline esters				
Choline esters					
Compound	Hydrolyzed by cholinesterases	Muscarinic activity	Nicotinic activity	Antagonism by atropine	Clinical uses
Acetylcholine	+++	+++	++	+++	No clinical use*
Carbachol	– – –	+++	+++	+	Glaucoma
Bethanechol	– – –	+++	– – –	+++	Postoperative urinary retention, Postoperative paralytic ileus

*Acetylcholine is not used clinically because of an extremely short duration of action.

Acetylcholine

Acetylcholine (ACh) is a quaternary ammonium compound that cannot penetrate the biological membranes. Hence, it has to be given intravenously.

ACh is not used clinically because when given intravenously, it has an extremely short duration of action as it is rapidly inactivated by plasma cholinesterases.

The actions of ACh are classified as either muscarinic or nicotinic, depending on the receptor subtype with which it interacts.

Muscarinic Actions

The muscarinic action of ACh are mentioned below:

Heart

The effects of ACh on the heart are similar to those produced by vagal stimulation. It stimulates M_2 receptors on the heart and produces negative chronotropic, inotropic and dromotropic effects (Figure 4).

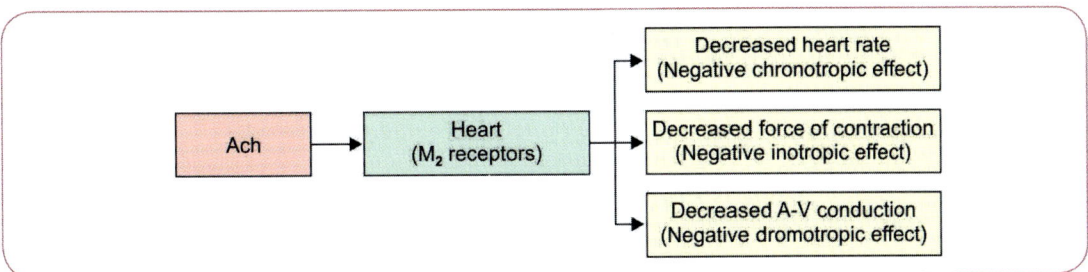

Figure 4: Effect of acetylcholine on the heart

Blood Vessels

ACh stimulates M_3 receptors on the vascular endothelial cells. This leads to the release of endothelium derived release factor (EDRF), also known as nitric oxide (NO). NO activates guanylyl cyclase resulting in increased cGMP. This results in vascular smooth muscle relaxation and vasodilatation (Figure 5).

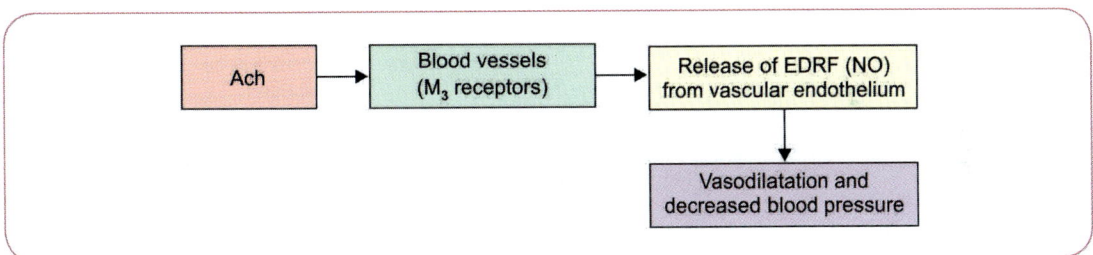

Figure 5: Effect of acetylcholine on the blood vessels

Gastrointestinal Tract (GIT)

ACh by stimulating M_3 receptors in the GIT, increases the tone and peristalsis of the GIT. The sphincters are relaxed, leading to defecation. The gastrointestinal secretions are increased (Figure 6).

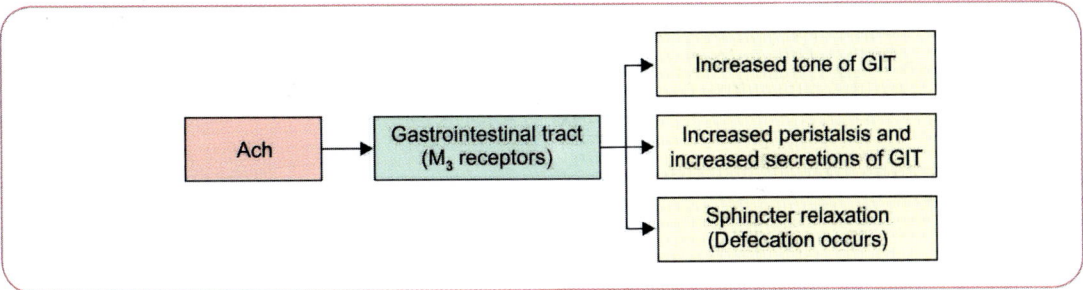

Figure 6: Effect of acetylcholine on the gastrointestinal tract

Urinary Bladder

ACh, by stimulating M_3 receptors in the urinary bladder, contracts the detrusor muscle and relaxes the trigone and sphincter leading to urination (Figure 7).

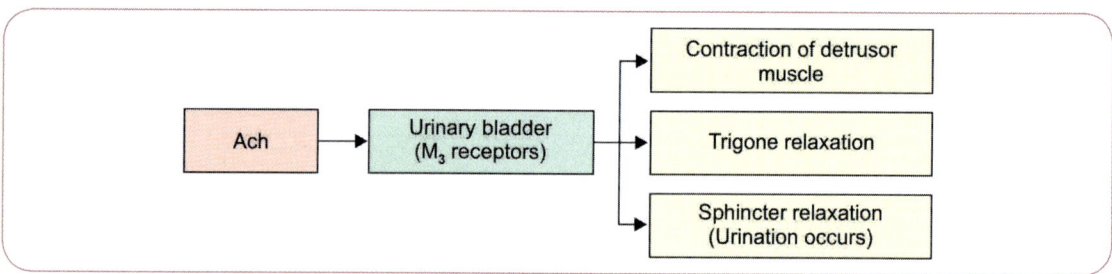

Figure 7: Effect of acetylcholine on the urinary bladder

Lungs

ACh, by stimulating M_3 receptors in the lungs, contracts the bronchial smooth muscle and increases the tracheobronchial secretions (Figure 8). This may result in precipitation of an attack of bronchial asthma.

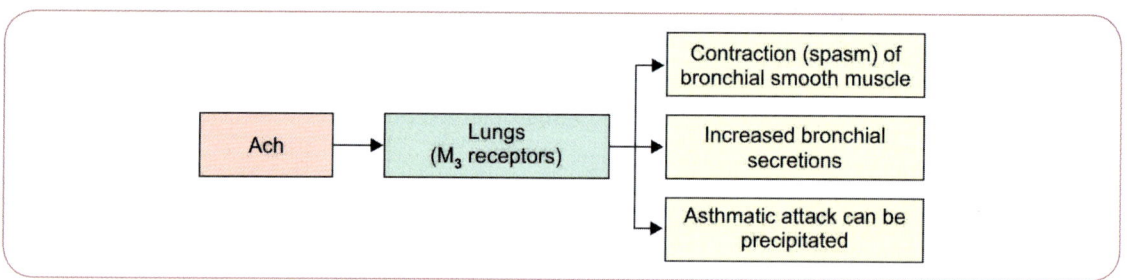

Figure 8: Effect of acetylcholine on lungs

Eyes

ACh, by stimulating M_3 receptors in the eyes, contracts the sphincter (circular) muscle of the iris resulting in miosis. It also contracts the ciliary muscle of the iris causing the lens to become more convex and leading to spasm of accommodation for near vision.

These effects result in opening of pores around the canals of Schlemm leading to drainage of aqueous humour and decrease of intraocular pressure in glaucomatous patients (Figure 9).

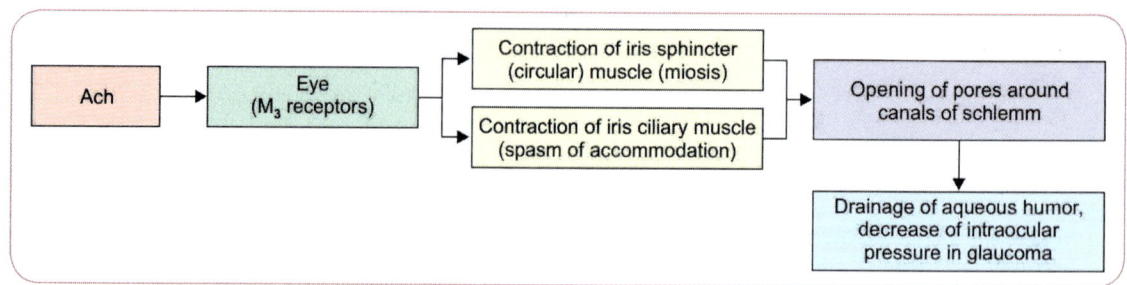

Figure 9: Effect of acetylcholine on eyes

Glands

ACh causes an increase in the secretions of sweat, salivary, lacrimal, gastric, bronchial and intestinal glands.

Nicotinic Actions

Higher doses of acetylcholine are required to produce the nicotinic actions.

Autonomic Ganglia

ACh, in higher doses stimulates both sympathetic and parasympathetic ganglia.

In cardiovascular system, the effects are mainly sympathetic; thus, tachycardia and rise in blood pressure occurs. In gastrointestinal and urinary system, the effects are mainly parasympathetic; thus, vomiting, diarrhea, and urination occurs.

Skeletal Muscles

ACh, in higher doses causes contraction of the muscle fibers, resulting in twitching and fasciculations.

Central Nervous System

ACh is a quaternary compound and therefore, does not cross the blood-brain barrier when injected intravenously.

Bethanechol

Bethanechol selectively stimulates the muscarinic receptors in the GIT and urinary bladder. It is used in post-operative urinary retention and paralytic ileus (when obstruction is ruled out) due to the following reasons:
- It has no effect on the nicotinic receptors
- Its muscarinic effects are completely antagonized by atropine
- It is not hydrolyzed by cholinesterases and therefore, has a long duration of action
- In urinary retention, it contracts detrusor and relaxes trigone and sphincter leading to voiding of urine
- In paralytic ileus, it increases tone and peristalsis of GIT and relaxes the sphincter leading to defecation

CHOLINOMIMETIC ALKALOIDS

PILOCARPINE

It is obtained from *Pilocarpus* plant. It is a tertiary amine; hence is stable to hydrolysis by cholinesterases. It is uncharged and can penetrate biological membranes (e.g. CNS).

It produces marked muscarinic effects. It has potent secretory activity (i.e. increases salivation, sweating and other secretions).

Clinical Uses

Ophthalmic Use

- Open angle (wide angle) glaucoma
  Pilocarpine (0.5–4%) eyedrops is used for open angle (wide angle) glaucoma. Applied topically to the eye, it penetrates cornea and rapidly causes miosis and ciliary muscle contraction. This leads to opening of pores around Schlemm's canal and facilitates the drainage of aqueous humor. This results in lowering of intraocular pressure.
  Pilocarpine acts rapidly (within few minutes) and the action lasts for 4–8 hours. The adverse effects include painful stinging sensation in the eye and spasm of accommodation.
- Break adhesions between iris and the lens (as in iridocyclitis)
  For this indication, it is given alternatively with a mydriatic.
- To counteract the mydriatic during refraction testing.
  It is used to reverse the pupillary dilatation that is caused by a mydriatic during refraction testing.

As Sialagogue (an agent that promotes the flow of saliva)

Pilocarpine (5–20 mg) orally is used to promote salivation in xerostomia (i.e. dry mouth) resulting from Sjögren syndrome and from radiation to head and neck.

Adverse Effects

The adverse effects include salivation, sweating, bronchospasm, vasodilation, bradycardia and diarrhea.

MUSCARINE

It is obtained from poisonous mushroom *Amanita muscaria* and *Inocybe* species. It only has muscarinic actions. It is not used therapeutically; however, toxicity may result from consuming mushrooms of *Inocybe* species.

Some common type of mushroom poisonings (mycetism) are mentioned in Table 3.

TABLE 3	Types of mushroom poisonings
Muscarinic type (Early onset)	• Caused by *Inocybe* species • Symptoms appear within 1 hour • Features include excessive muscarinic effects (salivation, sweating, bronchospasm, vasodilation, bradycardia, diarrhea etc.) • Treated effectively by IV atropine
Hallucinogenic type (Early onset)	• Caused by *Amanita muscaria* • Symptoms begin within 15–30 minutes • Produces mainly central effects; produces euphoria, enhanced imagination and hallucinations • Atropine is contraindicated • No effective treatment
Phalloidin type (Delayed onset)	• Caused by *Amanita phalloides* • Symptoms usually appear after 6–12 hours • Produces GIT, liver and kidney damage • Does not respond to atropine • Treatment is mainly supportive

ARECOLINE

It is an alkaloid found in areca or betel nut. It has both muscarinic and nicotinic actions. It has no clinical use.

ANTICHOLINESTERASES

Cholinesterases are enzymes that inactivate acetylcholine. There are two types of cholinesterases in the body (*see* Table 1).
- Acetyl cholinesterase (True cholinesterase)
- Butyryl cholinesterase (Pseudo or plasma cholinesterase)

Anticholinesterases are drugs that inhibit both acetylcholinesterase and butyrylcholinesterase. Hence, they extend the duration of acetylcholine availability following its release from the cholinergic nerve endings (Figure 10).

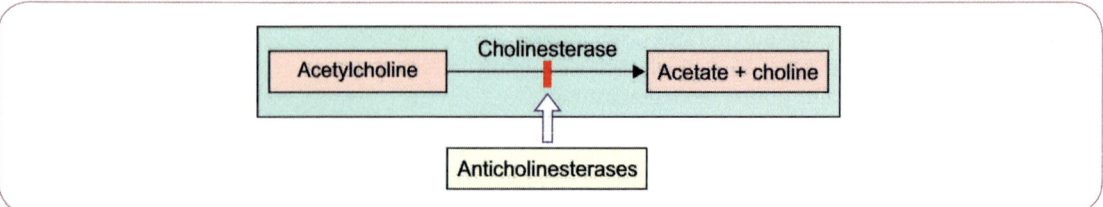

Figure 10: Anticholinesterases

CLASSIFICATION OF ANTICHOLINESTERASES

A classification of anticholinesterases is mentioned in Figure 11.

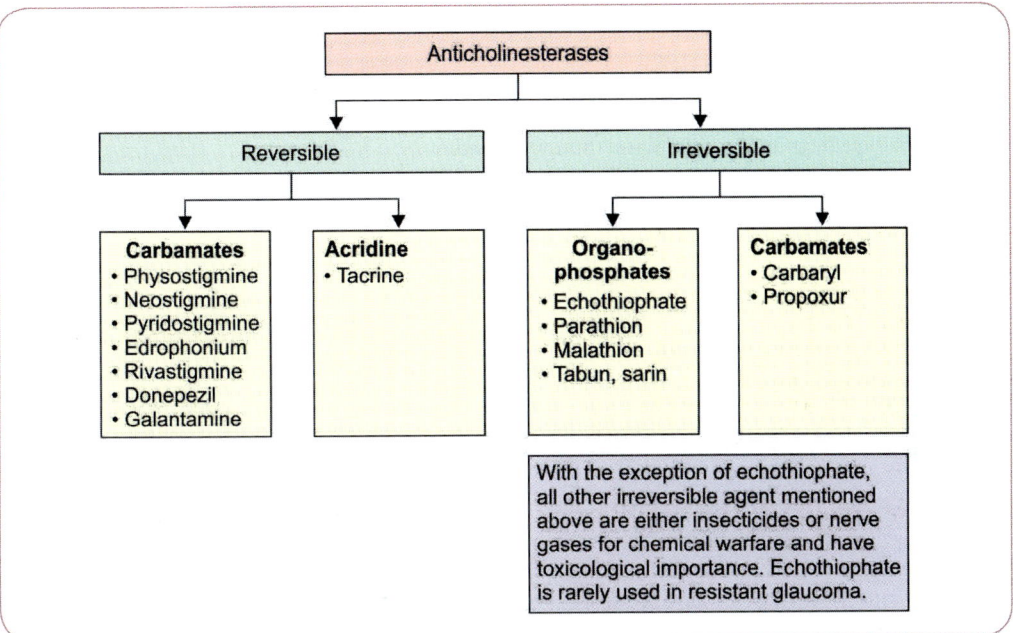

Figure 11: Classification of anticholinesterases

MECHANISM OF ACTION

The anticholinesterases bind to the cholinesterase enzyme and prolong the duration of acetylcholine availability.

Practically, the terms reversible and irreversible refer to the duration of cholinesterase enzyme inhibition (Figure 12).

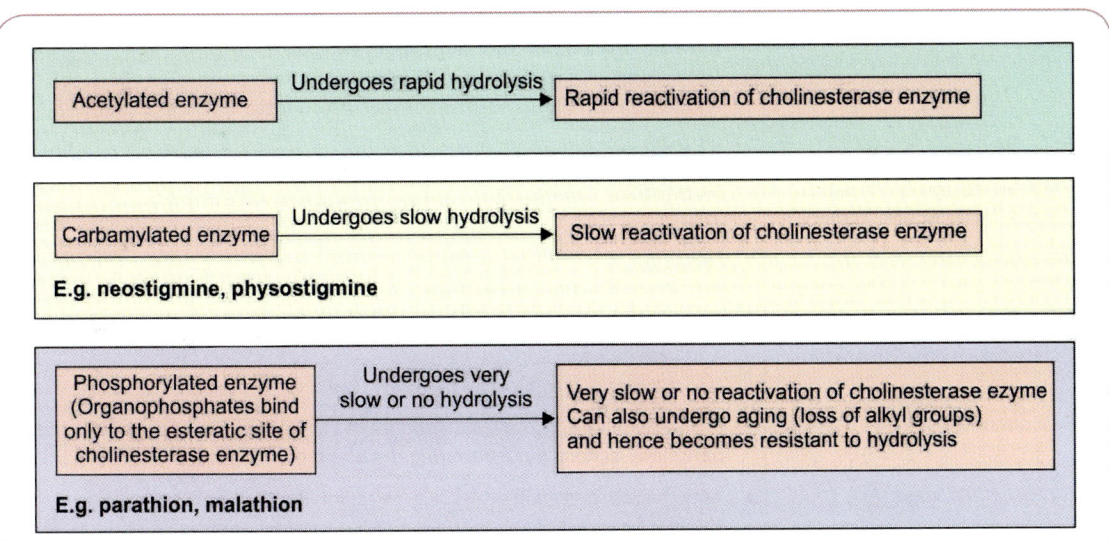

Figure 12: Mechanism of action of anticholinesterases

PHARMACOLOGICAL ACTIONS

The actions of anticholinesterases are similar to that of cholinergic agonists (e.g. acetylcholine).
1. Neuromuscular junction/Skeletal muscles
   - Increased concentration of ACh at the neuromuscular junction
   - ACh binds to nicotinic receptors and causes muscle contraction
   - Overdosage leads to persistent depolarization → weakness and paralysis
2. Cardiovascular system
   - Unpredictable effects and depend upon the specific agent
   - Muscarinic action can cause bradycardia, but ganglionic stimulation can cause tachycardia
3. Respiratory system
   - Bronchospasm, increased secretions
4. Gastrointestinal system
   - Increased motility
5. Eye
   - Miosis, blocking of accommodation reflex
   - Decreased intraocular pressure
6. Secretory glands
   - Stimulatory action

ADVERSE EFFECTS OF REVERSIBLE CHOLINESTERASES

Adverse effects are due to increased stimulation of cholinergic receptors (muscarinic and nicotinic) and can include tremors, muscle weakness, increased secretions (salivation), bronchospasm, diarrhea, abdominal cramps, bradycardia. Cholinergic crisis (in overdose) can result in exaggerated symptoms leading to respiratory paralysis, respiratory failure, cardiac arrest and fatalities.

CLINICAL USES OF REVERSIBLE CHOLINESTERASES

The clinical uses of reversible cholinesterases are mentioned in Table 4. Some of the uses are discussed subsequently.

TABLE 4	Clinical uses of reversible cholinesterases
1. As a miotic	• Glaucoma • Reversal of action of mydriatics after refraction testing • Used along with mydriatics to prevent formation of adhesions between iris and lens in conditions such as corneal ulcers, iritis
2. Myasthenia gravis	• Neostigmine along with other drugs such as corticosteroids can be used
3. Postoperative paralytic ileus or postoperative urinary retention	• Neostigmine can be used if there is not organic obstruction
4. Reversal of neuromuscular blockade due to skeletal muscle relaxants	• Neostigmine is commonly used • Administration of anticholinergics such as atropine or glycopyrrolate is done to block the muscarinic effects of neostigmine
5. Curare toxicity (e.g. cobra bite)	• Anti-snake venom is the antidote • Neostigmine + atropine can be used
6. Belladonna poisoning	• Physostigmine is the specific antidote. It can antagonize both central and peripheral actions by penetrating the blood brain barrier.
7. Alzheimer's disease (AD)	• Anticholinesterase inhibitors (e.g. rivastigmine, donepezil) can enhance the cholinergic transmission in the brain that can be beneficial in patients of AD

GLAUCOMA

Glaucoma is a group of eye disorders characterized by progressive optic nerve damage. This is usually associated with an increase in intraocular pressure (IOP).

The normal IOP is 10–20 mm Hg. Elevated IOP refers to a pressure >21 mm Hg. Glaucoma is the second most frequent cause of blindness worldwide.

AQUEOUS HUMOR DYNAMICS

The aqueous humor is produced by the ciliary body in posterior chamber of the eye. It passes between the lens and the iris to reach the pupil. It passes through the pupil to reach the anterior chamber of the eye.

In the anterior chamber, it passes between the iris and the cornea to reach the trabeculae. It leaves the eye by passing through the trabecular meshwork into the Schlemm's canal (Figure 13).

The angle (also called the irido-corneal angle) is defined as the angle formed between the iris and the cornea. This is the site of drainage of aqueous humor. At this site, trabeculae are present which drains into the Schlemm's canal.

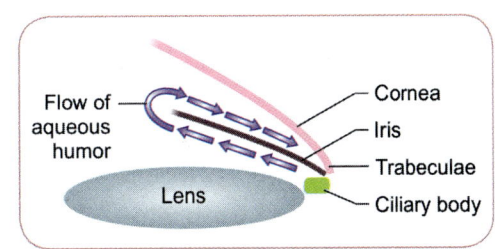

Figure 13: Aqueous humor dynamics in the eye

The aqueous drainage occurs through 2 routes:
- Majority (90%) occurs through trabecular route (trabeculae draining into Schlemm's canal)
- Minority (10%) occurs through uveoscleral route (connective tissue spaces in ciliary muscle draining into episcleral vessels)

The treatment of glaucoma is aimed at lowering the IOP. This is achieved by the following mechanisms:
- Decreasing the production (secretion) of aqueous humor
- Increasing the outflow (drainage) of aqueous humor

TYPES OF GLAUCOMA

Glaucoma are categorized in 2 main types, open-angle and closed-angle glaucoma (Table 5).

TABLE 5	Types of glaucoma	
Open-angle glaucoma (chronic simple glaucoma)		**Closed-angle glaucoma (acute congestive glaucoma)**
• Wide iridocorneal angle; normal anterior chamber		• Narrow iridocorneal angle; shallow anterior chamber
• Gradual condition; IOP rises slowly over years		• Acute condition; IOP rises very quickly
• Caused by loss of patency of trabecular meshwork		• Caused by blocking of draining canals, usually by a mydriatic
• Not a medical emergency		• Is a medical emergency
• Ocular hypotensive drugs usually is the definitive treatment: surgery usually is not required		• Surgery or laser irodotomy is the definitive treatment: ocular hypotensive drugs are used to terminate an attack

DRUGS USED IN GLAUCOMA

The various drugs used in the management of glaucoma are mentioned in Table 6.
- The treatment of open angle glaucoma is mainly by drug therapy; surgery is usually not required. The drugs mentioned in Table 6 are used in the treatment of open angle glaucoma.
- The treatment of acute congestive glaucoma is mainly surgical. The drugs are primarily used for terminating an acute attack. Only few of the drugs (from Table 6) are used in acute congestive glaucoma.

TABLE 6	Drugs used in the treatment of glaucoma

Beta-adrenergic blockers

| Topical β-blockers (Timolol, betaxolol, levobunolol, carteolol) | <ul><li>One of the preferred drugs for glaucoma</li><li>Act by decreasing the secretion of aqueous humor by ciliary body</li><li>Must be cautiously used in bronchial asthma and congestive heart failure</li><li>Advantages of topical β-blockers over miotics<ul><li>No change in pupil size</li><li>No decrease of vision in dim light</li><li>No spasm of accommodation</li><li>No fluctuations in IOP</li><li>Longer duration of action</li><li>Better tolerated</li></ul></li></ul>**Timolol**<ul><li>Is a nonselective β-blocker</li><li>Is the prototype of ocular hypotensives</li><li>Do not have intrinsic sympathomimetic or local anesthetic activity</li><li>Causes 20–35% decrease in IOP over baseline</li><li>High level of safety as the effect persists 2–3 weeks after discontinuation</li></ul>**Betaxolol and levobunolol**<ul><li>Betaxolol is a selective β_1-blocker</li><li>Betaxolol is less effective than timolol</li><li>Betaxolol has additional retinal protective effect</li><li>Levobunolol is longer acting, the other effects are similar to timolol</li></ul> |

Prostaglandin (PGF$_{2\alpha}$) analogues

| Topical PGF$_{2\alpha}$ analogues (Latanoprost, bimatoprost, tafluprost) | <ul><li>Are the first line drugs in the treatment of open angle glaucoma</li><li>Act by increasing the uveoscleral outflow of aqueous humor</li><li>High efficacy equivalent to timolol</li><li>Longer duration of action</li><li>Low incidence of adverse effects</li><li>Adverse effects include iris pigmentation, ocular irritation and blurring of vision</li></ul> |

Alpha-adrenergic agonists

| Epinephrine, dipivefrine, apraclonidine, brimonidine | Epinephrine, dipivefrine<ul><li>Dipivefrine is a prodrug of epinephrine. It penetrates cornea and is then converted to epinephrine.</li></ul>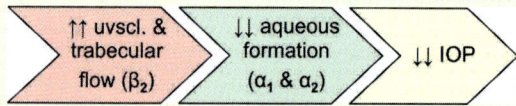<ul><li>Epinephrine is not used. Dipivefrine is used only as an add-on therapy in poorly controlled disease.</li></ul>**Apraclonidine, brimonidine**<ul><li>Apraclonidine and brimonidine are selective α_2-agonists. They act by the following mechanism:</li></ul>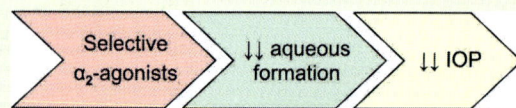<ul><li>They do not cross the blood-brain barrier; hence, there are no central effects.</li><li>Topical apraclonidine is used for:<ul><li>Prevention and treatment of IOP elevation post-surgery</li><li>As adjunctive therapy in patients who require additional reduction of IOP</li></ul></li></ul> |

Contd...

Cholinomimetic (Miotics)	
Directly acting (Pilocarpine) Indirectly acting (Physostigmine, echothiophate)	• Pilocarpine penetrates cornea and rapidly causes miosis and ciliary muscle contraction. This facilitates drainage of aqueous humor and lowers IOP. • It is used topically in open angle glaucoma as well as acute congestive glaucoma. • Physostigmine also increases outflow of the aqueous humor in the eye, making it useful in the treatment of glaucoma.
Carbonic anhydrase (CA) inhibitors	
Acetazolamide, dorzolamide, brinzolamide	• Acetazolamide is used orally or IV • Dorzolamide and brinzolamide are used topically • They act by the following mechanism: Inhibit CA enzyme → $\downarrow\downarrow HCO_3^-$ secretion in ciliary body → $\downarrow\downarrow$ aqueous formation & $\downarrow\downarrow$ IOP • The topical drugs are preferred as they have lesser systemic adverse effects • They are less efficacious and are used as add-on drugs to topical β-blockers/PG analogues
Osmotic solutions	
Mannitol (20%), Glycerol (50%)	• They induce fluid movement from the eye into the circulation by osmotic effect, thus reducing the IOP. • They are used mainly to terminate an acute attack in acute congestive glaucoma.

TREATMENT OF ACUTE CONGESTIVE GLAUCOMA

Acute congestive glaucoma (angle closure glaucoma) is an emergency; the IOP rapidly rises to a very high value (40–50 mm Hg). Failure to lower the IOP may result in rapid loss of sight.

For terminating an acute attack, the following drugs are used:

o **Osmotic solutions:** Hypertonic mannitol (20%), glycerol (50%) are infused to dehydrate/decongest the eye by their osmotic action.

o Acetazolamide (IV) may be employed followed by oral therapy.

o **Miotic:** Pilocarpine is started after few minutes only once the IOP starts falling by the above mentioned IV drugs.

o **Topical β-blocker:** Timolol can be instilled in the eye.

Drugs are only used to control an acute attack of angle closure glaucoma. Once the IOP decreases and an acute attack is controlled, surgery should be performed (partial iridectomy or laser irodotomy) as a definitive treatment.

MYASTHENIA GRAVIS

Myasthenia gravis is an autoimmune disorder.

There is formation of antibodies against postsynaptic acetylcholine receptors (nicotinic [N_M] receptors) and damage to the neuromuscular junction.

This leads to a disruption of neuromuscular transmission resulting in episodic muscle weakness and easy fatigability.

The clinical features worsen with muscle activity and improve with rest.

The following factors are considered for the diagnosis of myasthenia gravis:

o Clinical presentation including episodic muscle weakness, ptosis, diplopia, etc.

o Investigations such as measurement of acetylcholine receptor antibody levels, electromyography.

o Edrophonium challenge test (IV)—sometime used

  ❑ Injection (slow IV) of edrophonium in a patient with myasthenia gravis can lead to an improvement in muscle strength. This improvement is not seen in other muscular dystrophies.

❑ Complete resuscitative measures (including ventilatory support) should be available during the challenge test because worsening of weakness due to cholinergic crisis may occur.

Pharmacologic management of myasthenia gravis includes the following:

1. **Anticholinesterases (pyridostigmine, neostigmine)**
   - They inhibit the anticholinesterase enzyme and hence prevent the metabolism of acetylcholine. This causes an increase in the duration of acetylcholine availability following its release from the cholinergic nerve endings (Figure 14). Hence, more acetylcholine is available to act on the nicotinic receptors.
   - Neostigmine also directly stimulates the nicotinic receptors.
   - This leads to an improvement in the muscle strength and contraction.
   - Anticholinesterases offer symptomatic relief and do not have any effect on the underlying disease process.

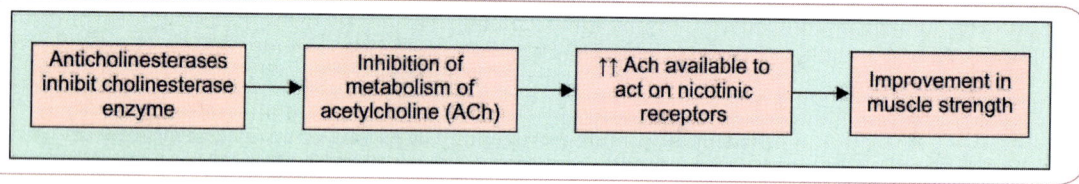

Figure 14: Anticholinesterases in myasthenia gravis

Cholinergic Crisis

It is caused due to persistent depolarization of the motor endplate.

Increased stimulation of cholinergic receptors (muscarinic and nicotinic) can result in symptoms such as tremors, muscle weakness, increased secretions (salivation), bronchospasm, diarrhea, abdominal cramps, bradycardia. It can lead to respiratory failure.

Management includes ventilatory support, administration of anticholinergic drugs (e.g. atropine), temporary stoppage of anticholinesterases (e.g. neostigmine, pyridostigmine).

Myasthenic Crisis

It is life threatening form of myasthenia gravis. It can present as respiratory muscle weakness leading to respiratory failure. Difficulty in swallowing may also be commonly observed.

Management includes ventilatory support, corticosteroids, immunoglobulins, and plasmapheresis.

Edrophonium can be used to differentiate the two types of crisis:
- ○ **Cholinergic crisis:** Worsening of muscle weakness upon administration of edrophonium
- ○ **Myasthenic crisis:** Improvement in muscle weakness upon administration of edrophonium

Complete resuscitative measures (including ventilatory support) should be available during edrophonium testing.

2. **Corticosteroids**
   - Prednisolone can be used as it has immunosuppressant activity and can inhibit the anti-receptor antibodies
3. **Other Immunosuppressants**
   - Azathioprine, cyclosporine
4. **Immunoglobulins**
5. **Plasmapheresis**
   - Plasma exchange can result in significant, but brief improvement
6. **Thymectomy**
   - Can result in gradual improvement in many patients

▌ SALIENT POINTS ABOUT ANTICHOLINESTERASE DRUGS

Physostigmine

- ○ It is a tertiary amine and can cross the blood brain barrier.
- ○ Clinical uses include glaucoma, belladonna (*Atropa belladonna*), atropine poisoning.

○ It is also used in atropine poisoning because it has cholinomimetic action. Hence, it can antagonize the anticholinergic effects of atropine.

○ It can also penetrate the blood brain barrier; hence, both the central and the peripheral effects of atropine are antagonized.

Neostigmine

○ It is a synthetic anticholinesterase drug.

○ Some of the clinical indications include myasthenia gravis, reversal of neuromuscular blockade due to skeletal muscle relaxants, postoperative paralytic ileus or postoperative urinary retention.

Some of the key differences between neostigmine and physostigmine are mentioned in Table 7.

TABLE 7	Physostigmine and neostigmine
Physostigmine	**Neostigmine**
• Natural alkaloid	• Synthetic
• Tertiary amine	• Quaternary compound
• Good oral absorption	• Poor oral absorption
• Crosses the blood brain barrier (BBB)—has CNS effects	• Does not cross the blood brain barrier—No CNS effects
• Penetrates cornea and hence used as a miotic	• Poor penetration into cornea and hence not used as a miotic
• Main action on the autonomic effectors • Does not directly stimulate N_M receptors	• Main action on skeletal muscles • Directly stimulates N_M receptors
• Key indication(s): glaucoma, atropine overdose	• Key indication(s): myasthenia gravis, reversal of neuromuscular blockade

• Physostigmine is used in atropine poisoning because it can antagonize the anticholinergic effects of atropine. It can penetrate the blood brain barrier, hence both the central and the peripheral effects of atropine are antagonized.
• Neostigmine is preferred over physostigmine for myasthenia gravis because neostigmine cannot cross the BBB and hence does not have CNS adverse effects.

Pyridostigmine

It is similar to neostigmine except that it is less potent and has a longer duration of action.

Pyridostigmine is preferred to neostigmine in myasthenia gravis because it has a longer duration of action and hence less frequent dosing is required.

ANTICHOLINESTERASE POISONING

Irreversible anticholinesterases are available as agricultural or household insecticides.

Organophosphorus (OP) compounds (irreversible anticholinesterases) are amongst the commonly used poisons. They can be absorbed through the skin, lungs and the GIT. Examples of organophosphorus compounds include parathion, malathion, etc.

MECHANISM OF ACTION

Organophosphorus compounds are irreversible inhibitors of cholinesterase enzymes and lead to an accumulation of acetylcholine at the nicotinic and muscarinic receptors.

They bind to the esteratic site of the cholinesterase enzyme and prevent the reactivation of the enzyme by causing its phosphorylation. Prolonged exposure to the organophosphorus compound can make the enzyme resistant to hydrolysis due to aging (loss of alkyl groups) (Figure 15).

Phosphorylated enzyme (Organophosphates bind only to the esteratic site of cholinesterase enzyme)	Undergoes very slow or no hydrolysis	Very slow or no reactivation of cholinesterase ezyme Can also undergo aging (loss of alkyl groups) and hence becomes resistant to hydrolysis

E.g. parathion, malathion

Figure 15: Organophosphorus (OP) poisoning

CLINICAL FEATURES

Clinical feature result from the effects of accumulation of acetylcholine at the muscarinic or nicotinic receptors (Figure 16).

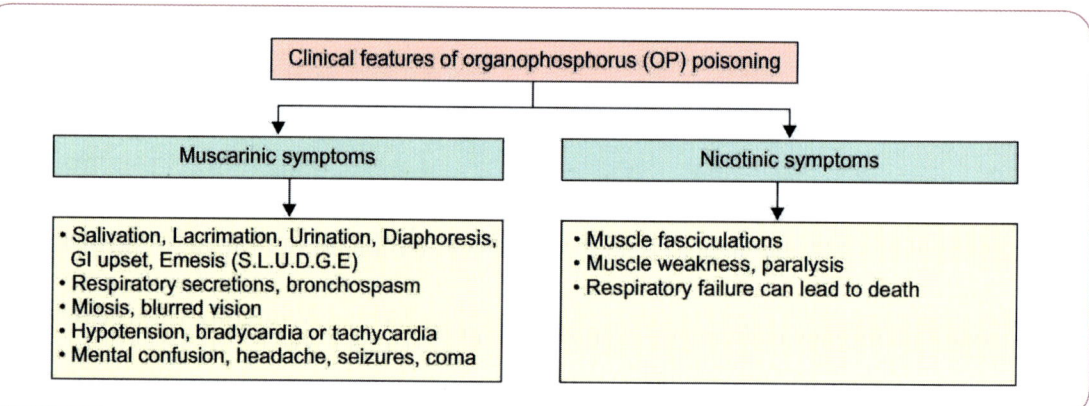

Figure 16: Clinical features of organophosphorus poisoning

MANAGEMENT

The management includes the following:
1. Supportive treatment
   - ❑ Airway management, adequate oxygenation and ventilatory support
   - ❑ Hemodynamic support including vitals and blood pressure, acid base and electrolyte balance
   - ❑ Control of seizures by judicious use of anticonvulsants such as diazepam
2. Termination of further exposure to the poison
   - ❑ Decontamination measures such as exposure to fresh air, removal of contaminated clothing, washing the skin and mucus membranes
   - ❑ Gastric lavage (if considered appropriate)
3. Specific measures
   - ❑ Atropine
   - ❑ Cholinesterase reactivators (Oximes-pralidoxime)

Atropine in Organophosphorus Poisoning

- ○ Atropine has anticholinergic actions (antimuscarinic) and hence is able to counteract the muscarinic symptoms of organophosphorus compounds.
- ○ Atropine does not have antinicotinic action and hence it is unable to reverse the muscular paralysis. This is because muscular paralysis is due to nicotinic action of the organophosphorus compounds (Figure 17).
- ○ Atropine is administered intravenously to patients of OP poisoning. Dosage may be repeated or increased till the pulmonary secretions are dried and the patient has adequate oxygenation.
- ○ Maintenance dosage of atropine may be required for 1–2 weeks.

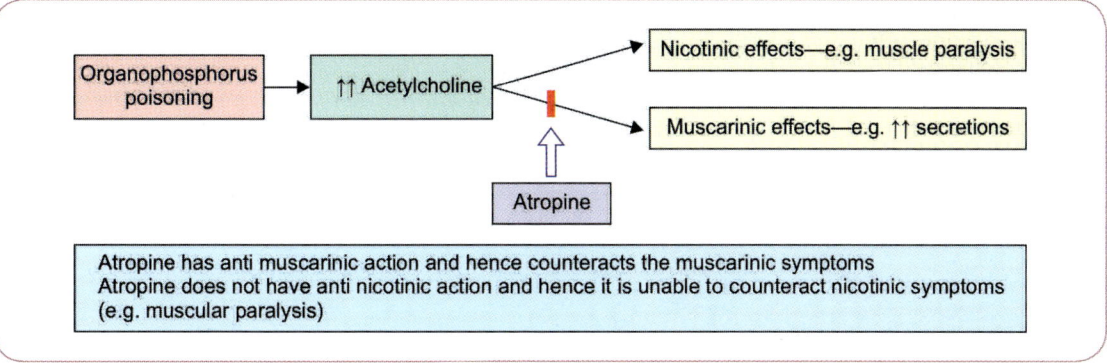

Figure 17: Atropine in organophosphorus poisoning

Cholinesterase Reactivators (Oximes – Pralidoxime) in Organophosphorus Poisoning

○ Pralidoxime binds to the unoccupied anionic site of the phosphorylated cholinesterase enzyme and reactivates it.

○ Hence, it restores the neuromuscular transmission by causing reactivation of the phosphorylated cholinesterase enzyme (Figure 18).

○ Therapy with pralidoxime needs to be initiated early (usually within 24 hours) before the phosphorylated cholinesterase enzyme undergoes aging (loss of alkyl) groups. Aging makes the enzyme resistant to hydrolysis.

○ Pralidoxime therapy in OP poisoning is secondary to atropine therapy.

○ Pralidoxime therapy is not effective in carbamate overdose (e.g. neostigmine, physostigmine) because carbamates occupy the anionic site of the cholinesterase enzyme. Hence, pralidoxime is unable to bind to the cholinesterase enzyme. Also, pralidoxime has mild anticholinesterase activity.

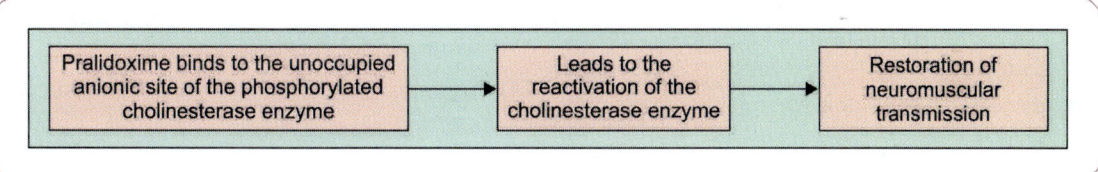

Figure 18: Pralidoxime in organophosphorus poisoning

CHRONIC ORGANOPHOSPHATE POISONING

It occurs due to prolonged or repeated exposure to the organophosphates. It can result in neurotoxicity such as polyneuritis and demyelination. Spasticity and upper motor neuron paralysis may also develop at a later stage. The mechanism is unknown and there is no specific treatment.

POSTOPERATIVE PARALYTIC ILEUS

Postoperative paralytic ileus is reduced or cessation of motility of the gastrointestinal tract.

Abdominal surgery (e.g. laparotomy) is one of the common causes of postoperative ileus.

Clinical features include nausea, vomiting, abdominal distension, minimal or absent bowel sounds. There is no flatus or bowel movement in the patient. It is imperative to rule out bowel obstruction.

Clinical management includes the following measures:

○ Exclude any bowel obstruction

○ Nasogastric suction and nil per oral status of the patient

○ Maintain adequate hydration, fluid and electrolyte balance

○ Pharmacotherapy
  ❑ Neostigmine → It is an acetylcholinesterase inhibitor. It increases tone and peristalsis of GIT and relaxes the sphincter.
  ❑ Bethanechol → It is a choline ester and it enhances the tone and peristalsis of GIT and relaxes the sphincter.
  ❑ Other drugs that can be considered include:
  Metoclopramide → prokinetic agent
  Erythromycin (antibiotic) → Promotes motility of the gastrointestinal tract by acting on the motilin receptors in the GIT.

ASSESS YOURSELF (Examination Questions of Various Universities)

1. Mechanism of action, therapeutic uses and adverse effects of neostigmine.

2. Pharmacological basis for uses of prostaglandin analogues in glaucoma.

3. Drug treatment of glaucoma.

4. Drug treatment of wide angle glaucoma, open angle glaucoma.

5. Management of organophosphorus poisoning.

6. Management of postoperative paralytic ileus.

7. Explain the rationale of using pilocarpine in wide angle glaucoma.

8. Explain the rationale of using apraclonidine in glaucoma.

9. Mechanism of action, therapeutic uses and adverse effects of physostigmine.

10. Explain why pyridostigmine is preferred to neostigmine for myasthenia gravis.

11. Why neostigmine is preferred for use in myasthenia gravis?

12. Explain why pralidoxime is ineffective as antidote to carbamate poisoning?

13. Rationale of oximes in insecticide poisoning.

14. Rationale of oximes in organophosphorus poisoning.

15. Pralidoxime in organophosphorus poisoning.

16. Edrophonium used in differentiating myasthenic crisis from cholinergic crisis while treating myasthenia gravis.

17. Explain the rationale of pilocarpine in xerostomia.

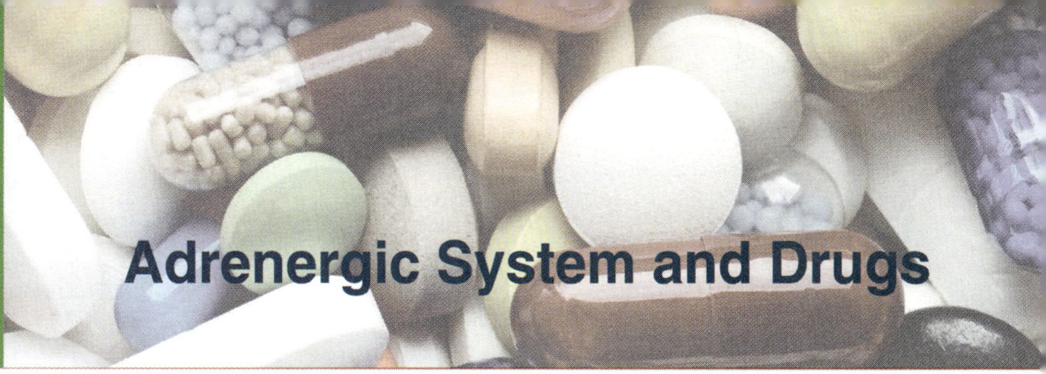

8

Adrenergic System and Drugs

The two major divisions of the autonomic nervous system are as follows:
- Sympathetic Nervous System → Dominant system in "Fight or flight" response
- Parasympathetic Nervous System → Dominant system in "Rest and digest" activities

Adrenergic agonists mimic the effects of sympathetic nervous system stimulation. Hence, they are also known as sympathomimetic drugs.

The major neurotransmitter of the adrenergic nervous system is noradrenaline. Adrenaline is secreted by the adrenal medulla and can be considered as a hormone since it is transported via blood to various target tissues. Dopamine is a metabolic precursor of noradrenaline and adrenaline (Figure 1).

Noradrenaline	Adrenaline	Dopamine
• Major neurotransmitter in the adrenergic nervous system • Acts on most postganglionic sympathetic sites and in some areas of brain	• Secreted by the adrenal medulla • Considered as a hormone as it is transported to act on different target organs	• Metabolic precursor of noradrenaline and adrenaline • Also acts via D_1 and D_2 receptors (apart from adrenergic receptors)

Figure 1: Catecholamines

ADRENERGIC NEUROTRANSMISSION

The neurotransmission in the adrenergic nervous system involves the following steps (Figure 2):
1. Synthesis and storage of catecholamines (including noradrenaline)
2. Release of catecholamines
3. Binding to receptors
4. Termination of action of catecholamines

Synthesis and Storage of Catecholamines (including noradrenaline)

The synthesis of catecholamines involves the following steps (Figure 3)
- Carrier mediated transport of tyrosine into the adrenergic neuron.
- Tyrosine gets hydroxylated to dihydroxyphenylalanine (DOPA) by the rate limiting enzyme tyrosine hydroxylase.
- DOPA gets decarboxylated to dopamine.
- Dopamine is then transported into the synaptic vesicles. It is then hydroxylated to form noradrenaline by the enzyme dopamine β hydroxylase. Noradrenaline is stored in the synaptic vesicles.

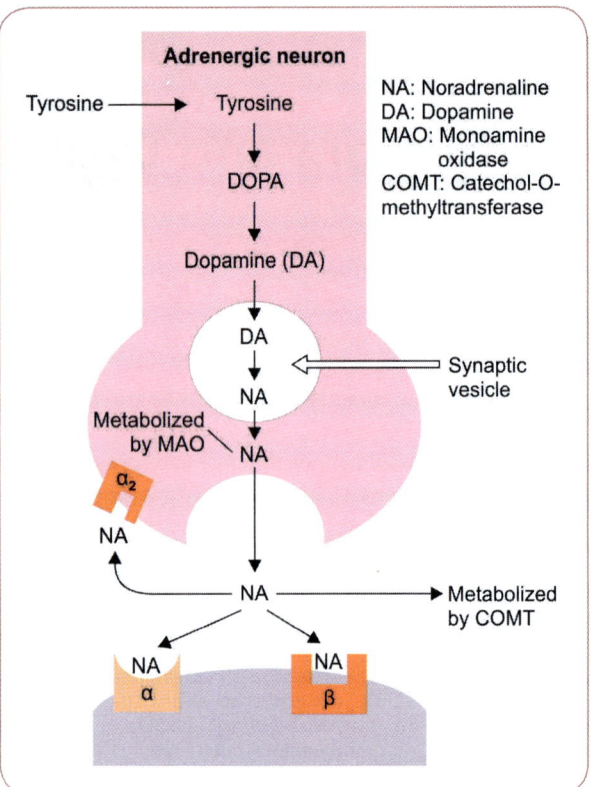

Figure 2: Adrenergic neurotransmission

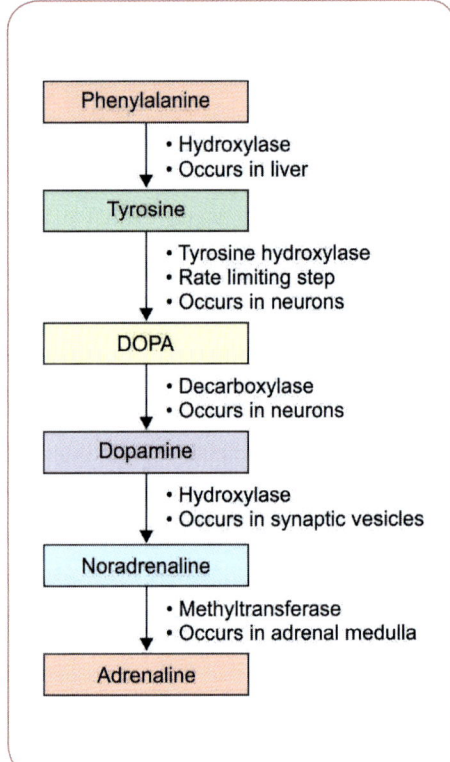

Figure 3: Synthesis of catecholamines

Release of Catecholamines

- The release of noradrenaline is triggered by an action potential that reaches the adrenergic neurons.
- An influx of calcium ions into the neuronal cytoplasm results in fusion of synaptic vesicles to the cell membrane.
- Release of noradrenaline into the synaptic space via exocytosis.

Binding to Receptors

- Noradrenaline released in the synaptic space binds to postsynaptic α and β receptors on the effector organs. This results in the formation of intracellular messengers and leads to various effects due to the stimulation of α and β receptors.
- Noradrenaline also binds to the presynaptic α_2 receptors. These receptors modulate the release of noradrenaline (activation of these receptors results in an inhibition of further release of noradrenaline from neurons).

Termination of Action of Catecholamines

Termination of action of noradrenaline can occur via the following mechanisms:
- Neuronal reuptake → reuptake back into the presynaptic neuron
  - Main mechanism for termination of action
  - Postneuronal reuptake, noradrenaline can either be stored in the synaptic vesicle or metabolized by the enzyme monoamine oxidase (MAO)
- Metabolized by the enzyme catechol-O-methyltransferase (COMT) in the synaptic cleft (*see* Figure 4)
- Enters the systemic circulation
  - Metabolized by the enzymes MAO and COMT present in the liver and other tissues

Adrenergic System and Drugs

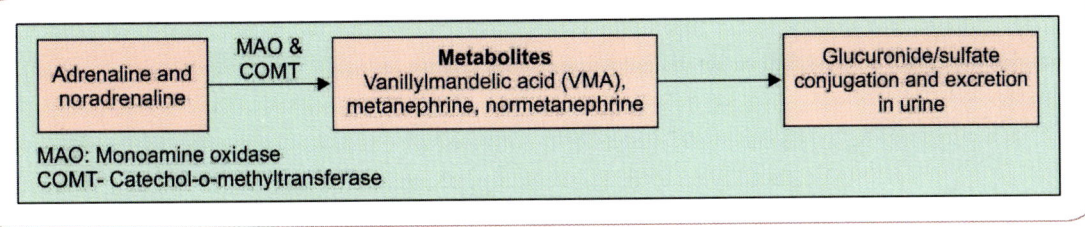

Figure 4: Metabolism of adrenaline and noradrenaline

ADRENERGIC RECEPTORS

Adrenergic receptors were classified by Ahlquist into two types:

- Alpha (α) receptors
- Beta (β) receptors

They are further subclassified into α_1, α_2 and β_1, β_2 and β_3 receptors (Figure 5).

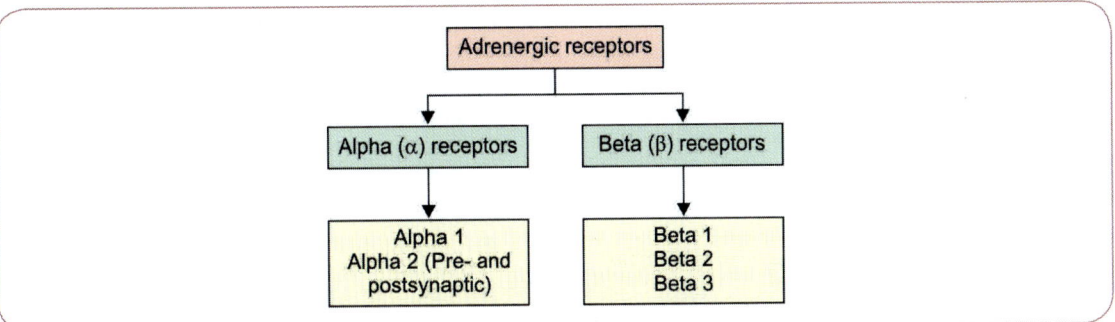

Figure 5: Adrenergic receptors

Some of the key actions of adrenergic receptors are mentioned in Figure 6.

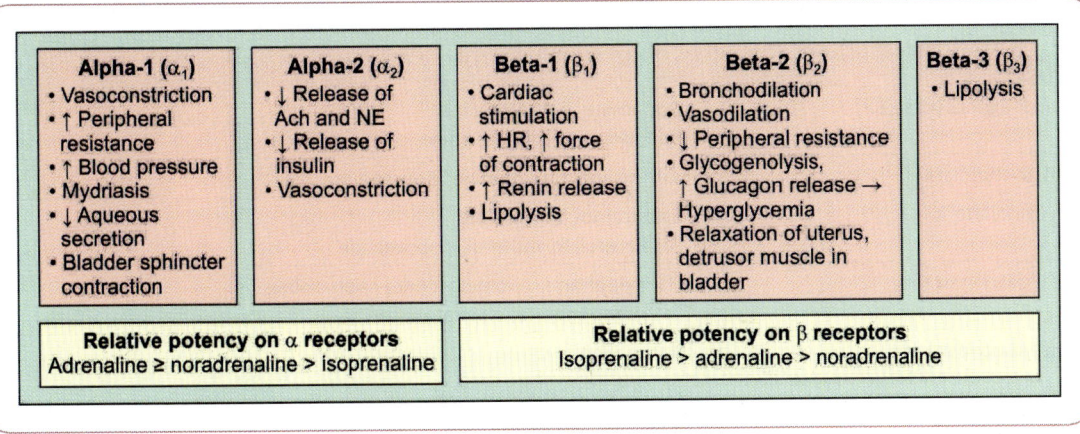

Figure 6: Key actions of adrenergic receptors

CLASSIFICATION OF ADRENERGIC DRUGS (SYMPATHOMIMETICS)

Adrenergic drugs can be classified as per the following criteria (Figure 7).
- Mechanism of action
- Chemical structure

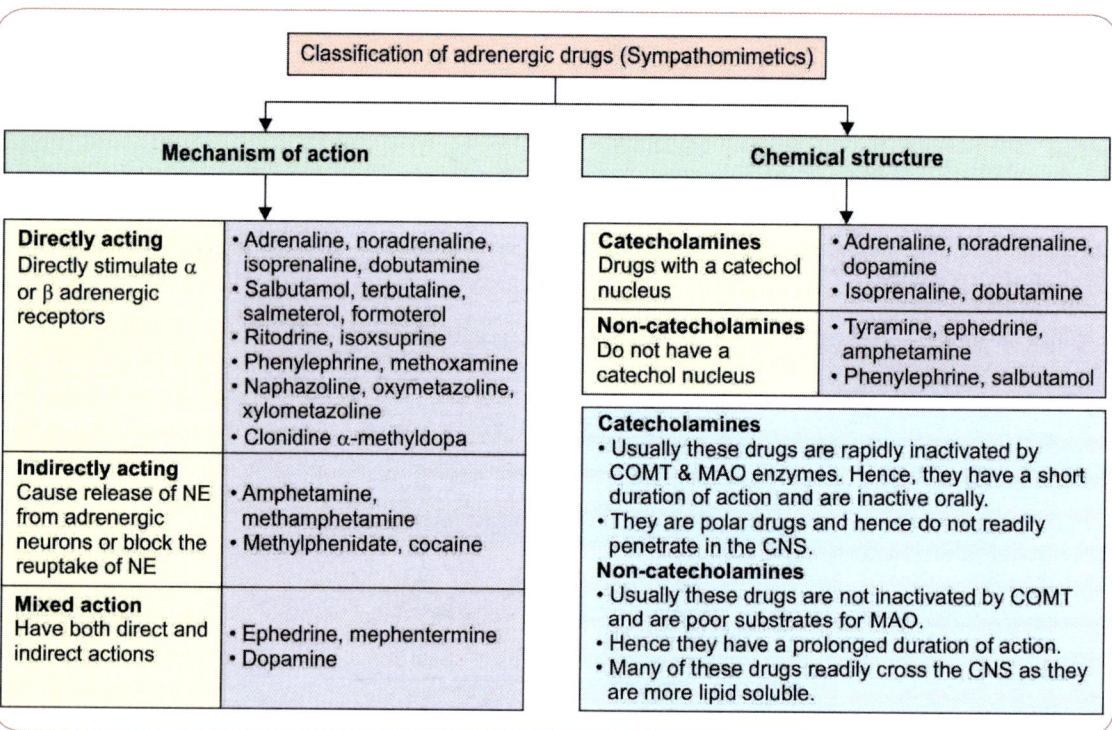

Figure 7: Classification of adrenergic drugs

Adrenergic drugs can also be tabulated as per their clinical use (Table 1).

TABLE 1	Clinical uses of adrenergic drugs (Sympathomimetics)
Pressor agents (raise BP)	• Dopamine, noradrenaline • Ephedrine, mephentermine, phenylephrine
Cardiac stimulants	• Adrenaline, dobutamine, isoprenaline
Bronchodilators	• Salbutamol, terbutaline • Salmeterol, formoterol, isoprenaline
Nasal decongestants	• Phenylephrine, xylometazoline, naphazoline • Pseudoephedrine, oxymetazoline
Local vasoconstrictor	• Adrenaline
Mydriatics	• Phenylephrine, ephedrine
Uterine relaxants	• Ritodrine, isoxsuprine
CNS stimulants	• Amphetamine, methamphetamine
Anorectics	• Sibutramine, fenfluramine • Dexamphetamine

INDIVIDUAL ADRENERGIC DRUGS (SYMPATHOMIMETICS)— DIRECTLY ACTING DRUGS

ADRENALINE (EPINEPHRINE)

It is a natural compound that is produced in the adrenal medulla following methylation of noradrenaline to adrenaline (*see* Figure 3).

The adrenal medulla releases about 80% adrenaline and 20% noradrenaline in the blood upon stimulation.

Adrenaline stimulates both α (α_1 and α_2) and β (β_1, β_2, and β_3) adrenergic receptors in the body. At low doses, β effects predominate, whereas at high doses, α effects are prominent.

Effects of adrenaline (like most catecholamines) depend upon the dose, rate and the route of administration.

Pharmacological Actions

Cardiovascular System

Adrenaline has a cardiac stimulant action. It acts on β_1 receptors to produce the following effects:
- Positive chronotropic effect ($\uparrow$ heart rate)
- Positive dromotropic effect ($\uparrow$ conduction velocity)
- Positive ionotropic effect ($\uparrow$ force of contraction)
- Increase in cardiac output and cardiac work $\rightarrow$ increase in cardiac oxygen demand
- Increase risk of arrhythmias

Adrenaline has the following effects on the blood vessels:
- α_1 stimulation $\rightarrow$ constriction of the blood vessels of the skin and mucus membranes
- β_2 stimulation $\rightarrow$ dilation of blood vessels in liver and skeletal muscles

Upon slow IV infusion, the general effect is an increase in the systolic blood pressure, fall in the diastolic blood pressure and a rise in the mean blood pressure.

Rapid IV administration of adrenaline (in animals) has a biphasic effect on the blood pressure.
- Initial increase in BP due to stimulation of α_1 receptors
- BP returns to normal followed by a fall in BP. This is due to reduced concentration of adrenaline (resulting from rapid uptake and metabolism) that is unable to act on the α receptors, but acts on the β_2 receptors. It causes vasodilation leading to a fall in BP.

However, if an α blocker has been administered prior to rapid IV administration of adrenaline (in animals), then only a fall in the BP is observed. This is because α receptor mediated vasoconstriction does not occur. This is known as vasomotor reversal of Dale.

Respiratory System

Adrenaline has the following effects on the respiratory system:
- β_2 stimulation $\rightarrow$ Potent bronchodilation and reduced release of inflammatory mediators from mast cells
- α_1 stimulation $\rightarrow$ Reduced secretions and relief of mucosal congestion

Eye

- α_1 stimulation $\rightarrow$ mydriasis and reduced secretion of aqueous humor
- However, this action is minimal upon topical application because adrenaline poorly penetrates the cornea

Urinary Bladder

- β_2 stimulation $\rightarrow$ relaxation of detrusor muscle
- α_1 stimulation $\rightarrow$ contraction of the sphincter
  The net result is difficulty in micturition.

Metabolic Effects

Adrenaline can cause hyperglycemia due to the following:
- β_2 stimulation → hepatic glycogenolysis
- α_1 stimulation → decreased section of insulin
- Reduced uptake of glucose by peripheral tissues

Other metabolic effects include increased lipolysis due to stimulation of the β receptors.

Skeletal Muscles

- Facilitation of neuromuscular transmission
- Tremors are an adverse effect of β_2 agonists such as salbutamol

CNS

- No significant effect is observed in clinically used doses because adrenaline does not readily cross the blood brain barrier
- Restlessness, headache, tremors may be observed in some patients

Other Effects

- β_2 stimulation → can lead to hypokalemia by facilitating the uptake of potassium in the cells

Pharmacokinetics

Catecholamines (adrenaline) are rapidly inactivated by MAO & COMT enzymes in tissues such as the liver and the GIT (*see* Figure 4). Hence, they have a short duration of action and are inactive orally. They are polar drugs and hence, do not readily penetrate in the CNS.

Adrenaline is administered parenterally. Intravenous or intramuscular route is preferred in cardiac arrest or in anaphylactic shock because absorption from subcutaneous route is poor.

Adverse Effects and Contraindications

The adverse effects of adrenaline are an extension of its pharmacological effects. These include:
- Hypertension, tachycardia, palpitations, arrhythmias including ventricular fibrillation
- Angina, myocardial infarction, cerebral hemorrhage

The contraindications of adrenaline should be considered as relative and not absolute in emergency life-threatening conditions. A benefit risk assessment should be considered prior to administration of adrenaline. Some of the contraindications include the following:
- Patients with organic heart disease, organic brain disease, hypertension, hyperthyroid, angina, and cerebral arteriosclerosis.
- Adrenaline should not be used in general anesthesia with halothane because of the risk of arrhythmias.
- Use of adrenaline as a vasoconstrictor is contraindicated for use in fingers, toes, ears, nose or genitalia.
- Adrenaline should not be used in patients on therapy with β blockers as significant rise in BP can occur due to unopposed α action.

Clinical Uses

1. **Anaphylactic shock**
   - Adrenaline is the drug of choice in patients of anaphylactic shock.
   - It can be injected via the intramuscular (IM) route on the anterolateral aspect of the middle third of thigh.
   - Subcutaneous administration of adrenaline in anaphylactic shock is not recommended as it is less effective.
   - The rationale for administering adrenaline in anaphylactic shock is mentioned in Figure 8.

Rationale of adrenaline in anaphylactic shock

Alpha-1 (α_1) receptor stimulation
• Vasoconstriction
• ↑ Peripheral resistance
• ↑ Blood pressure
• ↓ Mucosal edema (laryngeal edema)

Beta-2 (β_2) receptor stimulation
• Bronchodilation
• ↓ Release of mast cell mediators

Beta-1 (β_1) receptor stimulation
• Cardiac stimulation
• ↑ Heart rate
• ↑ Force of contraction

• Adrenaline is a physiological antagonist of histamine
• Adrenaline has a very rapid onset of action

Figure 8: Rationale of adrenaline in anaphylactic shock

2. **Bronchial asthma**
   - ❑ Adrenaline can be used in the management of acute severe asthma. The rationale of using adrenaline in acute severe asthma is mentioned in Figure 9.
   - ❑ Selective short-acting β_2 agonists (e.g. salbutamol) are commonly used for acute severe asthma.
   - ❑ The use of adrenaline in acute severe asthma has declined due to its cardiac adverse effects.

Rationale of adrenaline in acute severe asthma

Beta-2 (β_2) receptor stimulation
• Bronchodilation
• ↓ Release of mast cell mediators

Alpha-1 (α_1) receptor stimulation
• Reduced secretions
• Relief of mucosal congestion

Figure 9: Rationale of adrenaline in acute severe asthma

3. **Cardiopulmonary resuscitation**—used along with other measures
4. **Use along with local anesthetics**
   - ❑ The rationale, advantages and disadvantages of using vasoconstrictors along with local anesthetics (LA) are mentioned in Figure 10.

Rationale of using vasoconstrictors (e.g. adrenaline) with local anesthetics
• Vasoconstrictors (e.g. adrenaline) reduce the vasodilator effect of local anesthetics and decrease blood flow to the site of action
• This reduces the rate of absorption of the LA into the systemic circulation and hence prolongs the duration of action of the local anesthelic

Advantages
• Prolongs the duration of action of the local anesthetic
• Reduces the systemic toxicity of LA by decreasing the absorption of LA in the systemic circulation
• Reduces bleeding at the site of surgery

Disadvantages and contraindications
• Can lead to vasospasm and gangrene of the tissues. Hence use of vasoconstrictors is contraindicated for use in fingers, toes, penis, tip of nose, ear lobule
• Systemic toxicity can result from the absorption of adrenaline leading to cardiac complications such as hypertension, angina, myocardial infarction, arrhythmias etc.
• Hence vasoconstrictors should be avoided in patients with cardiac disorders such as hypertension, ischemic heart disease, arrhythmias etc.
• Reduction of the blood flow to the affected site may delay wound healing

Figure 10: Addition of vasoconstrictors (e.g. adrenaline) to local anesthetics

5. **Control epistaxis and other local bleeding**
   - ❑ Topical application is used
   - ❑ Control bleeding by causing vasoconstriction
6. **Glaucoma**
   - ❑ α_1 stimulation → mydriasis and reduced secretion of aqueous humor
   - ❑ However, this action is minimal upon topical application because adrenaline poorly penetrates the cornea
   - ❑ Hence, dipivefrine which is a prodrug of adrenaline is occasionally used in the management of glaucoma.

NORADRENALINE (NOREPINEPHRINE)

Noradrenaline is the main neurotransmitter in the adrenergic nervous system. It is a natural compound that is mainly produced in the synaptic vesicle of the adrenergic neurons. It is synthesized by hydroxylation of dopamine (*see* Figures 3 and 4).

Noradrenaline acts predominantly on α_1, α_2 and β_1 receptors and has minimal effect on the β_2 receptors.

Pharmacologic Actions

The main actions are on the cardiovascular system:

- ○ α_1 stimulation leads to vasoconstriction that causes a rise in the peripheral vascular resistance.
- ○ The extent of vasoconstriction is more than adrenaline because noradrenaline does not cause a compensatory vasodilation via stimulation of β_2 receptors.
- ○ The net result is a rise in the systolic and diastolic blood pressure.
- ○ An increase in the blood pressure leads to the stimulation of baroreceptors. This causes a rise in the vagal tone leading to reflex bradycardia.

Pharmacokinetics

Noradrenaline is rapidly inactivated by MAO and COMT enzymes in tissues such as the liver and the GIT (*see* Figure 4). Hence, it has a short duration of action and is inactive orally. It is a polar drug and hence does not readily penetrate in the CNS.

Adverse Effects

The adverse effects of noradrenaline are similar to that of adrenaline. Additionally, noradrenaline can cause tissue necrosis due to intense vasoconstriction action. Hence, it is given via intravenous (IV) infusion and not by intramuscular (IM) or subcutaneous (SC) route. Phentolamine can be used to treat ischemia due to extravasation of noradrenaline.

Intense vasoconstriction can also reduce the blood flow to the vital organs.

Clinical Uses

Noradrenaline is used for the emergency restoration of blood pressure in cases of acute hypotension. It causes a rise in the blood pressure due to intense vasoconstriction due to α_1 receptor stimulation. Noradrenaline not effective in acute severe asthma or anaphylaxis (Figure 11).

- Noradrenaline in not used in the treatment of acute severe asthma or anaphylaxis because it has minimal beta-2 (β_2) receptor stimulation action
- Hence it is less effective in causing bronchodilation and in inhibiting the release of mast cell inhibitors

Figure 11: Why is noradrenaline not effective in acute severe asthma or anaphylaxis

Some salient differences between adrenaline and noradrenaline are mentioned in Table 2.

TABLE 2	Adrenaline and noradrenaline	
	Adrenaline	Noradrenaline
Predominant function in body	• Hormone secreted by the adrenal medulla	• Neurotransmitter of the adrenergic nervous system
Main site of synthesis	• Synthesized from noradrenaline in the adrenal medulla	• Synthesized from dopamine in the synaptic vesicle (adrenergic neurons)
Action on adrenergic receptors (stimulates)	• α and β receptors	• α (α_1 and α_2) and β_1 receptors • No action on β_2 receptors
Effect on cardiac parameters	• HR ↑ • BP (↑↑ SBP, ↑↓ DBP, ↑ Mean BP) • CO ↑↑	• HR ↓ • BP (↓↓ SBP, ↑↑ DBP, ↑↑ Mean BP) • CO—
Bronchodilation	• Yes (Action on β_2 receptors)	• No (Does not act on β_2 receptors)
Administration	• Can be given IM, SC or IV	• Can cause tissue necrosis due to intense vasoconstriction • Hence, it is given via IV infusion and not by IM or SC route
Main clinical uses	• Anaphylactic shock • Cardiopulmonary resuscitation • Acute severe asthma	• Emergency restoration of blood pressure in cases of acute hypotension

ISOPRENALINE (ISOPROTERENOL)

○ Isoprenaline is a β receptor agonist and acts on β_1, β_2 and β_3 receptors.
○ Like all catecholamines, it is not effective orally as it is rapidly inactivated by MAO and COMT enzymes.
○ It is rarely used in clinical practice due to its non-selective action on all β receptors.
○ It has cardiac stimulant effect (β_1) as well as prominent bronchodilator (β_2) and vasodilator (β_2) effect.
○ Adverse effect profile is similar to that of adrenaline and includes cardiac arrhythmias.
○ Clinical uses include heart block and management of bronchospasm.

DOBUTAMINE

Dobutamine is a selective β_1 receptor agonist. It also has mild β_2 and α_1 adrenergic receptor agonist effects at therapeutic doses but the predominant effect is cardiac stimulation.

Dobutamine has a positive ionotropic effect on the heart.

The total peripheral resistance is not generally impacted due to the balancing of the β_2 (vasodilation) and α_1 (vasoconstriction) adrenergic receptor effects.

It increases cardiac output, but does not cause a significant increase in the myocardial oxygen requirements.

It is used for inotropic support in the short-term treatment of low output cardiac failure states (e.g. myocardial infarction, septic shock and cardiogenic shock). It is used in heart failure to increase cardiac output.

SALBUTAMOL (ALBUTEROL), TERBUTALINE, FORMOTEROL, SALMETEROL

These drugs are selective β_2 agonists.

Salbutamol (albuterol), terbutaline are *selective* short-acting β_2 agonists (SABAs)
○ Indicated as a reliever medication in bronchial asthma—relieve acute asthma exacerbations
○ Cause bronchodilation by stimulation of β_2 adrenergic receptors, decrease mast cell degranulation and histamine release, and promote mucociliary clearance (Figure 12).

○ Provide rapid relief in acute exacerbations of asthma and hence are called reliever or rescue medications

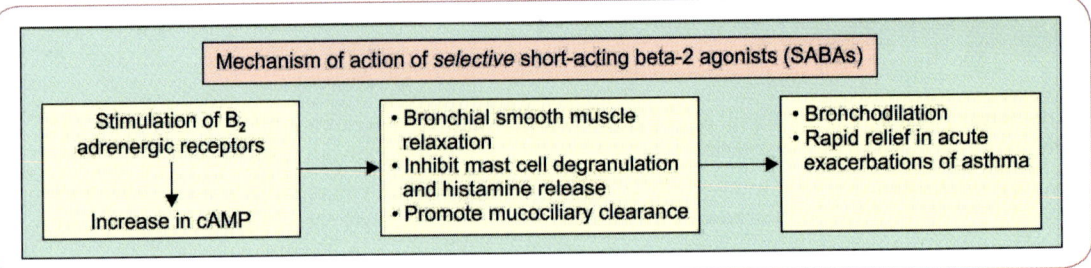

Figure 12: Mechanism of action of SABA in bronchial asthma

Salmeterol, formoterol are *selective* long-acting β_2 agonists (LABAs)

○ Indicated as a controller medication in bronchial asthma—regular, maintenance treatment of asthma

Selective β_2 agonists can also be used in short-term management of uncomplicated premature labor.

Adverse effects of selective β_2 agonists includes the following:

❑ Tremors → Due to stimulation of β_2 receptors in the skeletal muscles

❑ Hyperglycemia → Due β_2 receptor mediated hepatic glycogenolysis

❑ Tachycardia and palpitations → Due to stimulation of β_1 receptors in the heart

❑ Hypokalemia → Due to stimulation of β_2 receptors

❑ Ankle edema

PHENYLEPHRINE

Phenylephrine is a directly acting sympathomimetic drug. It acts predominantly on α_1 receptors and causes vasoconstriction. Vasoconstriction relieves nasal congestion. Hence, it is used as a nasal decongestant (Figure 13).

Other clinical uses include the treatment of hypotension in surgical/hospitalized patients. It is also used as a mydriatic.

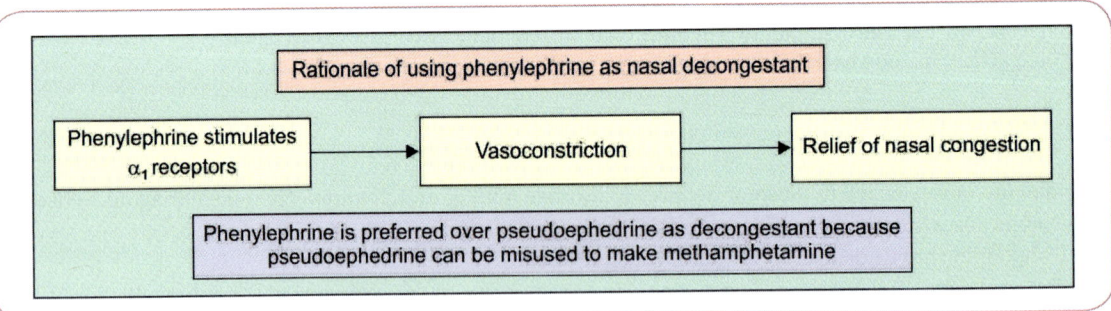

Figure 13: Phenylephrine as a nasal decongestant

MIRABEGRON

Mirabegron is a selective β_3-adrenoceptor agonist. It relaxes detrusor smooth muscle and enhances capacity of urinary bladder.

Clinical uses include symptomatic treatment of adult patients with overactive bladder (OAB) syndrome.

INDIVIDUAL ADRENERGIC DRUGS (SYMPATHOMIMETICS)— INDIRECTLY ACTING DRUGS

These drugs do not have a direct stimulant action on the adrenergic receptors. Instead, they either cause the release of noradrenaline (NA) from the adrenergic presynaptic neurons or they block the reuptake of NA into the presynaptic neurons.

AMPHETAMINE

Amphetamine has a potent central nervous system (CNS) stimulant action. Unlike adrenaline, it is effective orally and its effect lasts for several hours.

Pharmacological Actions

Amphetamine causes powerful CNS stimulation. The CNS effects occur due to cortical stimulation and possible stimulation of the reticular activating system. It produces the following effects (Figure 14).

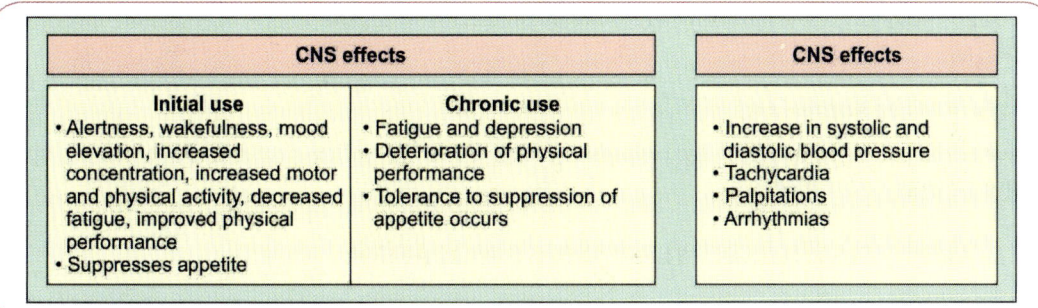

Figure 14: Pharmacological actions of amphetamine

Adverse Effects

The key adverse effects are mentioned in Figure 15.

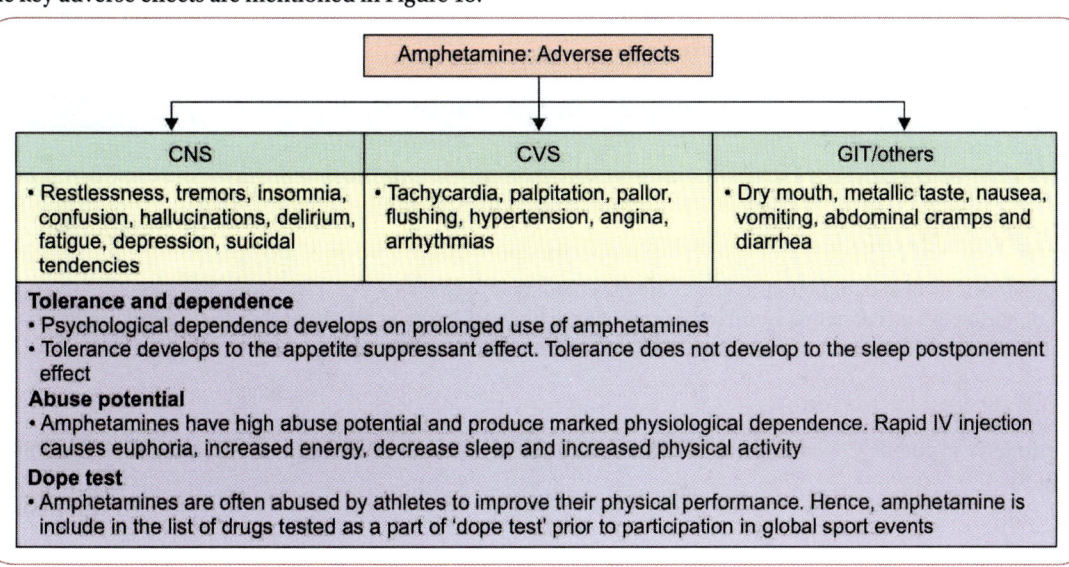

Figure 15: Adverse effects of amphetamines

Treatment of Acute Amphetamine Toxicity

The treatment involves the following measures:

- ○ Acidification of urine by ammonium chloride or ascorbic acid: This increases the ionization of amphetamine—prevents its reabsorption in the kidney—enhances the rate of elimination.
- ○ Sedatives (e.g. diazepam) are given for CNS symptoms and sodium nitroprusside is given for severe hypertension.

Clinical Uses

The clinical uses of amphetamine are mentioned below:

Narcolepsy

It is a sleep disorder characterized by an irresistible urge of falling asleep. Amphetamine prevents attacks of sleep due to CNS stimulant action.

Attention-Deficit Hyperactivity Disorder (ADHD)

Amphetamine paradoxically controls hyperactivity in children. The adverse effects may include insomnia and anorexia.

Weight Gain (As an Anorexiant)

Amphetamine reduces bodyweight by suppressing hypothalamic feeding center and decreasing appetite. Tolerance develops to this action.

METHAMPHETAMINE/METHYLPHENIDATE/MODAFINIL

- ○ Methamphetamine is related closely to amphetamine. In low doses, it has prominent central stimulant effects without significant peripheral effects. It has a high abuse potential.
- ○ Methylphenidate is structurally related to amphetamine. It has mild CNS stimulant action with more marked effects on mental than on motor activities. It is very effective in narcolepsy and ADHD. It has abuse potential similar to amphetamine. It is contraindicated in glaucoma.
- ○ Modafinil is the preferred drug for narcolepsy. It is not an amphetamine analogue. It promotes wakefulness but produces fewer other CNS stimulant effects.

INDIVIDUAL ADRENERGIC DRUGS (SYMPATHOMIMETICS)— MIXED ACTING DRUGS

EPHEDRINE

- ○ Ephedrine is an alkaloid obtained from the plant *Ephedra vulgaris*.
- ○ Ephedrine is a mixed acting sympathomimetic drug because it not only increases the release of noradrenaline from sympathetic neurons, but also directly stimulates both α and β receptors.

Pharmacological Actions

Ephedrine is a potent CNS stimulant. It also causes the following actions by stimulating α and β receptors (Table 3).

TABLE 3	Pharmacological actions of ephedrine
Receptor type stimulation	**Effects**
α receptors	• Vasoconstriction (α_1) • Mydriasis (α_1) • Urinary retention
β_1 receptors	• Cardiac stimulation (increased heart rate and cardiac output)
β_2 receptors	• Bronchodilation

Pharmacokinetics

○ It is not a catechol and hence is effective orally.
○ It is a poor substrate of MAO and COMT; hence has a long duration of action (half-life 3–6 hours).
○ It crosses the blood brain barrier and has a potent CNS stimulant action.

Adverse Effects

The adverse effects include hypertension (with parenteral use), insomnia, tachycardia, palpitation and urinary retention. Repeated administration may lead to tachyphylaxis.

Clinical Uses

Ephedrine is currently used in the following situations:
○ To treat hypotension that may occur during spinal anesthesia. It is used intravenously for this condition.
○ To treat mild chronic bronchial asthma. It is used orally for this condition.

It was previously also used for heart block, narcolepsy and bronchial asthma. However, the use has declined in these conditions due to the availability of higher efficacy and more selective drugs.

DOPAMINE

Dopamine is a catecholamine and is the immediate precursor of noradrenaline. Dopamine is inactivated by both MAO and COMT; hence, it is ineffective orally. It is therefore given only intravenously. It acts on D_1 dopaminergic as well as α_1 and β_1 adrenergic receptors.

Pharmacological Actions

The pharmacological actions of dopamine are mentioned in Table 4.

TABLE 4	Dose dependent actions of dopamine
Dopamine dose	**Effects**
Low doses (<2 µg/kg/min)	• Stimulates D_1 receptors and dilates renal, coronary and mesenteric blood vessels • Increases GFR and urine output
Moderate doses (2–5 µg/kg/min)	• Stimulates β_1 receptors in the heart and increases myocardial contractility and cardiac output • Stimulates D_1 receptors and dilates renal, coronary and mesenteric blood vessels • Improves cardiac and renal function
High doses (>5 µg/kg/min)	• Leads to α_1 receptor mediated vasoconstriction • Nullifies the beneficial effects of low/moderate doses of dopamine in heart failure

Adverse Effects and Precautions

The adverse effects of dopamine occur primarily due to sympathetic stimulation. These are nausea, vomiting, headache, tachycardia, hypertension, angina and arrhythmia.

Dopamine infusion should be given cautiously in a large vein because extravasation may lead to ischemic necrosis and sloughing of the surrounding tissue.

Clinical Uses

Dopamine is primarily used in the following conditions:
○ Cardiogenic and septic shock
○ Severe congestive heart failure with renal dysfunction

Dopamine is used in the above conditions as it increases blood pressure, improves cardiac/renal functions and increases blood flow to the renal, coronary and mesenteric blood vessels.

> **Note:**
> - Before dopamine is administered to a patient with shock, hypovolemia must be corrected by transfusion of plasma, blood or any other appropriate fluid.
> - During dopamine infusion, the patient should be continuously monitored for urine output, heart rate, blood pressure, myocardial function etc.

Some salient differences between dopamine and dobutamine are mentioned in Table 5.

TABLE 5	Dopamine and dobutamine	
	Dopamine	**Dobutamine**
Origin	• Natural catecholamine	• Synthetic catecholamine
Effect on receptors	• Low doses → Stimulates D_1 receptors • Moderate doses → Stimulates β_1 receptors • High Doses → Stimulates α receptors	• Selective β_1-adrenergic agonist • Mild β_2- and α_1-adrenergic receptor agonist
Clinical effect	• Predominant vasopressor effect	• Predominant ionotropic effect • Increase cardiac output • Does not significantly increase cardiac oxygen demand
Renal Blood Flow	• Direct effect on renal blood flow causing an increase in renal blood flow	• No direct effect on renal blood flow • May increase due to improved cardiac function
Main clinical uses	• Used predominantly to treat acute hypotension or shock, e.g. septic shock • Acute exacerbations of chronic heart failure where there is low cardiac output	• Used for inotropic support in the short-term treatment of low output cardiac failure states (e.g. myocardial infarction, septic shock and cardiogenic shock)

▌FENOLDOPAM

It is a selective agonist of peripheral D_1 receptors. It causes peripheral vasodilation leading to decrease in blood pressure.

It is used in the short-term management of severe hypertension, i.e. in hypertensive emergencies.

The adverse effects are mainly due to vasodilation and includes headache, flushing, reflex tachycardia, dizziness etc.

MEPHENTERMINE

It is a mixed action sympathomimetic drug.
- Direct action on the α and β receptors
- Also causes release of noradrenaline

It is used in the prevention and treatment of hypotension due to spinal anesthesia, surgical procedures and some hypotensive states.

NASAL DECONGESTANTS

Adrenergic α agonists are often used as nasal decongestants. These include:
- **Topical use:** Naphazoline, oxymetazoline, xylometazoline
- **Oral use:** Pseudoephedrine
- **Oral and topical use:** Phenylephrine

The rationale of using adrenergic α agonists is mentioned in Figure 16.

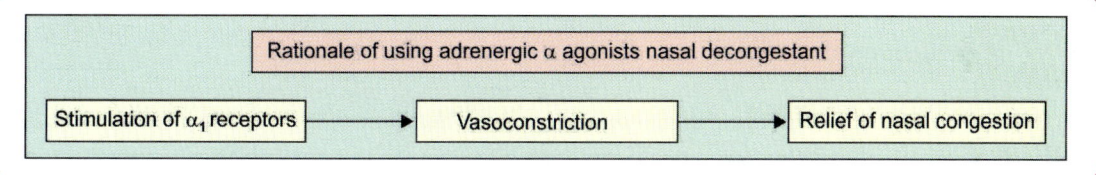

Figure 16: Nasal decongestants

- Information about phenylephrine, pseudoephedrine has been mentioned earlier.
- Prolonged therapy with nasal decongestants can lead to rebound congestion.
- These drugs should be used cautiously in patients with hypertension, cardiovascular disease, narrow angle glaucoma, hyperthyroidism or diabetes mellitus.
- Phenylpropanolamine is not currently used as a nasal decongestant because of the risk of hemorrhagic stroke.

ANTIOBESITY DRUGS

Obesity is defined as a body mass index (BMI) of ≥30 kg/m². Some of the antiobesity drugs are as follows:

ORLISTAT (LIPASE INHIBITORS)

- It inhibits intestinal lipase and reduces absorption of fat.
- Adverse effects include flatulence, diarrhea, and oily stools.
- Vitamin supplementation (A, D, E, K) should be done.
- Contraindications include malabsorption and cholestasis.

PHENTERMINE (ANOREXIANT)

- It is an anorexiant and is a centrally acting sympathomimetic amine. It increases the release of noradrenaline and dopamine and prevents their reuptake.
- All anorexiants have the potential for dependence or abuse.
- Adverse effects include headache, dry mouth, constipation, hypertension, and tachycardia.
- Phentermine should not be used in patients with uncontrolled hypertension, cardiovascular disease, hyperthyroidism or a history of drug abuse/addiction.

SECTION B ■ Drugs Acting on the Autonomic Nervous System

LORCASERIN (SEROTONIN AGONISTS)

- It is a selective agonist of serotonin (5-HT_{2C}) receptors in the hypothalamus.
- Stimulation of these receptors leads to suppression of appetite.
- Adverse effects include headache, nausea, fatigue, dry mouth, dizziness and constipation.
- Use of lorcaserin along with SSRI, SNRI and MAO inhibitors can lead to serotonin syndrome.
- Patients on lorcaserin should be monitored for the potential development of valvulopathy.

COMBINATION THERAPY OF PHENTERMINE AND TOPIRAMATE

- Phentermine is a centrally acting sympathomimetic amine and topiramate is an antiepileptic drug.
- Topiramate has been associated with congenital defects such as cleft palate; hence, the combination is contraindicated in pregnancy.
- Other adverse effects include paraesthesia, dizziness, insomnia, suicide ideation, hypertension, tachycardia, acute myopia and secondary angle closure glaucoma.

A summary of antiobesity drugs is mentioned in Table 6.

TABLE 6	Antiobesity drugs		
	Orlistat	**Lorcaserin**	**Phentermine**
Target organ	GIT	CNS	CNS
Target enzyme/receptor	Gastrointestinal lipase	5HT_{2C} receptor	Neurotransmitters (NA and 5-HT)
Mechanism of action	Decreases fat absorption	Suppresses appetite	Suppresses appetite
Key adverse effects	GIT: Flatulence, malabsorption, steatorrhea	Dry mouth headache, nausea, dizziness, serotonin syndrome	Dry mouth, headache, constipation, hypertension

Fenfluramine and dexfenfluramine have been withdrawn as they were associated with pulmonary hypertension and cardiac valve defects.

Sibutramine and rimonabant have been withdrawn because they were associated with cardiovascular toxicity.

ASSESS YOURSELF (Examination Questions of Various Universities)

1. Classify sympathomimetic agents. Describe therapeutic uses and adverse effects of adrenaline.
2. Pharmacological basis for the use of adrenaline in anaphylactic shock.
3. Mention rationale of combining adrenaline with local anesthetic agents.
4. Compare dopamine and dobutamine.
5. Explain the rationale of using adrenaline and lidocaine combination for local anesthesia.
6. Dopamine in cardiogenic shock.
7. Compare adrenaline and noradrenaline.
8. Drugs used in the treatment of obesity.
9. Orlistat.
10. Role of short acting β agonists in bronchial asthma.
11. Explain why noradrenaline not effective in acute severe asthma or anaphylaxis?

Anticholinergic drugs are those which block the actions of cholinergic drugs. The anticholinergic drugs can be subdivided into antimuscarinic drugs and antinicotinic drugs (Figure 1).

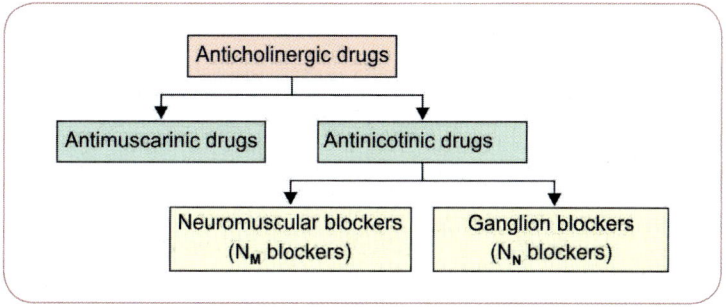

Figure 1: Anticholinergic drugs

ANTIMUSCARINIC DRUGS

The antimuscarinic drugs block the effects of acetylcholine (ACh) which are mediated by muscarinic receptors (e.g. on heart, smooth muscles, exocrine glands etc.).

Atropine and scopolamine are naturally occurring alkaloids extracted from belladonna plants. Atropine is obtained from *Atropa belladonna* and scopolamine from *Hyoscyamus niger*.

All antimuscarinic drugs are competitive antagonists i.e. they competitively inhibit the actions of ACh on muscarinic receptors (Figure 2).

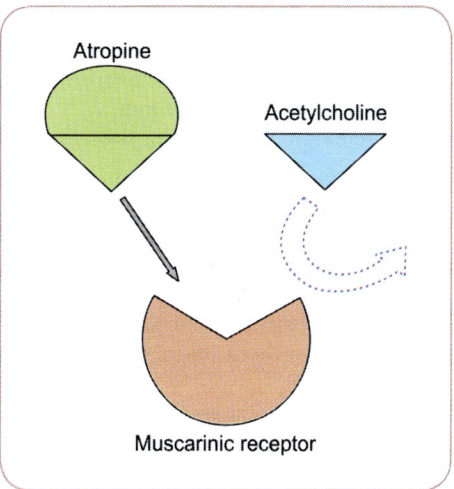

Figure 2: Competitive antagonism of ACh

Classification of Antimuscarinic Drugs

The classification of antimuscarinic drugs is mentioned in Figure 3.

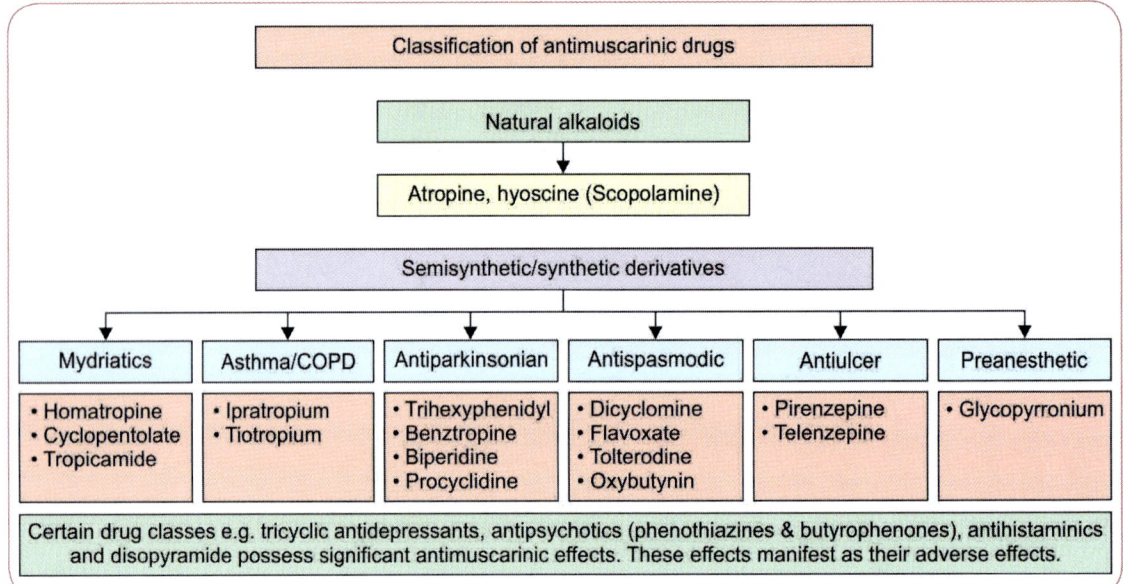

Figure 3: Classification of antimuscarinic drugs

ATROPINE

Atropine is the prototype drug of this class. It is a tertiary amine. It has high affinity for muscarinic receptors. It competitively binds to these receptors and prevents ACh from binding to it.

Pharmacological Actions

Central Nervous System

- At low doses, atropine has no significant CNS effect.
- At therapeutic doses, atropine has:
  - Mild CNS stimulant effect
  - Anti-parkinsonian effect—decreases cholinergic overactivity in basal ganglia
  - Anti-motion sickness effect—decreases vestibular excitation
- At high doses, it causes restlessness, excitation, hallucinations, delirium, paralysis, coma and death.

Cardiovascular System

- At low doses (0.5 mg), it causes transient initial bradycardia. This occurs due to blockade of presynaptic M_1 autoreceptors, thereby increasing ACh release.
- At higher (therapeutic) doses, it causes tachycardia due to blockade of M_2 receptors in the SA node. This is because of antagonization of vagal (parasympathetic) tone to the heart.
- Higher the vagal tone, more significant is the tachycardia (e.g. more in young adults and lesser in children and elderly). It also increases the AV conduction.
- In toxic (and rarely therapeutic) doses, atropine causes cutaneous vasodilatation occurs especially in blush area of the face (atropine flush).

Smooth Muscles

GIT

Atropine decreases tone and amplitude of contractions of stomach and intestines (acts as an antispasmodic).

It also decreases intestinal motility and increases the sphincter tone. This results in constipation. It has a weak antispasmodic action on the biliary tract and gallbladder.

Urinary Bladder

Atropine relaxes the detrusor muscle of urinary bladder and increases the tone of trigone and sphincter—can result in urinary retention in elderly males with enlarged prostate.

Lungs

Atropine relaxes the bronchial smooth muscle. It also reduces bronchial secretions as well as the mucociliary clearance. This results in mucus plug formation which may lead to dangerous airway obstruction that may also secondarily infect.

Hence, in chronic obstructive pulmonary disease (COPD), ipratropium/tiotropium (and not atropine) are the preferred drugs because they result in bronchodilatation but cause lesser drying of bronchial secretions. They also do not inhibit mucociliary clearance. Therefore, there are minimal chances of mucus plug formation.

Glands

o   All the body secretions (that are under cholinergic control) are decreased by atropine, e.g. sweat, salivary, lacrimal, tracheobronchial, gastric etc. This effect occurs due to blockade of M_3 receptors on the glands. There is no effect on bile as well as intestinal or pancreatic secretions.
o   The salivary secretions are particularly sensitive to atropine so that it rapidly produces dryness of mouth (xerostomia), making swallowing and talking difficult.

Eye

Atropine causes the following effects on the eye:
o   Relaxation of sphincter (circular) muscle leading to *Mydriasis*
o   Relaxation of ciliary muscle leading to *Cycloplegia*

The topical application of atropine causes cycloplegia lasting 5–6 days that results in photophobia and blurring of near vision.

Pharmacokinetics

Atropine, hyoscine and other synthetic tertiary amines are well absorbed from the GIT. They freely penetrate cornea. They are partly metabolized in the liver and are partly excreted unchanged by the kidneys.

Some of the salient differences between atropine and hyoscine are mentioned in Table 1.

TABLE 1	Comparison between atropine and hyoscine
Atropine	**Hyoscine (Scopolamine)**
• Obtained from *Atropa belladonna* and *Datura stramonium*	• Obtained from *Hyoscyamus niger*
• CNS effects are excitatory at low and high doses	• CNS effects are depressant at low doses and excitatory at high doses
• Lesser antimotion sickness property	• Higher antimotion sickness property

ATROPINE SUBSTITUTES

Many semisynthetic and synthetic derivatives of atropine have been developed, with the aim of producing relatively selective actions on certain organs and minimizing undesirable actions on the others.
The key features of some of the atropine substitutes are mentioned in Figure 4.

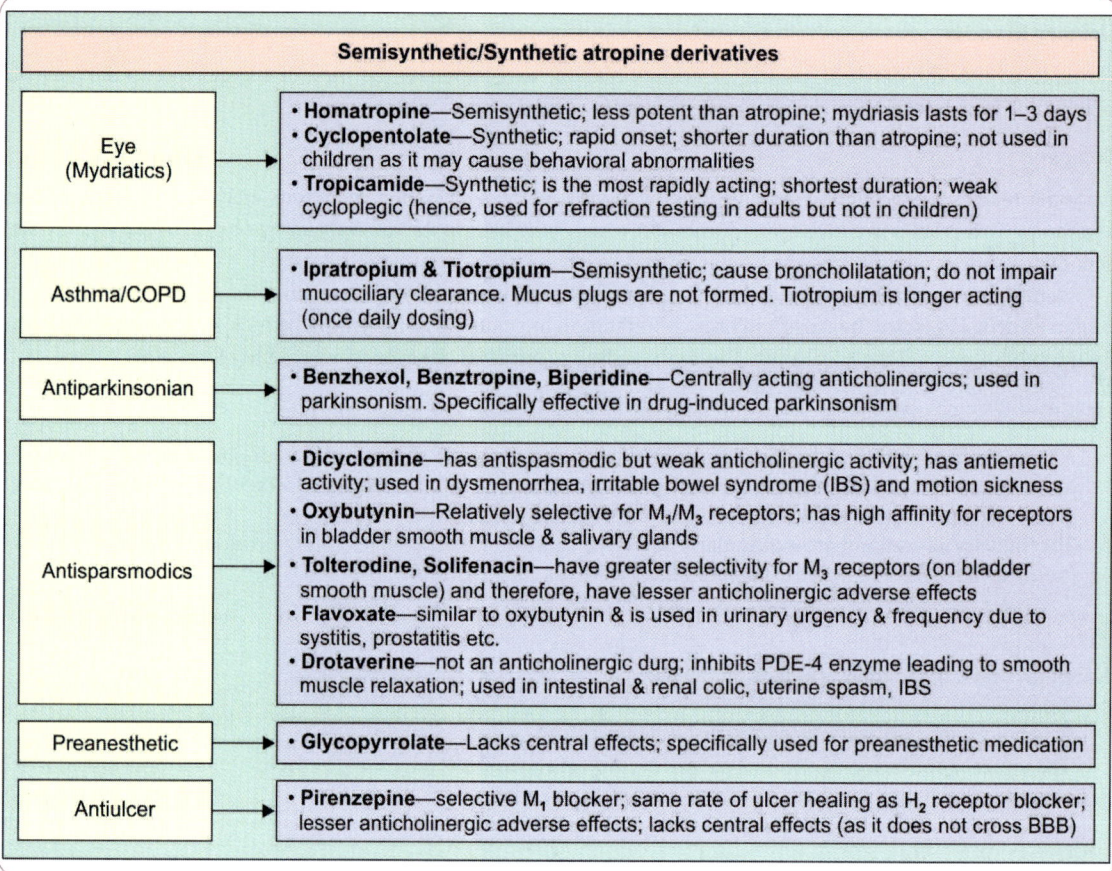

Figure 4: Semisynthetic/Synthetic atropine derivatives

Clinical Uses

Ophthalmic Uses

The ophthalmic uses of antimuscarinic drugs are mentioned in Figure 5.

COPD and Bronchial Asthma

Ipratropium and tiotropium cause bronchodilatation, but do not dry up the secretions and also do not impair mucociliary clearance. Mucus plugs are not formed. The chances of obstruction and infection are minimized. Hence, they are preferred over atropine for COPD and asthma.

Ipratropium and tiotropium are used by nebulizer or metered dose inhaler. Tiotropium is longer acting and needs once daily dosing, a major advantage over ipratropium which is to be given 4–5 times per day.

○ For COPD, they are used for regular maintenance therapy.
○ For asthma, they are used to control acute attacks, where they are given along with β_2-agonists such as salbutamol.

Ophthalmic uses	
Diagnostic	**Therapeutic**
Refraction testing • Both mydriatic and cycloplegia is required • Atropine, homatropine, cyclopentolate or tropicamide may be used • In adults, tropicamide is preferred due to shorter action* • In children, due to stronger muscles, potent cycloplegics such as atropine is required **Fundoscopic examination** • Only mydriasis is required; cycloplegia is not required • Antimuscarinic drugs are not used as they cause both mydriasis and cycloplegia. A short acting α-agonist (such as phenylephrine) is used	**Iridocyclitis** • Atropinic drugs (atropine, homatropine etc.) are used because of its long duration of action • They are useful in iritis, iridocyclitis, choroiditis, and relieve keratitis • They provide rest to the ocular muscles and relief painful spasms • They prevent adhesions between iris and lens & iris and cornea. They also break the adhesions if already formed. They are given alternatively with miotics for this purpose

* The duration of action of tropicamide is 15–60 minutes as compared to 5–6 days for atropine

• Atropine is preferred for refraction testing is children because the ocular muscles are stronger in children as compared to adults. Hence, potent cycloplegics such as atropine are preferred.
• Phenylephrine (short acting α-agonist) is preferred over atropine for fundoscopic examination because cycloplegia is not required for fundoscopy and only mydriasis is required. Hence antimuscarinic drugs such as atropine are not used for fundoscopy.

Figure 5: Ophthalmic uses of antimuscarinic drugs

Antiparkinsonian

The parkinsonian symptoms occur due to a relative imbalance between dopamine deficiency and cholinergic overactivity in the basal ganglia. Hence, anticholinergics are often used along with dopaminergic agonists for the treatment.

Centrally acting anticholinergic drugs (such as trihexyphenidyl (benzhexol), benztropine, biperidine and procyclidine) are used for the treatment of parkinsonism. They are the drugs of choice in drug-induced (phenothiazine-induced) parkinsonism. They are also effective in idiopathic parkinsonism but in this situation, they are less efficacious than levodopa.

Motion Sickness

Hyoscine (scopolamine) is the preferred drug in motion sickness. It inhibits vestibular disturbances and prevents motion sickness. The features of hyoscine in motion sickness are mentioned in Figure 6.

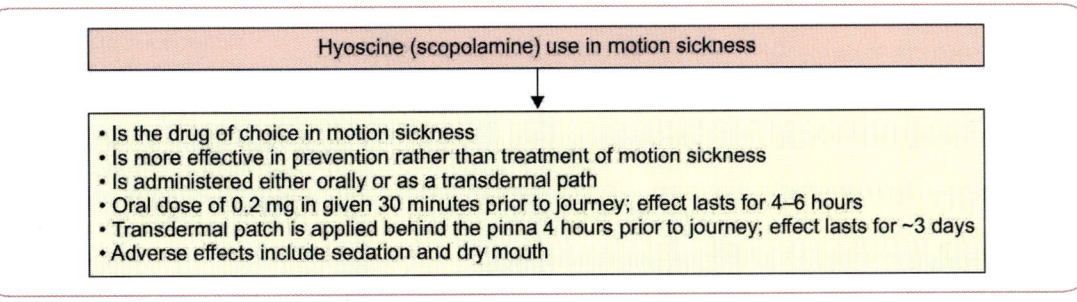

Hyoscine (scopolamine) use in motion sickness

• Is the drug of choice in motion sickness
• Is more effective in prevention rather than treatment of motion sickness
• Is administered either orally or as a transdermal path
• Oral dose of 0.2 mg in given 30 minutes prior to journey; effect lasts for 4–6 hours
• Transdermal patch is applied behind the pinna 4 hours prior to journey; effect lasts for ~3 days
• Adverse effects include sedation and dry mouth

Figure 6: Hyoscine use in motion sickness

Preanesthetic Medication

Glycopyrrolate or atropine are used in the following situations:

- ○ Prior to general anesthesia:
  - ❑ To reduce laryngospasm by decreasing secretions (salivary & tracheobronchial)
  - ❑ To prevent vagal bradycardia during surgery

  Glycopyrrolate is often preferred over atropine for preanesthetic medication because it does not readily cross the blood brain barrier and hence it does not produce CNS effects. It also causes relatively less tachycardia.
- ○ To protect against the peripheral muscarinic actions of anticholinesterases (neostigmine). The anticholinesterases are given to reverse residual neuromuscular blockade produced by nondepolarizing muscle relaxants.

Antispasmodic

Antimuscarinic drugs are used as antispasmodics in the conditions such as intestinal and renal colics, irritable bowel syndrome, dysmenorrhea etc.

Urinary Disorders

Oxybutynin is relatively selective for M_1/M_3 receptors. It has high affinity for receptors in bladder smooth muscle and salivary glands.

Hence, oxybutynin is used to relieve bladder spasm after urologic surgery (e.g. prostatectomy). It is also used to reduce involuntary voiding in children with neurologic disease.

Tolterodine, darifenacin and solifenacin have greater selectivity for M_3 receptors (on bladder smooth muscle) than oxybutynin and therefore, have lesser anticholinergic adverse effects. Darifenacin and solifenacin are longer acting than oxybutynin and have the advantage of once-daily dosing.

These drugs are preferable for use in urinary incontinence.

Peptic Ulcer

Pirenzepine and telanzepine are relatively selective M_1 receptor blockers. They decrease gastric secretion and afford symptomatic relief. It produces the same rate of ulcer healing as H_2 receptor blockers. Effective doses mostly produce some antimuscarinic adverse effects.

However, H_2 receptor blockers and proton pump blockers are considered the drug of choice in the treatment of peptic ulcers.

Cholinergic Poisoning

Antimuscarinic drugs are used in cholinergic poisonings in the following situations (Figure 7):

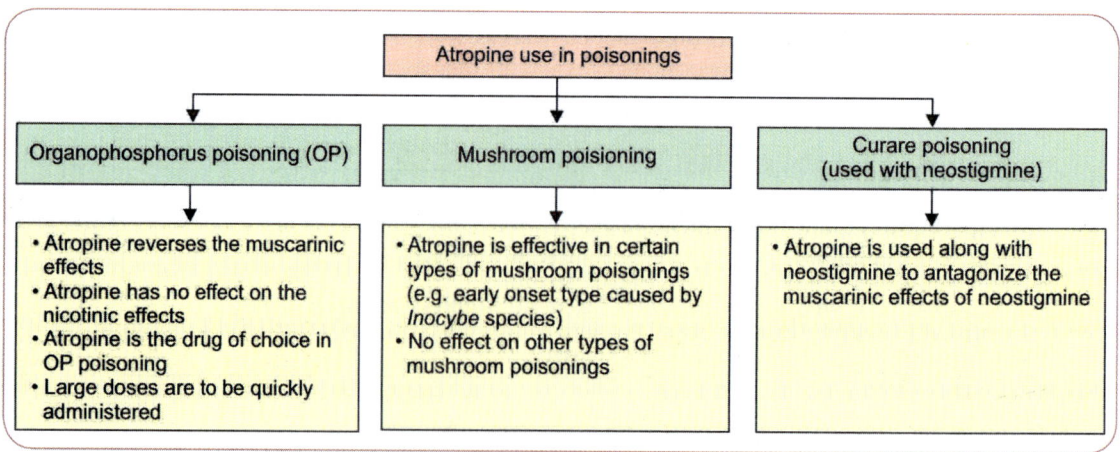

Figure 7: Atropine use in poisonings

Drug Interactions

Some key drug interactions of atropine are mentioned below:
- Tricyclic antidepressants, antipsychotics (phenothiazines/butyrophenones), and H_1 antihistaminics have anticholinergic activity—administration with atropine potentiates the anticholinergic effects of atropine.
- Atropine delays gastric emptying. This leads to delayed absorption of most drugs.
  - In case of levodopa, it may lead to its greater degradation and decreased bioavailability
  - In case of tetracyclines and digoxin, it may lead to increased absorption due to increased transit time in the GIT

Adverse Effects and Contraindications

The treatment by atropine on one organ system almost always induces undesirable effects on the other organ system. For example, mydriasis and cycloplegia are desirable effects on eye examination but they become undesirable effects when atropine is used for renal colic.

The adverse effects of atropine can be judged from its pharmacological actions. The key adverse effects are mentioned below:

1. **Eye:** Blurring of vision, photophobia, headache, precipitation of acute congestive glaucoma in patients with shallow anterior chamber (angle closure glaucoma)
2. **GIT:** Dryness of mouth (xerostomia), difficulty in swallowing, constipation
3. **Urinary tract:** Difficulty in urination and urinary retention in elderly males with enlarged prostate gland
4. **CVS:** Tachycardia and palpitation
5. **CNS:** In high doses, restlessness, excitation, hallucinations, delirium

Hence, the contraindications for atropine use are angle closure glaucoma, GIT obstruction, urinary tract obstruction, benign prostatic hyperplasia.

ATROPINE (BELLADONNA) POISONING

The atropine effects are manifested in an exaggerated form. Some of the common manifestations in poisoning patients are dry mouth, hot and flushed skin, mydriasis, tachycardia, increased body temperature, agitation and delirium. These effects are commonly referred by the proverb mentioned in Figure 8.

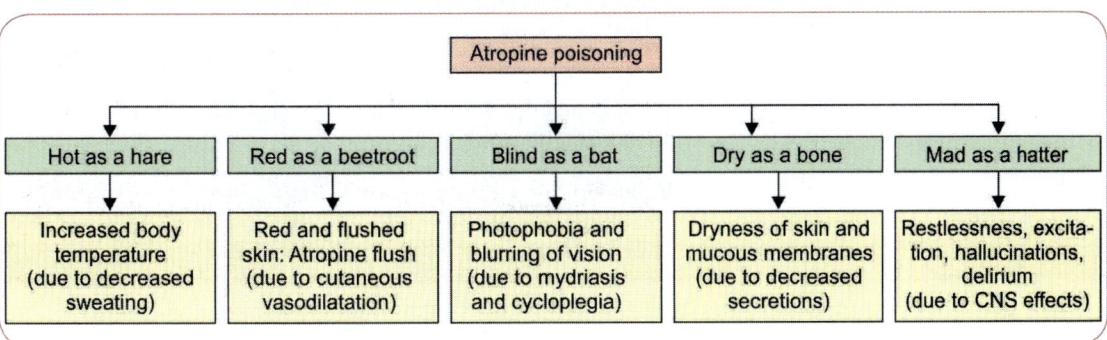

Figure 8: Atropine poisoning: Manifestations

Treatment of Atropine Poisoning

- Hospitalization
- Gastric lavage with tannic acid
- Cold sponging with ice bags to reduce body temperature
- Diazepam IV for sedation and control of convulsions
- Physostigmine IV to reverse central as well as peripheral effects of atropine (neostigmine does not reverse the central effects)
- Other supportive measures for circulation and respiration

GANGLION BLOCKERS

The ganglion blockers primarily act on the N_N receptors of the autonomic ganglia. They act both on sympathetic and parasympathetic ganglia.

The effects of ganglion blockers on various body systems are mentioned in Table 2.

TABLE 2	Effect of ganglion blockers at various organ sites	
Organ	Major tone	Effect of ganglion blockade
Heart	Parasympathetic	Tachycardia
Iris and ciliary muscle	Parasympathetic	Mydriasis and cycloplegia
GIT	Parasympathetic	Constipation, distension
Bladder	Parasympathetic	Urinary retention
Salivary gland	Parasympathetic	Xerostomia (dry mouth)
Sweat gland	Sympathetic	Anhidrosis (↓ sweating)
Blood vessels	Sympathetic	Vasodilatation

There are no selective ganglion blockers available. The ganglion blockers are very rarely used for therapeutic purpose. Some significant features of a few ganglion blockers are mentioned below:

NICOTINE

Nicotine is a component of cigarette (tobacco) smoke and has many undesirable effects. It produces harmful effects in all the body organs including lung, oral cavity and heart. It does not have any therapeutic benefit and is harmful for the health.

It initially produces stimulation, followed later by a prolonged inhibition of the autonomic ganglia. It does not have any clinical value except (in the form of transdermal patch application) for the treatment of nictotine dependence.

TRIMETHAPHAN

It is an ultrashort acting ganglion blocker. It acts by competing with ACh for the ganglion nicotinic receptors. It is used only to produce controlled hypotension (for reducing bleeding during neurosurgery), and to treat hypertensive emergencies.

ASSESS YOURSELF (Examination Questions of Various Universities)

1. Enumerate anticholinergic agents. Discuss their adverse effects and give their therapeutic uses based on their pharmacological actions. Illustrate with the help of suitable examples.

2. Enumerate anticholinergic agents. Discuss their uses giving specific example. Write the adverse effects of atropine.

3. Atropine substitutes.

4. Explain the role of glycopyrrolate as a preanesthetic medication.

5. Why phenylephrine and not atropine is used for fundoscopic examination?

6. Atropine (belladonna) poisoning.

10

Alpha Adrenergic Blockers

Alpha adrenergic blockers (α blockers) are drugs that block the effects mediated by α receptors in response to sympathetic stimulation or responses to α agonist drugs (Figure 1).

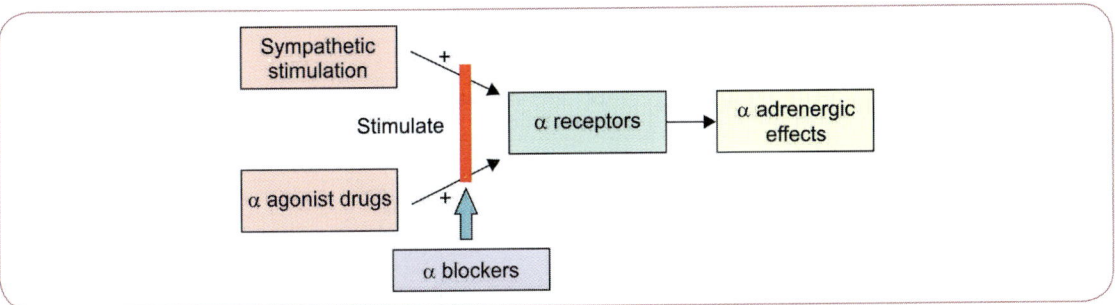

Figure 1: Alpha adrenergic blockers (α blockers)

CLASSIFICATION OF ALPHA ADRENERGIC BLOCKERS (α BLOCKERS)

A classification of alpha adrenergic blockers (α blockers) is mentioned in Figure 2.

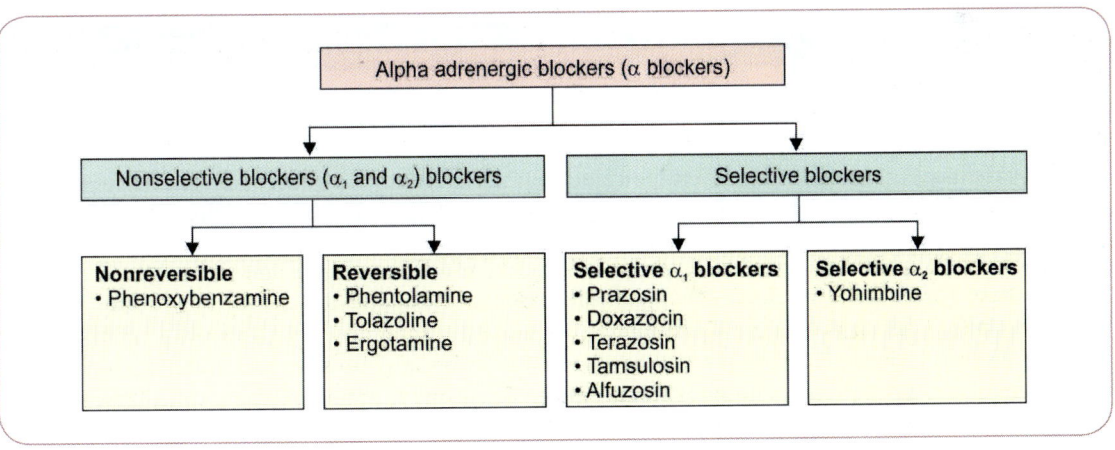

Figure 2: Classification of alpha adrenergic blockers (α blockers)

PHARMACOLOGICAL ACTIONS OF ALPHA ADRENERGIC BLOCKERS (α BLOCKERS)

The pharmacological actions of alpha adrenergic blockers (α blockers) are mentioned in Table 1 and Figure 3.

TABLE 1	Effects of α blockers
Organ system	**Effects of α blockers**
Eye	• Miosis
Nose	• Stuffiness
Blood vessels	• Reduced blood pressure • Reflex tachycardia (Figure 3)
GIT	• Increased intestinal motility, diarrhea
Urinary bladder	• Relaxation of muscle in trigone and sphincter (α_{1A} effect) • Improved urine flow
Vas deferens	• Inhibition of ejaculation

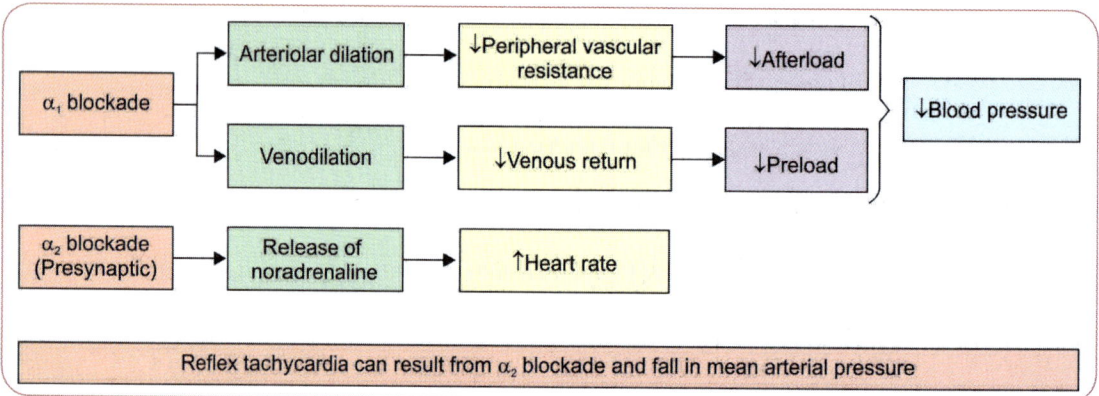

Figure 3: Effect of α blockers on blood vessels and blood pressure

NONSELECTIVE α BLOCKERS

PHENOXYBENZAMINE

Phenoxybenzamine is a non selective, irreversible α blocker. It blocks both α_1 and α_2 receptors. It has a long duration of action because it irreversibly blocks α receptors and it takes some time for the body to synthesize new receptors. Phenoxybenzamine has the following vascular effects:

○ α_1 blockade → Venodilation and reduced peripheral vascular resistance → reduction in blood pressure
○ α_2 blockade (presynaptic) → Release of noradrenaline leads to cardiac stimulation and tachycardia

It is administered orally or via slow IV infusion.

Adverse effects include postural hypotension with reflex tachycardia, dizziness, nasal stuffiness, inhibition of ejaculation, miosis, gastrointestinal upset. Postural hypotension is due to more prominent venodilator effect as compared to arteriolar dilation.

Phenoxybenzamine is used to manage hypertensive episodes in patients of pheochromocytoma.

PHENTOLAMINE

Phentolamine is a non selective, reversible α blocker. It blocks both α_1 and α_2 receptors. It has a rapid onset with a short duration of action.

Adverse effects are similar to that of phenoxybenzamine and includes postural hypotension with reflex tachycardia, arrhythmias and anginal pain. It is contraindicated in patients of coronary artery disease.

Clinical uses include management of hypertensive episodes in pheochromocytoma, clonidine withdrawal and cheese reaction. It is also used locally to counteract vasoconstriction due to extravasation of noradrenaline or dopamine following IV infusion Some key differences between phenoxybenzamine and phentolamine are mentioned in Table 2.

TABLE 2	Phenoxybenzamine and phentolamine
Phenoxybenzamine	**Phentolamine**
Irreversible α blocker	Reversible α blocker
Prolonged duration of action and slow onset	Short duration of action and rapid onset

SELECTIVE α₁ BLOCKERS

PRAZOSIN

Prazosin is a selective α_1 adrenergic blocker.

It causes a decrease in blood pressure by selectively blocking the α_1 receptor mediated vasoconstriction, thereby reducing the total peripheral vascular resistance (*see* Figure 3).

Other pharmacological effects of α adrenergic blockers are mentioned in Table 1.

It causes minimal reflex tachycardia.

Adverse effects include postural hypotension, blurred vision, palpitations, dizziness, lack of energy, impotence. Prazosin should preferably be taken at bedtime to reduce the incidence of first dose effect. (Figure 4).

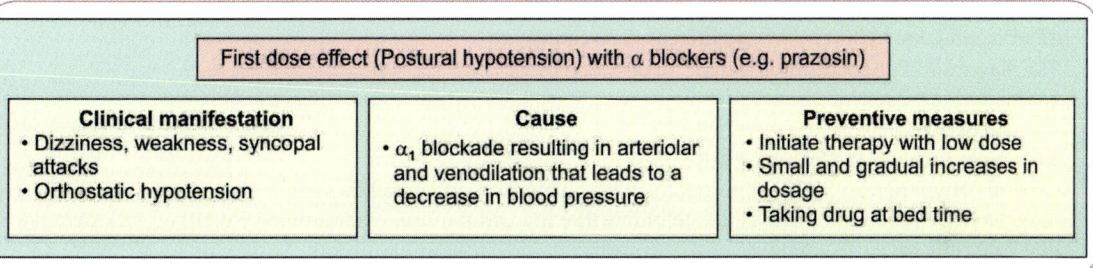

Figure 4: First dose effect with α blockers (e.g. Prazosin)

Clinical uses include the following:

- Management of hypertension (essential and secondary)
- Raynaud's phenomenon and Raynaud's disease
- Benign prostatic hyperplasia (BHP)—symptomatic management of urinary retention

Some of the key differences between phentolamine and prazosin are mentioned in Table 3.

TABLE 3	Phentolamine and prazosin	
	Phentolamine	**Prazosin**
Mechanism of action	• Nonselective, reversible α blocker	• Selective α_1 adrenergic blocker
Incidence of reflex tachycardia	• Higher incidence (presynaptic α_2 blockade leads to release of noradrenaline resulting in cardiac stimulation and tachycardia)	• Lower incidence
Clinical uses	• Management of hypertensive episodes in pheochromocytoma, cheese reaction, clonidine withdrawal • Used locally to counteract vasoconstriction due to extravasation of noradrenaline or dopamine following IV infusion	• Management of hypertension (essential and secondary) • Raynaud's phenomenon and Raynaud's disease • BHP

TERAZOSIN

It is similar to prazosin, but has a longer duration of action. It is preferred for use in BHP due to the requirement of a single daily dose.

DOXAZOSIN

It is a longer acting α blocker that is used for hypertension and BHP.

TAMSULOSIN

It is a uroselective α blocker (α_{1A} and α_{1D}) that has a higher affinity for the α_{1A} receptor subtype.

The α_{1A} receptor subtype predominates in the bladder and prostate and hence, tamsulosin is preferred for the symptomatic management of BHP.

Tamsulosin does not cause significant alterations in the heart rate or blood pressure because it has a lower affinity to α_{1B} receptors which are the predominant receptors in the blood vessels.

Adverse effects include dizziness and ejaculation disorders (e.g. retrograde ejaculation).

CLINICAL USES OF α BLOCKERS

Pheochromocytoma

It is a catecholamine-secreting tumor of the adrenal medulla.

Clinical features include persistent or paroxysmal hypertension. Other features include severe headache, tachycardia, postural hypotension and increased sweating.

The diagnosis of pheochromocytoma can be made by:
- Estimation of plasma or urinary metanephrines
- CT scan or MRI

Treatment includes the following measures:
- Control of hypertension with combination of alpha blockers and beta blockers
- Surgical resection of tumor—it is the definitive therapy and requires careful management of perioperative BP and volume status

Pharmacotherapy for Pheochromocytoma

- **Phenoxybenzamine:** It is used in the preoperative and intraoperative period to control hypertension and restore blood volume. It has the following actions:
  - Therapy with α blocker restores the blood volume that has been shifted from the vascular to the extravascular compartment by the catecholamines.
  - Restoration of the blood volume can also prevent the fall in blood pressure that can occur following removal of the tumor.
  - Significant increase in the intraoperative blood pressure may occur due to release of catecholamines resulting from the handling of the tumor. Phenoxybenzamine can prevent the rise in the blood pressure that can occur intraoperatively by handling of the tumor.
- **Other drugs that can be used for the management of hypertension in pheochromocytoma are:**
  - Phentolamine (α blocker)
  - Sodium nitroprusside (vasodilator)
  - Propranolol (β blocker) → It is also used for intraoperative control of tachyarrhythmias. Beta-blockers should not be used until adequate alpha-blockade has been achieved. This is because blockade of β_2 receptors can result in unopposed α_1 mediated vasoconstriction that can cause a severe rise in BP that may be fatal.

Hypertension Emergencies

- Phentolamine IV can be used to manage hypertensive episodes/emergencies in pheochromocytoma (intraoperative), cheese reaction and clonidine withdrawal.

Essential Hypertension

- Selective α_1 adrenergic blockers such as prazosin, terazosin and doxazosin can be used.

Benign Hyperplasia of Prostate

- α_1 adrenergic blockers reduce the tone of bladder neck/prostatic smooth muscle and increase the urinary flow rate. It leads to a more complete emptying of the urinary bladder.
- Selective α_1 adrenergic blockers such as prazosin, terazosin and doxazosin can be used.
- Tamsulosin is preferred because it is a uroselective α blocker (α_{1A} and α_{1D}) that has a higher affinity for the subtype α_{1A}. Hence, it does not cause significant alterations in the heart rate or the blood pressure because it has a lower affinity for α_{1B} receptors which are the predominant receptors in blood vessels.
- Refer to Figure 5.

Benign hyperplasia of prostate (BHP)

Clinical features
- It is a nonmalignant overgrowth of the prostate gland
- Symptoms include those of bladder outlet obstruction
- Weak stream, urinary hesitancy, frequency, nocturia, urge incontinence, urinary retention

Pharmacotherapy
- **α_1 blockers**
  - Reduce tone of bladder neck/prostatic smooth muscle → improve urinary flow rate → more complete emptying of the urinary bladder
  - E.g. Terazosin, doxazosin, tamsulosin, alfuzosin
- **5 alpha-reductase inhibitors**
  - Reduce size/growth of prostate gland
  - E.g. Finasteride, dutasteride
- **Phosphodiesterase type 5 inhibitor**
  - Patients with erectile dysfunction
  - E.g. Tadalafil

- Avoid drugs such as opioids, anticholinergics and sympathomimetics
- Surgical management including transurethral resection of the prostate (TURP)

Figure 5: Benign hyperplasia of prostate (BHP)

Peripheral Vascular Disease (Raynaud's Phenomenon and Raynaud's Disease)

- α blockers can increase the blood flow by relieving vasoconstriction
- E.g. Prazosin

Congestive Cardiac Failure

- Prazosin can have a short-term benefit

Male Sexual Dysfunction

- Local injection of papaverine along with phentolamine can be used

Phentolamine can be used Locally to Counteract Vasoconstriction due to Extravasation of Noradrenaline or Dopamine following IV Infusion

---

ASSESS YOURSELF (Examination Questions of Various Universities)

1. Rationale of tamsulosin in benign prostatic hypertrophy.
2. Drug therapy of benign hyperplasia of prostate.
3. First dose effect with prazosin.
4. Why prazosin should be preferably taken at bedtime?
5. Pharmacotherapy for pheochromocytoma.
6. Difference between phenoxybenzamine and phentolamine.

11

Beta Adrenergic Blockers

Beta adrenergic blockers (β-blockers) are competitive antagonists of β receptors. They block the β-receptor mediated effects of catecholamines and other adrenergic agonists (Figure 1). Propranolol is the prototype drug.

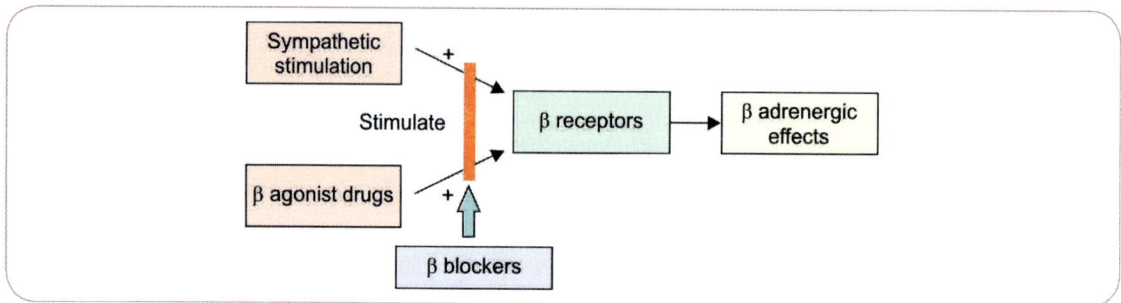

Figure 1: Beta blockers

CLASSIFICATION OF BETA BLOCKERS

A classification of β-blockers is mentioned in Figure 2.

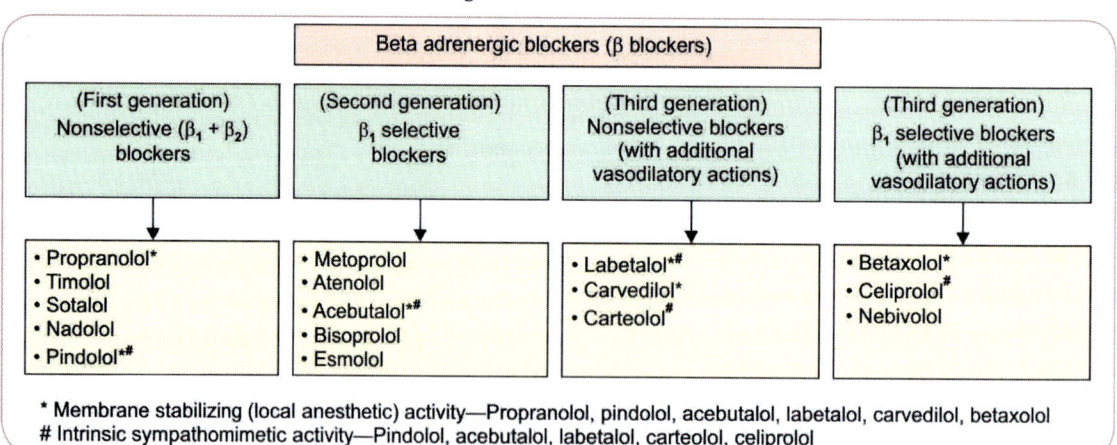

Figure 2: Classification of beta blockers

PHARMACOLOGICAL ACTIONS

The major clinical effects of β-blockers are on the cardiovascular system. The pharmacological actions of β-blockers are mentioned below:

Heart

Beta blockers depress most of the cardiac actions. The cardiac actions of β-blockers are mentioned in Figure 3.

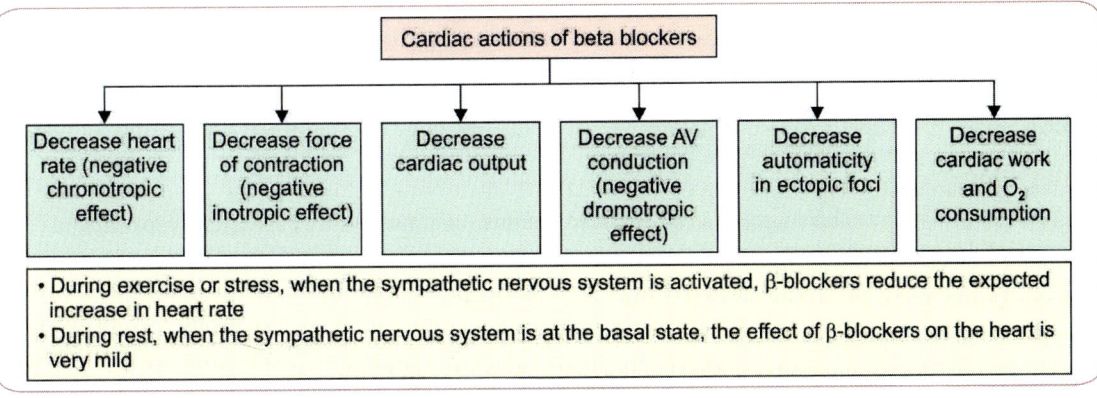

Figure 3: Beta blockers—actions on the heart

Blood Vessels

On propranolol administration, the following sequence of events occur (Figure 4):

Initially, blockade of β_2 receptors in the blood vessels leads to unopposed α_1 action. Also, reduction in cardiac output (CO) elicits a reflex compensatory response leading to activation of vascular α_1 receptors. Both these actions lead to vasoconstriction and an increase in peripheral vascular resistance (PVR).

However, on continuous administration, the resistance blood vessels gradually adapt to the decreased CO. This results in a decrease in PVR and reduction in both systolic and diastolic blood pressure.

It also decreases renin release from the juxtaglomerular cells of the kidney. This action is mediated by blockade of β_1 receptors.

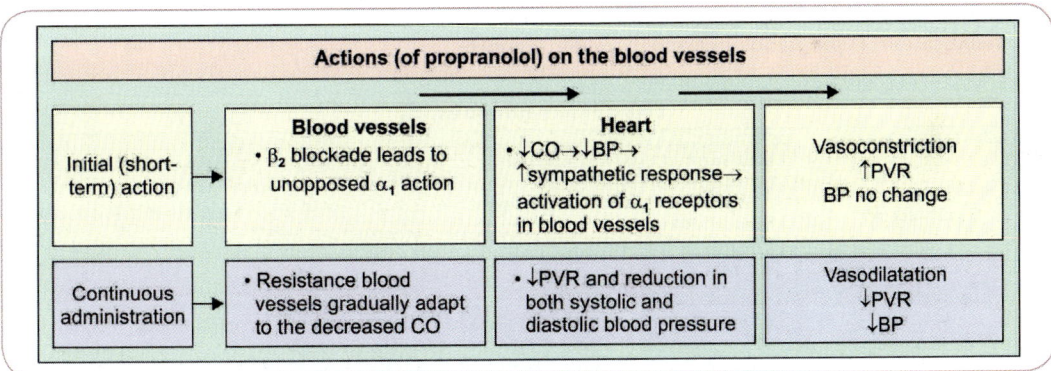

Figure 4: Propranolol—actions on the blood vessels

Respiratory System

Blockade of β_2 receptors in bronchial smooth muscle can result in life-threatening bronchospasm in patients with asthma or COPD. Hence, β-blockers (particularly nonselective ones) are contraindicated in patients with asthma or COPD.

Cardioselective β-blockers and those with intrinsic sympathomimetic activity (e.g. betaxolol, celiprolol) are less likely to cause bronchospasm.

Metabolic Effects

The following metabolic effects of β-blockers are noteworthy:
- Beta blockers inhibit glycogenolysis. They delay recovery from hypoglycemia in type 1 diabetes mellitus.
- Beta blockers decrease the normal warning signs and symptoms of hypoglycemia. Hence, they decrease the perception of hypoglycemia symptoms such as tremors, nervousness, tachycardia etc. Therefore, in diabetic patients with frequent hypoglycemic episodes, β-blockers should be cautiously used.

○ In patients with insulin resistance, nonselective β-blockers decrease insulin sensitivity, while β-blockers with vasodilatory action increase insulin sensitivity. Hence, in patients with diabetes, if β-blockers are required, β_1-selective blockers or β-blockers with vasodilatory action are preferred.

○ Prolonged use of nonselective β-blockers may decrease HDL cholesterol and increase LDL cholesterol and triglycerides. In contrast, β_1-selective blockers reportedly improve the plasma lipid profile of dyslipidemic patients.

Skeletal Muscle

Beta blockers inhibits catecholamine or stress-induced tremors. They also reduce the exercise capacity and cause tiredness by blocking the β_2 receptors in skeletal muscles, which results in decreased blood flow.

Eye

Propranolol applied topically, decreases the formation of aqueous humor and reduces IOP. However, it is rarely used for this purpose because of its local anesthetic action on cornea and lesser potency.

Timolol is the preferred β-blocker in glaucoma.

▌ PHARMACOKINETICS

Propranolol is highly lipophilic and is almost completely absorbed after oral administration. However, the bioavailability is only around 30% because of high first-pass metabolism in the liver.

The metabolism of propranolol is dependent on hepatic blood flow. On prolonged use, it decreases hepatic blood flow resulting in decreased hepatic extraction and increased oral bioavailability and half-life.

It is highly plasma protein bound and is widely distributed throughout the body. It crosses the blood brain barrier. The metabolites are excreted by the kidney.

▌ ADVERSE EFFECTS AND CONTRAINDICATIONS

The adverse effects of β-blockers are mostly extension of their pharmacological actions. The key adverse effects and contraindications of propranolol are mentioned in Figure 5.

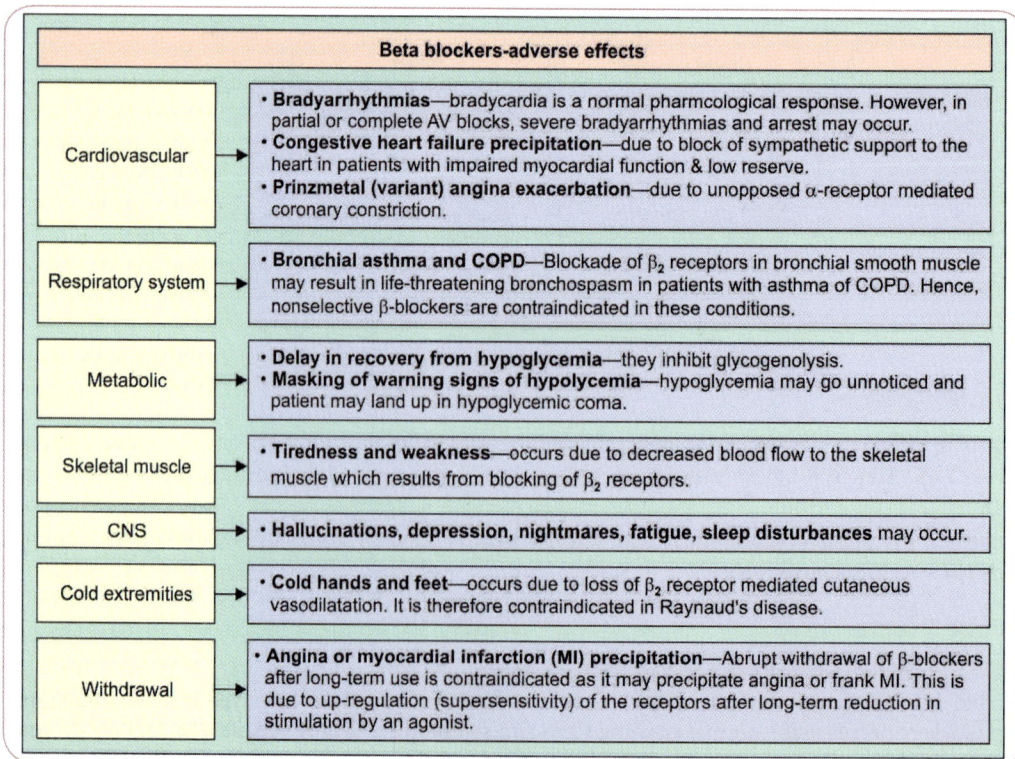

Figure 5: Adverse effects of beta blockers

DRUG INTERACTIONS

Some of the key drug interactions of beta blockers are mentioned in Figure 6.

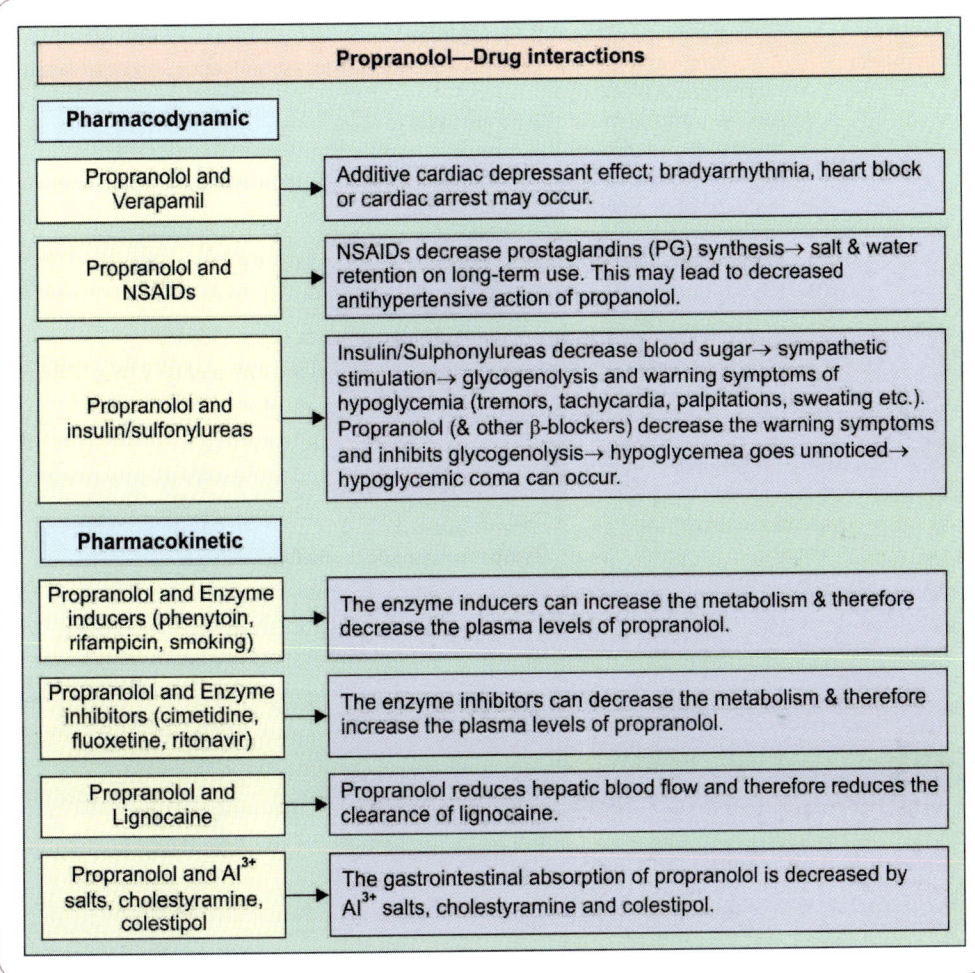

Figure 6: Drug interactions of beta blockers

MEMBRANE STABILIZING, INTRINSIC AGONIST ACTIVITY AND LIPID SOLUBILITY OF B BLOCKERS

Some salient features regarding membrane stabilizing activity, intrinsic agonist (sympathomimetic) activity and lipid solubility are mentioned in Tables 1 and 2.

TABLE 1	Membrane stabilizing, intrinsic agonist activity and lipid solubility
Membrane stabilizing activity	• Postulated to contribute towards the antiarrhythmic properties of β blockers • However, it occurs at high doses and is not of clinical significance • E.g. Propranolol, carvedilol
Intrinsic agonist (sympathomimetic) activity	• Some β blockers activate β_1/β_2 receptors • Bradycardia and reduced cardiac contractility is less prominent, exercise induced tachycardia is blocked • May be useful in patients who are likely to have severe bradycardia (e.g. elderly) or those with reduced cardiac reserve • Reduced likelihood of withdrawal induced exacerbation of hypertension or angina • Reduced or no worsening of lipid profile • Not effective in prophylaxis of migraine as they cause cerebral vasodilation • Inappropriate for secondary prophylaxis of myocardial infarction (MI) • E.g. Acebutolol, celiprolol
Lipid solubility	• Highly lipid soluble drugs are more likely to produce central effects • Metabolism of lipid soluble drugs occurs mainly in the liver and they have shorter $t_{1/2}$ • E.g. Propranolol

TABLE 2	Properties of β blockers		
	Membrane stabilizing activity	Intrinsic agonist (sympathomimetic) activity	Lipid solubility
Classical nonselective β blockers (First generation)			
Propranolol	++	Nil	High
Timolol	Nil	Nil	Low to moderate
Nadolol	Nil	Nil	Low
Cardioselective β_1 blockers (Second generation)			
Atenolol	Nil	Nil	Low
Acebutolol	+	+	Low
Esmolol	Nil	Nil	Low
Nonselective β blockers with additional actions (Third generation)			
Carvedilol	++	Nil	Moderate
Labetalol	+	+	Low
β_1 selective blockers with additional actions (Third generation)			
Celiprolol	Nil	+	Low
Nebivolol	Nil	Nil	Low

CARDIOSELECTIVE β_1 ADRENERGIC BLOCKERS

Cardioselective β_1 blockers preferentially block the β_1 receptors as compared to β_2 receptors.

Hence, they minimize the undesired effects associated with blockade of β_2 receptors (such as bronchoconstriction) that may be seen with nonselective β blockers (such as propranolol).

The ability to preferentially block β_1 receptors is relative and is lost at high doses.

The key differences between cardioselective β_1 blockers and nonselective β blockers are mentioned in Tables 3 and 4.

TABLE 3	Nonselective and cardioselective β blockers	
	Nonselective β blockers	Cardioselective β₁ blockers
Propensity to cause bronchoconstriction	• Higher	• Lower
Interference with carbohydrate metabolism	• Higher	• Lower
Incidence of cold hands and feet	• Higher	• Lower
Tendency to precipitate Raynaud's phenomenon	• Higher	• Lower
Harmful effects on lipid profile	• More	• Less
Suppression of essential tremor	• Yes	• No
Impairment of exercise tolerance	• Higher	• Lower
Examples	• Propranolol, sotalol, timolol, pindolol	• Metoprolol, atenolol, acebutolol, bisoprolol, esmolol, celiprolol

TABLE 4	Propranolol and atenolol	
	Propranolol	Atenolol
Classification	Nonselective β blocker (First generation)	Cardioselective β₁ blocker (Second generation)
Membrane stabilizing activity	Yes (High doses)	Nil
Intrinsic agonist (sympathomimetic) activity	Nil	Nil
Lipid solubility	High → higher incidence of CNS adverse effects	Low → lower incidence of CNS adverse effects

Atenolol

- Cardioselective β₁ blocker
- Long duration of action → once daily dosing is required
- Commonly used for angina and hypertension

Esmolol

- Cardioselective β₁ blocker
- Does not have membrane stabilizing or intrinsic agonist (sympathomimetic) activity
- Low plasma protein binding
- Rapid onset and short duration of action
- Rapidly inactivated by plasma esterases
- Used for supraventricular tachycardia and for the rapid control of ventricular rate in patients of atrial fibrillation or atrial flutter. It can be used in perioperative, postoperative, or other situations where short-term control of the ventricular rate with a short acting agent is required.

Nebivolol

- Highly selective β₁ blocker
- Is a nitric oxide (NO) donor and has mild vasodilating properties
- Used in hypertension and chronic heart failure

Labetalol

- Blocks both α and β receptors
- Has intrinsic agonist (sympathomimetic) activity
- Hence, it blocks $(\alpha_1 + \beta_1 + \beta_2)$ receptors and also has mild β_2 agonist activity
- Used in hypertension (including hypertension in pregnancy) and angina pectoris with existing hypertension
- Can be used intravenously for severe hypertension
- Labetalol should only be used during the first trimester of pregnancy if the potential benefits are likely to outweigh the potential risk to the fetus
- Adverse effects include postural hypotension, hepatotoxicity and failure of ejaculation

Carvedilol

- Blocks $\alpha_1 + \beta_1 + \beta_2$ receptors
- It also has calcium channel blocking and antioxidant properties
- Used in essential hypertension, chronic stable angina pectoris and as an adjunct in the therapy of moderate to severe stable chronic heart failure

▊ CLINICAL USES

The clinical uses of beta blockers can be classified into cardiovascular uses and other uses.

Cardiovascular Uses

Hypertension

Beta blockers are effective in the treatment of all grades of hypertension. Despite pharmacokinetic differences, all β-blockers are equally effective.

These are highly preferred drugs in patients with hypertension who have associated conditions such as MI, ischemic heart disease or congestive heart failure.

The advantages of beta blockers are as follows:
- Do not usually cause salt and water retention—hence, a diuretic is not always required to prevent edema or development of tolerance
- Have a sufficiently long duration of action
- Well tolerated

Angina Pectoris

Beta blockers decrease myocardial O_2 demand (be reducing heart rate, contractility and blood pressure), increase exercise tolerance and decrease frequency of angina attacks.

They are useful in patients with stable angina. They are contraindicated in Prinzmetal (variant) angina because this condition occurs due to coronary vasospasm; β-blockers, if given, will result in unopposed α-receptor mediated vasoconstriction. Hence, they will further aggravate the coronary spasm.

Myocardial Infarction (MI)

Beta blockers in MI are useful in the following 2 situations:
- **Acute MI:** β-blockers if initiated within the initial 4–6 hours of an attack (and then continued) limit the size of the infarct and prevents the occurrence of arrhythmia
- **Long-term use:** Prevents the chances of reinfarction and decreases mortality/prolongs survival.

Congestive Heart Failure

The use of beta blockers can acutely worsen heart failure. However, chronic use provides beneficial hemodynamic actions in patients with heart failure.

β-receptor stimulation has been shown to promote unfavorable cardiac remodeling in heart failure patients.

Therefore, certain β-blockers (such as metoprolol, bisoprolol, carvedilol), if introduced gradually and then used for long-term, retard the progression of heart failure, reduces mortality and prolongs life.

Cardiac Arrhythmias

Beta blockers are primarily used in atrial arrhythmia (atrial fibrillation, atrial flutter and PSVT) especially those associated with high levels of circulating catecholamines (e.g. during anaesthesia, thyrotoxicosis).

The benefits are mainly due to a decrease in AV nodal conduction and an increase in effective refractory period. The commonly used β-blockers include atenolol, esmolol, propranolol and metoprolol.

Noncardiovascular Uses

Pheochromocytoma

○ β blockers (e.g. propranolol) are used for intraoperative control of tachyarrhythmias. Beta-blockers should not be used until adequate alpha-blockade has been achieved. This is because blockade of β_2 receptors can result in unopposed α_1 mediated vasoconstriction that can cause a severe rise in blood pressure that may be fatal.

Hyperthyroidism

○ Propranolol is used in hyperthyroidism because of the following:
  - Used to control sympathetic symptoms such as palpitations, nervousness, tremors etc.
  - Inhibits peripheral conversion of $T_4 \rightarrow T_3$
  - It is also used during thyroid storm

Hypertrophic Obstructive Cardiomyopathy

○ β blockers reduce left ventricular outflow obstruction and improve cardiac output in these patients during exercise

Migraine

○ Propranolol is effective in the prophylaxis of migraine
○ It can reduce the frequency and severity of attacks in many patients
○ The mechanism of action is unclear

Anxiety

○ Propranolol blocks the peripheral manifestations of anxiety such as tremors, palpitations, tachycardia, sweating etc

Essential Tremor

○ Nonselective β blockers such as propranolol are used.

Glaucoma

○ Topical β blockers such as timolol are used
○ They reduce the intraocular pressure by decreasing the formation of aqueous humor

Clinical uses of beta blockers	
Cardiovascular	**Noncardiovascular**
1. Hypertension	1. Pheochromocytoma
2. Angina pectoris	2. Hyperthyroidism
3. Myocardial infarction	3. Hypertrophic obstructive cardiomyopathy
4. Congestive heart failure	4. Migraine
5. Cardiac arrhythmias	5. Anxiety
	6. Essential tremor
	7. Glaucoma

Figure 7: Clinical uses of beta blockers

Some of the clinical uses of beta blockers are summarized in Figure 7.

ASSESS YOURSELF (Examination Questions of Various Universities)

1. Describe therapeutic uses, adverse effects and contraindications of propranolol.
2. Cardioselective β1 blockers.
3. Adverse effects of β blockers

NOTES

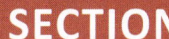

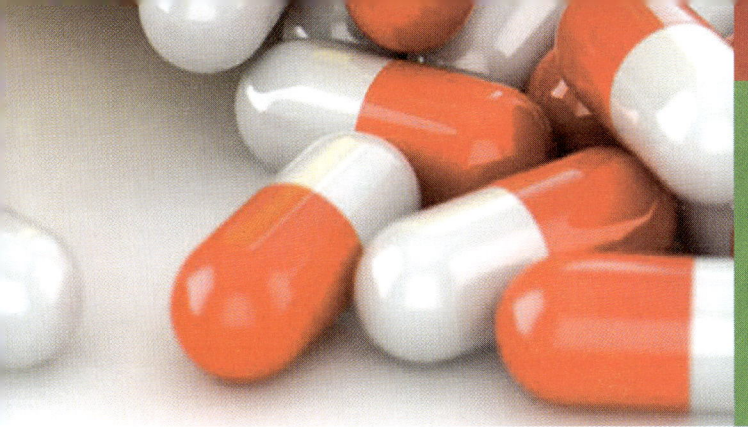

Drugs Acting on the Cardiovascular System

12

Antihypertensive Drugs

Hypertension is sustained increase of resting systolic blood pressure (≥140 mm Hg), diastolic blood pressure (≥90 mm Hg), or both.

The classification, etiology and complications of hypertension are mentioned in Figure 1.

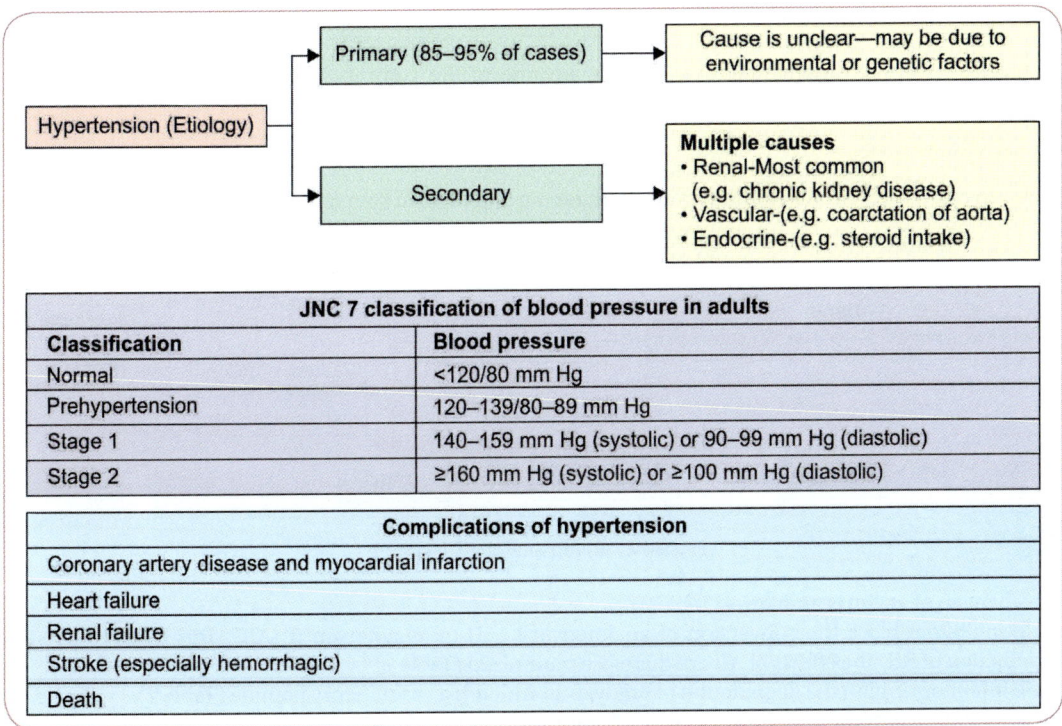

Figure 1: Hypertension

CLASSIFICATION OF ANTIHYPERTENSIVE DRUGS

The classification of drugs used for hypertension is mentioned in Table 1.

TABLE 1	Classification of antihypertensive drugs
Drug class	**Examples**
Angiotensin converting enzyme inhibitors (ACEI)	• Captopril, enalapril, lisinopril, perindopril, ramipril
Angiotensin receptor blockers (ARB)	• Losartan, candesartan, irbesartan, valsartan, telmisartan
Diuretics	• Thiazides—hydrochlorothiazide, chlorthalidone, indapamide • Loop diuretics—furosemide, bumetanide • Potassium sparing diuretics—spironolactone, triamterene, amiloride

Contd...

Calcium channel blockers (CCB)	• Verapamil, diltiazem, nifedipine, amlodipine
Beta blockers	• Cardioselective—metoprolol, atenolol, esmolol, acebutolol, celiprolol, nebivolol • Nonselective—propranolol, sotalol, nadolol
Alpha blockers	• Nonselective $(\alpha_1 + \alpha_2)$—phentolamine, phenoxybenzamine • Selective α_1—prazosin, terazosin, doxazosin
Beta + alpha blockers	• Labetalol, carvedilol
Vasodilators	• Arteriolar → Hydralazine, minoxidil • Arteriolar + Venous → Sodium nitroprusside
Central sympatholytics	• Clonidine, methyldopa

■ ANGIOTENSIN CONVERTING ENZYME INHIBITORS

Angiotensin converting enzyme (ACE) inhibitors are one of the commonly used drugs in the treatment of hypertension.

Mechanism of Action

Angiotensin converting enzyme inhibitors act on the renin angiotensin system (Figure 2).

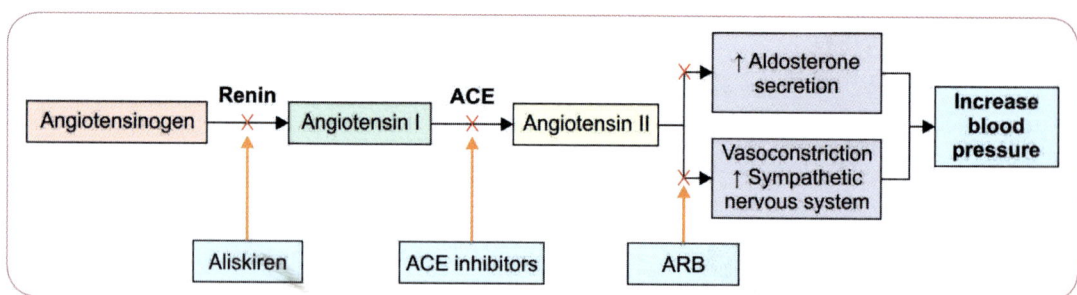

Figure 2: Renin angiotensin system

The mechanism of action is as follows (Table 2):
- ACE inhibitors block the conversion of angiotensin I (AI) to angiotensin II (AII). This leads to decreased production of AII. The effects of AII are therefore minimized (Table 2).
- ACE inhibitors inhibit the degradation of bradykinin which is a vasodilatory peptide (Table 2).
- ACE inhibitors prevent cardiac and vascular hypertrophy following myocardial infarction.

TABLE 2	Mechanism of action of ACE inhibitors

Inhibit angiotensin II generation
- Vasodilatation → ↓ peripheral resistance → ↓ BP
- Decreased aldosterone production → ↓ salt and water retention → ↓ BP
- Decreased sympathetic nervous system activity

Inhibit bradykinin breakdown
- ↑ Bradykinin levels → vasodilatation → ↓ peripheral resistance → ↓ BP
- ↑ Bradykinin levels → ↑ prostaglandin synthesis → vasodilatation → ↓ peripheral resistance → ↓ BP

Pharmacokinetics

All the ACE inhibitors are given orally except **E**nalaprilat which is the only drug in this class given intravenously for hypertensive emergencies.

All ACE inhibitors (except **C**aptopril and **L**isinopril) are prodrugs and require hepatic conversion to active metabolites. So, captopril and lisinopril may be preferred in severe hepatic impairment.

All ACE inhibitors (except **F**osinopril) are excreted mainly by the kidneys. Fosinopril is eliminated by both liver and kidneys.

The pharmacological features are similar for various members of this class. The various ACE inhibitors however, differ with regards to pharmacokinetic parameters (Table 3).

TABLE 3	**Pharmacokinetic properties of ACE inhibitors**				
	Captopril	**Lisinopril**	**Enalapril**	**Perindopril**	**Ramipril**
Activity	Active	Active	Prodrug	Prodrug	Prodrug
Time to peak action (hours)	1	6–8	4–6	6	3–6
Duration of action (hours)	8–12	≥24	24	>24	>24
Route of elimination	Kidney	Kidney	Kidney	Kidney	Kidney

Adverse Effects and Contraindications

The key adverse effects and contraindications of ACE inhibitors are mentioned in Table 4.

TABLE 4	**Adverse effects and contraindications of ACE inhibitors**
Cough (Dry cough)	• Occurs in 5–20% of patients • Is due to accumulation of bradykinin in the lungs • Disappears within 4 days of stopping the drug
Hypotension	• Sharp fall in BP may occur after the 1st dose of ACE inhibitor • More prominent in patients with volume depletion, heart failure
Hyperkalemia	• More likely in patients with renal insufficiency, diabetes and use of K+ sparing diuretics, β blockers and NSAIDs • Rare in other patients
Angioedema	• Rapid swelling in nose, throat, mouth, larynx, tongue, lips • Disappears within hours once ACE inhibitors are withdrawn • Airway protection is to be done and epinephrine, antihistaminics and/or glucocorticoids may be required

Acute renal failure	• ACE inhibitors are **contraindicated in bilateral renal artery stenosis** due to the following:
	  ▪ Normally, angiotensin II (by constricting efferent arteriole) helps to maintain the glomerular filtration pressure (GFR) in conditions of low perfusion pressure (e.g. bilateral renal artery stenosis, renal artery stenosis in a single kidney, volume depletion, heart failure, etc.)
	  ▪ If ACE inhibitors are given in situations of low perfusion pressure, the angiotensin II level decreases, and acute renal failure may be precipitated

Teratogenic effect	• ACE inhibitors are contraindicated in pregnancy (2nd and 3rd trimester) as it may lead to:
	  ▪ Fetal hypotension
	  ▪ Anuria
	  ▪ Renal failure
	  ▪ Fetal malformations and death

Skin rashes and itching	• Maculopapular rash may occur that may be associated with itching • May resolve spontaneously or with antihistaminics • More common with captopril
Dysgeusia (loss of taste sensation)	• Reversible loss or alteration of taste sensation may rarely occur • More common with captopril
Other rare effects	• Neutropenia, hepatotoxicity, glycosuria

Drug Interactions

The key drug interactions with ACE inhibitors are mentioned below:

○ *ACE inhibitors and NSAIDs*
  ❑ NSAIDs ↓↓ the antihypertensive effect of ACE inhibitors by blocking prostaglandin-induced vasodilatation
○ *ACE inhibitors and K+ sparing diuretics/K+ supplements*
  ❑ K+ sparing diuretics/K+ supplements may exacerbate ACE inhibitor-induced hyperkalemia
○ *ACE inhibitors and antacids*
  ❑ Antacids ↓↓ the bioavailability of ACE inhibitors
○ *ACE inhibitors and lithium*
  ❑ ACE inhibitors ↑↑ the level of lithium by decreasing its renal elimination; may lead to lithium toxicity

Clinical Uses

Hypertension

ACE inhibitors are used in all grades of hypertension.

They lower blood pressure mainly by decreasing peripheral vascular resistance. The cardiac output and heart rate are not significantly altered.

Unlike directly acting vasodilators, ACE inhibitors do not result in reflex sympathetic stimulation; therefore, can be used safely in ischemic heart disease.

Hypertension with Diabetes and Chronic Kidney Disease

ACE inhibitors are particularly useful as they decrease proteinuria, stabilize renal function and prevent renal complications.

ACE inhibitors are also particularly useful in diabetes, and are preferred in diabetes even in the absence of hypertension.

These benefits are achieved due to intrarenal effects such as decreased efferent arteriolar pressure leading to decrease in intraglomerular pressure.

Other Situations

ACE inhibitors are also extremely useful in hypertensive patients who have coexisting myocardial infarction and heart failure.

Acute Myocardial Infarction (MI)

Unless contraindicated (e.g. in severe hypotension or cardiogenic shock), ACE inhibitors should be immediately started (within 24 hours of an attack of MI) and continued for 6 weeks. They reduce early as well as long-term mortality in these patients.

Congestive Heart Failure

Unless contraindicated, ACE inhibitors should be given to all patients of symptomatic or asymptomatic heart failure.

ACE inhibitors prevent or delay the progression of heart failure, decrease the chances of myocardial infarction or sudden death and improve quality of life.

Diabetic Nephropathy

ACE inhibitors and angiotensin receptor blockers (ARB) are the preferred drugs in patients with diabetic nephropathy (both hypertensive and normotensive).

Scleroderma Renal Crisis

ACE inhibitors considerably improve survival in patients with scleroderma renal crisis.

ANGIOTENSIN RECEPTOR BLOCKERS

There are 2 types of angiotensin receptors: AT_1 and AT_2.

The angiotensin receptor blockers (ARBs) selectively block AT_1 receptors.

The ARBs therefore competitively inhibit the binding of angiotensin II to AT_1 receptor and blocks most of the actions of angiotensin II.

All the physiological effects of angiotensin II (including aldosterone release) are blocked by ARBs. ARBs produce similar type of effects as those of ACE inhibitors.

ARBs do not increase bradykinin levels (do not inhibit the degradation of bradykinin). Hence, cough and angioedema do not occur with ARBs.

Adverse Effects

ARBs are better tolerated than ACE inhibitors.

○ Like ACE inhibitors, they may cause hypotension, hyperkalemia when given with K^+ sparing diuretics, renal failure in patients with bilateral renal artery stenosis, teratogenicity, rashes, neutropenia and hepatotoxicity.

○ Unlike ACE inhibitors, they do not cause cough, angioedema and dysgeusia.

Clinical Uses

ARBs provide benefits similar to those of ACE inhibitors. The clinical utility of ARBs is similar to that of ACE inhibitors. ARBs are useful in:

○ hypertension
○ myocardial infarction
○ heart failure
○ diabetic nephropathy

Currently, ARBs are commonly used in patients who are intolerant to and experience adverse effects with ACE inhibitors (mainly cough).

The combination of ARBs and ACE inhibitors is not to be used together, as toxicity has been demonstrated in recent clinical trials.

DIURETICS

Thiazides

As per the JNC 7 guidelines, diuretics were the preferred initial agents in the absence of compelling indications.

However, as per the JNC 8 guidelines, ACE inhibitors, ARBs, CCBs and thiazide diuretics are equally effective in hypertensive nonblack populations, whereas CCBs and thiazide diuretics are preferred in black patients with hypertension.

(JNC: Joint National Committee of Prevention, Detection, Evaluation, and Treatment of High Blood Pressure)

Mechanism of Action

The mechanism of action of thiazide diuretics is mentioned in Figure 3.

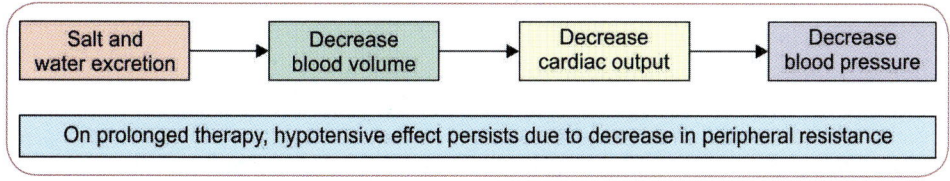

Figure 3: Mechanism of action of thiazides

Adverse Effects

○ Hypokalemia, hypercalcemia, hypomagnesemia, hypochloremic alkalosis, hyperuricemia, hyperglycemia and hyperlipidemia

- Avoided in patients with diabetes mellitus, gout, hyperlipidemia and renal insufficiency
- Can enhance digitalis toxicity due to hypokalemia

Advantages of Thiazides

- Inexpensive and well tolerated by elderly patients
- Prolonged duration of action; hence multiple dosing can be minimized
- Reduce excretion of calcium; hence can decrease fracture incidence in elderly patients
- Synergistic effect when used in combination with other antihypertensive drugs

Loop Diuretics

They are not used in mild to moderate hypertension, as they can cause significant decrease in blood volume and lead to electrolyte imbalance.

They are used in severe hypertension with underlying renal or cardiac disease. They are also used in heart failure to reduce pulmonary edema.

Potassium Sparing Diuretics

The salient features of these drugs are:

- Prevent excessive depletion of potassium; hence they are usually given along with thiazides
- Augment the antihypertensive effect of diuretics
- Spironolactone is an aldosterone receptor antagonist; therefore, antagonizes the sodium retaining and potassium excreting effects of aldosterone

CALCIUM CHANNEL BLOCKERS

Calcium channel blockers (CCBs) are used in the treatment of hypertension, in addition to their uses in angina and arrhythmia.

Mechanism of Action

Hypertension generally occurs due to an increase in peripheral vascular resistance.

The increase in peripheral vascular resistance occurs due to an increase in calcium concentration in vascular smooth muscle cells.

The CCBs block the inward movement of calcium into vascular smooth muscle cells. This results in decreased concentration of calcium inside the cells leading to smooth muscle relaxation, vasodilatation and decreased peripheral vascular resistance.

In dihydropyridines (e.g. nifedipine), a decrease in peripheral resistance leads to an increase in sympathetic discharge resulting in reflex tachycardia. This reflex tachycardia is minimal or absent with verapamil or diltiazem because both these drugs have direct cardiac depressant actions (verapamil > diltiazem) (Figure 4).

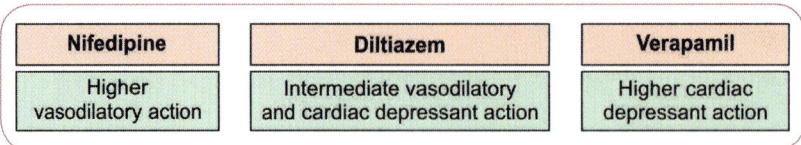

Nifedipine	Diltiazem	Verapamil
Higher vasodilatory action	Intermediate vasodilatory and cardiac depressant action	Higher cardiac depressant action

Figure 4: Calcium channel blockers

The other adverse effects of dihydropyridines (due to their vasodilatory action) are headache, flushing, palpitation and ankle edema. These effects can be reduced by using sustained release formulations and those with longer half-lives.

Clinical Uses

The CCBs are used in the treatment of hypertension, angina and arrhythmia.

They are particularly useful in elderly and in patients with asthma, hyperlipidemia and diabetes with kidney disease.

They decrease proteinuria and slow the renal disease progression in diabetic patients.

The dihydropyridines available for intravenous use (nicardipine and clevidipine) are useful in hypertensive emergencies.

BETA BLOCKERS

Beta blockers are effective antihypertensive drugs in mild to moderate hypertension.

Mechanism of Action

The mechanism of action of beta blockers in hypertension is mentioned in Figure 5.

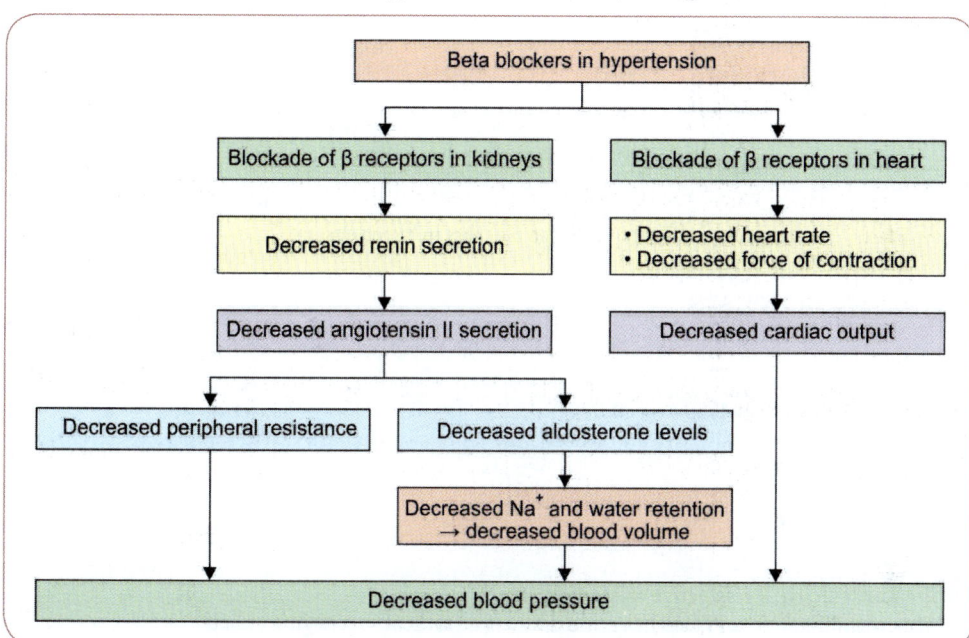

Figure 5: Beta blockers—mechanism of action

Adverse Effects

- CNS-fatigue, lethargy, insomnia
- CVS-bradycardia, hypotension
- Bronchospasm
- Masking of hypoglycemic symptoms
- Erectile dysfunction, loss of libido
- Altered lipid metabolism – ↑ triglycerides, ↓ HDL cholesterol
- Contraindicated in patients with severe peripheral arterial circulatory disease, severe asthma, severe chronic obstructive pulmonary disease, sick sinus syndrome, second- or third-degree heart block, uncontrolled heart failure
- Abrupt withdrawal may lead to angina, myocardial infarction and sudden death

Clinical Uses

- Hypertensive patients with cardiovascular risk factors including supraventricular tachyarrhythmias, chronic heart failure, postmyocardial infarction, angina pectoris
- May be used in young hypertensive patients with high renin levels

ALPHA BLOCKERS

The mechanism of action of alpha blockers in hypertension is mentioned in Figure 6.

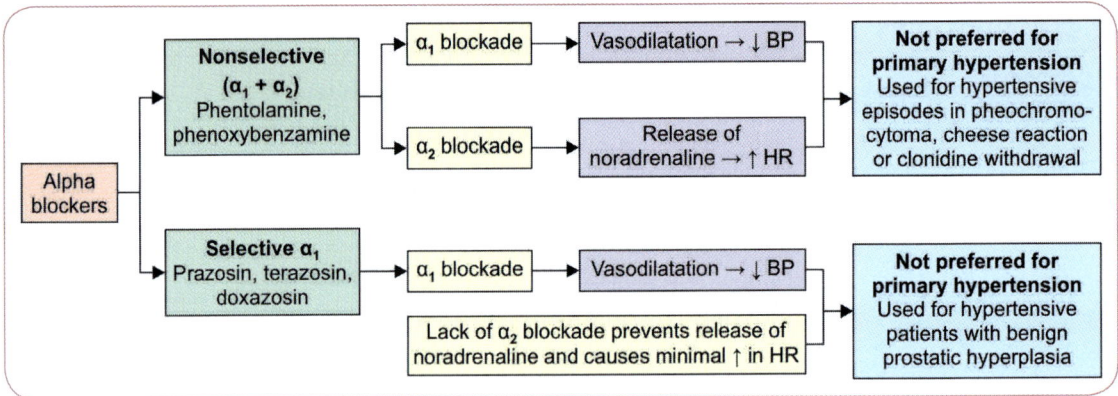

Figure 6: Alpha blockers in hypertension

BETA + ALPHA BLOCKERS

Labetalol

Labetalol is a nonselective β + selective α$_1$ blocker.

It reduces total peripheral resistance and is used intravenously in hypertensive emergencies, in cheese reaction and in clonidine withdrawal.

It is also used for hypertension in pregnant women.

Carvedilol

Carvedilol is a nonselective β + selective α$_1$ blocker.

It produces vasodilatation and also has antioxidant/free radical scavenging effects.

It is used in mild to moderate heart failure.

It has been reported to reduce mortality in heart failure patients (with systolic dysfunction), when used along with ACE inhibitors and diuretics.

VASODILATORS

Hydralazine

It is a directly acting arteriolar vasodilator. It has no effect on the veins.

It reduces peripheral vascular resistance. Reflex sympathetic discharge occurs which lead to tachycardia, increase cardiac output and renin release. This results in aldosterone secretion and salt and water retention. This leads to a hyperdynamic circulatory state which may result in precipitation of angina.

All of these effects counteract the antihypertensive effects of hydralazine.

To avoid such a situation, **hydralazine is always given in combination with drugs that block the compensatory mechanisms, i.e. with a β blocker and a diuretic**.

Hydralazine is well-absorbed orally and is metabolized by acetylation in the liver. The rate of acetylation is genetically determined so that there are slow acetylators and fast acetylators.

Adverse Effects

There are 2 types of adverse effects:

Extensions of Pharmacological Effects

Headache, flushing, hypotension, palpitations, tachycardia, angina pectoris

Immunological Reactions

- Drug-induced lupus syndrome (most common)
- Serum sickness, vasculitis

Clinical Uses

- Hypertension
  - Moderate to severe hypertension not controlled by first line drugs; not used alone
- Hypertension during pregnancy
- Hypertensive emergencies
- Heart failure
  - May be given with nitrates in patients with hypertension and heart failure

Minoxidil

It is an orally acting arteriolar vasodilator. Its effect results from opening of K^+ channels in the smooth muscle cell membrane. This leads to hyperpolarization of smooth muscle cells, resulting in smooth muscle relaxation and decrease in blood pressure.

Like hydralazine, it dilates arterioles but not veins. The pharmacological effects and reflex compensatory mechanisms resemble that of hydralazine. It is also used along with a β blocker and a diuretic to block the compensatory mechanisms.

The adverse effect profile resembles hydralazine except that minoxidil promotes hair growth (hypertrichosis). Minoxidil is used topically to promote hair growth in male pattern baldness.

Sodium Nitroprusside

It is a potent arteriolar and venodilator. It is used in hypertensive emergencies and in patients with severe CHF (to improve cardiac output). (Figure 7).

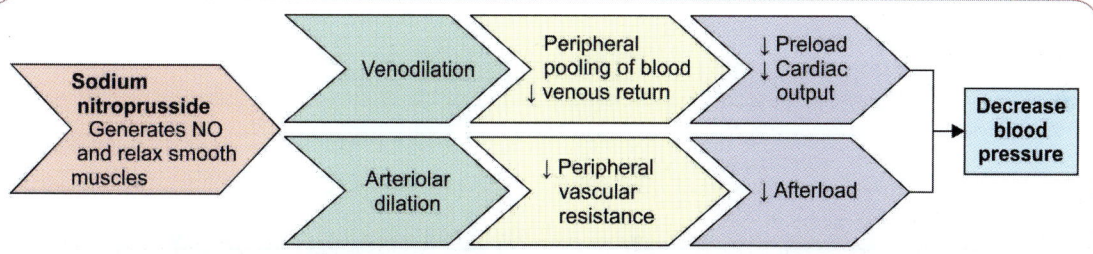

- Rapidly acting (onset within seconds); brief duration of action (2–5 minutes). Hence, given via IV infusion.
- It is unstable and rapidly decomposes on exposure to sunlight; hence, it is always freshly prepared and the infusion bottle is covered with black paper.
- Nitroprusside is split in the RBC/endothelial cells to release nitric oxide (NO) and cyanide:
  - NO increases cGMP and relaxes smooth muscle
  - Cyanide is converted in the liver to thiocyanate, which is excreted slowly in urine
- Adverse effects are related to accumulation of cyanide and may include nausea, vomiting, palpitation, arrhythmias, disorientation, toxic psychosis, metabolic acidosis and death.
- Unlike nitrates, tolerance does not develop to its actions.

Figure 7: Sodium nitroprusside

CENTRAL SYMPATHOLYTICS

Clonidine and methyldopa are centrally acting antihypertensive drugs that cross the blood brain barrier and decrease the sympathetic outflow from the vasomotor center.

The key features of central sympatholytic drugs are mentioned in Figure 8.

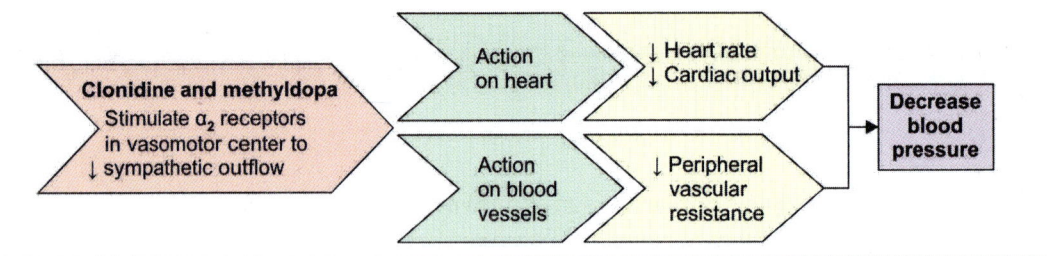

Clonidine
- Has a relatively short half-life. Also available as a transdermal patch.
- Adverse effects include sedation, dry mouth, constipation, disturbed sleep, depression and bradycardia.
- ***Withdrawal syndrome*** may occur following sudden stoppage of drug after prolonged use: alarming rise in BP, tachycardia, sweating, palpitation and vomiting. It occurs due to:
  - ♦ Increased sensitivity of α receptors to catecholamines
  - ♦ Sudden release of large amount of stored catecholamine

The withdrawal syndrome is treated by combined α + β blocker (labetalol) or by sodium nitroprusside.

Methyldopa
- Analogue of L-dopa. It is a prodrug.
- Converted to α methyldopamine and α methylnorpeinephrine.
- Preferred drug for treatment of hypertension in pregnancy.
- Adverse effects include positive Coomb's test, hemolytic anemia, hepatotoxicity, sedation, lethargy, dry mouth, nasal stuffiness, fluid retention, weight gain.

Figure 8: Central sympatholytics

MANAGEMENT OF HYPERTENSION

The management of hypertension includes both nonpharmacological and pharmacological measures (Figure 9).

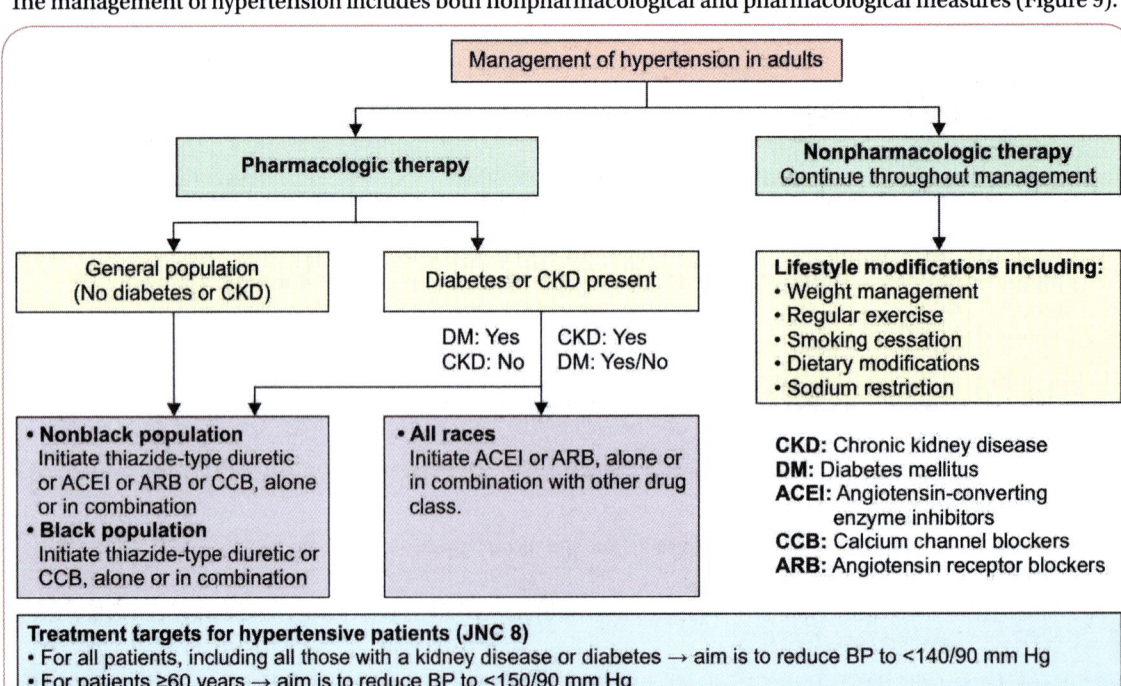

Figure 9: Management of hypertension

Source: 2014 Guideline for Management of High Blood Pressure JNC 8 (JAMA February 5, 2014 Volume 311, Number 5)

The commonly used antihypertensive drugs for patients with specific co-existing conditions are mentioned in Table 5.

TABLE 5	Drugs for specific co-existing conditions
Commonly used drugs for patients with specific co-existing conditions	
Postmyocardial infarction	ACE inhibitors, β blockers
Heart failure	ACE inhibitors, ARB, β blockers, K$^+$-sparing diuretics
Diabetes mellitus	ACE inhibitors, ARB, CCB, diuretics
Chronic kidney disease	ACE inhibitors, ARB
Cardiovascular risk factors	ACE inhibitors, β blockers, CCB, diuretics
Benign prostatic hyperplasia	α blockers
Pregnancy	Methyldopa, labetalol

HYPERTENSIVE EMERGENCY

Hypertensive emergency is severe hypertension with evidence of end organ damage (mainly brain, cardiovascular system and kidneys).

Hypertensive emergency may occur in patients with:

- Hypertensive encephalopathy
- Unstable angina or myocardial infarction with elevated BP
- Cerebrovascular accident (hemorrhage) or head trauma
- Dissecting aortic aneurysm
- Eclampsia
- Acute renal failure with hypertension
- Hypertensive episodes in pheochromocytoma, cheese reaction or clonidine withdrawal
- Hypertensive acute left ventricular failure and pulmonary edema

The management of hypertensive emergency requires rapid control of blood pressure in the intensive care unit using various drugs (Table 6).

TABLE 6	Drugs for hypertensive emergencies
Drug	**Comments**
Clevidipine	• Ultrashort acting calcium channel blocker • Used cautiously in patients with acute heart failure
Nicardipine	• Calcium channel blocker • Can cause reflex tachycardia
Labetalol	• Beta + alpha blocker • Not used in acute left ventricular failure, patients with asthma
Esmolol	• Short acting beta blocker • Suitable for perioperative hypertension in aortic dissection
Hydralazine	• Arteriolar vasodilator • Suitable for eclampsia
Phentolamine	• Alpha blocker • Suitable for hyperadrenergic states—hypertensive episodes in pheochromocytoma, cheese reaction or clonidine withdrawal
Sodium nitroprusside	• Needs a special delivery system (e.g. infusion pump)
Nitroglycerine	• Suitable for patients of myocardial ischemia, heart failure

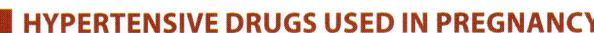

HYPERTENSIVE DRUGS USED IN PREGNANCY

The aim of treating chronic hypertension in pregnancy is to reduce the maternal risk; however, the choice of antihypertensive drugs is mainly governed by fetal safety (Table 7).

TABLE 7	Antihypertensive drugs in pregnancy
Antihypertensive drugs in pregnancy	
Preferred first line drug (Due to better safety profile)	Methyldopa
Other drugs that can be considered	Labetalol, cardioselective beta blockers, hydralazine, prazosin, nifedipine
Drugs to be avoided (Due to risk of fetal toxicity)	ACE inhibitors and ARBs

ASSESS YOURSELF (Examination Questions of Various Universities)

1. Classify and enumerate antihypertensive drugs. Discuss the mechanism of action, adverse effects, contraindications and clinical uses of angiotensin converting enzyme (ACE) inhibitors.

2. Mention three drugs used in hypertensive emergencies. Discuss the mechanism of action, pharmacological actions and adverse effects of sodium nitroprusside.

3. Write short notes on:
   a. Central sympatholytics
   b. Methyldopa
   c. Enalapril
   d. Angiotensin receptor blockers

4. Explain why:
   a. ACE inhibitors cause dry hackling cough
   b. Clonidine should not be stopped suddenly

MULTIPLE CHOICE QUESTIONS

1. Not a centrally acting antihypertensive:
   (Recent Question Dec 2016)
   a. Methyldopa   b. Clonidine
   c. Minoxidil   d. Guanabenz

2. Which of the following drug is contraindicated in a case of B/L renal artery stenosis?
   (Recent Question Dec 2016)
   a. Methyldopa   b. Enalapril
   c. Hydralazine   d. Dopamine

3. Which of the following is drug of choice for pregnancy-induced hypertension?
   (AIIMS Nov 2015)
   a. Atenolol   b. α-methyl dopa
   c. Enalapril   d. Nitroprusside

4. Which of the following antihypertensive is absolutely contraindicated in pregnancy?
   (AIIMS May 2015)
   a. Enalapril   b. Methyldopa
   c. Nifedipine   d. Labetalol

5. The most significant adverse effect of ACE inhibition is: *(AIIMS May 2006)*
   a. Hypotension   b. Hypertension
   c. Hypocalcemia   d. Hypercalcemia

6. ACE inhibitors should not be used with:
   (Recent Question 2016)
   a. Amiloride
   b. Calcium channel blockers
   c. Chlorthalidone
   d. Spironolactone

7. Antihypertensive drug contraindicated in pregnancy is: *(Recent Question 2016)*
   a. Enalapril
   b. Cardio selective beta blockers
   c. Methyldopa
   d. Hydralazine

8. ACE inhibitors cause: *(Recent Question 2016)*
   a. Hyperkalemia   b. Hypokalemia
   c. Hypocalcemia   d. Hypernatremia

9. Alpha methyldopa is primarily used for:
   (Recent Question 2016)
   a. Pregnancy induced hypertension
   b. Endovascular hypertension
   c. First line agent in hypertension
   d. Refractory hypertension

10. Which of the following ACE inhibitor is not a prodrug?   *(Recent Question 2016)*
    a. Fosinopril   b. Enalapril
    c. Ramipril   d. Lisinopril

11. Not an adverse effect of ACE inhibitors:
    (Recent Question 2016)
    a. Cough   b. Hypokalemia
    c. Angioneurotic edema   d. Skin rash

12. The antihypertensive agent that should be avoided in young females and is used topically to treat alopecia is: *(Recent Question 2016)*
    a. Hydralazine   b. Prazosin
    c. Minoxidil   d. Indapamide

Ans.

1.	(c)	2.	(b)	3.	(b)	4.	(a)	5.	(a)	6.	(a, d)
7.	(a)	8.	(a)	9.	(a)	10.	(d)	11.	(b)	12.	(c)

13. **Which antihypertensive is a prodrug and is converted to its active form in brain?**
    (Recent Question 2016)
    a. Clonidine
    b. Methyldopa
    c. Minoxidil
    d. Nitroprusside

14. **Which of the following drug is used in severe hypertensive emergencies, is very short acting and must be given by IV infusion?**
    (Recent Question 2016)
    a. Diazoxide
    b. Hydralazine
    c. Labetolol
    d. Nitroprusside

15. **Sodium-nitroprusside act by activation of:**
    (Recent Question 2016)
    a. Guanylate cyclase
    b. K⁺ channels
    c. Ca⁺⁺ channels
    d. Cyclic AMP

16. **Cough is an adverse reaction seen with intake of:** *(Recent Question 2016)*
    a. Thiazide
    b. Nifedipine
    c. Enalapril
    d. Prazosin

17. **An antihypertensive drug that causes positive Coombs test is:** *(Recent Question 2016)*
    a. Methyldopa
    b. Clonidine
    c. Hydralazine
    d. Sodium-nitropruside

18. **ACE inhibitors are contraindicated in:**
    (Recent Question 2016)
    a. Diabetes mellitus
    b. Hypertension in old age groups
    c. Scleroderma
    d. Bilateral renal artery stenosis

19. **Cough and angioedema in a patient receiving ACE inhibitors is due to** *(Recent Question 2016)*
    a. Bradykinin
    b. Renin
    c. Angiotensin-II
    d. All

20. **Treatment of choice in hypertension with diabetes mellitus is:** *(Recent Question 2016)*
    a. Beta blockers
    b. Thiazides
    c. ACE inhibitors
    d. Calcium channel blockers

21. **Which of the following antihypertensive causes sedation:** *(Recent Question 2016)*
    a. Clonidine
    b. Hydralazine
    c. Losartan
    d. Amlodipine

22. **ACE inhibitor not to be given along with:**
    (Recent Question 2016)
    a. Amiloride
    b. Xipamide
    c. Hydrochlorothiazide
    d. Chlorthalidone

23. **Enalapril is a/an:** *(Recent Question 2016)*
    a. Angiotensin receptor blocker
    b. Angiotensin converting enzyme inhibitor
    c. Renin inhibitor
    d. Calcium channel blocker

24. **SLE like reaction is caused by:**
    (Recent Question 2016)
    a. Hydralazine
    b. Rifampicin
    c. Paracetamol
    d. Furosemide

Ans.

13.	(b)	14.	(d)	15.	(a)	16.	(c)	17.	(a)	18.	(d)
19.	(a)	20.	(c)	21.	(a)	22.	(a)	23.	(b)	24.	(a)

13

Antianginal Drugs

Angina pectoris refers to chest pain or discomfort due to coronary heart disease. It is the result of myocardial ischemia caused by an imbalance between myocardial oxygen supply and demand.

The pathophysiology and treatment of angina pectoris is mentioned in Figure 1.

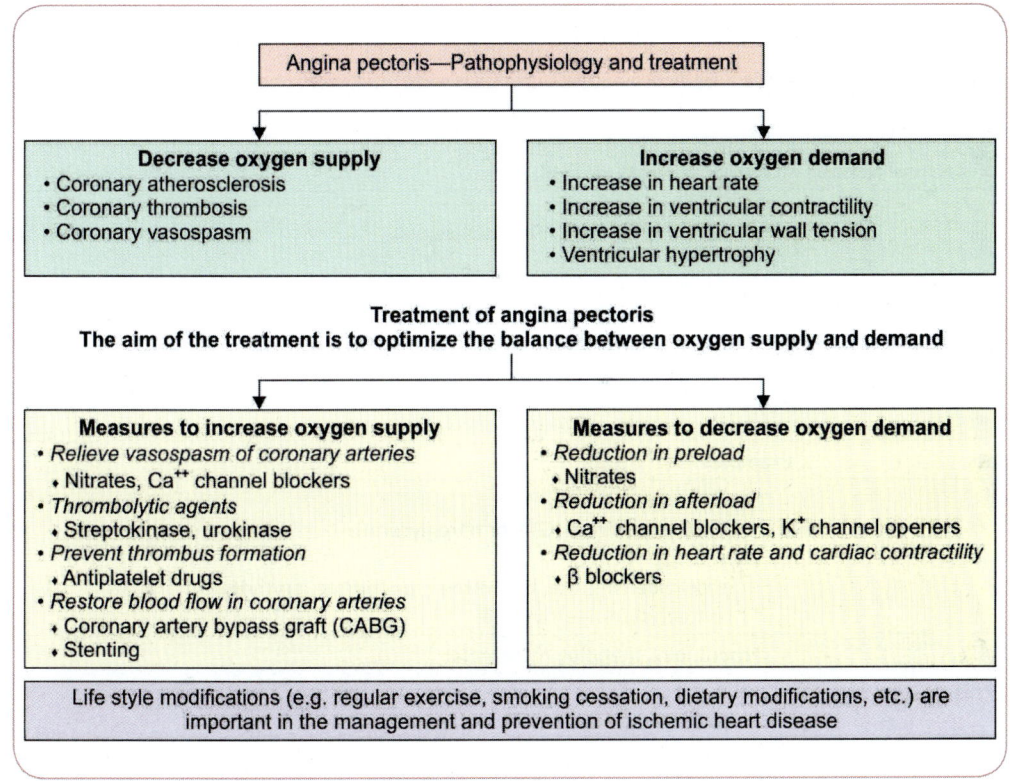

Figure 1: Pathophysiology and treatment of angina pectoris

TYPES OF ANGINA PECTORIS

The various types of angina pectoris are mentioned in Figure 2.

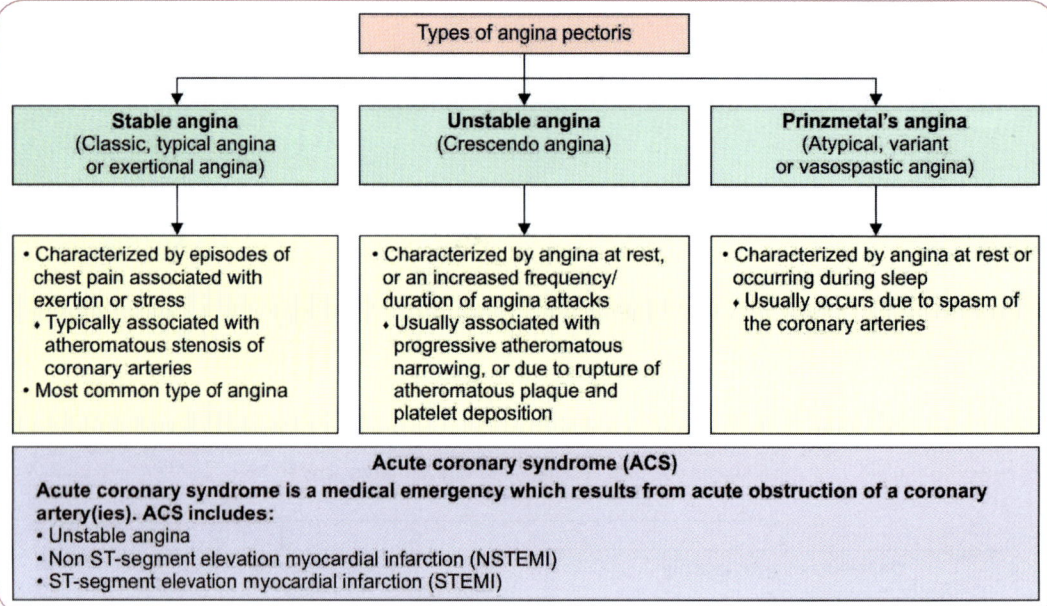

Figure 2: Types of angina

CLASSIFICATION OF ANTIANGINAL DRUGS

The classification of drugs used in angina is mentioned in Table 1.

TABLE 1	Antianginal drugs
Drug class	**Examples**
Nitrates	• Short acting 　▪ Glyceryl trinitrate (GTN or nitroglycerin) • Long acting 　▪ Isosorbide dinitrate, isosorbide mononitrate, erythrityl tetranitrate, pentaerythritol tetranitrate
Beta blockers	• Propranolol, atenolol, metoprolol
Calcium channel blockers	• Phenylalkylamine 　▪ Verapamil • Benzothiazepine 　▪ Diltiazem • Dihydropyridine 　▪ Amlodipine, nicardipine, nifedipine, nimodipine, felodipine, lercanidipine
Sodium channel blocker	• Ranolazine
Potassium channel opener	• Nicorandil
Others	• Antiplatelets 　▪ Low dose aspirin, clopidogrel • Statins 　▪ Simvastatin • Trimetazidine, ivabradine

NITRATES

Organic nitrates are prodrugs and they act by releasing nitric oxide (NO). They are very useful in the management of angina.

Mechanism of Action

Nitrates release NO that activates the enzyme guanylyl cyclase leading to an increase in cGMP levels, resulting in relaxation of vascular smooth muscles (Figure 3).

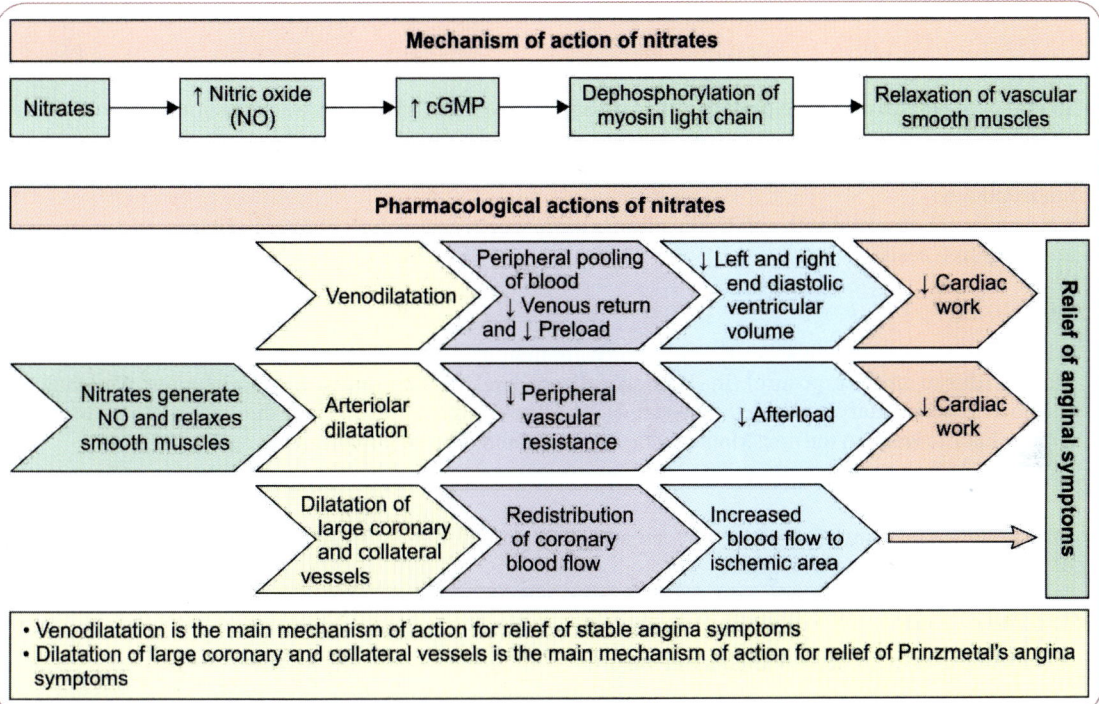

Figure 3: Mechanism of action of nitrates

Pharmacokinetics

Organic nitrates are well absorbed from the buccal mucous membrane, skin and the intestines.

All nitrates undergo extensive first-pass metabolism in liver, except isosorbide mononitrate. Therefore, isosorbide mononitrate has excellent bioavailability after oral administration and a significantly longer duration of action than isosorbide dinitrate.

- ○ **Sublingual nitroglycerin** has a rapid onset (within 2–3 minutes) and a short duration of action. The sublingual tablet is used for managing an acute attack of angina.
- ○ **Isosorbide dinitrate** can be used sublingually for an acute attack of angina as well as orally for prophylaxis of angina. It has a low oral bioavailability due to high first-pass metabolism in the liver.
- ○ **Isosorbide mononitrate** is used and preferred over dinitrate for prophylaxis because it has minimal first-pass metabolism and therefore, a longer duration of action.

The various nitrates used in the treatment of angina are mentioned in Table 2.

TABLE 2	Nitrates used in angina	
Drug	**Dosage and route**	**Duration of action**
Glyceryl trinitrate (nitroglycerin)	0.5 mg, sublingual 0.4–0.8 mg, sublingual spray	10–30 minutes 10–30 minutes
Isosorbide dinitrate	5–10 mg, sublingual 5–40 mg, oral	20–40 minutes 6–10 hours
Isosorbide mononitrate	20–40 mg, oral	6–10 hours
Erythrityl tetranitrate	15–60 mg, oral	4–6 hours

Adverse Effects

These are mainly due to vasodilatation: throbbing headache, flushing, postural hypotension, tachycardia and dizziness.

Methemoglobinemia may occur at higher doses.

Tolerance

○ Tolerance to nitrates occurs on prolonged use. This tolerance weans off rapidly when the body is free of nitrates. Hence, an 8-hour nitrate-free period per day is required to prevent tolerance.

○ Tolerance is mostly seen with long acting preparations (oral, transdermal) or continuous IV infusions without interruptions.

○ It is usually not observed with sublingual nitrates as they have a very short duration of action and are used on an as required basis.

Monday Disease

○ It is seen in workers in industries where nitrates are manufactured. The workers typically get headaches on Monday (due to nitrate exposure). The headache disappears by Friday due to the development of tolerance.

○ Due to a drug free interval during the weekend (Saturday/Sunday), the tolerance diminishes. Therefore, upon coming back to work on the next Monday, the headache and other symptoms recur again.

Drug Interactions

Phosphodiesterase inhibitors (e.g. sildenafil) can potentiate the vasodilatory effects of nitrates leading to increased risk of profound hypotension and death.

Therapeutic Uses

The therapeutic uses of nitrates are mentioned below:

Angina Pectoris

Classic Angina

(By reducing myocardial oxygen demand)

Nitrates are useful in both an acute attack and prophylaxis of angina (Figure 4).

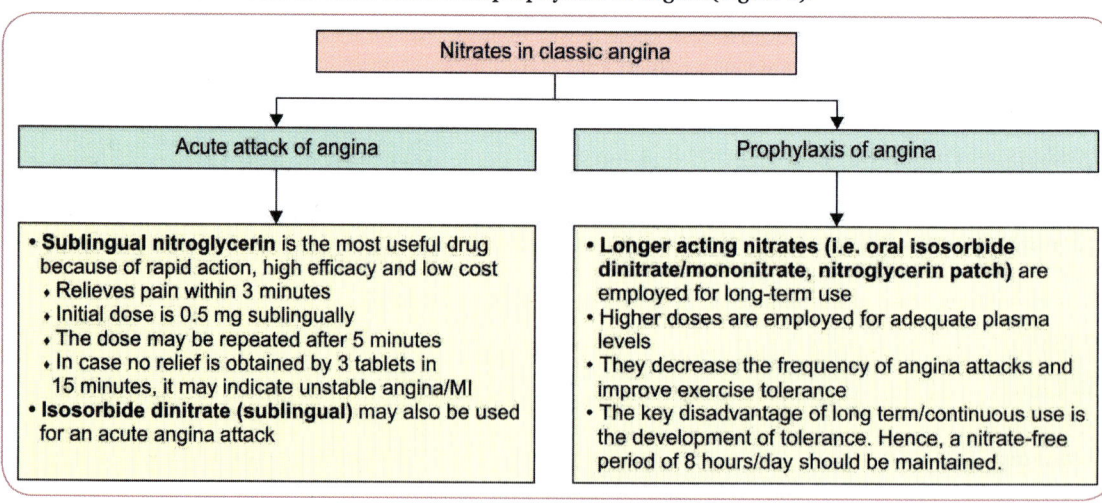

Figure 4: Nitrates in classic angina

Unstable Angina

(By dilating epicardial coronary arteries and lowering myocardial oxygen demand)

Unstable angina is a type of acute coronary syndrome and represents worsening of angina status of the patient. It requires aggressive therapy by multiple medications:

- Nitrates
  - ➤ Sublingual nitroglycerin is usually started. If the pain is not relieved after 3 doses within 15 minutes, IV nitroglycerin may be employed.
  - ➤ Nitrates are useful as they decrease myocardial oxygen demand and increase coronary blood flow
- Beta blockers
  - ➤ β blockers are usually employed in all cases of unstable angina, unless contraindicated
- Antiplatelet drugs
  - ➤ Along with nitrates and β blockers, antiplatelet drugs (e.g. aspirin, clopidogrel, prasugrel) are the mainstay of therapy in unstable angina
- Glycoprotein IIb/IIIa receptor antagonists
  - ➤ For example, eptifibatide, tirofiban, abciximab
- Anticoagulants
  - ➤ For example, low molecular weight heparin, unfractionated heparin
- Calcium channel blockers
  - ➤ For example, amlodipine, verapamil and diltiazem

Prinzmetal's (Variant) Angina

(By relaxation/dilatation of smooth muscles of epicardial coronary arteries and decreasing coronary spasm)

The coronary vasospasm in variant angina is treated with IV nitroglycerin. In some patients, nitrates are required to be combined with calcium channel blockers for total control.

Myocardial Infarction (MI)

Intravenous nitroglycerin is frequently used in initial stages of MI, as it relieves chest pain, pulmonary congestion and limits the area of necrosis.

It is to be avoided in MI if there is hypotension, or if the patient has taken sildenafil/tadalafil in the previous 24 hours.

Congestive Heart Failure (CHF)

Intravenous nitroglycerin is frequently used in CHF. Nitrates provide relief by decreasing preload, leading to decrease in end diastolic volume, improvement in left ventricular function and subsequently decrease in pulmonary congestion.

Biliary Colic

Nitrates provide relief by relaxing smooth muscles.

Cyanide Poisoning

Nitrates are useful in cyanide poisoning due to the following mechanism (Figure 5):

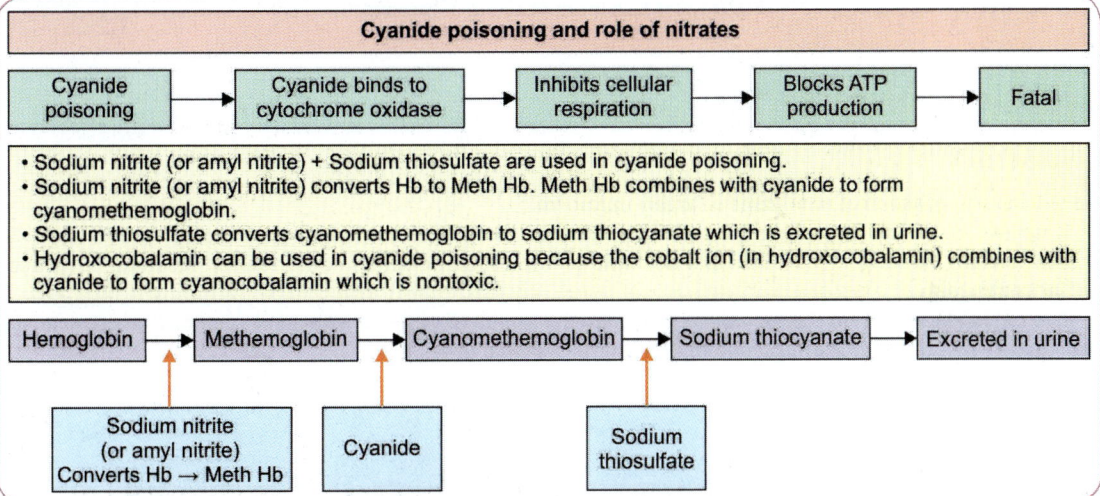

Figure 5: Nitrates in cyanide poisoning

BETA BLOCKERS

Beta blockers are beneficial in angina as they decrease heart rate and contractility by acting on β_1 receptors of the heart. This results in a decrease in cardiac work, cardiac output and myocardial oxygen demand.

At rest, this effect is modest. However, the more important facet of action is that β blockers limit the increase in heart rate, contractility, etc. during exercise, anxiety and stress.

The following are noteworthy regarding beta blocker use in angina patients:
- They are used along with nitrates for chronic prophylaxis of angina. They also improve exercise tolerance and decrease the frequency of anginal attacks.
- Use of cardioselective beta blockers (β_1 - metoprolol, atenolol, etc.) is preferred in classic angina.
- **Use of β blockers is contraindicated in variant angina** because blockade of β_2 receptors can aggravate coronary spasm due to unopposed α_1 receptor mediated coronary vasoconstriction.
- β blockers reduce cardiac output; hence cause an increase in the left ventricular end diastolic volume. This leads to an indirect increase in the myocardial oxygen requirement. Hence, use of β blockers as single drug therapy for angina can reduce their beneficial effects. Therefore, they are combined with nitrates to counteract this increase in the left ventricular end diastolic volume.
- Adverse effects include:
  - Bradycardia, hypoglycemia, heart block and bronchospasm
  - Abrupt withdrawal can precipitate myocardial infarction due to sudden increase in sympathetic tone

POTASSIUM CHANNEL OPENER

Nicorandil

Nicorandil is used for prevention and long-term treatment of chronic stable angina pectoris. The mechanism of action is shown in Figure 6.

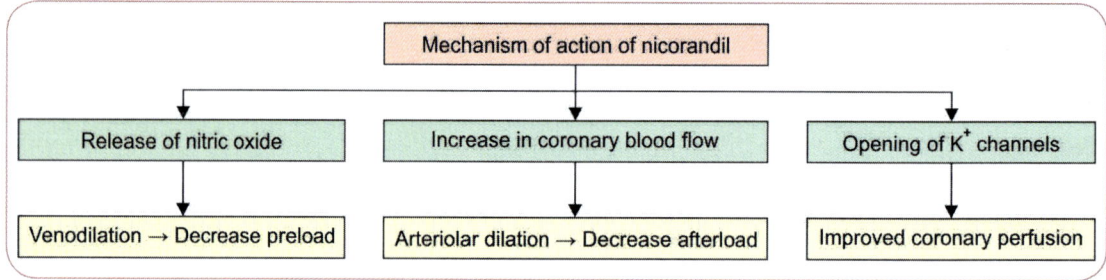

Figure 6: Mechanism of action of nicorandil

SODIUM CHANNEL BLOCKER

Ranolazine

The mechanism of action of ranolazine is largely unknown.

It appears to act by decreasing the sodium current in cardiac cells, which is involved in calcium entry by sodium-calcium exchanger. This leads to a decrease of intracellular calcium concentration resulting in reduced cardiac contractility.

It is indicated as add-on therapy for symptomatic treatment of patients with stable angina pectoris who are inadequately controlled or are intolerant to first-line antianginal drugs.

OTHER DRUGS

Trimetazidine, Ivabradine

Trimetazidine

It is known as a metabolic modulator.

It acts by partially inhibiting the fatty acid oxidation pathway in cardiac cells; hence also known as 'pFOX inhibitor'.

In ischemic tissue, the metabolism shifts to fatty acid oxidation. This requires a higher amount of O_2 as compared to glucose metabolism. Trimetazidine, by inhibiting fatty acid oxidation shifts back the metabolism to glucose oxidation; thereby decreasing the O_2 requirement in ischemic tissue.

It is used as an add-on therapy for angina pectoris when it is not adequately controlled by first-line antianginal drugs.

THERAPY FOR ACUTE MYOCARDIAL INFARCTION

The drugs used in the management of acute myocardial infarction are mentioned in Table 3.

TABLE 3	Acute myocardial infarction—drug therapy
Therapy for acute myocardial infarction	
Antiplatelet drugs	• Aspirin (165–325 mg) given to all patients at presentation unless contraindicated • Maintenance dose daily to be continued • Chewable aspirin is preferred because it promotes quick absorption to achieve therapeutic levels faster • Clopidogrel can be given to patients who are allergic to aspirin
Analgesia	• Morphine used to treat severe or refractory pain
ACE inhibitors or ARBs	• Reduce incidence of CHF, have long-term survival benefits • For example, lisinopril, ramipril, valsartan
Anticoagulants	• Prevent thromboembolic complications and thrombus extension • For example, heparin or LMW heparin (dalteparin or enoxaparin)
Beta blockers	• Administered in the early stages of MI, unless contraindicated • They decrease size of infarct, prevent reinfarction, decrease incidence of arrhythmias and decrease mortality • For example, metoprolol
Nitrates	• Reduce cardiac chest pain related to ischemia by causing coronary vasodilatation
Oxygen therapy	• Low flow oxygen therapy if there is reduced oxygen saturation or dyspnea
Thrombolysis	• Drugs—streptokinase, alteplase, reteplase, urokinase • Primary percutaneous coronary intervention
Others	• Hypolipidemic drugs—statins (e.g. simvastatin, lovastatin) • Correction of acidosis—sodium bicarbonate
Mnemonic (MONA-BT) • **M** Morphine • **O** Oxygen, others • **N** Nitrates • **A** Aspirin, ACE inhibitors/ARBs, anticoagulants • **B** β blockers • **T** Thrombolysis	

Passing MBBS Series

DRUG COMBINATIONS IN ANGINA

There are three main classes of antianginal drugs:
- Nitrates
- β blockers
- Calcium channel blockers (CCBs)

The rationale for their use in various combinations is mentioned in Figures 7, 8, 9 and 10.

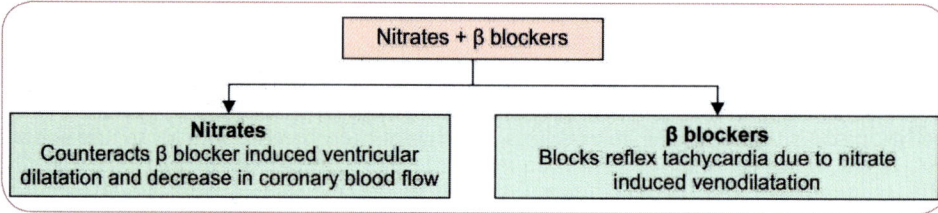

Figure 7: Rationale of nitrates + β blockers in angina

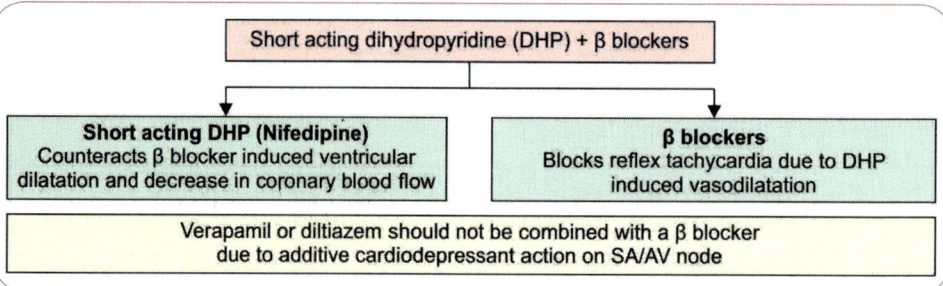

Figure 8: Rationale of short acting DHP + β blockers in angina

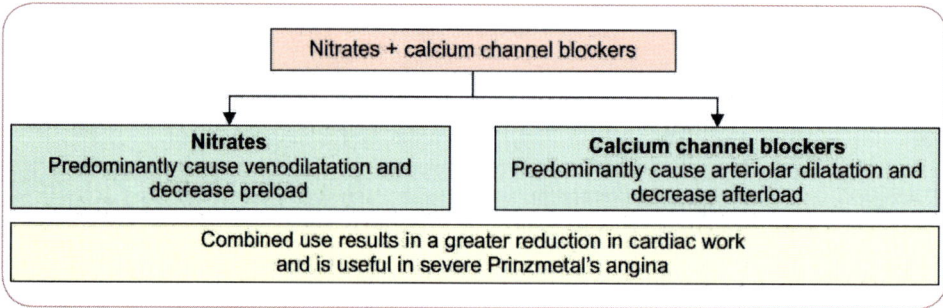

Figure 9: Rationale of nitrates + CCBs in angina

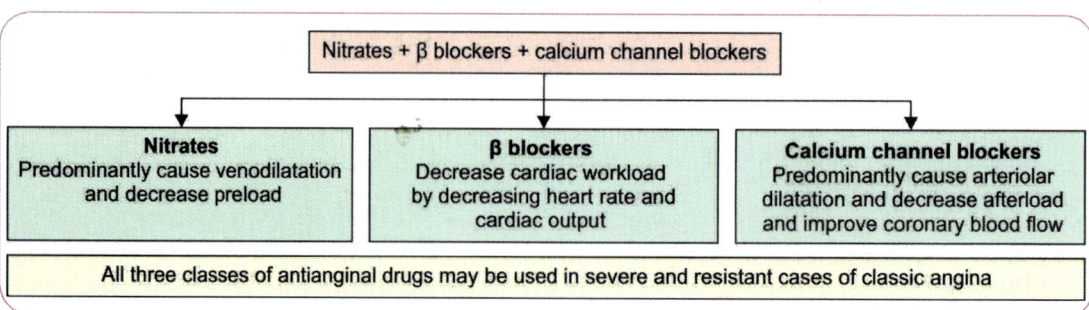

Figure 10: Rationale of nitrate + β blockers + CCBs in angina

144

ASSESS YOURSELF (Examination Questions of Various Universities)

1. Classify antianginal drugs. Discuss the mechanism of action, pharmacokinetics, adverse effects and clinical uses of organic nitrates.

2. Discuss the drug therapy of acute myocardial infarction.

3. Write short notes on:
   a. Potassium channel opener
   b. Nitroglycerine
   c. Monday morning sickness

4. Explain why:
   a. Beta blockers are contraindicated in patients with variant angina
   b. Nitrates are not given continuously in patients with stable angina
   c. Sildenafil should not be prescribed to patient taking nitrates
   d. Beta blockers should not be stopped abruptly in patients with angina pectoris
   e. Nitrates are effective in cyanide poisoning

MULTIPLE CHOICE QUESTIONS

1. Ranolazine is a: *(Recent Question 2016)*
   a. Vasodilator   b. Antianginal
   c. Antihypertensive   d. Antiarrhythmic

2. Nitroglycerin can be administered by all of the following routes, except:
   (Recent Question 2016)
   a. Oral   b. Sublingual
   c. Intramuscular   d. Intravenous

3. Potassium channel opener with anti-anginal activity is:
   a. Nicorandil   b. Dipyridamole
   c. Trimetazidine   d. Oxyfedrine

4. Drug of choice for prinzmetal angina is:
   (Recent Question 2016)
   a. Nifedipine   b. Propranolol
   c. CCB   d. GTN

5. Drug not used in prinzmetal angina is:
   a. Propranolol   *(Recent Question 2016)*
   b. Verapamil
   c. Nitrites
   d. Isosorbide dinitrate

6. Nitroglycerin causes all except: *(AI 2009)*
   a. Hypotension and bradycardia
   b. Methemoglobinemia
   c. Hypotension and tachycardia
   d. Vasodilatation

7. The nitrate which does not undergo first-pass metabolism is: *(AI 2000)*
   a. Isosorbide mononitrate

   b. Nitroglycerin
   c. Pentaerythritol tetranitrate
   d. Isosorbide dinitrate

8. Mechanism of action of sodium nitrite in cyanide poisoning is: *(PGI June 2005)*
   a. Produces methemoglobinemia
   b. Increased blood flow to liver
   c. Increased blood flow to heart
   d. Increased blood flow to kidney

9. Glyceryl trinitrate is given by sublingual route because of: *(Recent Question 2016)*
   a. Short half-life in plasma
   b. High hepatic first-pass metabolism
   c. Extensive protein binding
   d. High bioavailability by oral route

10. Drug not to be given in ischemic heart disease is: *(Recent Question 2016)*
    a. ACE inhibitor   b. Atenolol
    c. Isoproterenol   d. Streptokinase

11. Mechanism of action of NO is:
    (Recent Question 2016)
    a. $\uparrow$ cGMP   b. $\uparrow$ cAMP
    c. $\uparrow$ PGD$_2$ d. $\uparrow$ PGE$_2$

12. Treatment of choice for cyanide poisoning:
    (Recent Question 2016)
    a. KMNO$_4$
    b. NaCl
    c. NaHCO$_3$
    d. Sodium nitrite + sodium thiosulfate

Ans.

1.	(b)	2.	(c)	3.	(a)	4.	(d)	5.	(a)	6.	(a)
7.	(a)	8.	(a)	9.	(b)	10.	(c)	11.	(a)	12.	(d)

Cardiac arrhythmias are group of conditions in which the heartbeat can be:
- Irregular
- Too fast (tachyarrhythmias)
- Too slow (bradyarrhythmias)

Figure 1 mentions the main types of arrhythmias with a few examples.

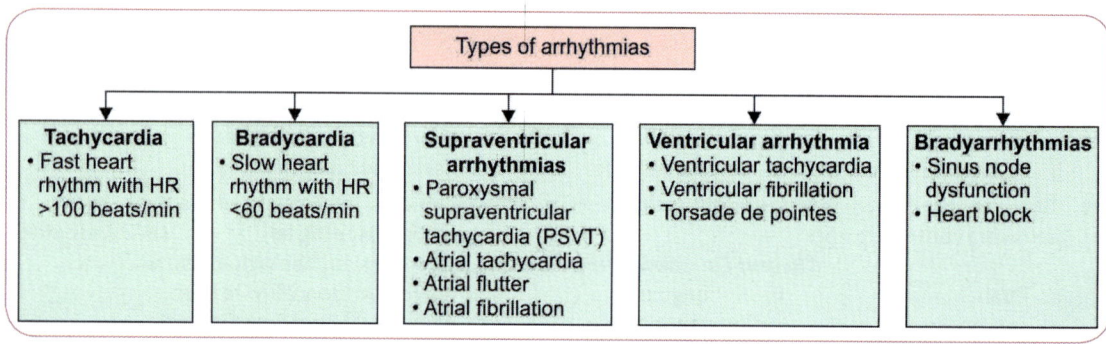

Figure 1: Types of arrhythmias

CARDIAC PHYSIOLOGY

The relevant terminology relating to cardiac physiology is mentioned in Table 1.

TABLE 1	Cardiac terminology
Cardiac systole	• Both the ventricles contract and eject blood into the aorta (left ventricle) and pulmonary artery (right ventricle)
Cardiac diastole	• Both the ventricles are relaxed
Cardiac cycle	• It is the sequence of electrical and mechanical events that repeats with each heartbeat. It includes the phase of cardiac systole and the phase of cardiac diastole.
Heart rate (HR)	• Number of cardiac contractions per minute—normal range 60–100 beats/min
Stroke volume (SV)	• Volume of blood pumped by the ventricle in a single contraction • Normal range is 60–130 mL
Cardiac output (CO)	• Volume of blood pumped by the ventricle in one minute • CO = HR × SV • Normal range is 4–8 L/min
Preload	• It is the stretch or the volume of the ventricular myocardium at the end of diastole • Also known as the left ventricular end diastolic pressure (LVEDP)
Afterload	• It is the amount of resistance which the left ventricle must overcome during systole to eject blood into the circulation • Also known as the systemic vascular resistance (SVR)

Action Potential of Cardiac Muscle Fiber

The transmembrane potential (TMP) of a cardiac cell is –90 mV. It is the electrical potential difference between the inside and the outside of a cell. The following ions are the key determinants of TMP:

o   Sodium, calcium and chloride—more in extracellular fluid
o   Potassium—more in intracellular fluid

Figure 2 depicts the transmission of electrical impulses in the cardiac muscle.

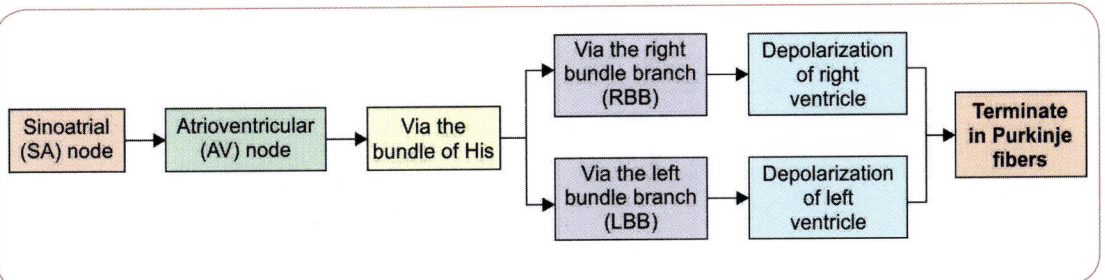

Figure 2: Transmission of electrical impulses

The action potential in the cardiac muscle consists of 5 phases (0–4) (Figure 3).

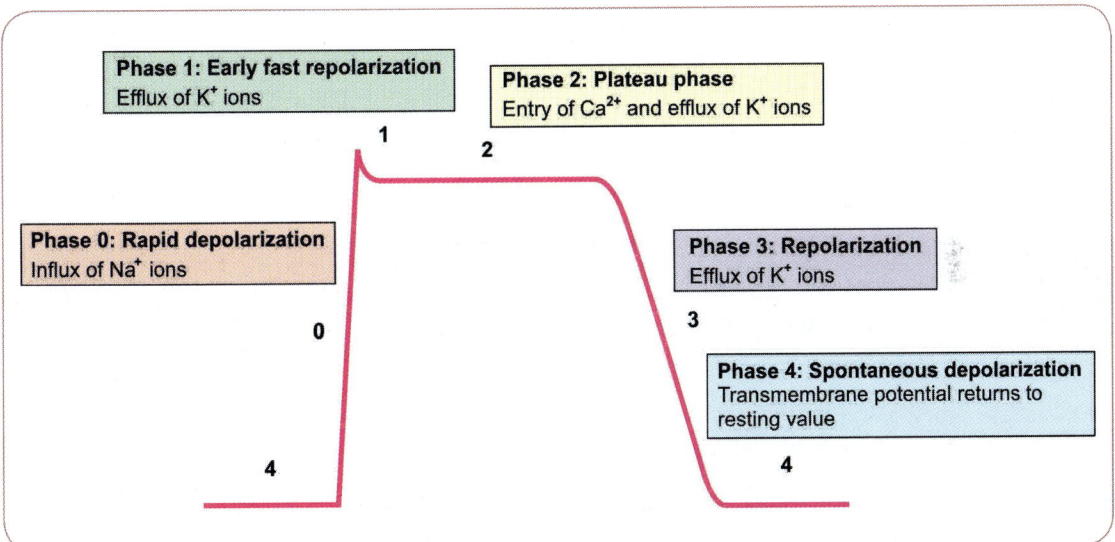

Figure 3: Cardiac action potential

CLASSIFICATION OF ANTIARRHYTHMIC DRUGS

The classification of antiarrhythmic drugs is mentioned in Figure 4.

SECTION C ■ Drugs Acting on the Cardiovascular System

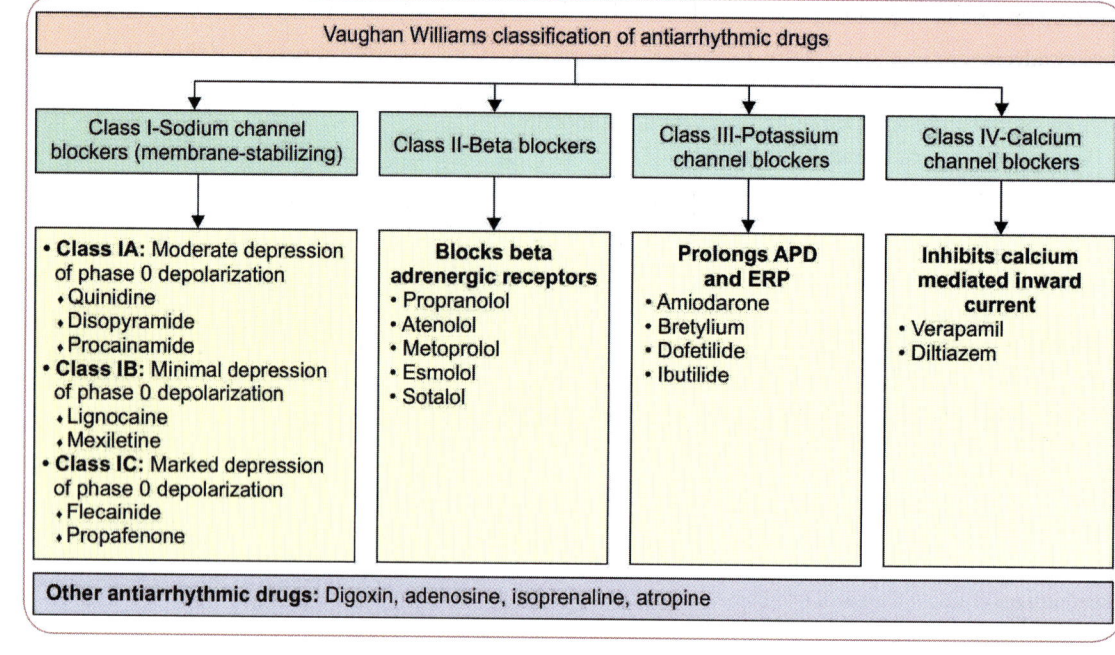

Figure 4: Vaughan Williams classification of antiarrhythmic drugs

CLASS IA ANTIARRHYTHMICS

These drugs block Na⁺ channels in the open state. They moderately delay channel recovery.

Quinidine

It is a stereoisomer of the antimalarial alkaloid quinine, obtained from cinchona bark.

Pharmacological Actions

The key pharmacological actions of quinidine are mentioned in Figure 5.

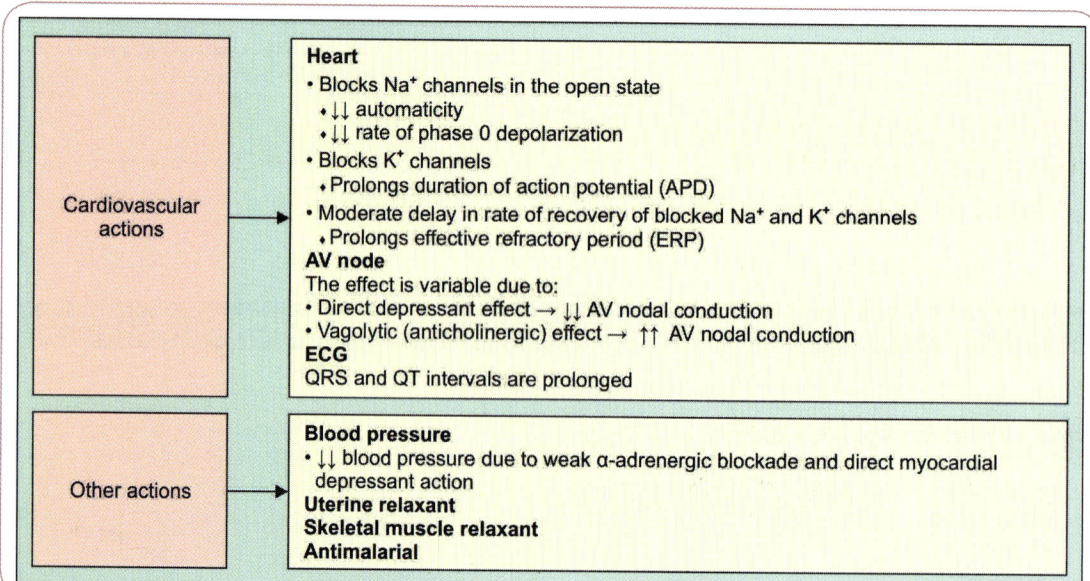

Figure 5: Pharmacological actions of quinidine

Adverse Effects

The key adverse effects of quinidine are mentioned in Table 2.

TABLE 2	Adverse effects of quinidine
Noncardiac	**Cardiac**
Diarrhea-most common adverse effect	Torsades de pointes
Immunological reactions • Thrombocytopenia • Hepatitis • Bone marrow depression • Lupus syndrome	Marked QT prolongation
	Ventricular tachycardia at very high doses
Cinchonism: It is a syndrome that occurs in toxic doses and is characterized by headache, tinnitus, deafness, ringing in ears, vertigo, visual disturbances, mental changes, etc.	

Drug Interactions

Some of the drug interactions with quinidine are mentioned in Table 3.

TABLE 3	Drug interactions with quinidine
Quinidine and β blockers/verapamil	Additive cardiac depressant actions
Quinidine and digoxin	Quinidine inhibits P-glycoprotein and digoxin is a substrate for P-glycoprotein. Hence, digoxin toxicity can occur.
Quinidine and CYP2D6 substrates	Quinidine is a potent inhibitor of CYP2D6. It may lead to increased levels of drugs metabolized through CYP2D6 e.g. codeine, propafenone
Quinidine and diuretics	Hypokalemia caused by diuretics may lead to an increased risk of torsades de pointes

Clinical Uses

Although quinidine is effective in a wide range of atrial and ventricular arrhythmias, it is not commonly used to terminate them because of high risk of adverse effects and availability of better alternative drugs.

It may occasionally be used to maintain sinus rhythm in patients with atrial flutter or fibrillation, and to prevent recurrence of ventricular tachycardia or fibrillation.

Procainamide

It is an analogue of local anesthetic procaine.
The cardiac electrophysiologic actions are similar to quinidine, but have the following differences:
○ No vagolytic (anticholinergic) action
○ No α adrenergic blocking action

Pharmacokinetics

It is well absorbed after oral administration. It can also be given intravenously. The plasma half-life is 3–4 hours; therefore, frequent dosing is required.

It is metabolized in the liver by acetylation. The major metabolite N-acetyl procainamide (NAPA) lacks Na^+ channel blocking activity but has K^+ channel blocking activity and prolongs APD. There are 'fast' and 'slow' acetylators of procainamide (similar to that for isoniazid).

Both procainamide and its metabolite NAPA are excreted by the kidneys; hence, dose reduction may be required in patients with renal failure.

Adverse Effects

The important adverse effects are mentioned in Figure 6.

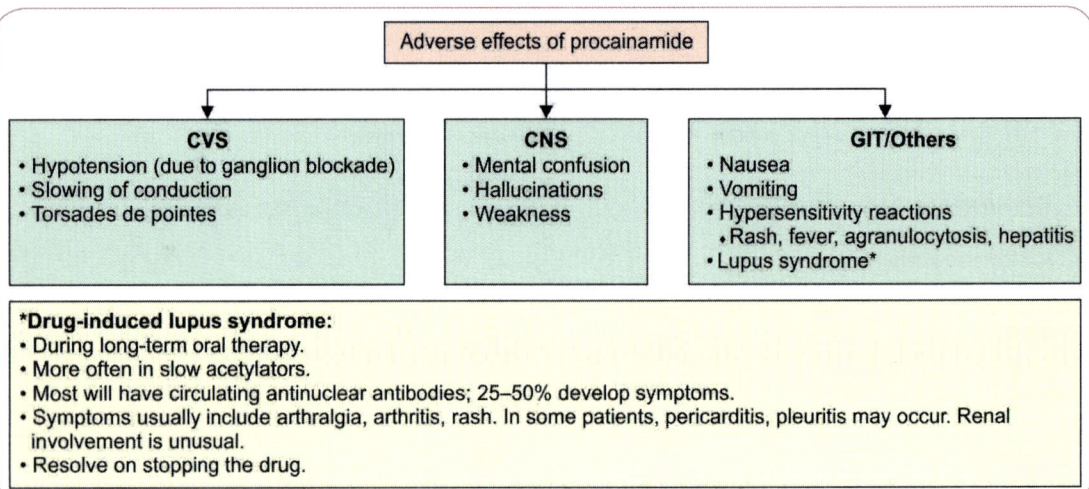

Figure 6: Adverse effects of procainamide

Clinical Uses

It is used for the treatment of ventricular arrhythmias associated with acute MI.

It is not used for long-term oral therapy because of high risk of adverse effects (lupus syndrome) and the need for frequent dosing (due to short half-life).

Disopyramide

The cardiac electrophysiologic actions are similar to quinidine, but have the following differences:
- No α adrenergic blocking action
- More marked anticholinergic action

Pharmacokinetics

It is well absorbed after oral administration. It is partly metabolized by the liver and partly excreted unchanged by the kidneys. The plasma half-life is 6–8 hours.

Adverse Effects

The toxic concentration can lead to electrophysiologic disturbances similar to that of quinidine.

Disopyramide commonly depress myocardial contractility, which may precipitate heart failure and may also lead to torsades de pointes. It should therefore not be used in patients with heart failure.

The symptomatic adverse effects are predominantly due to its anticholinergic actions and include the following:

Dry mouth, blurred vision, constipation, urinary retention (in benign prostatic hyperplasia) and worsening of pre-existing glaucoma.

Clinical Uses

It is used in the following situations:
- To prevent recurrences of ventricular tachycardia or fibrillation
- To maintain sinus rhythm in patients with atrial flutter or fibrillation

CLASS IB ANTIARRHYTHMICS

These drugs block Na$^+$ channels more in the inactivated state than in the open state. They do not delay channel recovery.

Lignocaine (Lidocaine)

Lignocaine is a local anesthetic that is also highly effective in the treatment of ventricular arrhythmias associated with acute MI. It is used only by the intravenous route.

Pharmacological Actions

Lignocaine blocks inactivated Na$^+$ channels more than the open channels. It exerts greater effect on partially depolarized (ischemic) tissue.

- The most important cardiac action is decrease of automaticity in ectopic foci. Lignocaine decreases automaticity by reducing the slope of phase 4 depolarization and altering the threshold for excitability. However, SA node automaticity is not decreased.
- Action potential duration is usually unaffected. It causes minimal depression of contractility and there are no autonomic actions.
- It has minimal effect on normal ECG (no significant effect on PR, QRS or QT).

Pharmacokinetics

Lignocaine is not effective orally due to extensive first-pass metabolism in the liver. It is therefore administered only by IV route. It has a short half-life of 1–2 hours. It is metabolized in the liver and excreted by the kidneys.

Lignocaine is given by IV infusion in a loading dose of 150–200 mg over 15 minutes followed by a maintenance dose of 2–4 mg/minute. The following points are noteworthy:

- *In heart failure patients*, both the volume of distribution and total body clearance of lignocaine are decreased. Therefore, both the loading and maintenance doses should be reduced.
- *In hepatic disease patients*, volume of distribution is increased and plasma clearance is decreased. Hence, maintenance doses should be reduced but loading doses can be normally given.

Drug Interactions

Lignocaine and Propranolol/Cimetidine

Propranolol and cimetidine decrease hepatic blood flow. The clearance of lignocaine is hepatic blood flow dependent; hence its clearance is decreased. This leads to an increase in lignocaine levels which may increase the risk of toxicity.

Adverse Effects

Lignocaine is one of the least cardiotoxic Na$^+$ channel blocker. It has practically no proarrhythmic effects. The adverse effects (like most other LAs) are mainly neurologic. It may cause the following:
Nystagmus (early indicator of toxicity), headache, drowsiness, paresthesia, tremor, slurred speech and convulsions.

Clinical Uses

- Lignocaine is the *preferred drug for the treatment of ventricular arrhythmias associated with acute MI or cardiac surgery*.
- It is used in digoxin toxicity because it does not worsen AV block during treatment of ventricular arrhythmia.
- It is not a preferred drug in atrial arrhythmia because atrial action potentials are of a very short duration; hence, the Na$^+$ channels are in the inactivated state for only a brief period of time.

Note: Routine prophylactic use to prevent ventricular arrhythmia after MI in every patient, has shown to increase mortality. Hence, it is recommended to use lignocaine for the treatment of ventricular arrhythmia and not for the prevention of arrhythmia in every case of MI.

Mexiletine

It is an orally active analogue of lignocaine. The pharmacological actions are similar to lignocaine.

The main adverse effects are dose related nausea, tremors, lethargy and blurred vision.

It is available in both oral and IV formulations. It is used in the treatment of ventricular arrhythmias as an alternative to lignocaine.

CLASS IC ANTIARRHYTHMICS

These drugs are the most potent Na^+ channel blockers. They have more potent action on the open state of the channels. They markedly delay channel recovery.

Propafenone and Flecainide

They are the most potent Na^+ channel blockers. They markedly suppress phase 0 depolarization in Purkinje and myocardial fibers. This leads to marked slowing of conduction throughout the heart.

Propafenone additionally has β blocking property.

Adverse Effects

Both the drugs can lead to exacerbation of cardiac arrhythmias and may precipitate heart failure, especially in patients with pre-existing arrhythmias or myocardial infarction.

Propafenone may cause metallic taste, constipation, bradycardia and bronchospasm. It should be avoided in asthma.

Flecainide may cause blurred vision, dizziness and nausea.

Clinical Uses

They are used for the maintenance of sinus rhythm in supraventricular tachycardia. They are also used in the treatment of ventricular arrhythmias with modest efficacy.

CLASS II ANTIARRHYTHMICS—BETA BLOCKERS

Beta blockers inhibit ectopic activity mediated by adrenergic stimulation.

They have the following actions:
- Predominantly affect the sinoatrial (SA) and atrioventricular (AV) nodes
- Decrease the rate of automaticity
- Prolong the effective refractory period of AV node and reduce conduction velocity

Propranolol also has a quinidine like (membrane-stabilizing) action at higher doses.

Sotalol

- Nonselective β blocker that also has a Class III (potassium channel blocking) action
- It prolongs the duration of action potential, decreases AV conduction and reduces automaticity
- Has a risk of causing torsades de pointes, since it prolongs the duration of action potential and QT interval

Esmolol

- Cardioselective $β_1$ blocker
- Quick and short acting drug; very short elimination half-life (~9 minutes) as it is metabolized by erythrocyte esterases
- Used intravenously
- Used in conditions where immediate control of ventricular rate is required, e.g. rapid control of ventricular rate in patients with atrial fibrillation or atrial flutter in perioperative, postoperative, or other situations
- Also used in patients of supraventricular tachycardia

CLASS III ANTIARRHYTHMICS—POTASSIUM CHANNEL BLOCKERS

Amiodarone

Amiodarone is an iodine containing drug which is structurally related to thyroxine.

Mechanism of Action

Amiodarone exhibits multiple antiarrhythmic effects and shows Class I, II, III and IV actions along with some α blocking activity. The main actions include the following:
- Prolongs the action potential duration
- Prolongs the effective refractory period

Pharmacokinetics

It is strongly protein bound and has a long plasma half-life (3–8 weeks). Following oral ingestion, the action develops over several days to weeks. However, the action develops rapidly following IV injection.

Adverse Effects

Amiodarone has a complex adverse effect profile (Figure 7).

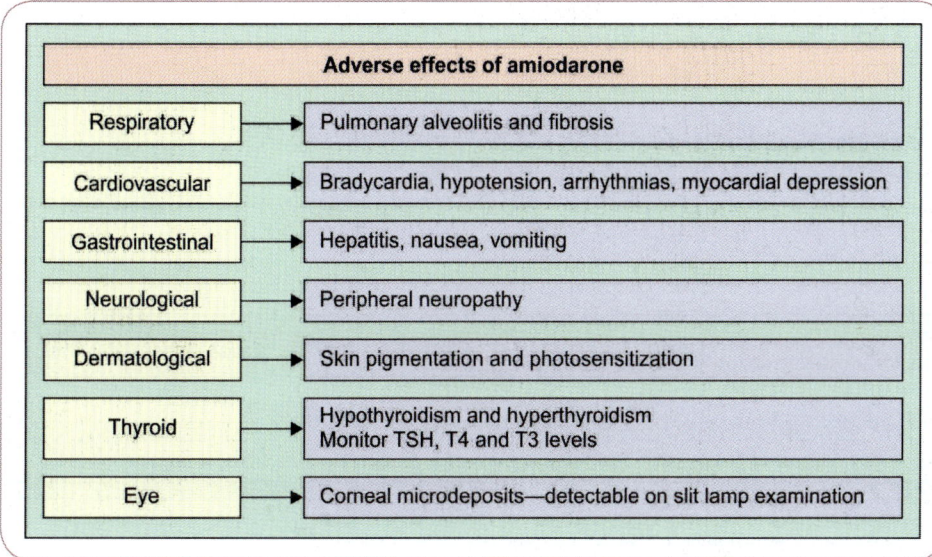

Adverse effects of amiodarone	
Respiratory	Pulmonary alveolitis and fibrosis
Cardiovascular	Bradycardia, hypotension, arrhythmias, myocardial depression
Gastrointestinal	Hepatitis, nausea, vomiting
Neurological	Peripheral neuropathy
Dermatological	Skin pigmentation and photosensitization
Thyroid	Hypothyroidism and hyperthyroidism Monitor TSH, T4 and T3 levels
Eye	Corneal microdeposits—detectable on slit lamp examination

Figure 7: Amiodarone—adverse effects

Clinical Uses

Amiodarone is useful in a broad range of ventricular and supraventricular arrhythmias. These include resistant ventricular tachycardia and recurrent ventricular fibrillation.

Drug Interactions

- Amiodarone decrease the renal clearance of digoxin and warfarin; hence leads to a rise in digoxin and warfarin levels
- Amiodarone given along with β blockers or calcium channel blockers may result in additive A-V block

Ibutilide

Ibutilide is used for immediate conversion of atrial flutter and atrial fibrillation to normal sinus rhythm; however, it is more effective in atrial flutter.

It may cause QT prolongation and torsades de pointes; hence, it is given in the hospital setup with ECG monitoring for 4 hours after infusion or until QT interval becomes normal.

Dofetilide

It is used for the maintenance of normal sinus rhythm in patients with atrial fibrillation.
It may cause QT prolongation and torsades de pointes; hence, it is given in the hospital setup.

CLASS IV ANTIARRHYTHMICS—CALCIUM CHANNEL BLOCKERS

The drugs in this class include verapamil (prototype drug) and diltiazem. The dihydropyridines (e.g. nifedipine) are not antiarrhythmic but may precipitate arrhythmias.

The mechanism of action is to block L-type calcium channels and delay their recovery. They also have the following actions:
- Reduce automaticity
- Prolong refractoriness (especially of the AV node)

The clinical uses include:
- Decrease ventricular rate in atrial flutter and atrial fibrillation
- Treatment of paroxysmal supraventricular tachycardia (PSVT)

OTHER ANTIARRHYTHMIC DRUGS

Adenosine

It is a naturally occurring purine nucleoside.
It slows conduction through the AV node and increases the refractory period.
The duration of action is short (approx 10–15 seconds) due to rapid uptake by RBCs and endothelial cells.

Mechanism of Action and Clinical Uses (Figure 8)

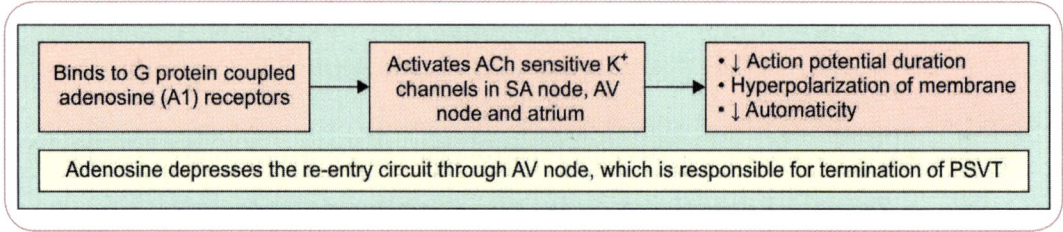

Figure 8: Mechanism of adenosine

The advantages of adenosine in the treatment of paroxysmal supraventricular tachycardia (PSVT) are as follows:
- Highly effective (equivalent to or more effective than verapamil)
- Short duration of action (10–15 seconds) → transient adverse effects
- Does not cause hemodynamic deterioration → can be administered in CHF or in patients on β blockers

Adverse Effects
- Transient chest pain, dyspnea, flushing, hypotension, transient ventricular standstill
- Precipitation of bronchospasm in asthmatics

Drug Interactions
- Dipyridamole inhibits uptake and metabolism of adenosine and potentiates its action
- Aminophylline, theophylline and other xanthines antagonize the action of adenosine by blocking adenosine receptors

Atropine

It is used in cases of AV block occurring due to vagal overactivity, as seen in digoxin toxicity or in some patients of myocardial infarction.

ANTIARRHYTHMIC THERAPY FOR VARIOUS ARRHYTHMIAS

The therapies employed for some of the cardiac arrhythmias are mentioned in Table 4.

TABLE 4	Cardiac arrhythmias
Cardiac arrhythmias	**Therapy**
Paroxysmal supraventricular tachycardia (PSVT)	• Adenosine • Verapamil
Atrial flutter	• Cardioversion • Esmolol
Atrial fibrillation	• Cardioversion • Esmolol
Ventricular tachycardia	• Lignocaine • Cardioversion
Ventricular fibrillation	• Electrical defibrillation • Lignocaine

ASSESS YOURSELF (Examination Questions of Various Universities)

1. Classify antiarrhythmic drugs. Discuss the mechanism of action, pharmacokinetics, adverse effects and clinical uses of lignocaine.

2. Write short notes on:
   a. Adenosine
   b. Amiodarone
   c. Drugs used in paroxysmal supraventricular tachycardia (PSVT)

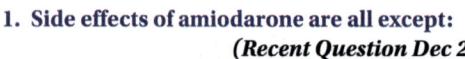

MULTIPLE CHOICE QUESTIONS

1. Side effects of amiodarone are all except:
   (Recent Question Dec 2016)
   a. Pulmonary fibrosis   b. Hepatotoxicity
   c. Hypothyroidism   d. Nephrotoxicity

2. All are toxicities seen with amiodarone therapy except: *(AIIMS May 2009)*
   a. Pulmonary fibrosis
   b. Corneal microdeposits
   c. Cirrhosis of liver
   d. Productive cough

3. Which of the following antiarrhythmic agents does not belong to class IC? *(AIIMS Nov 2006)*
   a. Tocainide   b. Encainide
   c. Flecainide   d. Propafenone

4. Patient on verapamil should not be given beta blocker as: *(Recent Question 2016)*
   a. Conduction block
   b. Bronchospasm
   c. Neurogenic shock
   d. Anaphylaxis

5. All of the following are used in atrial arrhythmias except: *(Recent Question 2016)*
   a. Digoxin   b. Verapamil
   c. Quinidine   d. Lignocaine

6. Adverse effects of quinidine are all except:
   (Recent Question 2016)
   a. SLE
   b. Diarrhea
   c. Bradycardia
   d. Torsades de pointes

7. The antiarrythmic drug which causes myocardial depression is:
   (Recent Question 2016)
   a. Sotalol   b. Quinine
   c. Amiodarone   d. None of these

8. Beta blockers are antiarrhythmic agents of type: *(Recent Question 2016)*
   a. I   b. II
   c. III   d. IV

9. Which drug can cause thyroid dysfunction?
   (Recent Question 2016)
   a. Amiodarone   b. Ampicillin
   c. Ibutilide   d. Acyclovir

10. Which of the following drugs can cause torsades de pointes? *(Recent Question 2016)*
    a. Quinidine   b. Lignocaine
    c. Esmolol   d. Flecainide

11. The antiarrhythmic drug of choice in most of the cases of acute paroxysmal supraventricular tachycardia is: *(Recent Question 2016)*
    a. Adenosine   b. Amiodarone
    c. Propranolol   d. Quinidine

12. Which of the following has the maximum half-life? *(Recent Question 2016)*
    a. Adenosine   b. Amiodarone
    c. Esomolol   d. Lidocaine

13. Dofetilide is which class of antirrhythmic drug?
    (Recent Question 2016)
    a. Class 1   b. Class 2
    c. Class 3   d. Class 4

Ans.												
1.	(d)	2.	(d)	3.	(a)	4.	(a)	5.	(d)	6.	(c)
7.	(c)	8.	(b)	9.	(a)	10.	(a)	11.	(a)	12.	(b)
13.	(c)										

14. Procainamide is a class___antiarrhythmic drug. *(Recent Question 2016)*
    a. I
    b. II
    c. III
    d. IV

15. MOA of verapamil is: *(PGI May 2012)*
    a. Inhibition of Ca^{+2} channel
    b. Inhibition of Na^+ channel
    c. Inhibition of K^+ channel
    d. Block membrane repolarization
    e. Membrane stabilization

16. Verapamil belongs to which Class of Anti-arrhythmic drugs? *(NIMHANS 2013)*
    a. I
    b. II
    c. III
    d. IV

17. Ventricular fibrillation is treated by: *(TN PG 2007)*
    a. Esmolol
    b. Flecainide
    c. Ibutilide
    d. Lignocaine

Ans.

| 14. | (a) | 15. | (a) | 16. | (d) | 17. | (d) |

15 Drugs Used for Heart Failure

Heart failure is a disorder in which the heart is not able to pump adequate blood to meet the requirements of the body. This results in the following:

○ Inadequate blood to the tissues due to inadequate cardiac contraction
○ Organ congestion caused by elevated pulmonary or systemic venous pressures

The body compensates for the failing heart by utilizing the mechanisms shown in Figure 1.

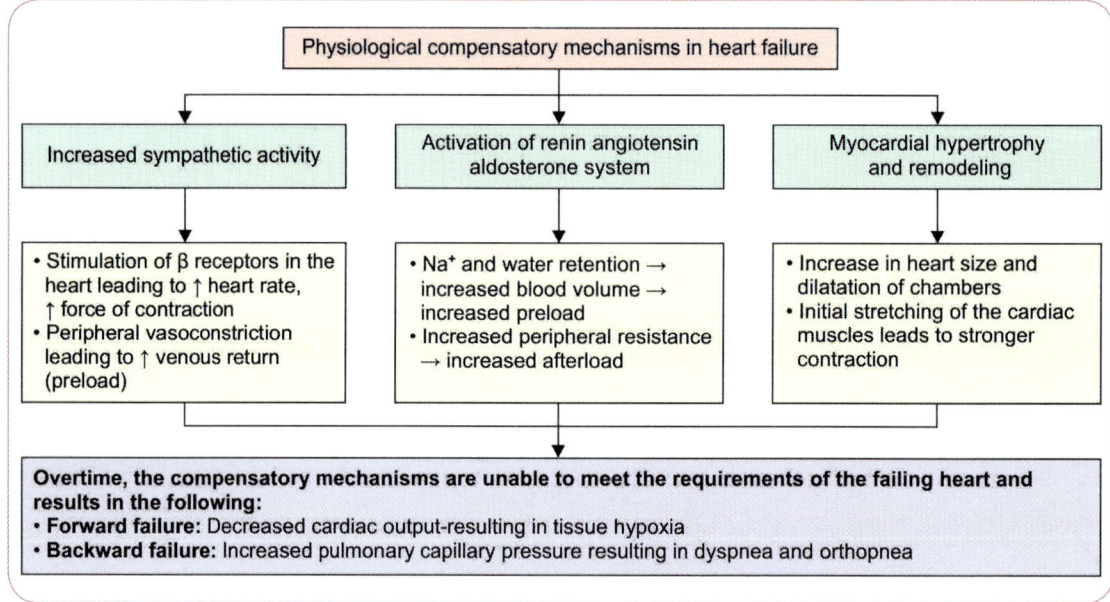

Figure 1: Compensatory mechanisms in heart failure

DRUGS USED FOR HEART FAILURE—CLASSIFICATION

The drugs employed in the management of heart failure are mentioned in Table 1.

TABLE 1	Drugs used for heart failure

Diuretics	• Loop diuretics
	  ▪ Furosemide, bumetanide
	• Thiazides
	  ▪ Chlorothiazide, hydrochlorothiazide, metolazone
	• Aldosterone antagonists
	  ▪ Spironolactone, eplerenone

Contd...

Vasodilators	• Arteriolar and venodilators
	▪ ACE inhibitors—enalapril, lisinopril, ramipril, fosinopril
	▪ Angiotensin receptor blockers (ARBs)—losartan, candesartan
	▪ Sodium nitroprusside
	• Arteriolar dilators
	▪ Hydralazine, minoxidil, nicorandil
	• Venodilators
	▪ Nitroglycerin, isosorbide dinitrate
Sympathomimetic amines	Dobutamine, dopamine
Beta blockers	Carvedilol, metoprolol, bisoprolol
Cardiac glycosides	Digoxin
Others	• Phosphodiesterase-3 inhibitors
	▪ Milrinone, inamrinone
	• Natriuretic peptide
	▪ Nesiritide

TREATMENT STRATEGIES FOR HEART FAILURE

The treatment strategies for the management of heart failure employ drugs that have actions on the following (Figure 2):

○ Renin angiotensin aldosterone system
○ Increased sympathetic activity
○ Myocardial hypertrophy and remodeling

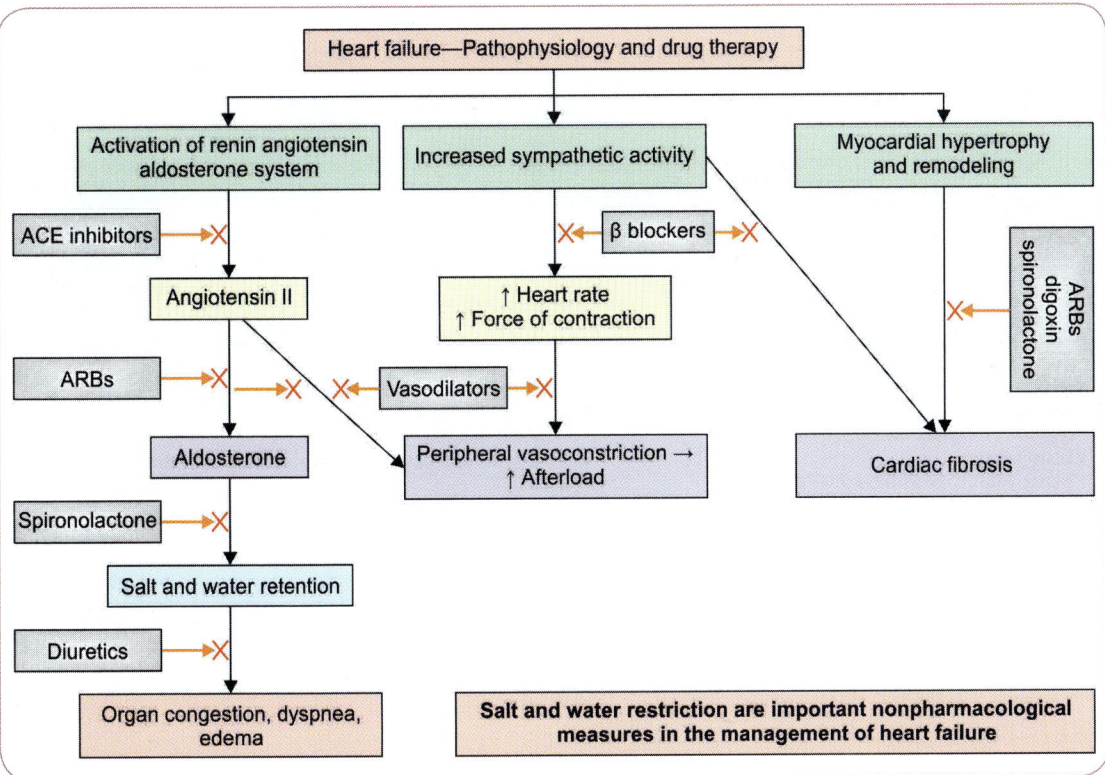

Figure 2: Heart failure—pathophysiology and drug therapy

Drugs Acting on the Cardiovascular System ■ SECTION C

DIURETICS

Diuretics (particularly furosemide) are the preferred drugs for management of congestive symptoms in heart failure.

Diuretics reduce circulating fluid volume by promoting salt (Na$^+$) and water excretion (Figure 3).

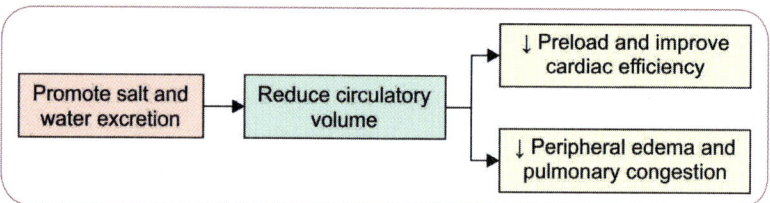

Figure 3: Diuretics in heart failure

An important adverse effect is hypokalemia; hence potassium monitoring should be performed.

The risk of severe volume contraction, hypotension, hyponatremia and hypomagnesemia should also be considered during therapy.

Aldosterone antagonists such as spironolactone and eplerenone are used to counteract hypokalemia caused by loop diuretics.

Aldosterone antagonists also decrease morbidity and mortality in patients of severe heart failure (on therapy with other heart failure drugs, e.g. ACE inhibitors).

VASODILATORS

Vasodilators, especially ACE inhibitors, have a central role in the management of heart failure (Figure 4).

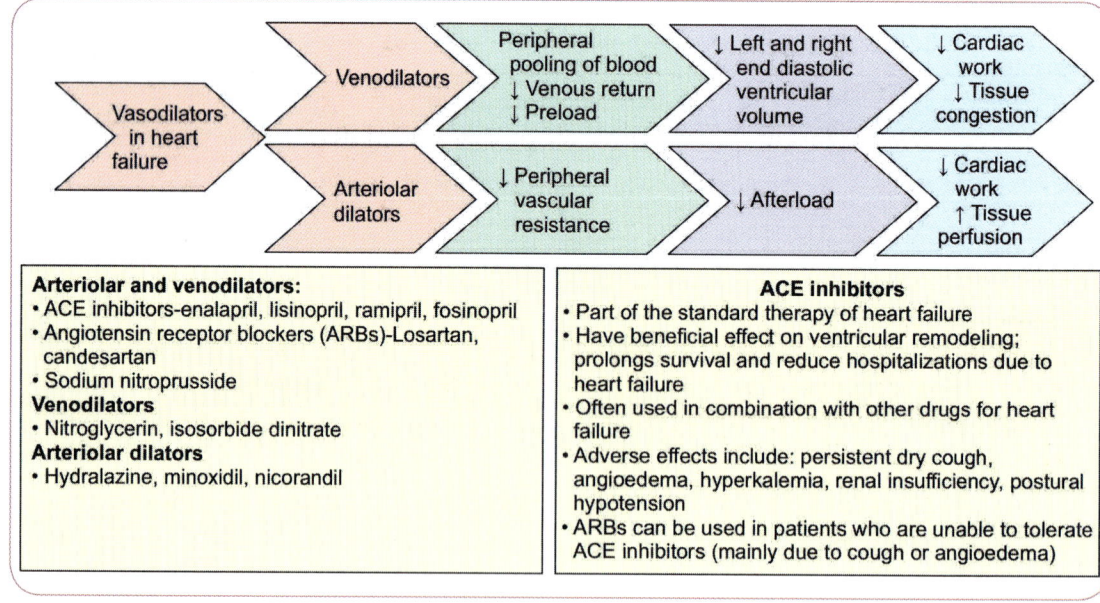

Figure 4: Vasodilators in heart failure

BETA BLOCKERS

Beta blockers are useful in heart failure because they can improve ejection fraction, reduce mortality and decrease hospitalization.

The beta blockers used in heart failure include bisoprolol, carvedilol and metoprolol.

They have the following actions:
- Decrease production of renin
- Decrease heart rate
- Prevent harmful effects of sympathetic stimulation on cardiac muscles; reduce remodeling and hypertrophy
- Reduce frequency of arrhythmias

They are contraindicated in patients with severe peripheral arterial circulatory disturbances, severe asthma, severe chronic obstructive pulmonary disease, sick sinus syndrome, second- or third-degree heart block and uncontrolled heart failure. Abrupt withdrawal may lead to angina, myocardial infarction and sudden death.

CARDIAC GLYCOSIDES

The glycosides consist of an aglycone (steroid nucleus linked to a lactone ring at the 17 position) to which one or more sugar moieties are attached (at the carbon 3).

The sources of some cardiac glycosides are mentioned in Table 2.

TABLE 2	Sources of cardiac glycosides
Source	**Glycosides**
Digitalis purpurea (leaf)	Digitoxin
Digitalis lanata (leaf)	Digoxin, digitoxin
Strophanthus gratus (seed)	Ouabain

By convention, 'Digitalis' has been used as a collective term for 'Cardiac glycosides' because most of the drugs are obtained from digitalis (foxglove) plant.

William Withering, an English scientist, first described the usefulness of cardiac glycosides in heart failure.

Digoxin is the prototype drug and is more widely used than the other cardiac glycosides.

Mechanism of Action

Digoxin inhibits the sodium pump (Na$^+$, K$^+$-ATPase) and has a positive inotropic action on the heart (i.e. increase myocardial contractility) (Figure 5).

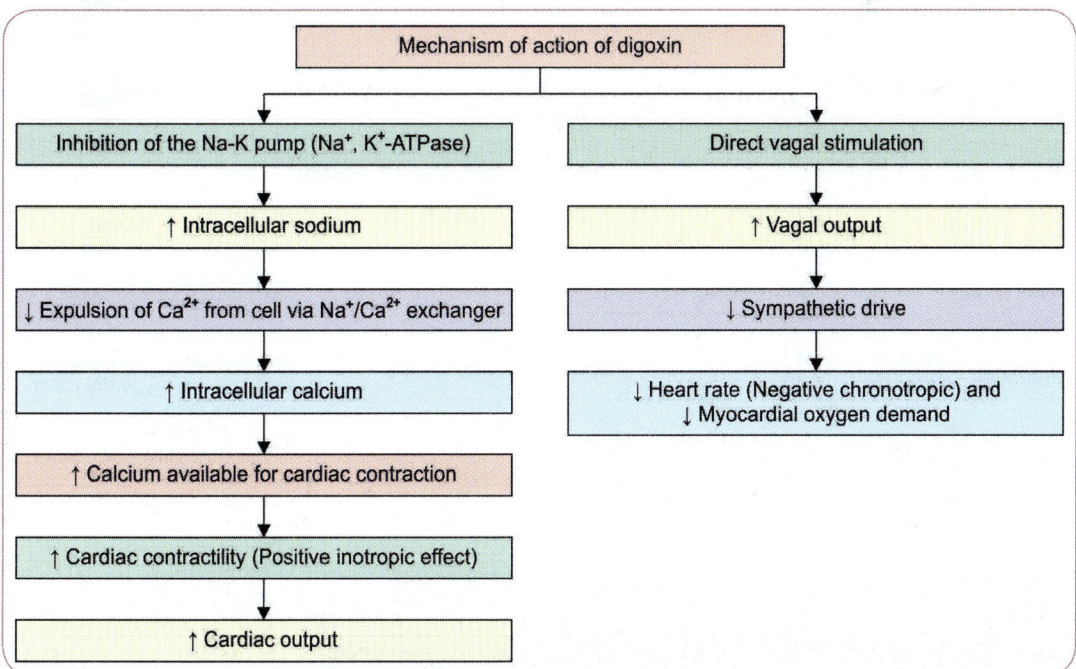

Figure 5: Digoxin—mechanism of action

Pharmacological Actions

The pharmacological actions of digoxin can be divided into cardiac and extracardiac:

Cardiac Effects

- Myocardial contractility
  - Increase cardiac contractility (positive inotropic effect)
  - Results in complete emptying of ventricles during systole and increase in cardiac output
  - Reduction in the size of the heart also reduces the myocardial oxygen requirement
- Heart rate
  - Decrease heart rate (negative chronotropic effect) and reduce myocardial oxygen demand
- Electrophysiological effects
  - Complex effects on conduction velocities and refractory periods in the cardiac muscle
  - Therapeutic doses → prolongs effective refractory period and decreases conduction velocity in the AV node; can lead to bradycardia and AV block
  - Higher doses → may increase automaticity in cardiac tissue; can lead to arrhythmias

Extracardiac Effects

- Gastrointestinal system
  - Anorexia, nausea and vomiting
  - Mediated via a direct action on the GIT and via central action on the CNS (stimulation of CTZ)
- Central nervous system
  - Disorientation, mental confusion and visual disturbances including blurred vision

Pharmacokinetics

Digoxin is the most commonly used glycoside. It is available in oral and IV formulations. It is usually given orally. Food delays absorption. It is widely distributed in the body and is concentrated in heart, skeletal muscle, liver and kidney.

The main tissue reservoir is skeletal muscle and not adipose tissue; therefore, dosing should be based on lean body mass of the patient.

Digoxin is excreted unchanged by the kidneys. Its renal clearance is proportionate to the creatinine clearance. Hence, dose reduction is required in patients with renal failure.

The elimination half-life is around 36–40 hours, allowing once daily dosing.

Adverse Effects

Digoxin has a **narrow margin of safety,** i.e. there is a small difference between a therapeutic dose and a toxic dose. The key adverse effects of digoxin are mentioned in Figure 6.

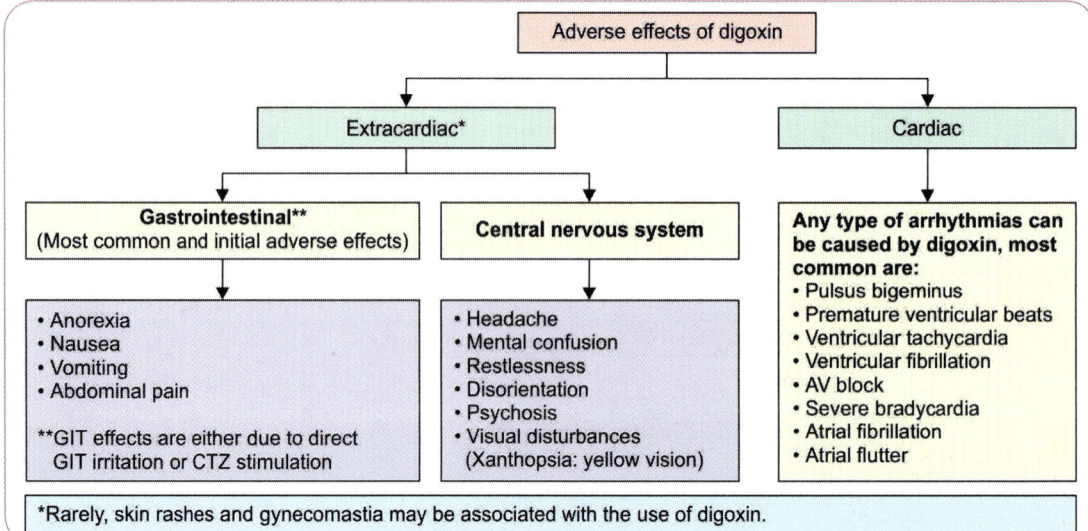

Figure 6: Adverse effects of digoxin

Digoxin Toxicity

The following measures are undertaken in various scenarios of digoxin toxicity:

- **Extracardiac manifestations** (e.g. gastrointestinal toxicity or visual changes)
  - Reduce the dose of digoxin
  - Stop digoxin therapy, if required
- **Tachyarrhythmias**
  - Stop digoxin and diuretics (both cause hypokalemia)
  - KCl administration oral or IV (K^+ decreases binding of digoxin to Na^+, K^+-ATPase and reduce digoxin-induced automaticity)

> **Note:** Digoxin may also lead to hyperkalemia (in acute intake of large doses). Hence, serum electrolyte levels, digoxin levels, and ECG should always be monitored during treatment of digoxin toxicity, and appropriately managed.

- **Ventricular arrhythmias**
  - The drug of choice is **IV lignocaine**. It has the advantage of suppressing enhanced automaticity while it does not precipitate AV block.
  - Intravenous phenytoin may also be used
- **Supraventricular arrhythmias**
  - Oral or IV propranolol may be given for treatment
- **AV block and bradyarrhythmia**
  - Atropine or cardiac pacing may be employed for treatment

Digoxin antibodies (Digibind): In serious life-threatening digoxin toxicity, K^+ levels are usually elevated, automaticity is frequently depressed, and the use of antiarrhythmic drugs may cause cardiac arrest.

In such a scenario, digoxin antibodies (digoxin immune Fab) are used along with a temporary cardiac pacemaker.

It neutralizes circulating digoxin and is rapidly excreted by the kidneys. It is extremely useful in rapidly reversing severe toxicity by most glycosides.

Clinical Uses

Congestive Heart Failure

Heart failure is mainly due to either systolic dysfunction or diastolic dysfunction. Digoxin is mainly used to improve the systolic dysfunction in heart failure.

- Systolic dysfunction occurs when the ventricles are dilated and the ventricular muscle is unable to generate sufficient wall tension to pump adequate blood. It occurs in ischemic heart disease, dilated cardiomyopathy, valvular incompetence, etc.
- Diastolic dysfunction occurs when the ventricular wall is thickened and the ventricle is unable to completely relax during diastole. Hence, the output is low because the ventricular filling is inadequate. It occurs in hypertension, aortic stenosis, hypertrophic cardiomyopathy, etc.

Digoxin provides benefit in the failing heart by improving circulation and perfusion leading to correction of hypoxia (Figure 7).

Atrial Fibrillation

Atrial fibrillation (AF) is the most common abnormal heart rhythm. The incidence of AF increases with age.

In AF, the atria beat at a very high rate. The high atrial rate leads to an excessively high ventricular rate.

Digoxin depresses AV node by increasing its effective refractory period (ERP) and decreasing its conduction velocity. It therefore reduces ventricular rate in AF by decreasing the number of electrical impulses passing down the AV node.

The other drugs beneficial in this condition are β blockers and verapamil.

Atrial Flutter

Digoxin controls the ventricular rate by slowing AV conduction.

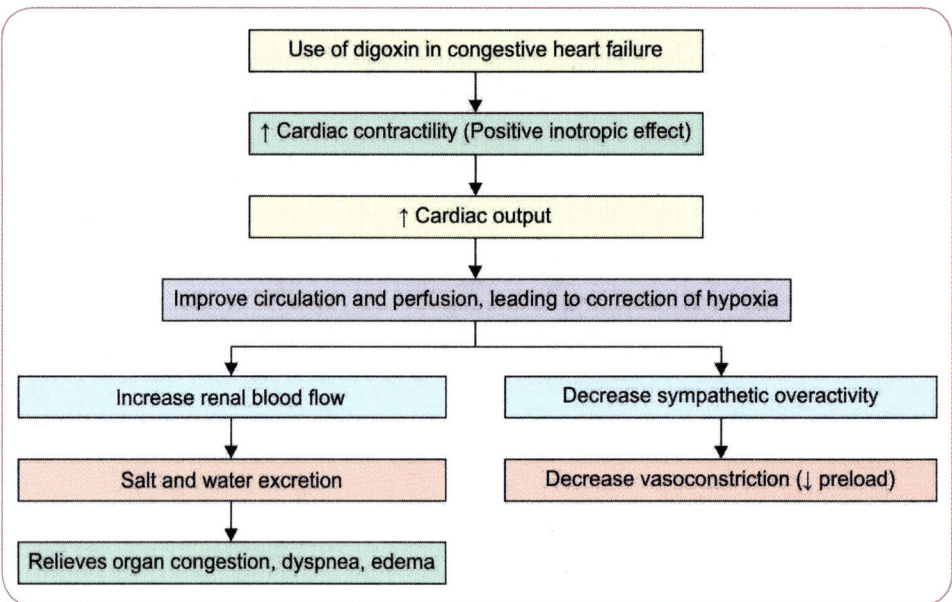

Figure 7: Use of digoxin in congestive heart failure

Paroxysmal Supraventricular Tachycardia

Adenosine is the drug of choice. Verapamil is also frequently employed. Digoxin is the reserve drug for this condition.

Drug Interactions

The key drug interactions with digoxin are mentioned in Table 3.

TABLE 3	Drug interactions with digoxin
Digoxin and β blocker/verapamil/diltiazem	Additive depressant action on SA and AV node; AV block may be precipitated
Digoxin and thiazide/loop diuretics	• Hypokalemia caused by diuretics may precipitate digoxin toxicity • This is because digoxin normally competes with K^+ for same binding site on Na^+, K^+-ATPase • Hence, hypokalemia may lead to increased binding of digoxin to Na^+, K^+-ATPase
Digoxin and antacids/cholestyramine	Antacids/cholestyramine decrease the GIT absorption of digoxin
Digoxin and calcium	Calcium accelerates the filling of intracellular stores and synergizes with digoxin; precipitates digoxin toxicity
Digoxin and verapamil/amiodarone/clarithromycin	Digoxin is a substrate for P-glycoprotein. Thus, inhibitors of P-glycoprotein (e.g. verapamil/amiodarone/clarithromycin) may ↑ concentration of digoxin by ↓ renal clearance.

SYMPATHOMIMETIC AMINES

Dopamine and dobutamine can be used via intravenous infusion in the management of acute heart failure.

Dopamine

It is a catecholamine and has dose dependent actions (Table 4).

TABLE 4	Dose dependent actions of dopamine
Dopamine dose	**Effects**
Low doses (<2 µg/kg/min)	• Stimulates D_1 receptors and dilates renal, coronary and mesenteric blood vessels • Increases GFR and urine output
Moderate doses (2–5 µg/kg/min)	• Stimulates β_1 receptors in the heart and increases myocardial contractility and cardiac output • Stimulates D_1 receptors and dilates renal, coronary and mesenteric blood vessels • Improves cardiac and renal function
High doses (>5 µg/kg/min)	• Leads to α receptor mediated vasoconstriction • Nullifies the beneficial effects of low/moderate doses of dopamine in heart failure

Dobutamine

Dobutamine is indicated as inotropic support in CHF patients with systolic dysfunction. It is administered via IV infusion.

Dobutamine directly stimulates β_1-adrenergic receptors leading to a positive inotropic effect on the heart, resulting in increased myocardial contractility, stroke volume and cardiac output.

It also has mild β_2- and α_1-adrenergic agonist effects at therapeutic doses but the predominant effect is cardiac stimulation. The total peripheral resistance is not generally impacted due to the balancing of the β_2 (vasodilatation) and α_1 (vasoconstriction) adrenergic effects.

OTHER DRUGS

- Phosphodiesterase-3 inhibitors
  - Milrinone, Inamrinone
- Natriuretic peptide
  - Nesiritide

Inamrinone and Milrinone (Phosphodiesterase-3 inhibitors)

These are selective phosphodiesterase-3 (PDE-3) inhibitors.

PDE-3 inhibition leads to an increase of cAMP levels. This further results in an increase in contractility (positive inotropic) and vasodilator actions. Hence, they are called 'inodilator' drugs.

These are administered only intravenously.

The adverse effects of inamrinone include nausea, vomiting, arrhythmia, thrombocytopenia and increase in liver enzymes. Milrinone is less likely to cause thrombocytopenia and hepatotoxicity but it causes arrhythmia.

PDE-3 inhibitors are used only for short-term circulatory support in acute heart failure and severe exacerbation of chronic heart failure.

Nesiritide (Natriuretic peptide)

Nesiritide is the recombinant form of the brain natriuretic peptide, which is normally produced by the ventricular myocardium.

It is approved for use in acute (not chronic) heart failure.

It is a vasodilator and also causes diuresis. It is administered only intravenously. It has a short half-life of 18 minutes.

The most common adverse effect is excessive hypotension. It has also been reported to cause renal damage.

ASSESS YOURSELF (Examination Questions of Various Universities)

1. Mention different categories of drugs used in the treatment of congestive heart failure.

   Give one example in each category.

2. Discuss the mechanism of action, adverse effects and clinical uses of digoxin.

3. Explain the rationale of using:

   a. Spironolactone in congestive heart failure (CHF)

   b. Beta blockers in the management of CHF

   c. Digoxin in the management of CHF

   d. Digoxin in the management of atrial fibrillation with heart failure

   e. Enalapril in the management of CHF

   f. Clonidine should not be stopped suddenly

MULTIPLE CHOICE QUESTIONS

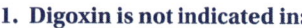

1. Digoxin is not indicated in:

   (Recent Question 2016)

   a. Atrial flutter   b. Atrial fibrillation
   c. High output failure d. PSVT

2. Digoxin toxicity is enhanced by all of the following except:

   (AIIMS May 2010, 2009, Nov 2008)

   a. Hyperkalemia   b. Hypercalcemia
   c. Hypomagnesemia   d. Renal failure

3. Which of the following is a monovalent cation that can reverse a digitalis induced arrhythmia?

   (Recent Question 2016)

   a. Digibind antibodies b. Lignocaine
   c. Magnesium   d. Potassium

4. Half-life of digoxin is: *(Recent Question 2016)*

   a. 12 hours   b. 24 hours
   c. 36 hours   d. 48 hours

5. Most effective method of treatment of digitalis toxicity is: *(Recent Question 2016)*

   a. Hemodialysis   b. Cardioversion
   c. Digoxin antibody d. Atropine

6. All of the following drugs are used for the treatment of congestive heart failure except:

   (Recent Question 2016)

   a. Nitroglycerine   b. Spironolactone
   c. Nesiritide   d. Trimetazidine

7. All of the following statements about nesiritide are true except: *(Recent Question 2016)*

   a. It is a BNP analogue
   b. It can be used in decompensated CHF

   c. It can be administered orally
   d. It causes loss of Na^+ in the urine

8. Digibind is used to: *(Recent Question 2016)*

   a. Potentiate the action of digoxin
   b. Decrease the metabolism of digoxin
   c. Treat digoxin toxicity
   d. Rapidly digitalize the patient

9. Digitalis toxicity can cause:

   (Recent Question 2016)

   a. Hyperkalemia   b. Nausea
   c. Arrhythmias   d. All of the above

10. Drug used in heart failure:

    (Recent Question 2016)

    a. Celiprolol   b. Carteolol
    c. Carvedilol   d. All of the above

11. Digoxin increases refractoriness at:

    (Recent Question 2016)

    a. SA node   b. AV node
    c. Ventricular cells d. Atrial cells

12. Drug used in the treatment of congestive heart failure is: *(NIMHANS 2013)*

    a. ACE inhibitor   b. Beta blocker
    c. ART blocker   d. All of the above

13. Digoxin acts by inhibiting:*(MH CET 2014, 2007)*

    a. $Na^+ K^+$ ATPase   b. $H^+ K^+$ ATPase
    c. $NA^+–K^+–2C1$ channel
    d. $Na^+ – H^+$ ATPase

14. Which inotropes act on both D receptor and alpha receptor: *(PGI May 2018)*

    a. Dopamine   b. Epinephrine
    c. Isoprenaline d. Nor-epinephrine
    e. Phenylephrine

Ans.

1.	(c)	2.	(a)	3.	(d)	4.	(c)	5.	(c)	6.	(d)
7.	(c)	8.	(c)	9.	(d)	10.	(c)	11.	(b)	12.	(d)
13.	(a)	14.	(a)								

16 Drug Therapy for Dyslipidemia (Hyperlipidemia)

Dyslipidemia (hyperlipidemia) refers to an increase in the levels of plasma cholesterol and/or triglycerides (TGs), or a decrease in the levels of high-density lipoproteins.

These contribute to the development of atherosclerosis which is associated with the development of ischemic cardiovascular and cerebrovascular diseases. These diseases are a major cause of morbidity and mortality (Figure 1).

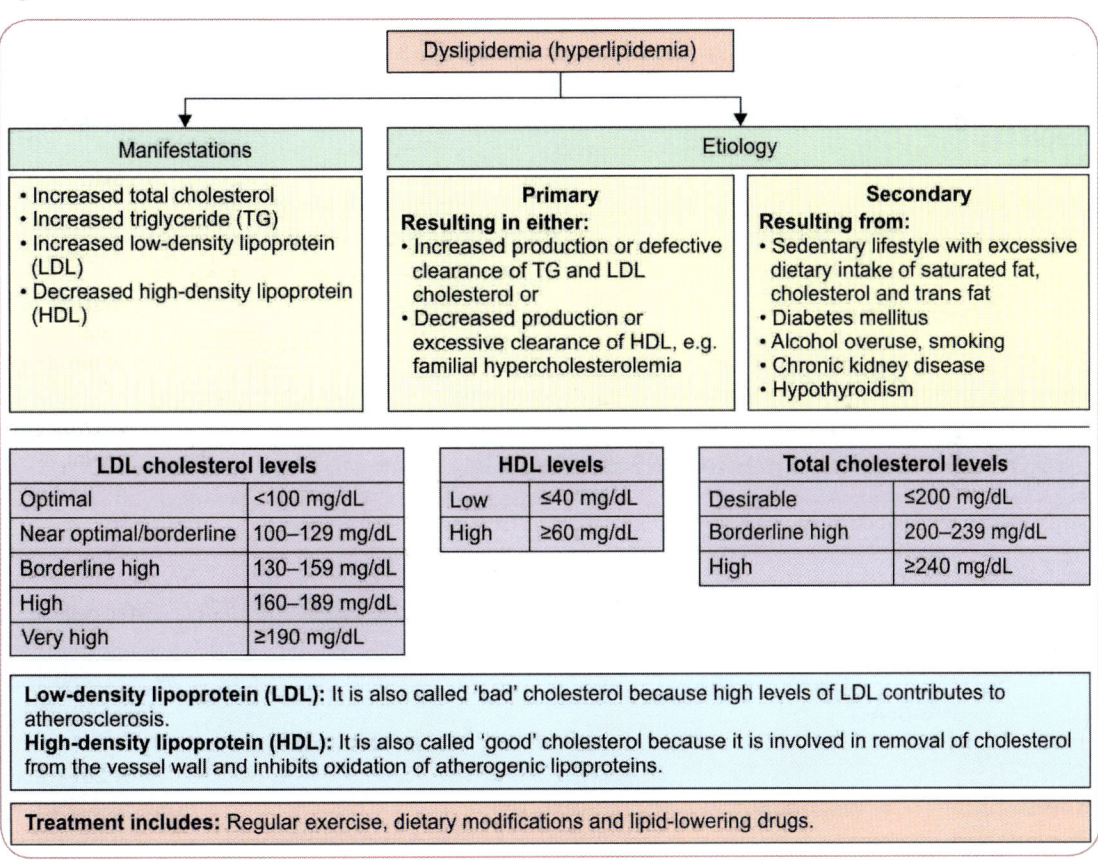

Figure 1: Dyslipidemia

The various types of lipoproteins involved in the transport of lipids in the circulation is mentioned in Table 1.

TABLE 1	Lipoproteins
Chylomicrons and very low density lipoprotein (VLDL)	• Triglyceride rich lipoproteins • Transport triacylglycerol to cells in the body
Low density lipoprotein (LDL)	• Transport cholesterol to cells in the body
High density lipoprotein (HDL)	• Removal of cholesterol from the vessel walls

The classification of hyperlipoproteinemia is mentioned in Table 2.

TABLE 2	Fredrickson classification of hyperlipoproteinemia	
Phenotype	**Lipoprotein(s) increased**	**Lipids elevated**
I	Chylomicrons	Triglycerides
II A	LDL	Cholesterol
II B	LDL and VLDL	Triglycerides and cholesterol
III	VLDL and chylomicron remnants	Triglycerides and cholesterol
IV	VLDL	Triglycerides
V	Chylomicrons and VLDL	Triglycerides and cholesterol

CLASSIFICATION OF DRUGS USED FOR DYSLIPIDEMIA

The classification of drugs used for dyslipidemia is mentioned in Table 3.

TABLE 3	Drugs for dyslipidemia
HMG-CoA reductase inhibitors (Statins)	Lovastatin, simvastatin, pravastatin, atorvastatin, rosuvastatin, fluvastatin, pitavastatin
Lipoprotein lipase activators (Fibrates)	Clofibrate, gemfibrozil, fenofibrate, bezafibrate
Inhibit lipolysis and triglyceride synthesis	Niacin (Nicotinic acid)
Bile acid sequestrants (Resins)	Cholestyramine, colestipol
Inhibitors of intestinal cholesterol absorption	Ezetimibe
Newer drug for treatment of dyslipidemia	Lomitapide

HMG-CoA REDUCTASE INHIBITORS (STATINS)

Statins are the most effective and best tolerated drugs in the treatment of dyslipidemia.

Mechanism of Action

Statins competitively inhibits the enzyme HMG-CoA reductase, which catalyzes the rate limiting step in cholesterol synthesis (Figure 2).

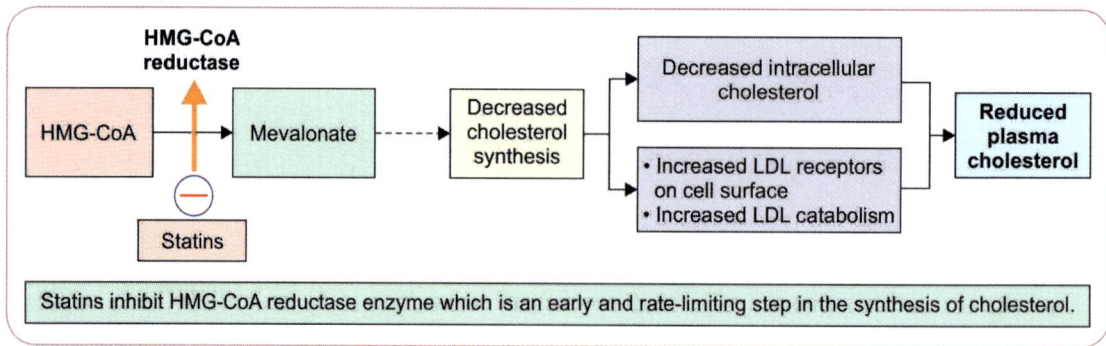

Figure 2: Mechanism of action of statins

The inhibition of cholesterol synthesis (by statins) leads to depletion of intracellular supply of cholesterol.

The decrease in intracellular cholesterol results in a compensatory increase in the number of LDL receptors at the cell surface. The LDL receptors bind to the circulating LDL molecules resulting in an increased uptake of the circulating LDL and finally its catabolism inside the cells.

Hence, statins are highly effective in decreasing plasma LDL cholesterol. They also cause a modest decrease in plasma TG levels and a small increase in plasma HDL cholesterol.

Other beneficial effects of statins include:
- Atherosclerotic plaque stabilization
- Anti-inflammatory and antioxidant actions
- Improvement of coronary endothelial function
- Decreased platelet aggregation

Pharmacokinetics

Among statins, **L**ovastatin and **S**imvastatin are Prodrugs and are converted in the liver to their active forms. The rest of the statins are administered in their active forms.

The below mentioned points is noteworthy regarding various statins:
- All statins have high first pass metabolism in the liver. The excretion occurs mainly through bile and feces.
- The half-lives of most statins range from 1 to 3 hours except atorvastatin (14 hours), pitavastatin (12 hours) and rosuvastatin (19 hours).
- As hepatic cholesterol synthesis occurs predominantly in the midnight, the statins should be administered at night to achieve maximum effectiveness. However, this is not required for atorvastatin, pitavastatin and rosuvastatin because of their longer half-lives.
- Regarding potency, pitavastatin, rosuvastatin and atorvastatin are the most potent statins followed by simvastatin and pravastatin, which are further followed by lovastatin and fluvastatin.

Adverse Effects

The key adverse effects of statins are mentioned in Figure 3.

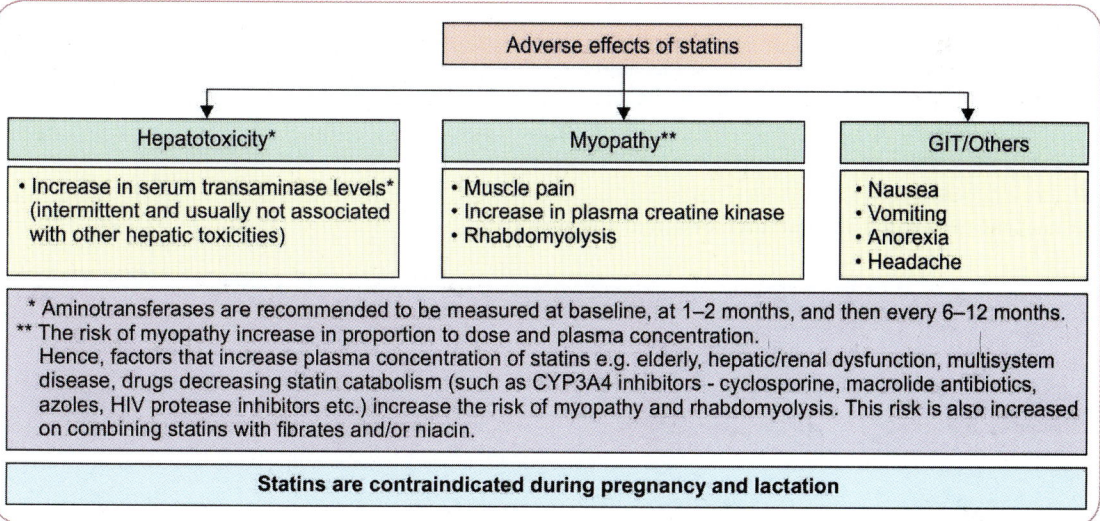

Figure 3: Adverse effects of statins

Drug Interactions

The key drug interactions with statins are mentioned in Figure 4.

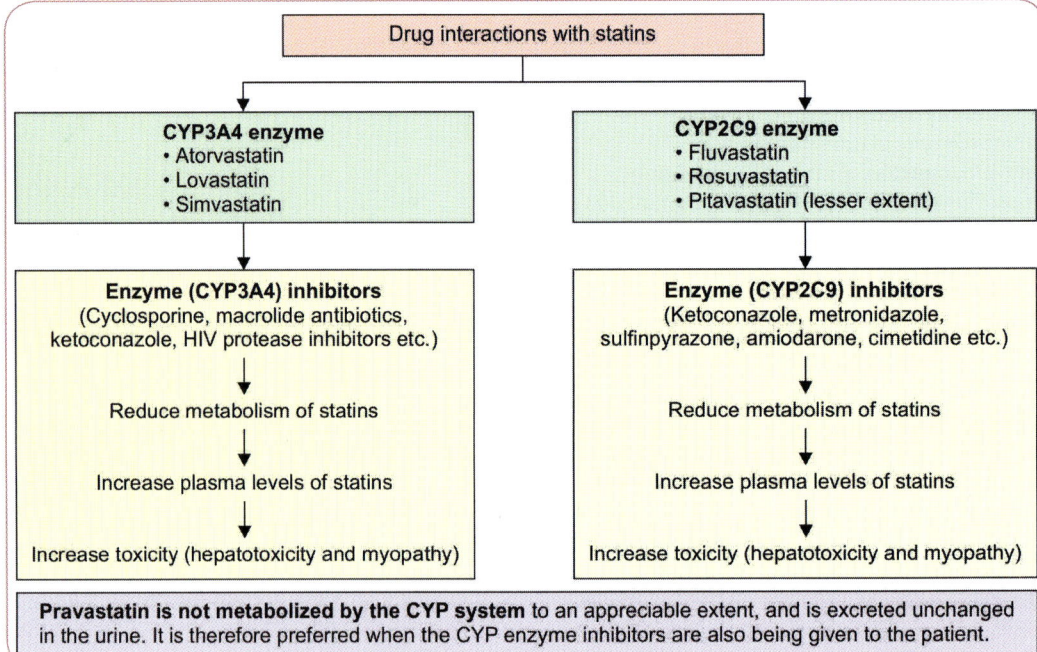

Figure 4: Drug interactions with statins

Clinical Uses

○ Primary hyperlipidemia with increased LDL and total cholesterol levels
○ Secondary hypercholesterolemia (due to diabetes, nephrotic syndrome etc.)

▌ LIPOPROTEIN LIPASE ACTIVATORS (FIBRATES)

The mechanism of action of fibrates is mentioned in Figure 5.

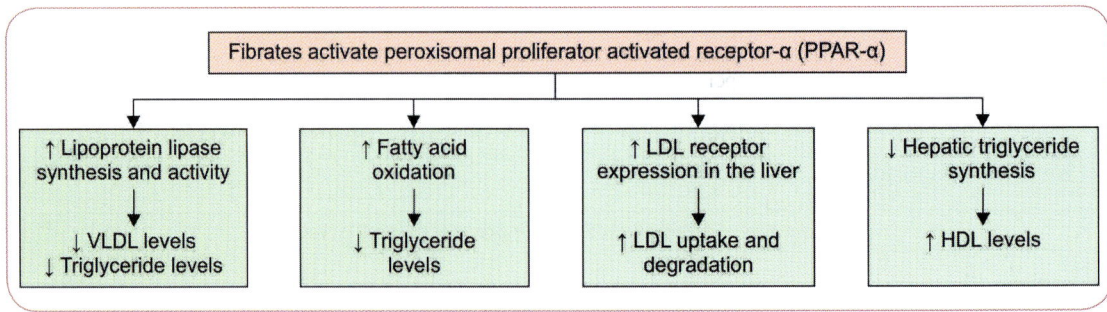

Figure 5: Fibrates—mechanism of action

Adverse Effects

○ Epigastric distress, diarrhea
○ Skin rashes, bodyache, blurred vision

- Cholelithiasis
- Myositis, myopathy, rhabdomyolysis
- Risk of myopathy is increased when fibrates are given along with statins
- May potentiate the effects of coumarin type anticoagulants such as warfarin, acenocoumarol or phenprocoumon. Careful INR monitoring is required.

Clinical Uses

- Treatment of severe hypertriglyceridemia with or without low HDL cholesterol
- Mixed hyperlipidemia when a statin is contraindicated or not tolerated

INHIBITS LIPOLYSIS AND TRIGLYCERIDE SYNTHESIS

Niacin is a water-soluble B-complex vitamin. It has hypolipidemic effects at much higher doses than that required for vitamin effects.

The hypolipidemic actions of niacin are mentioned in Figure 6.

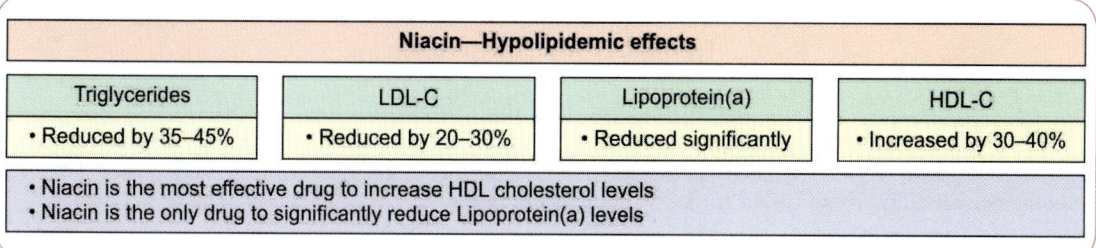

Figure 6: Niacin—hypolipidemic effects

Mechanism of Action (Figure 7)

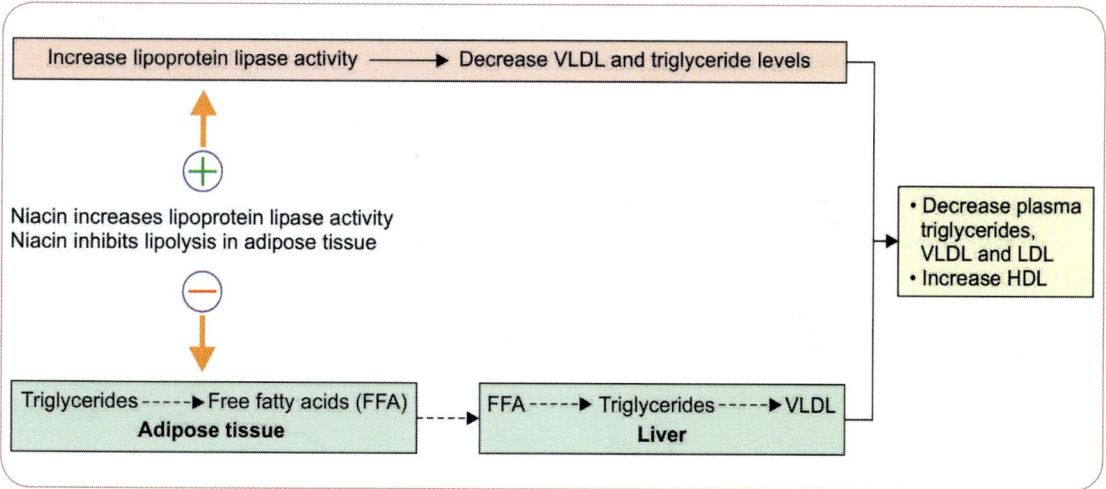

Figure 7: Niacin—mechanism of action

Adverse Effects

The common adverse effects that limit patient's compliance are flushing and dyspepsia.
The key adverse effects of niacin are mentioned in Figure 8.

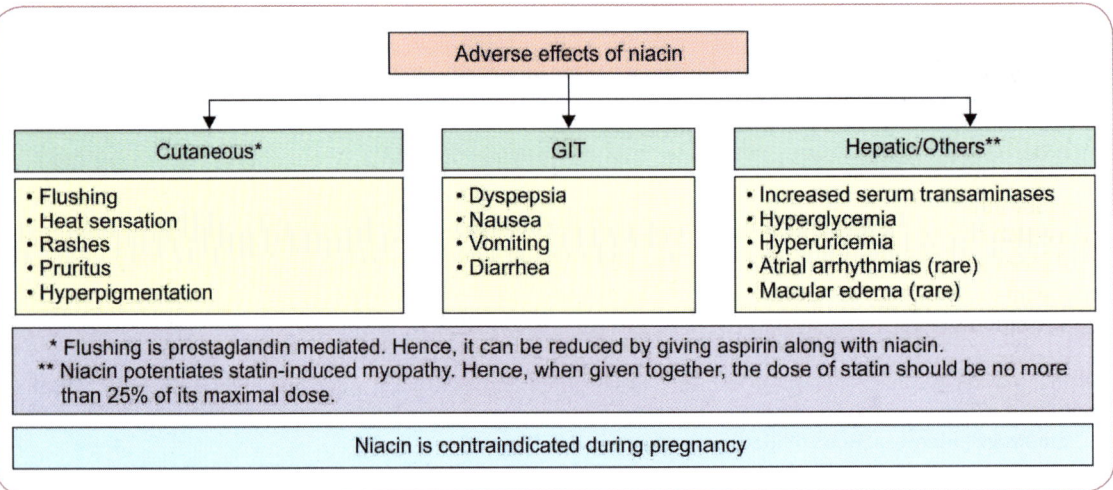

Figure 8: Adverse effects of niacin

Clinical Uses

Niacin is used mainly in patients with hypertriglyceridemia. It is mostly used for lowering VLDL and raising HDL levels. It is usually administered as an adjunct to statins or fibrates.

BILE ACID SEQUESTRANTS (RESINS)

The resins are large molecules that are not absorbed from the intestine. The resins bind bile acids in the intestine and interrupt their absorption.

Normally, more than 95% of bile acids are absorbed from the intestine. The resins interrupt this absorption. This leads to an increase in excretion of bile acids in the stools and a decrease pool of bile acids in the liver. This results in an increase in hepatic bile acid synthesis from cholesterol.

The hepatic cholesterol content therefore decreases leading to an increased expression of LDL receptors on the cell surface. This results in an increased LDL clearance from the plasma and a decrease in plasma LDL cholesterol (LDL-C) levels.

Rationale for Combining Resins with Statins

The resins decrease bile acid absorption which results in a reduction in hepatic cholesterol content. However, this leads to a compensatory upregulation of HMG-CoA reductase enzyme activity in the liver resulting in increased cholesterol synthesis.

Hence, combining statins with resins prevents the increase in HMG-CoA reductase enzyme activity induced by resins. This substantially increases the effectiveness of resins.

Adverse Effects

As the resins are not absorbed from the intestine, they do not lead to systemic adverse effects.

The adverse effects commonly seen with resins are bloating, dyspepsia, nausea, flatulence and constipation.

Resins may impair the absorption of fat soluble vitamins (A, D, E and K).

Resins bind to and reduce the absorption of many drugs in the intestine. These include digoxin, warfarin, thiazides, furosemide, thyroxine, aspirin, phenylbutazone etc. Therefore, other medications should be given at least 1–2 hours before or 4–6 hours after resins.

Resins may lead to an increase in triglycerides; therefore, they are contraindicated in patients with significant triglyceridemia (>400 mg/dL).

Clinical Uses

As statins are very effective for use as monotherapy, resins are used as second choice drugs if statins do not effectively lower the LDL-C levels.

INHIBITORS OF INTESTINAL CHOLESTEROL ABSORPTION

Ezetimibe inhibits intestinal cholesterol absorption. It inhibits both dietary and biliary cholesterol absorption. The main action outcome is reduction in LDL-C levels.

If given alone, the maximal efficacy of ezetimibe for decreasing LDL-C is 15–20%. This decrease in LDL-C is equivalent to, or less than what is achieved by using 10–20 mg of statins.

The rationale for combining ezetimibe with statins is mentioned in Table 4.

TABLE 4	Ezetimibe with statins
• Statins inhibit cholesterol synthesis in the liver. This leads to a compensatory increase in intestinal cholesterol absorption. • Ezetimibe inhibits intestinal cholesterol absorption. This leads to a compensatory increase in cholesterol synthesis in the liver. Combining ezetimibe with statins prevents both the increase in cholesterol synthesis induced by ezetimibe, and the increase in intestinal cholesterol absorption induced by statins.	

The combination of highest simvastatin dose (80 mg) and ezetimibe (10 mg) produced LDL-C reduction by 60%, which is greater than what can be achieved by any statin as monotherapy.

Adverse Effects

There are no specific adverse effects except for rare allergic reactions and a low incidence of reversible hepatic dysfunction. Myositis has rarely been noted.

NEWER DRUG FOR TREATMENT OF DYSLIPIDEMIA

Lomitapide

Lomitapide is a selective inhibitor of microsomal triglyceride transfer protein (MTP).

MTP plays a key role in the assembly of ApoB containing lipoproteins in the liver and intestines. Inhibition of MTP decreases the secretion of VLDL and reduces the accumulation of LDL in plasma.

Lomitapide use is restricted to adults with homozygous familial hypercholesterolemia, as an adjunct to a low-fat diet and other lipid lowering drugs.

Lomitapide can cause elevations in alanine aminotransferase, aspartate aminotransferase and hepatic steatosis. Monitoring of liver function tests is recommended.

EFFECTS OF ANTIDYSLIPIDEMIC DRUGS ON LIPOPROTEINS

Table 5 summarizes the effects of various antidyslipidemic drugs on the levels of triglycerides, HDL and LDL.

TABLE 5	Effects of antidyslipidemic drugs		
Drug class	Triglycerides	HDL	LDL
HMG-CoA reductase inhibitors (Statins)	↓↓	↑↑	↓↓↓↓
Lipoprotein lipase activators (Fibrates)	↓↓↓↓	↑↑	↓
Inhibits lipolysis and triglyceride synthesis (Niacin)	↓↓↓	↑↑↑	↓↓
Bile acid sequestrants (Resins)	↑	↑	↓↓↓
Inhibitors of intestinal cholesterol absorption (Ezetimibe)	↓	↑	↓

ASSESS YOURSELF (Examination Questions of Various Universities)

1. **Enumerate hypolipidemic drugs. Discuss the mechanism of action, pharmacokinetics, adverse effects and clinical uses of statins.**

2. **Describe the mechanism of action, therapeutic uses and adverse effects of atorvastatin.**

3. **Write short notes on:**
   a. HMG CoA reductase inhibitors
   b. Rosuvastatin
   c. Ezetimibe

4. **Explain why statins are given in the night.**

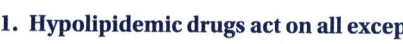

MULTIPLE CHOICE QUESTIONS

1. **Hypolipidemic drugs act on all except:**
   (Recent Question 2016)
   a. HMG CoA reductase
   b. Lipoprotein lipase
   c. Acyl CoA, cholesterol acyl transferase 1
   d. Peripheral decarboxylase

2. **Drug that decreases LpA in blood:**
   (Recent Question 2016)
   a. Statin   b. Nicotinic acid
   c. Ezetimibe   d. CETP inhibitors

3. **Mechanism of action of fibrates in treatment of hyperlipidemia is:** *(Recent Question 2016)*
   a. Activator of lipoprotein lipase
   b. PPAR alpha agonist
   c. Decreased synthesis of VLDL
   d. Inhibitor of CETP

4. **Mechanism of action of cholestyramine is:**
   (Recent Question 2016)
   a. Bind to bile acid
   b. Decrease HMG-COA
   c. Increase excretion of cholesterol
   d. Decrease utilization of cholesterol

5. **Drug that inhibits absorption of cholesterol from intestine:** *(Recent Question 2016)*
   a. Resins   b. Ezetimibe
   c. Niacin   d. Orlistat

6. **Competitive inhibition of rate limiting step in cholesterol synthesis is by:**
   (Recent Question 2016)
   a. Bile acid sequestrants
   b. Fibric acid derivatives
   c. Statins
   d. Nicotinic acid

7. **Mechanism of action of lovastatin is by:**
   (Recent Question 2016)
   a. Competitive inhibition of rate limiting step in cholesterol synthesis
   b. Bile acid sequestration
   c. Activate lipoprotein lipase
   d. Inhibits lipolysis and triglyceride

8. **The vitamin which in large doses decreases triglycerides and cholesterol levels:**
   (Recent Question 2016)
   a. Vitamin B_{12} b. Nicotinic acid
   c. Vitamin B_1 d. Retinol

9. **Mechanism of action of clofibrate:**
   (Recent Question 2016)
   a. Inhibit HMG CoA reductase
   b. Inhibit HMG CoA synthase
   c. Inhibit absorption of cholesterol
   d. Stimulates lipoprotein lipase

10. **Drug contraindicated in severe hypertrigly ceridemia is:** *(JIPMER 2010)*
    a. Fibrates   b. Simvastatin
    c. Niacin   d. Cholestyramine

11. **HDL is specifically increased by:** *(WB PG 2007)*
    a. Lovastatin   b. Niacin
    c. Gemfibrozil   d. Probucol

12. **Drug possessing highest efficacy to increase plasma HDL is:** *(MH CET 2009)*
    a. Ezetimibe   b. Nicotinic acid
    c. Gemfibrozil   d. Rosuvastatin

13. **HMG CoA reductase acts by inhibiting:**
    (MH CET 2005)
    a. Ezetimibe   b. Gemfibrozil
    c. Clofibrate   d. Lovastatin

Ans.

1.	(d)	2.	(b)	3.	(b)	4.	(a)	5.	(b)	6.	(c)
7.	(a)	8.	(b)	9.	(d)	10.	(d)	11.	(b)	12.	(b)
13.	(d)										

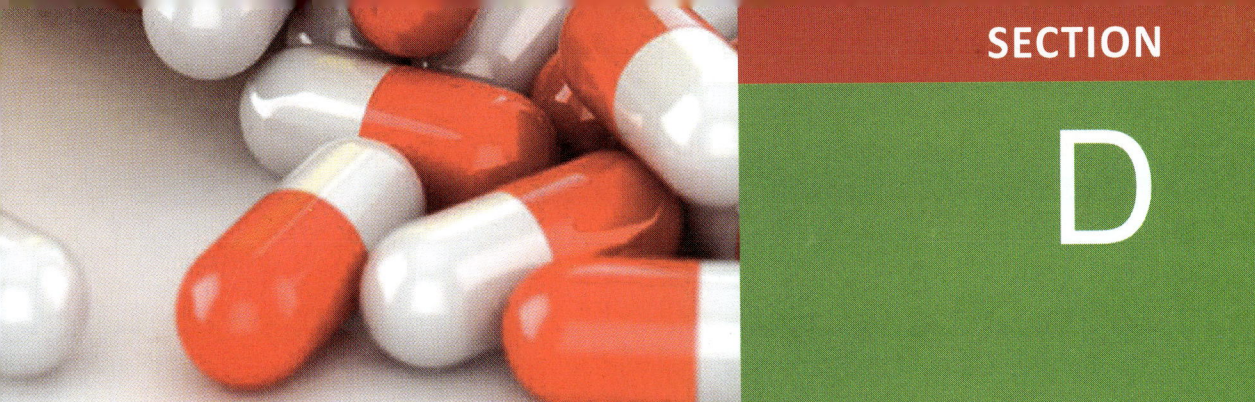

Drugs Acting on the Central Nervous System

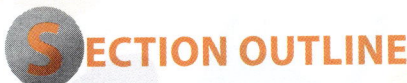

SECTION OUTLINE

17 Alcohol (Ethyl and Methyl Alcohol)

ETHYL ALCOHOL (ETHANOL)

Alcohol, mainly in the form of ethyl alcohol, is produced from the fermentation of sugars (Figure 1).

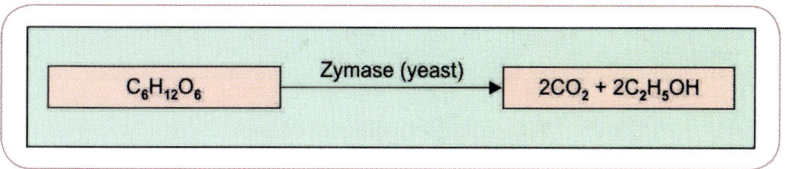

$$C_6H_{12}O_6 \xrightarrow{\text{Zymase (yeast)}} 2CO_2 + 2C_2H_5OH$$

Figure 1: Fermentation of sugars

Pharmacological Actions

The key effects of alcohol are mentioned in Table 1.

TABLE 1	Effects of alcohol
Topical/Local	• Astringent (precipitates surface proteins) • Antiseptic • Counterirritant
Central nervous system (CNS)	• CNS depressant → higher doses can lead to loss of consciousness, medullary paralysis and death • Slowing of reflexes • Initially CNS excitement is observed (due to behavioral disinhibition), that progresses to CNS depression as the plasma concentration increases
Cardiovascular system	• Dose dependent effects • Low to moderate doses → cutaneous vasodilatation (flushing), tachycardia • Higher doses → depression of myocardium and vasomotor center, decrease in blood pressure
Hematological	• Regular consumption of small amounts → increase HDL cholesterol → decrease risk of coronary artery disease • Chronic alcoholics → megaloblastic anemia due to interference with folate metabolism
Body temperature	• Increase heat loss due to vasodilatation • Decrease body temperature

Liver	• Chronic alcohol intake results in:
	  ▪ Alcoholic fatty liver disease
	  ▪ Alcoholic hepatitis
	  ▪ Cirrhosis

Respiratory system	• Depression of respiratory center

Contd...

Gastrointestinal tract	• Increase gastric acid secretion, gastritis • Acute pancreatitis
Renal	• Diuresis due to ingestion of water along with alcohol and inhibition of ADH release
Glucose metabolism	• Moderate intake can lead to hyperglycemia • Acute intoxication can lead to hypoglycemia

Metabolism of Ethanol

Ethanol is mainly metabolized in the liver by the enzyme alcohol dehydrogenase (Figure 2). Some amount of ethanol is also oxidized by hepatic microsomal enzymes.

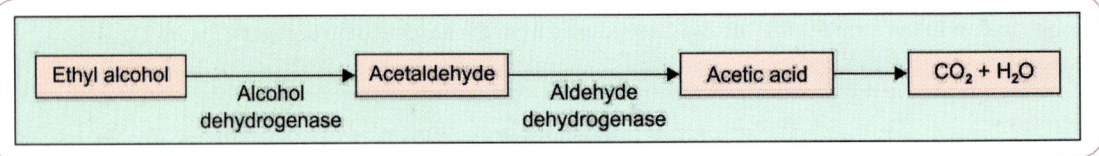

Figure 2: Metabolism of ethanol

Ethanol undergoes zero order elimination kinetics. This means that a constant amount of the drug is metabolized per unit of time. If the plasma concentration increases, the rate of metabolism does not proportionately increase. A constant amount of alcohol continues to be metabolized in the body (Table 2).

TABLE 2	Zero order kinetics—ethanol

- A constant amount of ethanol is metabolized per unit of time.
- The rate of alcohol metabolism is constant and does not depend on its plasma concentration.
- If the plasma concentration of ethanol increases, the rate of metabolism does not proportionately increase. A constant amount of the alcohol continues to be metabolized.

Clinical Uses

The clinical uses of alcohol are mentioned below:

Antiseptic

○ Ethanol (in concentration 40–90%) is effective as an antiseptic and cleansing agent. The antiseptic efficacy varies with ethanol concentration as follows:
  - 20–70% → efficacy increases
  - 70–90% → efficacy remains constant
  - >90% → efficacy decreases
○ Generally, ethanol (in concentration of 70%) is used for disinfection of the skin before invasive procedures
○ It is an irritant and should not be used on open wounds, ulcers, mucus membranes and sensitive skin (scrotum)
○ It does not kill spores but promotes rusting → considered a poor disinfectant for instruments

Methanol Poisoning

Ethanol competes with methanol for the metabolizing enzyme alcohol dehydrogenase, and saturates it. This results in reduced formation of toxic metabolites of methanol such as formaldehyde and formic acid.

Prevention of Bedsores

Alcohol is topically applied in bedridden patients for the prevention of bedsores.

Pyrexia

Alcohol sponges can be used.

Neuralgias

Trigeminal and other neuralgias, cancer pain → injection of alcohol near the nerves or ganglia can lead to analgesia.

ACUTE ALCOHOL INTOXICATION (ACUTE ETHANOL OVERDOSE)

Acute alcohol intoxication is a medical emergency. There is a risk of fatality due to conditions such as respiratory depression, aspiration etc.

The clinical features include the following:
- Hypotension, arrhythmias, hypoglycemia
- Gastritis, emesis, aspiration
- Respiratory and cardiac depression
- Sedation, drowsiness, unconsciousness, coma, death

The management of acute alcohol intoxication include the following:
- Airway protection is vital
  - Endotracheal intubation and ventilatory support including mechanical ventilation
- Maintenance of fluid and electrolyte balance including correction of acidosis by sodium bicarbonate
- Circulatory management including adequate hydration
- Correction of hypoglycemia by glucose
- Thiamine administration to treat or prevent Wernicke's encephalopathy
- Hemodialysis, gastric lavage may be considered in specific situations, if deemed appropriate

MANAGEMENT OF CHRONIC ALCOHOLISM

The management of chronic alcoholism requires a multipronged approach consisting of the following:
- Counseling including psychiatric care, occupational therapy etc.
- Specialist consultation for any alcohol-induced complications
- Medications
  - Disulfiram (aldehyde dehydrogenase inhibitor)
  - Acamprosate
  - Naltrexone
  - Ondansetron, topiramate

Disulfiram (Aldehyde Dehydrogenase Inhibitor)

Disulfiram is used as an alcohol avoidance therapy.

It causes an irreversible inhibition of the enzyme aldehyde dehydrogenase. This leads to an increase in the levels of acetaldehyde (in blood and tissues) in patients taking alcohol. Increased levels of acetaldehyde cause distressing symptoms in the patient (aldehyde syndrome) (Figure 3).

These symptoms include headache, flushing, sweating, nausea, vomiting, confusion, fainting, blurring of vision, seizures, hypotension, circulatory collapse, arrhythmias, coma etc.

Due to these distressing symptoms that occur when alcohol is consumed by a patient on disulfiram, the patient develops an aversion towards alcohol.

However, a careful review should be performed to confirm if it is appropriate to administer disulfiram in a particular patient.

Adverse effects of disulfiram include drowsiness, fatigue, nausea, vomiting and skin rashes. Fatalities have also been reported following alcohol intake in patients on disulfiram therapy.

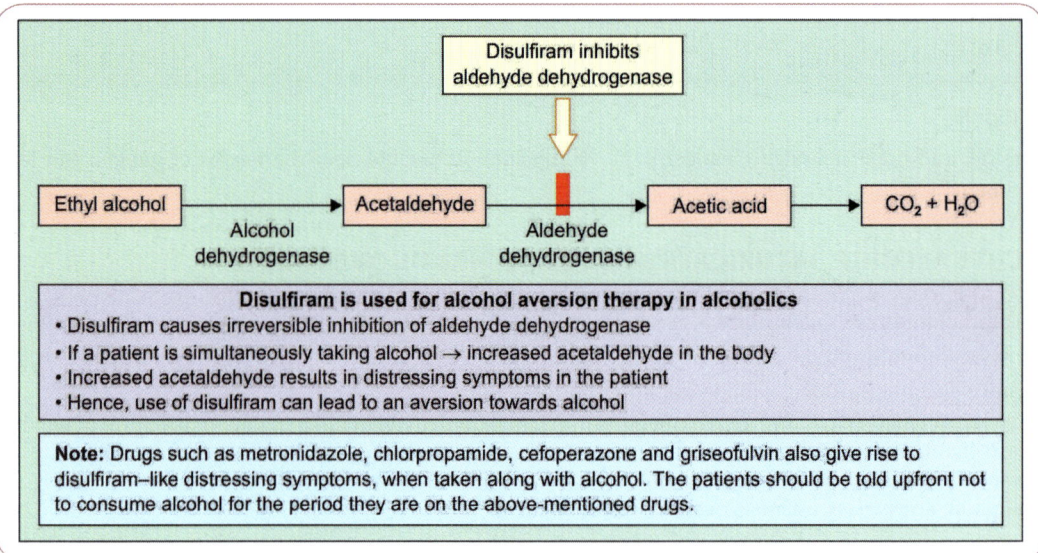

Figure 3: Disulfiram as alcohol aversion therapy

Acamprosate

Acamprosate is a GABA analogue. It is used as maintenance therapy to reduce relapse drinking in abstinent alcoholics. In this regard, its efficacy is similar to naltrexone.

A possible mechanism of action is stimulation of inhibitory GABAergic neurotransmission and inhibition of excitatory amino acids, such as glutamate.

It is administered in a dose of 666 mg thrice a day. It is well tolerated. The main adverse effect is diarrhea. It is mainly excreted unchanged in the urine.

Naltrexone

It is a long acting opioid antagonist that can reduce the craving to alcohol. It is useful in preventing relapse in alcoholics.

It is administered in a dose of 50 mg once a day for several months. The main adverse effect is nausea. It can cause dose-dependent hepatotoxicity.

ALCOHOL WITHDRAWAL

Alcohol withdrawal can occur following sudden cessation of alcohol intake in chronic alcoholics. The clinical manifestations include the following:
- Tremors, restlessness, weakness, sweating, hyperreflexia
- Hallucinations–visual or auditory
- Delirium tremens, anxiety attacks, ataxia, vestibular abnormalities, collapse

The management include the following measures:
- Intensive care management may be required in severe cases
- Thiamine is administered to prevent Wernicke-Korsakoff syndrome
- Benzodiazepines (e.g. diazepam, chlordiazepoxide) are often used. They help in the management of symptoms such as anxiety, mental confusion, seizures, abnormal sleep, palpitations etc.
- Counseling including psychiatric care, occupational therapy etc.
- Specialist consultation for any alcohol-induced complications

METHYL ALCOHOL (METHANOL, WOOD ALCOHOL)

Methyl alcohol is a component of various industrial solvents (e.g. antifreeze, paint removers). It is also a constituent of illegally manufactured/adulterated alcoholic beverage.

Methyl alcohol only has toxicological importance.
Methyl alcohol is metabolized to toxic compounds such as formaldehyde and formic acid (Figure 4).

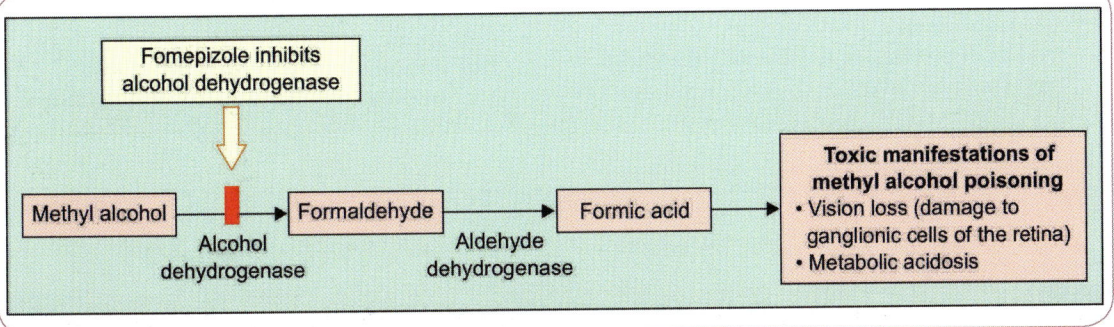

Figure 4: Metabolism of methyl alcohol

Clinical Manifestations of Methyl Alcohol Intoxication

It is a medical emergency and fatalities can occur in patients of methyl alcohol intoxication. The key clinical manifestations are mentioned in Table 3.

TABLE 3	Clinical manifestations of methyl alcohol intoxication
Neurologic features	• Drowsiness, sedation, seizures, coma
Vision loss	• Flashes of light, blurring of vision, blindness (occurs due to formic acid induced damage to the ganglionic cells of the retina)
Others	• Nausea, vomiting, epigastric pain • Metabolic acidosis • Respiratory depression, dyspnea • Pancreatic necrosis

Management of Methyl Alcohol Intoxication

- Airway protection is essential
  - Endotracheal intubation and ventilatory support including mechanical ventilation
- Maintenance of fluid and electrolyte balance including correction of acidosis by sodium bicarbonate. Bicarbonate may reverse the visual damage and reduce the amount of formic acid.
- Circulatory management including adequate hydration
- Protection of the eyes from light by keeping the patient in a dark room
- Ethanol (10%) is administered through nasogastric (Ryle's) tube. The rationale of using ethanol in methanol poisoning is as follows:
  - Ethanol has a higher affinity than methanol for alcohol dehydrogenase.
  - Ethanol administration results in saturation of alcohol dehydrogenase. Hence, the metabolism of methanol is inhibited.
  - This leads to reduced formation of toxic metabolites of methanol, such as formaldehyde and formic acid.
- Fomepizole (4-methylpyrazole)
  - It is an inhibitor of alcohol dehydrogenase. It leads to inhibition of metabolism of methanol. This results in reduced formation of toxic metabolites of methanol, such as formaldehyde and formic acid (*see* Figure 5).
  - Fomepizole does not lead to inebriation (seen with ethanol) and has a longer half-life.
  - Limited availability and cost can be an issue with fomepizole.
- Hemodialysis
  - It can remove formic acid and methanol from the body
- Calcium leucovorin
  - It can enhance the metabolism of formic acid and reduce its concentration

ASSESS YOURSELF (Examination Questions of Various Universities)

1. Discuss the drug treatment of acute methyl alcohol poisoning.
2. Explain the rationale for the use of ethanol in methanol poisoning.

3. Write short notes on:
   a. Disulfiram
   b. Management of chronic alcoholism
   c. Management of acute alcohol intoxication

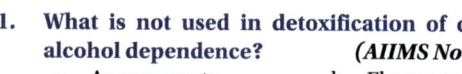

MULTIPLE CHOICE QUESTIONS

1. What is not used in detoxification of chronic alcohol dependence? *(AIIMS Nov 2015)*
   a. Acamprosate   b. Flumazenil
   c. Naltrexone   d. Disulfiram

2. Anticraving agents for alcohol dependence are all except: *(Recent Question 2016)*
   a. Lorazepam   b. Acamprosate
   c. Topiramate   d. Naltrexone

3. Which of the following is used to maintain abstinence in alcohol dependence?
   (Recent Question 2016)
   a. Naltrexone   b. Clonidine
   c. Disulfiram   d. Naloxone

4. The combination of alcohol and disulfiram results in nausea and hypotension as a result of accumulation of: *(Recent Question 2016)*
   a. Acetaldehyde   b. Acetate
   c. Methanol   d. NADH

5. Disulfiram like reaction is not seen with:
   (Recent Question 2016)
   a. Amoxicillin   b. Metronidazole
   c. Cefoperazone   d. Disulfiram

6. Administration of disulfiram in an alcoholic can cause all these side effects except:
   (JIPMER 2014)
   a. Flushing   b. Headache
   c. Hypertension   d. Nausea

7. Ethanol is used in ethylene glycol poisoning. What is the mechanism of action?
   (JIPMER 2013)
   a. Competitive inhibition of alcohol dehydrogenase
   b. Competitive inhibition of aldehyde dehydrogenase
   c. Competitive inhibition of NADPH oxidase
   d. Noncompetitive inhibition of aldehyde dehydrogenase

8. Disulfiram is used in the Rx of: *(TNPG 2011)*
   a. Mania   b. Schizophrenia
   c. Alcohol abuse   d. Psychosis

9. Disulfiram with acamprosate is used for:
   (TNPG 2008)
   a. Maintenance therapy of alcohol abstinence
   b. Acute opioid poisoning
   c. Cannabis over dosage
   d. Neuroleptic malignant syndrome

Ans.

| 1. (b) | 2. (a) | 3. (a) | 4. (a) | 5. (a) | 6. (c) |
| 7. (a) | 8. (c) | 9. (a) | | | |

18

Antidepressant and Antianxiety Drugs

Depression and anxiety are the most common mental disorders. Approximately 10–15% of population experience an episode of major depression at some point in their lifetime.

Depression is twice as common in females as compared to males, and the incidence increases with age in both sexes.

Depression may be classified into either major depression (unipolar depression) or manic-depressive illness (bipolar depression) (Figure 1).

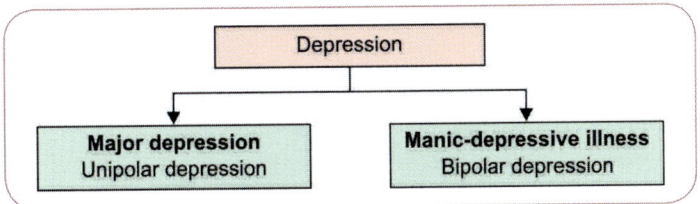

Figure 1: Types of depression

Major depression is characterized by the presence of following features (on most days for a period of at least 2 weeks):

o Depressed or sad mood for most parts of the day
o Markedly diminished interest or pleasure in most activities
o Significant weight loss or weight gain (due to altered eating or activity patterns)
o Sleep disturbance–increase or loss of sleep
o Psychomotor agitation or retardation
o Fatigue or loss of energy
o Feeling of guilt or worthlessness
o Diminished ability to think or concentrate
o Suicidal ideation

Manic-depressive illness (bipolar depression) is characterized by alternate cycles of mania (elevated mood) and depression (sad mood).

Major depression is primarily treated by antidepressant drugs. Manic-depressive illness is primarily treated by lithium, several antiepileptic and antipsychotic drugs.

ANTIDEPRESSANT DRUGS

MECHANISM OF ACTION

Multiple hypothesis have been proposed for the pathogenesis of depression. The key hypothesis are monoamine hypothesis and neurotrophic hypothesis (Figure 2).

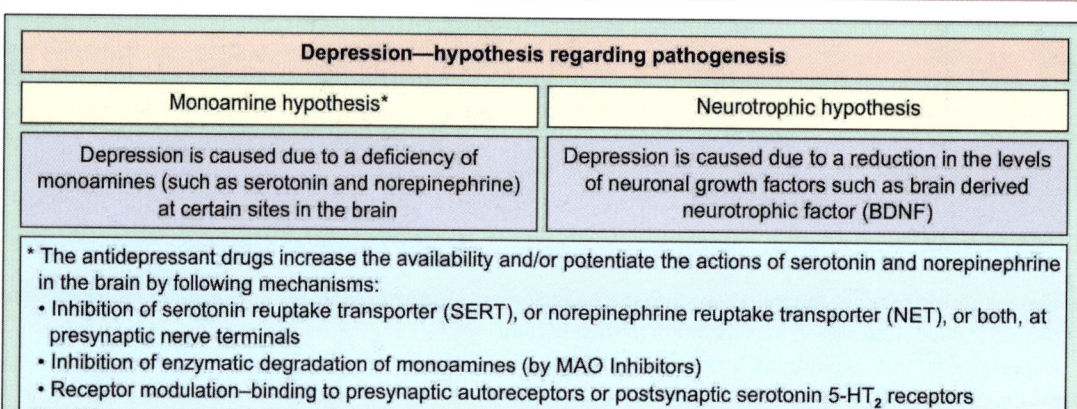

Figure 2: Mechanism of action of antidepressant drugs

CLASSIFICATION

The classification of antidepressant drugs is mentioned in Figure 3.

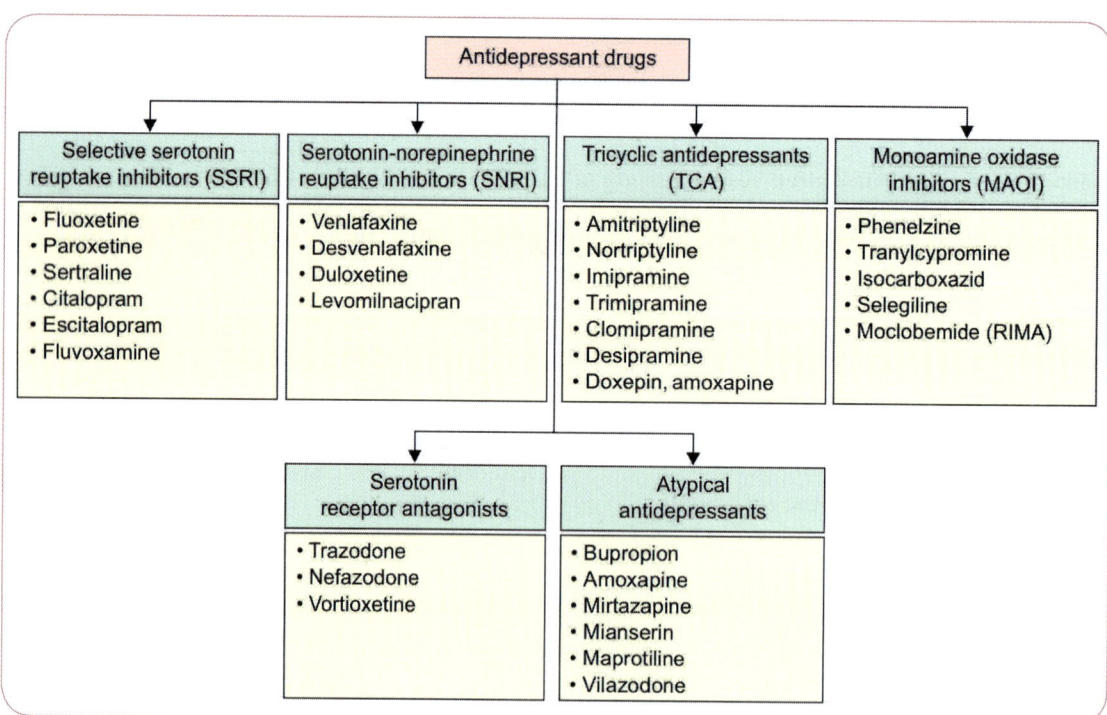

Figure 3: Classification of antidepressant drugs

SELECTIVE SEROTONIN REUPTAKE INHIBITORS

Selective serotonin reuptake inhibitors (SSRI) are a class of drugs whose primary action is to increase serotonin levels in the synaptic cleft.

The commonly used SSRIs are fluoxetine, paroxetine, sertraline, citalopram, escitalopram and fluvoxamine.

Mechanism of Action

The SSRIs selectively inhibit the serotonin reuptake transporter (SERT) in the presynaptic membrane thereby preventing the clearance (reuptake) of serotonin (Figure 4).

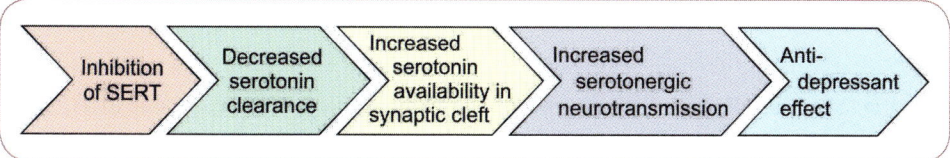

Figure 4: Mechanism of action of SSRI

Pharmacokinetics

All SSRIs are orally active. The peak plasma levels are reached within 2–8 hours. Most SSRIs have elimination half-lives between 16 and 36 hours. Hence, they are given in a once-daily dosing schedule.

Fluoxetine is an exception to the above because it has a much longer half-life and is given in a once-weekly dosing schedule (Figure 5).

Fluoxetine: Exceptional pharmacokinetics

- Fluoxetine is different from other SSRIs in that it has a much longer half-life (approx. 50 hours versus 16–36 hours for other SSRIs). Additionally, fluoxetine is metabolized (by CYP2D6) to an active compound norfluoxetine, which has a very long half-life of around 10 days.
- This has 2 important implications:
  1. Fluoxetine is given in a once-weekly dosing schedule.
  2. Fluoxetine needs to be discontinued at least 4 weeks prior to the introduction of MAO inhibitors (as compared to 2 weeks for other SSRIs).

Figure 5: Fluoxetine: Pharmacokinetics

Most SSRIs are metabolized by the cytochrome enzyme CYP2D6. The SSRIs are also moderate to potent inhibitors of CYP2D6.

This results in a significant potential for interactions with various drugs that are substrates of CYP2D6, e.g. TCAs, certain antipsychotics, antiarrhythmics etc.

Note:
- Paroxetine and fluoxetine are potent inhibitors of CYP2D6. Most of the other SSRIs are moderate CYP2D6 inhibitors.
- CYP1A2, CYP2C19 and CYP3A4 are also involved in SSRI metabolism and these may also be inhibited to certain extent by various SSRIs.

Adverse Effects

The SSRIs have mostly replaced the TCAs and MAOIs, and are now considered the first-line drugs in the treatment of depression.

The SSRIs have a favorable adverse effect profile that results in a much better patient acceptability and tolerability. The SSRIs are relatively safe even in overdose.

The SSRIs, unlike the TCAs, have very little blocking activity on cholinergic, alpha-adrenergic and H_1-histaminic receptors. The SSRIs, therefore do not cause the adverse effects that result from the blockade of these receptors (Table 1).

TABLE 1	Adverse effects NOT caused by SSRI	
Do not cause	Anticholinergic (Atropine like)	• Dry mouth, constipation • Urinary retention, blurred vision • Cognitive dulling, tachycardia
Do not cause	Anti α-adrenergic	Orthostatic hypotension, tachycardia
Do not cause	Antihistaminic	Sedation, weight gain

However, the SSRIs are not free of adverse effects. The adverse effects of SSRIs are due to an increase in the serotonergic tone at the following body locations (Table 2).

TABLE 2	Adverse effects of SSRI
Brain	Insomnia, irritability, anxiety, decreased libido, headache
Spinal cord	Sexual side effects (erectile dysfunction, delayed orgasm and ejaculation)
Gastrointestinal tract	Nausea, vomiting, diarrhea, GIT disturbance

SEROTONIN-NOREPINEPHRINE REUPTAKE INHIBITORS

Serotonin-norepinephrine reuptake inhibitors (SNRI) are a class of drugs whose primary action is to increase the level of serotonin and norepinephrine in the synaptic cleft.

The commonly used SNRIs are venlafaxine, desvenlafaxine, duloxetine and levomilnacipran.

Mechanism of Action

The SNRIs inhibit the serotonin reuptake transporter (SERT) and norepinephrine reuptake transporter (NET) in the presynaptic membrane thereby preventing the clearance (reuptake) of serotonin and norepinephrine (Figure 6).

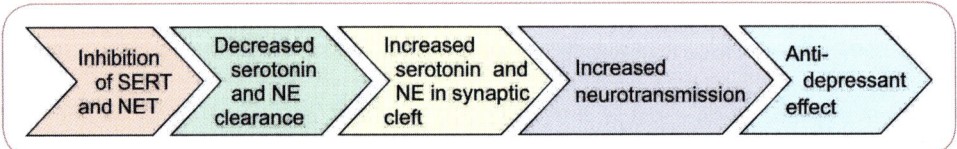

Figure 6: Mechanism of action of SNRI

The SNRIs are often effective in patients (with depression) in whom SSRIs are ineffective. Additionally, depression that is accompanied by chronic painful symptoms (including backache, myalgia) often responds to SNRIs.

Adverse Effects

The SNRIs (like the SSRIs) have a favorable adverse effect profile that results in much better patient acceptability and tolerability. The SNRIs are also relatively safe in overdose.

The SNRIs, unlike the TCAs, have very little blocking activity on cholinergic, alpha-adrenergic and H_1-histaminic receptors. The SNRIs, therefore do not cause the adverse effects that result from the blockade of these receptors (Table 3).

TABLE 3	Adverse effects NOT caused by SNRI	
Do not cause	Anticholinergic (Atropine like)	• Dry mouth, constipation • Urinary retention, blurred vision • Cognitive dulling, tachycardia
Do not cause	Anti α-adrenergic	Orthostatic hypotension, tachycardia
Do not cause	Antihistaminic	Sedation, weight gain

The following adverse effects however, are reported with the use of SNRIs (Figure 7).

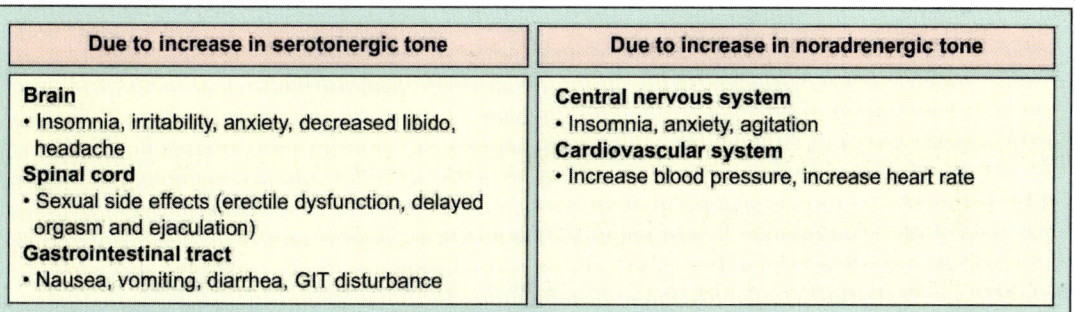

Due to increase in serotonergic tone	Due to increase in noradrenergic tone
Brain • Insomnia, irritability, anxiety, decreased libido, headache **Spinal cord** • Sexual side effects (erectile dysfunction, delayed orgasm and ejaculation) **Gastrointestinal tract** • Nausea, vomiting, diarrhea, GIT disturbance	**Central nervous system** • Insomnia, anxiety, agitation **Cardiovascular system** • Increase blood pressure, increase heart rate

Figure 7: Adverse effects of SNRI

Safety Considerations Regarding SSRIs and SNRIs

The key safety considerations regarding SSRIs and SNRIs are mentioned below:

○ **Use in children and adolescents:** The USFDA has issued a black box warning for the use of antidepressants in children and adolescents, due to an increased risk of suicidality (suicidal ideation or suicide attempts). These drugs should be used cautiously and the pediatric patients should be kept under observation.

○ **Overdose:** The patients with SSRI or SNRI overdose alone, usually have a mild course as compared to patients with TCA overdose. However, the following are noteworthy regarding overdose with SSRIs/SNRIs.

  ❑ SSRI/SNRI overdose usually do not lead to cardiac arrhythmias. The TCA overdose, in contrast has a significant risk of serious arrhythmias including ventricular tachycardia and ventricular fibrillation.

  ❑ Seizures are a potential risk with antidepressant drugs. Hence, as with other antidepressants, SSRI/SNRI overdose may lead to the occurrence of seizures.

  ❑ SSRI/SNRI may lead to 'serotonin syndrome' when they are used in association with MAOIs or any other highly serotonergic drugs. Serotonin syndrome may include symptoms of hyperthermia, sweating, muscle rigidity, myoclonus and changes in mental status and vital signs.

○ **Discontinuation syndrome:** Most of the SSRIs/SNRIs, if abruptly withdrawn, can lead to discontinuation syndrome.

The syndrome is most prominent with SSRIs having shorter half-lives and those with no active metabolites, such as paroxetine. On the other hand, only few patients experience discontinuation syndrome on withdrawing fluoxetine. This is because of a long half-life (approx. 10 days) of fluoxetine's active metabolite norfluoxetine.

When stopping treatment with SSRI/SNRI, the dose should be gradually reduced over a period of at least 1–2 weeks to reduce the risk of withdrawal reactions.

▌ TRICYCLIC ANTIDEPRESSANTS

Tricyclic antidepressants were the first line of treatment for depression until the introduction of SSRIs during 1984-1997.

Currently, the TCAs are used in the treatment of depression that does not respond to SSRIs or SNRIs. This is because TCAs have poor tolerability, narrow therapeutic window and cause fatality in overdose (Figure 8).

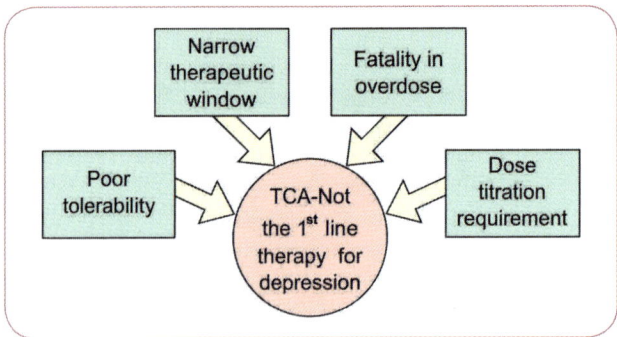

Figure 8: Disadvantages of TCAs as compared to SSRIs/SNRIs

The primary action of TCAs is to increase the level of serotonin and norepinephrine in the synaptic cleft.

The TCAs used are amitriptyline, nortriptyline, imipramine, trimipramine, clomipramine, desipramine, doxepin and amoxapine.

Mechanism of Action

The TCAs inhibit the serotonin reuptake transporter (SERT) and norepinephrine reuptake transporter (NET) in the presynaptic membrane thereby preventing the clearance (reuptake) of serotonin and norepinephrine (Figure 9).

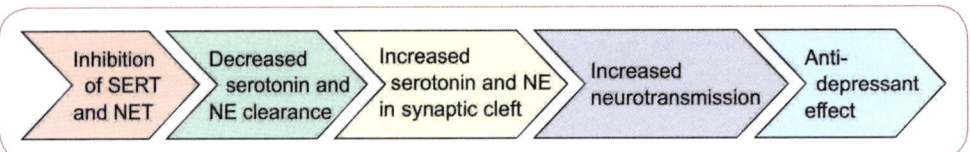

Figure 9: Mechanism of action of TCA

There is considerable variability in the affinity for SERT versus NET across various TCAs. For example, clomipramine has higher affinity for SERT as compared to that for NET.

Pharmacokinetics

The TCAs are well absorbed orally and have a long half-life (~8–80 hours). This allows for once-daily dosing. They are highly plasma protein bound and have a large volume of distribution.

They are mainly metabolized in the liver by cytochrome isoenzymes (CYP2D6, CYP3A4, CYP1A2), and the metabolites are excreted in the urine. Some of the TCAs produce active metabolites (e.g. imipramine to desipramine, amitriptyline to nortriptyline).

A narrow therapeutic window has been observed with the TCAs. An optimal antidepressant effect is observed within a narrow plasma concentration range of 50–200 ng/mL of imipramine, amitriptyline and nortriptyline. There is suboptimal effect both above and below this concentration range.

Titration and individualization of TCA doses is therefore required, as there is significant pharmacokinetic variation observed in different individuals administered the same dosage.

Adverse Effects

The key adverse effects of TCAs are mentioned in Table 4.

TABLE 4	Adverse effects of TCA		
Due to increase in serotonergic tone	**Due to increase in noradrenergic tone**	**Due to blockade of muscarinic, α-adrenergic and histaminic receptors**	**Due to quinidine like action on cardiac conduction**
Brain • Insomnia, irritability, anxiety, decreased libido, headache **Spinal cord** • Sexual side effects (erectile dysfunction, delayed orgasm and ejaculation) **Gastrointestinal tract** • Nausea, vomiting, diarrhea, GIT disturbance	**Central Nervous System** • Insomnia, anxiety, agitation **Cardiovascular System** • Increased blood pressure, increased heart rate	**Anticholinergic** • Dry mouth, constipation, urinary retention, blurred vision, cognitive dulling, tachycardia **Anti α-adrenergic** • Orthostatic hypotension, tachycardia **Antihistaminic** • Sedation, weight gain	**Cardiac arrhythmias** • TCAs have a quinidine like action on cardiac conduction. This can be life-threatening in TCA overdose. • Hence, TCAs are not indicated in patients with ischemic heart disease – sudden deaths may occur

TCA Overdose

Suicide attempts are a frequent occurrence in major depression. Overdose of drugs is a commonly employed method in suicide attempts. Antidepressants (particularly the TCAs) are commonly used in intentional overdose.

The clinical features of TCA overdose are an extension of their adverse effects. Cardiac abnormalities (including arrhythmias, cardiac failure) and neurological disturbances (including seizures, coma) are the main complications. TCA overdose may be fatal and should be immediately managed.

Treatment is mainly symptomatic and supportive. Following measures should be considered:
○ Respiratory support including securing of the airway
○ Gastric lavage and forced emesis
○ Intensive care with continuous monitoring and maintenance of cardiac function, blood gases and electrolytes
○ Diazepam for controlling seizures
○ Lignocaine for controlling cardiac arrhythmias, but it should be used cautiously to avoid precipitating seizures

Drug Interactions

The key drug interactions of the TCAs are mentioned in Figure 10.

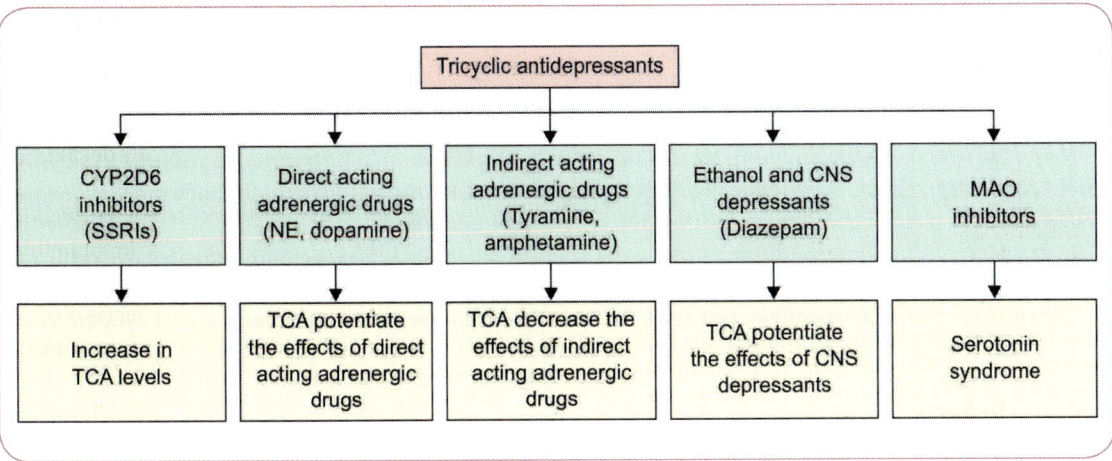

Figure 10: Drug interactions of TCA

Drugs Acting on the Central Nervous System

SECTION D

MONOAMINE OXIDASE INHIBITORS

Monoamine oxidase (MAO) is a mitochondrial enzyme that degrades the biogenic amines such as norepinephrine, dopamine and serotonin. MAO is found in nerves and other tissues such as intestinal wall and liver.

There are two types of MAO enzymes: MAO-A and MAO-B (Figure 11).

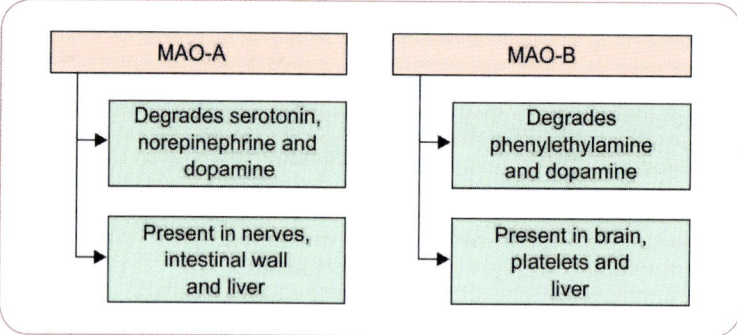

Figure 11: Types of MAO enzymes

Inhibitors of MAO enzymes prevent the degradation of biogenic amines and thereby cause an increase in the levels of norepinephrine, dopamine and serotonin.

The MAO inhibitors are classified based on the selectivity of inhibition of different MAO enzymes (Figure 12):

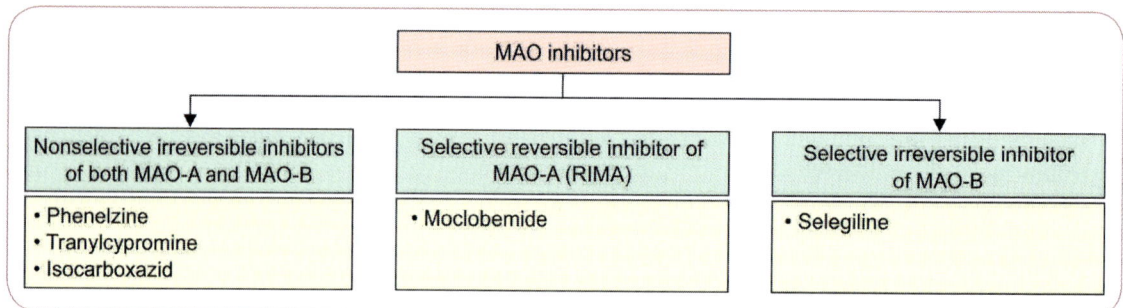

Figure 12: Types of MAO inhibitors

Cheese Reaction

It is a severe hypertensive reaction (hypertensive crisis) resulting from a drug interaction when MAO inhibitors are taken along with foods rich in tyramine (such as cheese, fish, meat, red wine etc.)

Normally, tyramine is broken down by MAO enzymes in the liver and GIT. However, in patients taking MAO inhibitors, the degradation of tyramine does not occur. This leads to increased tyramine levels in the blood that results in displacement of norepinephrine from the sympathetic nerve endings.

Increased levels of norepinephrine in the blood leads to increased blood pressure, hypertensive crisis and possibly, cerebrovascular accidents (Figure 13).

Treatment includes phentolamine and prazosin, apart from supportive management.

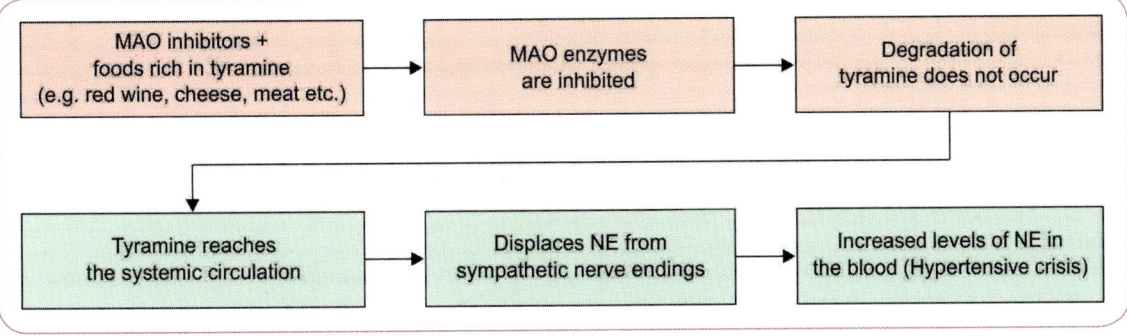

Figure 13: Cheese reaction

Salient Features of MAO Inhibitors

The salient features of some MAO inhibitors are mentioned below:

Selegiline

- Irreversibly inhibits MAO-B at lower doses; but inhibits both MAO-A and MAO-B at higher doses
- Lower doses are used to treat Parkinson's disease
- Higher doses are used to treat major depressive disorder
- Only antidepressant available as a transdermal patch.

Moclobemide

- Reversible and selective MAO-A inhibitor (RIMA)
- Due to reversible and competitive MAO inhibition, excess tyramine levels displace moclobemide from the MAO enzymes. This greatly decreases the risk of food interactions (e.g. cheese reactions).
- Does not have anticholinergic, antiadrenergic, antihistaminic and cardiovascular adverse effects. Further, it is relatively safe in overdose. Hence, it is a suitable drug in elderly and those with heart disease.
- It is an alternate drug for mild to moderate depression and social phobia.

ATYPICAL ANTIDEPRESSANT DRUGS

The salient features of some atypical antidepressant drugs are mentioned below:

Bupropion

- Weak dopamine and serotonin reuptake inhibitor.
- Indicated for depression as well as smoking cessation in combination with motivational support.
- Very low incidence of sexual dysfunction.
- No sedative action.
- Adverse effects include dry mouth, sweating, nervousness and an increased risk of seizures at higher doses

Mirtazapine

- Blocks presynaptic α_2 autoreceptors and α_2 heteroreceptors leading to an increase in the release of norepinephrine (NE) and serotonin (5-HT) respectively.
- It has strong antihistaminic activity that leads to sedation. Therefore, it is useful when depression is associated with difficulty in sleeping.
- It does not have anticholinergic activity.
- Adverse effects include sedation and weight gain.
- It is also known as NaSSA i.e. noradrenergic and specific serotonergic antidepressant (Table 5).

TABLE 5	Mirtazapine: NaSSA antidepressant

- It is an antagonist of presynaptic α2 autoreceptors on noradrenergic neurons. This results in an increase of norepinephrine release.
- It is an antagonist of presynaptic α2 heteroreceptors on serotonergic neurons. This results in an increase of serotonin release.
- It is also an antagonist of postsynaptic 5-HT2 and 5-HT3 receptors.
- It is an agonist of postsynaptic 5-HT1 receptors.

Net Result

- An increased noradrenergic activity (by norepinephrine in the cleft) + a specific increased serotonergic activity, at 5-HT1A receptors (by serotonin in the cleft).
- This mechanism of action results in an equivalent antidepressant efficacy, but minimizes many serotonergic adverse effects such as GIT symptoms, insomnia & sexual dysfunction (the adverse effects are presumed to be mediated by 5-HT2 and 5-HT3 receptors).

SEROTONIN RECEPTOR ANTAGONISTS

The salient features of serotonin receptor antagonists are mentioned below:

Trazodone and Nefazodone

- Blocks postsynaptic 5-HT$_{2A}$ receptors. They also block histaminic receptors and α-adrenergic receptors. They do not block cholinergic receptors.
- They cause sedation due to strong antihistaminic activity, and orthostatic hypotension due to antiadrenergic activity.
- Trazodone is associated with priapism.
- Nefazodone is associated with hepatotoxicity.

CLINICAL USES OF ANTIDEPRESSANT DRUGS

The clinical uses of antidepressant drugs are mentioned below:

Major Depression

- Antidepressants are used for acute as well as long-term treatment of major depression.
  - A successful initial treatment phase is usually followed by 6–12 months of maintenance phase, after which the treatment is gradually withdrawn.
  - If the patient has had 2 separate episodes of major depression, or is chronically depressed (>2 years), lifelong treatment is recommended.
    The SSRIs are currently the treatment of choice and are preferred over TCAs. This is because of poor tolerability, narrow therapeutic window and fatality (in overdose) associated with TCAs.
- **Therapeutic lag:** Following initiation of therapy, there is usually a lag period of 3–4 weeks before significant improvement in depressive symptoms occurs (Figure 14).
    However, the challenge during treatment initiation is that the adverse effects appear early during the lag period when the antidepressant effects have not fully become evident. This requires counseling that the patient persists with the treatment.
    During this lag period, electroconvulsive therapy (ECT) may be preferred for agitated, depressed patients with a high risk of suicide.

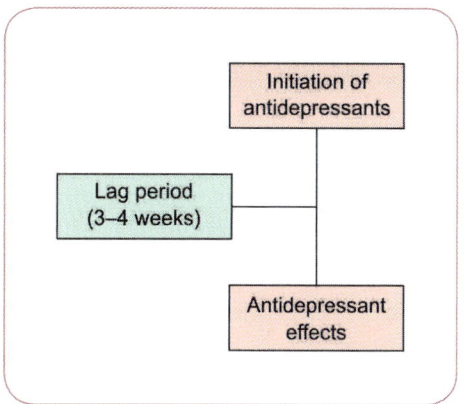

Figure 14: Therapeutic lag of antidepressants

Obsessive Compulsive Disorder (OCD)

o SSRIs (including fluvoxamine) and clomipramine are used in the treatment of OCD.

Anxiety Disorder

o SSRIs and SNRIs are the treatment of choice in various anxiety disorders.
o As SSRIs and SNRIs have a slower onset of action, benzodiazepines (BZD) are prescribed along with antidepressants for a short period of time. This is because BZDs act faster and provide rapid relief.

Attention Deficit Hyperactivity Disorder (ADHD)

o TCAs (such as imipramine, nortriptyline etc.) are used in the treatment of ADHD.
o Amphetamine like drugs (such as dextroamphetamine, methylphenidate etc.) may also be used.

Pain Disorders

o TCAs have been used in the treatment of neuropathic pain conditions (such as postherpetic, diabetic neuropathy, fibromyalgia etc.).
o SNRIs are also effective and are being increasingly used due to better tolerability.

Enuresis

o Imipramine is effective in reducing enuresis (bedwetting). However, desmopressin is currently the preferred drug for treating enuresis in children.

Migraine

o Amitriptyline may be used in the prophylaxis of migraine.

Atopic Dermatitis

o Topical doxepin has been employed for itching in atopic dermatitis.

ANTIANXIETY DRUGS

Anxiety is an unpleasant emotional state associated with discomfort or fear about any defined or undefined situation.

The drugs commonly used in the anxiety disorders are mentioned in Figure 15.

SECTION D ■ Drugs Acting on the Central Nervous System

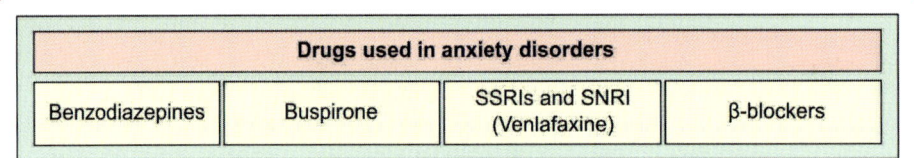

Figure 15: Antianxiety drugs

BENZODIAZEPINES

Benzodiazepines are one of the most widely used drugs in anxiety disorders. This is because they offer the following advantages:
- Rapid onset of action—they are very useful in acute anxiety states
- Relatively high therapeutic index—they are relatively safe in overdoses
- Negligible effects on autonomic and cardiovascular functions
- Availability of flumazenil to rapidly reverse effects, if required

The benzodiazepines commonly used in anxiety disorders include alprazolam, chlordiazepoxide, clonazepam, diazepam, lorazepam etc.

Benzodiazepines facilitate the inhibitory effects of GABA by acting on the GABA$_A$ receptors.

The adverse effects include sedation, confusion, memory impairment, decreased alertness, dependence and abuse.

They are the most widely used drugs for acute anxiety states as they have a rapid onset of action. They are also used, although less commonly, for long-term treatment of generalized anxiety disorders and panic disorders. Tolerance develops to its anxiolytic actions on prolonged use.

BUSPIRONE

Buspirone is a partial agonist at 5-HT$_{1A}$ receptors.

It does not have sedative, anticonvulsant or muscle relaxant action. It does not cause tolerance or physical dependence. It does not affect GABA transmission and does not potentiate the effects of alcohol or other CNS depressants.

The therapeutic effect is delayed; and it takes up to 2 weeks for the effects to fully develop.

Buspirone is only effective in cases of mild to moderate generalized anxiety disorders.

SSRIS AND SNRI (VENLAFAXINE)

These drugs are nowadays being preferred for the treatment of generalized anxiety disorders and certain types of phobias.

Since the response is delayed, they are not effective in acute anxiety states.

BETA BLOCKERS

Propranolol and other nonselective β-blockers are mainly used to reduce the sympathetic symptoms associated with anxiety (e.g. palpitations, tremors, tachycardia, sweating).

They are effective in acute anxiety states and performance anxiety (e.g. examination fear, public speaking phobia etc.)

Benzodiazepines and beta blockers are the only drugs effective in the treatment of acute anxiety states. The other drugs such as SSRIs, venlafaxine, bupropion etc. are effective in chronic anxiety conditions.

ASSESS YOURSELF (Examination Questions of Various Universities)

1. Classify antidepressant drugs. Discuss the mechanism of action, adverse effects and clinical uses of fluoxetine.
2. Write short notes on:
   a. Buspirone in anxiety
   b. Fluoxetine in endogenous depression
   c. Selective serotonin reuptake inhibitors
   d. Cheese reaction

   e. MAO inhibitors
   f. Imipramine
3. Discuss in brief the pharmacotherapy of:
   a. Depression
   b. Anxiety
4. Mention 2 advantages of fluoxetine over imipramine.

MULTIPLE CHOICE QUESTIONS

1. Which of the following drug increases serotonin and norepinephrine and is also an alpha 2 antagonist? *(Recent Question Dec 2016)*
   a. Venlafaxine   b. Mirtazapine
   c. Duloxetine   d. Fluoxetine
2. Fluoxetine is given for a patient and after 5 days there is no improvement in symptoms. What is the next step? *(Recent Question Dec 2016)*
   a. Double the doses
   b. Add lithium
   c. Wait as it takes 2–6 weeks to respond
   d. Change to TCA
3. Antidepressant drug that can be used in nocturnal enuresis is: *(Recent Question 2016)*
   a. Imipramine   b. Fluvoxamine
   c. Phenelzine   d. Bupropion
4. What is the drug of choice for obsessive compulsive disorder? *(Recent Question 2016)*
   a. Imipramine
   b. Fluoxetine
   c. Benzodiazepines
   d. Alprazolam
5. Which of the following is not a serotonin norepi-nephrine reuptake inhibitor?
   (Recent Question 2016)
   a. Venlafaxine
   b. Duloxetine
   c. Milnacipran
   d. Tianeptine
6. Which of the following is not a SSRI?
   (Recent Question 2016)
   a. Escitalopram   b. Sertraline
   c. Paroxetine   d. Amitriptyline

7. Which of the following drug-receptor pair(s) correctly matched: *(PGI May 2012)*
   a. Buspirone : 5HT-1 agonist
   b. Granisetron: 5HT-2 antagonist
   c. Cisapride: 5 HT-3 agonist
   d. Methysergide: 5 HT-4 antagonist
   e. Imipramine: TNF-α inhibitor
8. Escitalopram is a: *(NIMHANS 2011)*
   a. Selective serotonin reuptake inhibitor
   b. Nonspecific norepinephrine uptake inhibitor
   c. Atypical antidepressant
   d. MAO inhibitor
9. Selegiline is: *(NIMHANS 2010)*
   a. Dopa decarboxylase inhibitor
   b. MAO-B inhibitor
   c. COMT inhibitor
   d. MAO-A inhibitor
10. Moclobemide is: *(APPG 2006)*
    a. SSRI
    b. Antipsychotic drug
    c. MAO inhibitor
    d. Prevent recyclation of adrenalin
11. Tranylcypromine (MAO inhibitor) should be avoided with _____ as it causes dangerous drug interaction. *(MHCET 2007)*
    a. Sertraline   b. Amitriptyline
    c. Alprazolam   d. Any of the above
12. Bupropion *(WBPG 2011)*
    a. Antilipidemic   b. Antiepileptic
    c. AntiDM   d. Antismoking
13. Not a MAO inhibitor: *(WBPG 2009)*
    a. Tranylcypromine   b. Isocarboxazid
    c. Phenelzine   d. Maprotiline

Ans.

1. (b)	2. (c)	3. (a)	4. (b)	5. (d)	6. (d)
7. (a)	8. (a)	9. (b)	10. (c)	11. (a)	12. (d)
13. (d)					

Epilepsy is a disorder of the brain that is characterized by paroxysmal cerebral dysrhythmia. It refers to disordered, rhythmic firing of the brain neurons.

Epileptic seizures have been classified as **partial seizures** (originating at a focal site in cortex) or **generalized seizures** (involving both cerebral hemispheres right from the beginning).

The different types of epilepsy are mentioned in Table 1.

TABLE 1	Types of epilepsy
Generalized seizures	
Generalized tonic-clonic seizures (GTCS, grand mal)	• Manifests as aura → cry → loss of consciousness → tonic phase → clonic phase → CNS depression, postictal confusion
Absence seizures (Petit mal)	• Common in children • Involve brief changes in awareness, staring and transient loss of consciousness
Atonic seizures	• Loss of consciousness with muscle relaxation
Myoclonic seizures	• Sudden, short, shock like contractions that can involve a limb or the entire body
Partial seizures	
Simple partial seizures	• Can manifest as focal seizures, sensory abnormality, depending upon the involvement of a specific cortical region • There is no loss of consciousness
Complex partial seizures (Temporal lobe or psychomotor epilepsy)	• Abnormal behavior, aimless movements • There is impaired consciousness

CLASSIFICATION OF ANTIEPILEPTIC DRUGS (TABLE 2)

TABLE 2	Classification of antiepileptic drugs
Hydantoin	Phenytoin, fosphenytoin
Barbiturate	Phenobarbitone (phenobarbital)
Deoxybarbiturate	Primidone
Iminostilbene	Carbamazepine, oxcarbazepine
Aliphatic carboxylic acid	Sodium valproate (valproic acid), divalproex
Succinimide	Ethosuximide
Benzodiazepines	Clonazepam, diazepam, lorazepam
Phenyltriazine	Lamotrigine
Others	Gabapentin, pregabalin, vigabatrin, levetiracetam, tiagabine, topiramate, zonisamide

PHENYTOIN

Phenytoin is a hydantoin derivative and is one of the commonly used antiepileptic drug.

Mechanism of Action

Phenytoin has a stabilizing effect on the neuronal membrane and inhibits the spread of seizure discharge.

Phenytoin prolongs the inactivated state of the voltage sensitive Na^+ channels and thereby prevents the return of sodium channels to the active state. Therefore, it prevents the repetitive firing of the neurons.

At higher doses, phenytoin also enhances GABA-mediated inhibition, decreases glutamate levels and inhibits calcium channels.

Pharmacokinetics

Phenytoin is slowly absorbed from the GIT. It is highly (~80–90%) plasma protein bound and widely distributed in the body.

Metabolism of phenytoin occurs in the liver by hydroxylation and glucuronide conjugation.

The metabolism kinetics of phenytoin is capacity limited. It demonstrates dose dependent elimination kinetics (i.e. over the therapeutic dose range, the metabolism changes from first order to zero order kinetics).

At low plasma levels, phenytoin metabolism follows first order kinetics— i.e. rate of elimination is proportional to the plasma concentration. However, as the plasma concentrations increases, the capacity of liver to metabolize phenytoin becomes saturated, and any further increase in the doses results in significant increases in the plasma concentration. This can result in phenytoin toxicity.

Phenytoin precipitates in glucose solution and is administered intravenously in normal saline.

Adverse Effects

The key adverse effects of phenytoin are mentioned in Tables 3 and 4.

TABLE 3	Adverse effects with phenytoin (At therapeutic levels)
Gingival hyperplasia/Gum hypertrophy	• Due to overgrowth of tissue; probably involves altered collagen metabolism • Can be reduced by maintaining good oral hygiene
Coarsening of facial features, hirsutism, acne	• Can be problematic in young women
Hypersensitivity reactions	• Includes rashes, lymphadenopathy
Megaloblastic anemia	• Phenytoin reduces the absorption of folate and enhances its excretion
Hyperglycemia	• Due to inhibition of insulin release
Osteomalacia with hypocalcemia	• Due to altered metabolism of vitamin D and inhibition of intestinal absorption of calcium
Fetal hydantoin syndrome	• Phenytoin (used during pregnancy) can lead to a group of defects in the developing fetus due to its teratogenic effects • Can result in microcephaly, hypoplastic phalanges, cleft palate etc. • Possibly caused by the arene oxide metabolite of the drug

TABLE 4	Adverse effects with phenytoin (At high concentrations)
CNS	• Ataxia, vestibular and cerebellar symptoms, diplopia, nystagmus • Mental confusion, alterations in behavior, hallucinations, drowsiness
Cardiovascular	• Cardiac arrhythmias, decreased blood pressure can occur with IV administration • Intravenous injection can lead to soft tissue irritation (can result in necrosis)
GIT	• Nausea, vomiting, epigastric pain

Drug Interactions

○ Drugs that increase phenytoin levels → isoniazid, cimetidine, chloramphenicol, warfarin
○ Phenytoin and carbamazepine induce each other's metabolism
○ Induction of microsomal enzymes by phenytoin can lead to increased breakdown of steroids, oral contraceptive pills (OCP) → can lead to failure of OCPs

Clinical Uses

The clinical uses of phenytoin include:
○ Generalized tonic-clonic seizures (GTCS)
○ Partial seizures (simple and complex)
○ Status epilepticus (used intravenously via slow infusion)
○ Trigeminal neuralgia (preferred drug for this condition is carbamazepine)

FOSPHENYTOIN

○ It is a prodrug of phenytoin
○ It is less damaging to the blood vessels upon IV administration and can be infused at a faster rate, as compared to phenytoin
○ It can be infused via normal saline or glucose solution, unlike phenytoin
○ It can be used in patients of status epilepticus

PHENOBARBITONE (PHENOBARBITAL)

Phenobarbitone is a barbiturate that binds to the barbiturate binding site of $GABA_A$ receptor. It causes CNS depression and has GABA faciliatory and GABA mimetic actions.

The adverse effects include sedation, psychomotor slowing, poor concentration, depression, irritability, ataxia and decreased libido. Cognitive and behavior alterations can also occur. Prolonged use of phenobarbitone can also lead to osteomalacia and megaloblastic anemia.

Phenobarbitone is effective in a wide variety of seizures. It is effective in generalized tonic-clonic seizures and partial seizures. It can also be used in patients of status epilepticus, but the response can be slow. It is relatively inexpensive.

It is currently not popular due to the availability of better antiepileptic drugs.

CARBAMAZEPINE

It is an iminostilbene and is chemically related to imipramine.

Mechanism of Action

The mechanism of action is similar to phenytoin. It prolongs the inactivated state of the sodium channels and thereby prevents the return of sodium channels to the active state. Therefore, it prevents the repetitive firing of the neurons.

Pharmacokinetics

Carbamazepine is poorly water soluble and oral absorption is slow and erratic. It is metabolized extensively in the liver to an active metabolite (10–11 epoxy carbamazepine) as well as other inactive metabolites. It is approx. 75% bound to plasma proteins.

It can also cause autoinduction of metabolism.

Adverse Effects

The adverse effects of carbamazepine include the following:
- Neurotoxicity—diplopia, ataxia, sedation, vertigo
- Nausea, vomiting, diarrhea
- Hematological disorders—aplastic anemia, agranulocytosis
- Hypersensitivity reactions—skin rashes, lupus like syndrome
- Hepatic dysfunction, hepatitis
- Water retention and hyponatremia due to ADH release

Drug Interactions

- Induction of microsomal enzymes by carbamazepine can lead to decreased efficacy of oral contraceptives, haloperidol, topiramate, lamotrigine
- Metabolism of carbamazepine is inhibited by isoniazid and erythromycin
- Phenytoin, valproic acid, phenobarbitone increase the metabolism of carbamazepine
- Carbamazepine can induce the metabolism of phenytoin, valproic acid and phenobarbitone

Clinical Uses

The clinical uses of carbamazepine include the following:
- Generalized tonic-clonic seizures (GTCS)
- Partial seizures (simple and complex)
- Trigeminal neuralgia
- Mania and bipolar mood disorder

OXCARBAZEPINE

Oxcarbazepine is a congener of carbamazepine. It is a prodrug that is better tolerated, has fewer drug interactions and is less potent, as compared to carbamazepine.

The indications are similar to that of carbamazepine.

ETHOSUXIMIDE

Ethosuximide inhibits T type calcium current in the thalamus. It is effective against absence seizures.

The adverse effects include gastrointestinal toxicity and mood changes.

SODIUM VALPROATE (VALPROIC ACID)

Sodium valproate is a branched chain aliphatic carboxylic acid.

Mechanism of Action

The following mechanisms of action have been postulated:
- Prolongs the inactivated state of the sodium channels (like phenytoin)
- Inhibits T type calcium current in the thalamus (like ethosuximide)
- Increases release of GABA by:
  - Increasing the synthesis of GABA (stimulation of the enzyme glutamic acid decarboxylase)
  - Decreasing the degradation of GABA (inhibition of the enzyme GABA transaminase).

Pharmacokinetics

Sodium valproate has good oral absorption. It is metabolized in the liver and the metabolites are excreted via urine. It is highly bound to plasma proteins (~90%).

Adverse Effects

The adverse effects of sodium valproate include the following:
- Anorexia, nausea, vomiting, alopecia, curling of hair
- Tremor, ataxia, drowsiness
- Increased risk of bleeding
- Hypersensitivity including rashes
- Increase in liver enzymes → monitoring of liver function is recommended
- Fulminant hepatitis → observed in children
- Acute pancreatitis
- Teratogenicity → use during pregnancy can cause neural tube defects such as spina bifida

Drug Interactions

- Carbamazepine and sodium valproate induce each other's metabolism
- Sodium valproate can increase the levels of
  - Phenytoin → by inhibiting the metabolism of phenytoin and displacing it from protein binding sites
  - Phenobarbitone → by inhibiting the metabolism of phenobarbitone
- Increase risk of teratogenicity if sodium valproate and carbamazepine are administered together

Clinical Uses

Sodium valproate is a broad-spectrum antiepileptic drug and is used in the following conditions:
- Absence seizures
- Generalized tonic-clonic seizures (GTCS)
- Partial seizures (simple and complex)
- Myoclonic and atonic seizures
- Mania and bipolar disorders
- Prophylaxis of migraine

BENZODIAZEPINES

Benzodiazepines are GABA receptor agonists.

Clonazepam

- Clonazepam has significant anticonvulsant action.
- Clinically used in absence and myoclonic seizures.
- Adverse effects include sedation, dizziness, hypotonia, dysarthria. It may cause behavioral abnormalities in children.
- Tolerance develops to its therapeutic effect.

Diazepam

- Clinically used (intravenously) in emergency management of convulsions in patients with status epilepticus, febrile seizures, eclampsia, poisonings etc.
- Diazepam is not used for prolonged periods due to significant sedative effect and the development of tolerance.

Lorazepam

- Clinically used (intravenously) in emergency management of convulsions in patients with status epilepticus, eclampsia, etc.
- It has a longer duration of action as compared to diazepam.

LAMOTRIGINE

It is a phenyltriazine. The mechanism of action is prolongation of the inactivated state of sodium channels. It may reduce the release of neurotransmitters such as glutamate.

It is a broad-spectrum antiepileptic drug. Clinical uses include generalized tonic-clonic seizures, partial seizures (simple and complex), absence, myoclonic seizures and Lennox-Gastaut syndrome.

The adverse effects include somnolence, dizziness, rashes, ataxia, diplopia, vomiting and hypersensitivity reactions.

OTHER ANTIEPILEPTIC DRUGS

The salient features of gabapentin, pregabalin, vigabatrin, levetiracetam, tiagabine, topiramate and zonisamide are mentioned in Table 5.

TABLE 5	Other antiepileptic drugs
Drug	Comments
Gabapentin	• GABA derivative, increases the release of GABA • Clinically used as an adjunct in partial seizures (simple and complex) • Also used for analgesia in diabetic neuropathy and postherpetic neuralgia • The adverse effects include dizziness and fatigue
Pregabalin	• Increases the release of GABA • Clinically used in partial seizures and analgesia in diabetic neuropathy and postherpetic neuralgia
Vigabatrin	• Inhibits GABA transaminase (which is involved in GABA degradation), thus increasing the concentration of GABA in the brain • Clinically used as an adjuvant in refractory complex partial seizures • The adverse effects include visual field constriction, sedation, depression and psychosis • Due to permanent and progressive bilateral vision loss, vigabatrin is a reserve drug only in cases not responding to other antiepileptics
Levetiracetam	• Clinically used as an adjunctive therapy of generalized tonic-clonic, myoclonic and partial onset seizures in adults and children • Do not lead to drug interactions • The adverse effects include somnolence, dizziness and fatigue
Tiagabine	• Inhibits the GABA transporter-1 (GAT-1), thus increasing the activity of GABA • Clinically used as an adjuvant therapy in partial seizures • The adverse effects include sedation, amnesia, dizziness and abdominal pain

Topiramate	• Has multiple mechanisms of action
	  ▪ Prolongation of the inactivated state of sodium channels
	  ▪ Antagonism of glutamate receptors
	  ▪ Enhances GABA action
	  ▪ Weak carbonic anhydrase inhibitor
	• Clinically used for partial seizures, generalized tonic-clonic seizure, Lennox-Gastaut syndrome and prophylaxis of migraine
	• The adverse effects include ataxia, sedation, paresthesia and risk of renal stones

Zonisamide	• Structurally related to sulfonamide antibiotics • Causes inhibition of T type calcium currents as well as prolongation of the inactivated state of sodium channels • Clinically used as adjunctive therapy in partial seizures

A summary of the clinical uses of antiepileptic drugs is mentioned in Table 6.

TABLE 6	Clinical uses of antiepileptic drugs
Type of seizures	**Antiepileptic drug(s)**
Generalized tonic-clonic (Grand mal epilepsy)	• Phenytoin • Sodium valproate • Carbamazepine • Phenobarbitone
Partial seizures (Simple)	• Phenytoin • Carbamazepine • Sodium valproate
Partial seizures (Complex)	• Phenytoin • Carbamazepine • Sodium valproate
Myoclonic seizures	• Sodium valproate
Absence seizures (Petit mal)	• Sodium valproate • Ethosuximide • Lamotrigine
Atonic seizures	• Sodium valproate
Febrile seizures	• Diazepam (rectal administration)
Status epilepticus	• Diazepam • Lorazepam • Phenytoin • Fosphenytoin • Phenobarbitone

◼ STATUS EPILEPTICUS

It is a medical emergency and requires prompt medical treatment. The usual presentation is recurrent attacks of tonic-clonic convulsions without the recovery of consciousness in between.

The mortality rate is approx. 20%. The aim of therapy is to rapidly terminate the epilepsy, because the longer the epilepsy remains untreated, the greater are the chances of permanent brain injury.

The drugs are given by the intravenous route only.

Pharmacotherapy of status epilepticus is mentioned in Table 7.

TABLE 7	Pharmacotherapy of status epilepticus
• Benzodiazepines → intravenous diazepam or intravenous lorazepam	
• Intravenous fosphenytoin or phenytoin or phenobarbital	
• In resistant cases, anesthetic doses of either thiopental, midazolam, or propofol can be considered	
• General supporting measures of the airway, breathing, circulation, cardiac rhythm and oxygenation	

ASSESS YOURSELF (Examination Questions of Various Universities)

1. Classify antiepileptic drugs. Discuss the mechanism of action, pharmacokinetics, adverse effects and clinical uses of phenytoin.
2. Discuss the mechanism of action, adverse effects and clinical uses of sodium valproate.
3. Write short notes on:
   a. Carbamazepine
   b. Lamotrigine
   c. Status epilepticus
   d. Drug therapy of grand mal epilepsy

   e. Drug therapy of absence seizures
   f. Why diazepam is used in status epilepticus but not in the routine treatment of Grand mal epilepsy
   g. Name two antiepileptic drugs used in the treatment of petit mal epilepsy
4. Discuss the pharmacological basis for the use of the following:
   a. GABA agonists/facilitators in seizure control
   b. Sodium valproate in epilepsy

MULTIPLE CHOICE QUESTIONS

1. Drug for migraine which is antiepileptic
   (Recent Question Dec 2016)
   a. Topiramate   b. Lamotrigine
   c. Carbamazepine   d. Vigabatrin
2. Which drug can cause progressive visual field constriction?   *(AIIMS Nov 2015)*
   a. Phenobarbitone   b. Vigabatrin
   c. Ethosuximide   d. Valproate
3. Which statement is true about carbamazepine?
   (Recent Question 2016)
   a. Used in trigeminal neuralgia
   b. Carbamazepine is an enzyme inhibitor
   c. Can cause megaloblastic anemia
   d. It is the drug of choice for status epilepticus
4. Which among the following is the mechanism of action of carbamazepine? *(Recent Question 2016)*
   a. Prolongation of inactivated state of Na$^+$ channels
   b. Facilitates GABA
   c. Inhibition of Ca^{2+} channels
   d. NMDA receptor blockade
5. Cleft lip is caused by which of the following drug?   *(Recent Question 2016)*
   a. Levetiracetam   b. Phenytoin
   c. Sodium valproate   d. Phenobarbitone
6. Fetal hydantoin syndrome is seen if following drug is used in pregnancy?
   (Recent Question 2016)
   a. Phenytoin   b. Alcohol
   c. Ethosuximide   d. Phenobarbitone
7. Ethosuximide can be used for the treatment of:
   (Recent Question 2016)
   a. Generalized tonic-clonic seizures

   b. Absence seizures
   c. Complex seizures
   d. Myoclonic seizures
8. Which antiepileptic drug does not act via inhibition of sodium channels?
   (Recent Question 2016)
   a. Vigabatrin   b. Carbamazepine
   c. Lamotrigine   d. Phenytoin
9. Status epilepticus is managed best with the use of which of the following drugs?
   (Recent Question 2016)
   a. Intravenous diazepam
   b. Intravenous phenytoin sodium
   c. Intramuscular phenobarbitone
   d. Rectal diazepam
10. Osteomalacia is adverse effect of:
    (Recent Question 2016)
    a. Primidone   b. Phenytoin
    c. Carbamazepine   d. Valproic acid
11. Which drug is contraindicated in pregnancy?
    (Recent Question 2016)
    a. Phenytoin   b. Insulin
    c. Heparin   d. All
12. Valproic acid   *(Recent Question 2016)*
    a. It is an enzyme inducer
    b. It causes obesity
    c. It causes hirsutism
    d. It causes neural tube defects
13. Drug of choice for myoclonic seizures:
    (Recent Question 2016)
    a. Vigabatrin   b. Phenytoin
    c. Valproate   d. Carbamazepine

Ans.

1. (a)	2. (b)	3. (a)	4. (a)	5. (b)	6. (a)
7. (b)	8. (a)	9. (a)	10. (b)	11. (a)	12. (d)
13. (c)					

Sedatives and Hypnotics

Sedatives and hypnotics are drugs acting on the central nervous system.

Sedatives are drugs that reduce anxiety, calm the patient, and diminish responsiveness to stimulation. They do not induce sleep.

Hypnotics are drugs that induce or maintain sleep resembling normal sleep. The patient can be awakened by strong stimulation.

NEUROTRANSMITTERS IN THE CENTRAL NERVOUS SYSTEM

Neurotransmitters play a vital role in the transmission of signals in the body. Neurotransmitters can have excitatory or inhibitory effects on the central nervous system (CNS) (Figure 1).

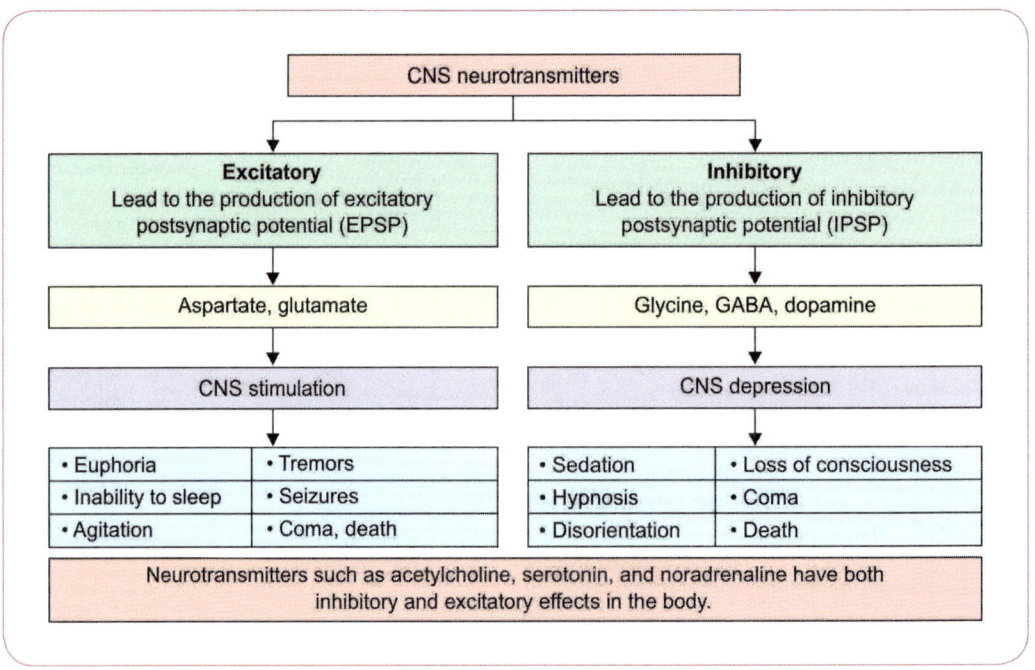

Figure 1: Central nervous system neurotransmitters

STAGES OF SLEEP

The stages of sleep and features of insomnia are mentioned in Table 1.

TABLE 1	Stages of sleep and insomnia
Nonrapid eye movement (NREM)	• Constitutes approx. 75-80% of the total sleep time in adults • Consists of four stages—1, 2, 3 and 4 • Stage 3 and 4 are known as deep sleep or slow wave sleep
Rapid eye movement (REM)	• Constitutes approx. 20-25% of the total sleep time in adults • Follows every cycle of NREM sleep • Associated with marked brain activity • Dreams occur in REM sleep
Generally, the sleep advances through stages 1, 2, 3 and 4 of NREM sleep, followed by a short duration of REM sleep. Usually, this pattern occurs approximately 5-6 times in a night.	
Insomnia is characterized by: • Problems in initiating or maintaining sleep • Early awakening • Poor quality of sleep or unrefreshing sleep	

CLASSIFICATION OF SEDATIVES AND HYPNOTICS

The classification of sedative and hypnotic drugs is mentioned in Table 2.

TABLE 2	Classification of sedatives and hypnotics					
Benzodiazepines		Barbiturates		Nonbenzodiazepines	Miscellaneous	
Long acting	• Diazepam • Chlordiazepoxide • Clonazepam	Long acting	• Phenobarbitone	• Zolpidem • Zopiclone • Zaleplon	• Melatonin • Ramelteon • Triclofos • Chloral hydrate • Orexin receptor antagonist - e.g. suvorexant"	
Intermediate acting	• Alprazolam • Lorazepam • Temazepam • Nitrazepam	Short acting	• Pentobarbitone			
Short acting	• Midazolam • Triazolam • Oxazepam	Ultra short acting	• Thiopentone • Methohexitone			

BENZODIAZEPINES

Benzodiazepines (BZD) are the preferred drugs for sedation and hypnosis, as compared to barbiturates.

Mechanism and Sites of Action

Benzodiazepines bind to a specific benzodiazepine site on the $GABA_A$ receptor. BZDs have a *GABA-facilitatory action* and enhance the binding to GABA to $GABA_A$ receptors.

In contrast to barbiturates, BZDs have no GABA-mimetic action.

Upon binding, BZDs increase the frequency of opening of GABA-gated chloride channels. This results in hyperpolarization of membranes leading to CNS depression (Figure 2).

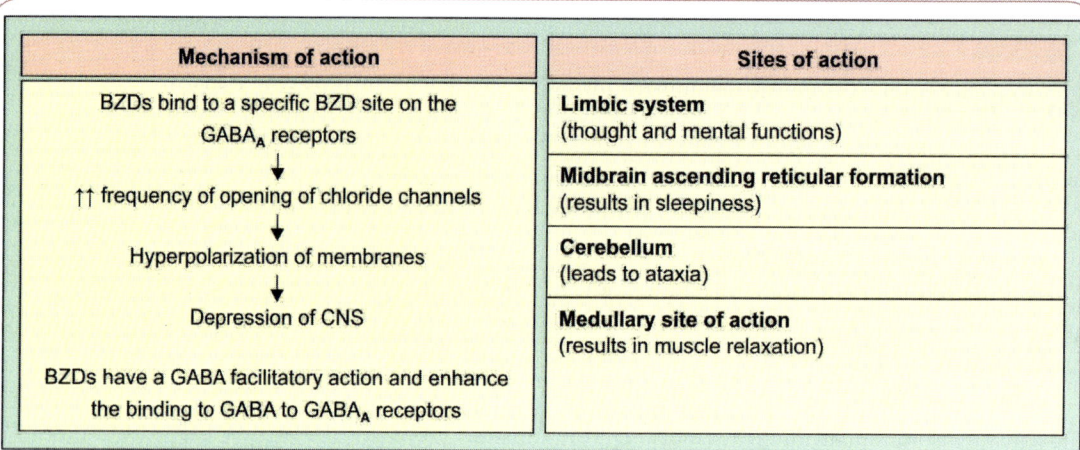

Figure 2: Benzodiazepines—mechanism and sites of action

Pharmacokinetics

There are significant pharmacokinetic variations amongst benzodiazepines.

All BZDs can be given orally except midazolam. Some of them can be given intravenously or intramuscularly e.g. diazepam, lorazepam, midazolam and chlordiazepoxide. Diazepam can also be given by rectal route in children.

Plasma protein binding is variable (e.g. flurazepam 10%, alprazolam 70%, diazepam ~99%). Despite high plasma protein binding of some BZDs, significant drug displacement reactions are usually not observed because BZDs have a large volume of distribution.

Metabolism of BZDs occur in the liver, initially by phase I processes (dealkylation, hydroxylation) and subsequently by phase II processes (conjugation). For some of the BZDs (e.g. diazepam, midazolam), active metabolites are generated after phase I metabolism.

Note: Oxazepam and lorazepam do not pass through phase I processes and are directly conjugated by phase II metabolic processes.

The short-acting BZDs do not have residual (hangover) effects due to rapid redistribution. The long-acting BZDs (and those with active metabolites) also do not have residual effects (due to rapid redistribution), if used for a short-term. However, on long-term use, they can cause cumulative and residual effects.

The water-soluble metabolites generated after phase II processes are excreted in the urine.

BZDs cross the placental barrier and are secreted in breast milk.

Adverse Effects

The margin of safety with BZDs is high; and they are generally well tolerated.

The adverse effects of BZDs include:
- Drowsiness, decreased alertness, confusion, tiredness, dizziness, muscular weakness, psychomotor impairment, blurred vision, amnesia, ataxia
- Respiratory depression
- Tolerance can develop to the sedative effect
- Dependence—physical and psychological dependence occur on chronic use
- Increased risk of drug dependence/abuse in patients with history of alcohol or drug abuse
- Withdrawal syndrome—abrupt discontinuation can lead to withdrawal symptoms such as headache, mood changes, anxiety, sleep disturbance including insomnia, irritability, tremors, seizures etc.

o Paradoxical reactions such as stimulation, aggression, excitement etc.
o Elderly patients are more susceptible to the CNS effects of benzodiazepines
o BZDs can potentiate the depressant effects of alcohol and other CNS depressants
o BZDs can have harmful effects on the neonate if used during late phase of pregnancy or during labor. These effects include hypothermia, hypotonia ("Floppy baby syndrome"), respiratory depression, cardiac rhythm abnormalities etc.

Clinical Uses

Sedation and Hypnosis (Treatment of Insomnia)

Benzodiazepines are useful in the management of insomnia due to the following actions:
o Reduce sleep latency (patient falls asleep faster)
o Increase total sleep duration and reduce intermittent awakenings
o Decrease duration of stage 3 and 4 of NREM sleep
o Increase duration of stage 2 NREM sleep
o Decrease duration of REM sleep
o Decrease night terrors and movements during sleep

Benzodiazepines are preferred over barbiturates for the treatment of insomnia because of the following:
o BZDs have a wide therapeutic index leading to a higher margin of safety. Risk of loss of consciousness is higher with barbiturates.
o BZDs cause less distortion of sleep pattern and result in near normal sleep
o BZDs have a lower incidence of hangover effects (drowsiness, headache)
o BZDs have a lower incidence of respiratory or cardiac depression
o BZDs have a lower incidence of tolerance, dependence and abuse liability
o BZDs have a lower incidence of drug interactions as they do not have enzyme inducing properties
o Flumazenil is a BZD antagonist that can be used in patients of BZD overdose. No such antagonist is available for barbiturate overdose.

The key differences between benzodiazepines and barbiturates are mentioned in Table 3.

TABLE 3	Differences between benzodiazepines and barbiturates	
Parameter	Benzodiazepines (BZD)	Barbiturates (BBT)
Mechanism of action	GABA-facilitatory action	GABA-mimetic action
Binding site on GABA receptor complex	Specific BZD site	Specific BBT (? Picrotoxin) site
Therapeutic index	High	Low
Risk of loss of consciousness	Low	High
Depression of CVS and respiratory function	Low	High
Distortion of sleep pattern	Less (produce near normal sleep pattern)	More
Hangover (drowsiness, headache on next morning)	Less	More
Tolerance, dependence	Low incidence	High incidence
Abuse liability	Low	High
Enzyme induction and chances of drug interactions	Low	High
Antagonist	Yes (Flumazenil)	No
Clinical use as sedative and hypnotic	Commonly used	Rarely used

The benzodiazepines are used in the management of following types of insomnia (Table 4).

TABLE 4	Insomnia
Transient insomnia	• Usual duration of insomnia is 1–3 days • Associated with conditions such as unfamiliar surroundings, jet lag, shift workers etc. • Shorter acting drugs such as triazolam or temazepam can be considered
Short-term insomnia	• Usual duration of insomnia is 1–3 weeks • Associated with conditions such as work-related stress, period of grief, physical pain etc. • Temazepam can be considered
Chronic insomnia	• Usual duration of insomnia is >3 weeks • Associated with underlying disease or personality disorder • Intermittent use of longer acting drugs such as nitrazepam can be considered • Treatment of the underlying disease or personality disorder is essential

Antianxiety

The BZDs exert antianxiety effect due to action on the limbic system. Drugs such as diazepam, chlordiazepoxide, alprazolam and lorazepam have antianxiety action.

Anticonvulsant

The BZDs such as diazepam are used for emergency control of seizures in status epilepticus, tetanus and febrile convulsions. Other BZDs having anticonvulsant actions include clonazepam, nitrazepam and flurazepam.

However, diazepam is not used for maintenance therapy in epileptic patients because tolerance can develop to the anticonvulsive actions.

Preanesthetic Medication and General Anesthesia

The BZDs have sedative, antianxiety and amnesic actions; hence, are used for preanesthetic medication and general anesthesia. Midazolam and diazepam are often used for this purpose.

Minor Operative Procedures Including Endoscopies

The BZDs have sedative, antianxiety, muscle relaxant and amnesic actions; hence, are used for minor operative procedures including endoscopies. Midazolam and diazepam are often used for this purpose.

Muscle Relaxant

The BZDs produce muscle relaxation by central action. Diazepam is used in patients of spinal trauma and tetanus to reduce muscle spasm.

Conscious Sedation

Conscious sedation is used for multiple procedures such as dental procedures, endoscopies, liver, breast and kidney biopsies. It is often useful in uncooperative and anxious patients.

Alcohol Withdrawal

The BZDs are used in the management of symptoms occurring due to alcohol withdrawal.

INDIVIDUAL FEATURES OF BENZODIAZEPINES

The important features of commonly used benzodiazepines are mentioned below:

Diazepam

- It is the prototypic benzodiazepine.
- It is a long-acting benzodiazepine.
- It is completely absorbed from the GI tract and undergoes extensive metabolism in the liver.
- On occasional use, there is no residual effect (due to redistribution).
- On prolonged use, accumulation occurs (leads to prolonged antianxiety effects).
- Withdrawal effects are mild.
- It has sedative, antianxiety, muscle relaxant, amnesic and anticonvulsant properties.
- Can be used rectally to control convulsions in children.
- Desmethyldiazepam is an active metabolite of diazepam that has a long duration of action.

Alprazolam

- It is clinically used for the short-term management of anxiety, and anxiety associated with depression
- Withdrawal effects are particularly severe

Midazolam

- It is a short-acting benzodiazepine; has rapid onset of action
- It is administered by IV or IM routes
- It is commonly used for conscious sedation, preanesthetic medication and general anesthesia

NONBENZODIAZEPINES

These drugs bind to a specific benzodiazepine site on the $GABA_A$ receptor complex. Upon binding, they increase the frequency of opening of GABA-gated chloride channels. This results in hyperpolarization of membranes leading to CNS depression.

These drugs are commonly referred to as 'Z' drugs as their names start with the letter 'Z'. The drugs available are zolpidem, zaleplon, zopiclone and eszopiclone.

The key features of these Z drugs are mentioned in Figure 3.

Z drugs: Common pharmacological features

- Agonist effect on the specific benzodiazepine site on the $GABA_A$ receptor.
- Less/no anticonvulsant and muscle relaxant action, as compared to BZDs.
- Less withdrawal effects and less rebound insomnia, as compared to BZDs.
- Shorter half-life, minimal disturbance of overall sleep architecture.
- Clinical manifestations of Z drugs' overdose is similar to BZD overdose.
- Flumazenil is effective in treating overdose of both Z drugs and BZDs.
Hence, Z drugs, are increasingly being preferred in the treatment of insomnia.

Figure 3: Nonbenzodiazepines—pharmacological features

Zolpidem

- It is used for the short-term treatment of insomnia in adults.
- It reduces sleep latency and prolongs sleep duration.
- It decreases frequency of awakenings and improves quality of sleep.
- It does not have muscle relaxant, antianxiety and anticonvulsant properties.
- It causes minimal rebound insomnia and minimal tolerance or dependence.
- It is well-absorbed orally, metabolized in the liver and excreted in the urine.
- It has a short half-life of 2 hours.
- It is very well tolerated. The adverse effects are mild and commonly include headache, GIT disturbance and confusion.
- It is currently one of the commonly prescribed hypnotic drug.

Zopiclone

- It is used for the short-term treatment of insomnia in adults. It is also used in weaning off insomniacs who are regularly taking BZDs.
- It does not cause a reduction of REM sleep; it prolongs stage 3 and 4 of sleep.
- The chances of rebound insomnia or hangover is less than BZDs.
- The adverse effects include impaired alertness, bitter taste, dry mouth and rarely dependence.
- Eszopiclone is an active enantiomer of zopiclone used orally for long-term treatment of insomnia and maintenance of sleep.

Zaleplon

- Amongst the nonbenzodiazepines, it is the shortest acting hypnotic drug.
- It is clinically used for the management of sleep onset insomnia.

BARBITURATES

Barbiturates are now rarely used as sedatives or hypnotics. They are predominantly used as anticonvulsants (phenobarbitone) and for the induction of anesthesia (thiopentone).

Mechanism of Action

Barbiturates cause non-selective depression of the CNS. They act by binding to a specific site on the $GABA_A$ receptor complex. The CNS depression is generally dose dependent, with smaller doses leading to sedation and higher doses leading to loss of consciousness, anesthesia and coma (Figure 4).

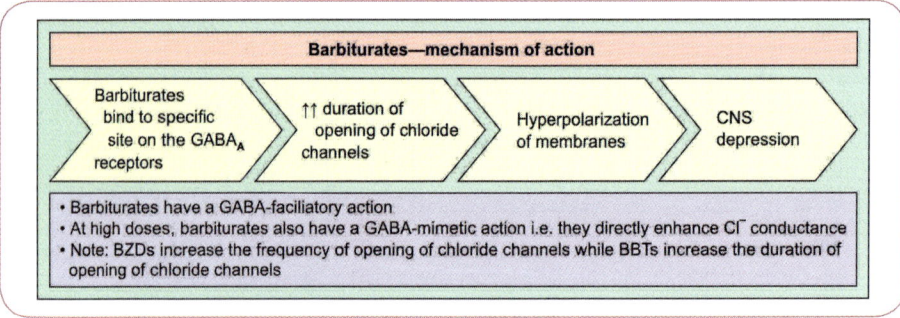

Figure 4: Mechanism of action of barbiturates

Pharmacological Actions

Some of the pharmacological actions of barbiturates are mentioned in Table 5.

TABLE 5	Pharmacological actions of barbiturates
Central nervous system	• Nonselective depression of the CNS • Sedation, hypnosis, loss of consciousness, coma, death • Anticonvulsant action • No analgesic property, may cause hyperalgesia
Cardiovascular system	• Higher doses can cause cardiac depression, leading to reduced blood pressure and heart rate
Respiratory system	• Higher doses can cause respiratory depression

The differences between barbiturates and benzodiazepines are mentioned in Table 3.

Clinical Uses

The clinical uses of barbiturates are mentioned below:
- **General anesthesia**
  - Ultrashort acting barbiturates such as thiopentone are used for induction of general anesthesia. Thiopentone is also used as an adjunct to provide hypnosis during balanced anesthesia with other anesthetic agents, such as analgesics and muscle relaxants.
- **Anticonvulsant**
  - Long acting barbiturates such as phenobarbitone are used in patients of epilepsy.
- **Neonatal hyperbilirubinemia**
  - Phenobarbitone is an enzyme inducer. Hence, it can enhance the activity of enzyme glucuronyl transferase. This leads to metabolism and excretion of bilirubin resulting in reduced levels of bilirubin in the body.
- **Sedative and hypnotic**
  - As compared to benzodiazepines, barbiturates are rarely used as sedatives-hypnotics. The reasons for the same are mentioned in Table 3.

Adverse Effects

The key adverse effects of barbiturates are mentioned below:
- Drowsiness, decreased alertness, confusion, ataxia, memory impairment
- Hypersensitivity reactions
- Physical and psychological dependence—have significant abuse liability
- Withdrawal symptoms following abrupt discontinuation
- Tolerance development
- Respiratory and cardiac depression
- Barbiturates (e.g. thiopentone) are contraindicated in patients of acute intermittent porphyria.
  - This is because barbiturates can induce microsomal enzymes (ALA synthetase) and cause an increase in porphyrins leading to precipitation of acute intermittent porphyria.
- Long-term administration of phenobarbitone may result in megaloblastic anemia due to interference of folate absorption from the GIT.
- **Acute barbiturate poisoning:** The clinical features are due to CNS depression and includes loss of consciousness, respiratory depression, cardiovascular depression with hypotension, cardiac arrest and coma.

  The management includes the following:
  - Maintenance of airway and breathing → endotracheal intubation and ventilatory support including mechanical ventilation
  - Maintenance of fluid and electrolyte balance
  - Circulatory management including adequate hydration. Vasopressor support may be required.
  - Gastric lavage with activated charcoal
  - Alkaline diuresis → Sodium bicarbonate is used to produce alkaline urine. Barbiturates (being weakly acidic drugs) become ionized in alkaline urine. Ionized form of barbiturates is not reabsorbed from the renal tubules. This leads to increased excretion of barbiturates in the urine.
  - Hemodialysis

MISCELLANEOUS DRUGS

Melatonin

- It is a hormone produced by the pineal gland.
- It has sleep promoting action and is involved in the control of circadian rhythms.
- It is clinically used in the short-term treatment of primary insomnia in adult patients (age 55 years or more).

Ramelteon

- It is a melatonin receptor agonist and has high affinity for MT_1 and MT_2 receptors.
- Ramelteon's activity on MT_1 and MT_2 receptors is possibly associated with its sleep promoting effects.

- ○ It has minimal abuse potential and does not cause dependence.
- ○ It is clinically used in the management of sleep-onset insomnia.
- ○ The adverse effects include nausea, fatigue, somnolence, dizziness and hyperprolactinemia.

Orexin Receptor Antagonist – e.g. Suvorexant

- ○ Orexin A and B are peptides in the hypothalamus neurons that are involved in the control of wakefulness. Orexin-receptor antagonist such as suvorexant is therefore, considered to suppress wakefulness and promote sleep-enabling effects.
- ○ Suvorexant is indicated for the treatment of insomnia, characterized by difficulties with sleep onset and/or sleep maintenance.

▋ BENZODIAZEPINE ANTAGONIST

Flumazenil is a competitive benzodiazepine antagonist that can reverse the effects of benzodiazepine agonists (e.g. diazepam) or inverse agonists (e.g. β-carboline).

Flumazenil is used intravenously.

It is used to reverse the CNS depressant effects in BZD poisonings/overdose (specific antidote).

It is also used to reverse the sedative/hypnotic effects of benzodiazepines (e.g. diazepam, midazolam), zolpidem and zaleplon occurring during anesthesia practice or in the intensive care unit.

It has a short half-life of 1 hour due to rapid hepatic clearance. As most BZDs have a duration of action longer than flumazenil, sedation frequently comes back after 1 hour or so. Hence, flumazenil has to be repeatedly administered for several hours.

The adverse effects include allergic reactions, dizziness, nausea, vomiting, agitation and withdrawal symptoms.

ASSESS YOURSELF (Examination Questions of Various Universities)

1. Classify sedatives and hypnotics. Discuss the mechanism of action, adverse effects and clinical uses of diazepam.
2. List important differences between barbiturates and benzodiazepines.
3. Write short notes on:
   a. Flumazenil
   b. Non-benzodiazepine hypnotics
   c. Clinical uses of diazepam
   d. Zolpidem in insomnia
4. Mention two advantages of benzodiazepines over barbiturates as hypnotic.

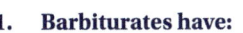

MULTIPLE CHOICE QUESTIONS

1. **Barbiturates have:** *(Recent Question Dec 2016)*
   a. GABA mimetic
   b. GABA facilitatory
   c. Both
   d. None
2. **Inverse agonist is:** *(Recent Question 2016)*
   a. Buspirone
   b. β carboline
   c. Flumazenil
   d. Zolpidem
3. **Antagonist of benzodiazepine is:**
   (Recent Question 2016)
   a. Naltrexone
   b. Flumazenil
   c. Naloxone
   d. N-Acetyl cysteine
4. **Agents not acting via GABA-A receptors:**
   (Recent Question 2016)
   a. Zopiclone
   b. Benzodiazepines
   c. Thiopentone
   d. Promethazine
5. **Increased tendency to fall asleep at night without causing central nervous system depression is a property exhibited by:** *(Recent Question 2016)*
   a. Pyridoxine
   b. Diphenhydramine
   c. Melatonin
   d. Ethanol
6. **Drug contraindicated in acute intermittent porphyria:** *(Recent Question 2016)*
   a. Thiopentone
   b. Ketamine
   c. Propofol
   d. Etomidate
7. **Long-acting benzodiazepines-A/E** *(TNPG 2010)*
   a. Diazepam
   b. Clonazepam
   c. Lorazepam
   d. Chlordiazepoxide

Ans.

1. (c)	2. (b)	3. (b)	4. (d)	5. (c)	6. (a)	
7. (c)						

21 Opioid Analgesics

Opioids have been used for many years for the management of pain.

Opium is a dark brown substance obtained from the capsule of poppy (*Papaver somniferum*). Opiate is a substance that is derived from opium (e.g. morphine).

CLASSIFICATION OF OPIOIDS AND OPIOID ANTAGONISTS

A classification of opioids and opioid antagonists is mentioned in Table 1.

TABLE 1	Opioid agonists and antagonists
Opioid agonists	**Natural opium alkaloids** • Phenanthrene derivatives → Morphine, codeine, thebaine • Benzoisoquinoline derivatives → Papaverine, noscapine *Thebaine, papaverine and noscapine are nonanalgesics*
	Semisynthetic opiates • Diacetylmorphine (heroin), pholcodine, hydromorphone
	Synthetic opioids • Pethidine, fentanyl, alfentanil, remifentanil, sufentanil, tramadol, methadone, dextropropoxyphene
Partial μ (mu) agonist and κ (kappa) antagonist	Buprenorphine
Opioid agonist-antagonists	Pentazocine, butorphanol, nalorphine
Pure antagonists	Naloxone, naltrexone, nalmefene

OPIOID RECEPTORS

Opioids produce their effects by interacting with opioid receptors. The opioid receptors are present in the brain (e.g. thalamus), spinal cord, peripheral nerves and tissues. Some of the salient features regarding the three main types of opioid receptors are mentioned in Table 2.

TABLE 2	Opioid receptors
μ (mu) receptor	• ↑↑ affinity for morphine • Functional subtypes are μ_1 (mu$_1$) and μ_2 (mu$_2$) • Key effects include supraspinal and spinal analgesia, respiratory depression, miosis, sedation, decreased gastrointestinal motility, euphoria, physical dependence
κ (kappa) receptor	• ↑↑ affinity for ketocyclazocine and dynorphin A • Functional subtypes are κ_1 (kappa$_1$) and κ_3 (kappa$_3$) • Key effects include supraspinal and spinal analgesia, respiratory depression, sedation, decreased gastrointestinal motility, dysphoria, psychomimetic, physical dependence
δ (delta) receptor	• ↑↑ affinity for leu/met enkephalins • Key effects include supraspinal and spinal analgesia, respiratory depression, decreased gastrointestinal motility, proconvulsant effect

OPIOID AGONISTS

NATURAL OPIOID AGONIST

Morphine

Morphine is the main alkaloid in opium and is a commonly used opioid. It acts mainly on the μ (mu) opioid receptor. It is considered as a prototype drug.

Pharmacological Effects

The pharmacological effects of morphine are mentioned below:

Central Nervous System (CNS)

Morphine has both stimulatory and depressant effects on the CNS.

CNS depressant effects are:
- Analgesia
  - Morphine is a potent analgesic drug
  - Produces analgesia through spinal and supraspinal sites
  - Has a better effect on dull visceral pain as compared to sharp somatic pain
  - Alters the perception of pain and the associated reaction (e.g. apprehension, fear)
- Subjective effects
  - Can result in mental confusion, reduced concentration, reduced apprehension, decreased anxiety
  - Can lead to euphoria
- Sedation
  - Can produce drowsiness; higher doses can lead to coma
- Respiratory depression
  - Causes depression of the respiratory center in the medulla
  - Death in morphine overdose is often due to respiratory failure
- Cough suppression
  - Due to suppression of the cough center
- Hypothermia
  - Depression of the temperature regulating center—can lead to hypothermia
- Depression of the vasomotor center
  - Can lead to hypotension

CNS stimulatory effects are:
- Nausea and vomiting
  - Due to stimulation of the chemoreceptor trigger zone (CTZ)
- Miosis
  - Due to stimulation of Edinger-Westphal nucleus of the IIIrd cranial nerve (oculomotor nerve)
- Bradycardia
  - Due to stimulation of the vagal center

Cardiovascular System

- Vasodilation—occurs due to the following:
  - Release of histamine
  - Depression of vasomotor center
  - Reduction in tone of blood vessels
- Increased vasodilation in the systemic circulation—leading to shift of blood from the pulmonary to systemic circulation

215

Gastrointestinal Tract

○ Constipation: Occurs due to the following:
  ❑ Direct action (on the intestines and the CNS) to increase tone and decrease motility
  ❑ Spasm of sphincters
  ❑ Reduction in GI secretions

Tolerance does not develop to the constipating effect of morphine.

Endocrine

○ Decrease levels of FSH, LH and ACTH
○ Increase levels of GH and prolactin
○ Decrease release of ADH

Other Effects

○ Urinary bladder → Increase tone of sphincter and detrusor muscle. Can lead to urinary retention.
○ Biliary tract → Increase intrabiliary pressure by causing spasm of sphincter of Oddi. Can lead to biliary colic.
○ Bronchoconstriction, pruritus → Due to release of histamine
○ Mild hyperglycemia
○ Physical and psychological dependence

A summary of the key pharmacological effects (of morphine) is mentioned in Table 3.

TABLE 3	Pharmacological effects of morphine
CNS depressant effects	• Analgesia, sedation • Respiratory depression, cough suppression • Hypothermia, depression of vasomotor center
CNS stimulatory effects	• Nausea, vomiting, miosis • Stimulation of vagal center ($\downarrow$ HR)
Cardiovascular system	• Hypotension • Shifting of blood from the pulmonary to systemic circulation
Gastrointestinal tract	• Constipation
Endocrine	• $\downarrow$ levels of LH, FSH, ACTH • $\uparrow$ levels of GH and prolactin • $\uparrow$ release of ADH
Other effects	• Urinary retention • $\uparrow$ intrabiliary pressure → biliary colic • Release of histamine → pruritus, bronchoconstriction • Physical and psychological dependence

Pharmacokinetics

Morphine has a high first pass metabolism with poor oral bioavailability; oral absorption is slow and unreliable.

Morphine is frequently administered parenterally (IM, IV). It is widely distributed in the body and crosses the placenta.

Morphine undergoes glucuronide conjugation in the liver. The metabolites morphine-6-glucuronide has analgesic effects, while morphine-3-glucuronide can cause neuroexcitatory effects.

Morphine is eliminated mainly in the urine.

Adverse Effects

The key adverse effects of morphine are mentioned in Table 4.

TABLE 4	Adverse effects of morphine
• Respiratory depression including apnea
• Respiratory depression can also occur in the newborn if morphine is administered to the mother during labor. It can lead to apnea.
• Constipation, nausea, vomiting
• Urinary retention, blurring of vision
• Sedation, drowsiness, confusion
• Pruritus
• Hypotension
• Reduced seizure threshold
• Allergic reactions → urticaria, rashes, anaphylaxis
• Acute morphine poisoning
• Drug tolerance → develops to many effects of morphine; however, minimal or no tolerance develops to the miotic and constipating effect. Opioids also exhibit cross tolerance.
• Drug dependence (physical and psychological)

ACUTE MORPHINE POISONING

Clinical Features

○ Respiratory depression, constricted or pinpoint pupils, coma
○ Confusion, dizziness, hypotension, shock, pulmonary edema
○ Death is often due to respiratory failure

Management

○ Management of airway, breathing and circulation.
○ Establishment of a patent airway along with assisted or controlled ventilation
○ Fluid and electrolyte balance
○ Gastric lavage with potassium permanganate
○ Naloxone is the specific antidote. It is administered intravenously.

Drug Dependence (Physical and Psychological)

Morphine can produce physical and psychological drug dependence. It can lead to addiction and drug abuse.

Clinical features of morphine withdrawal include the following:
○ Drug seeking behavior
○ Yawning, salivation, lacrimation, irritability, sweating, diarrhea, increased blood pressure, mydriasis
○ Cardiovascular collapse can occur.

Management of morphine dependence includes the following:
○ Requires care in a specialized center
○ Withdrawal of morphine → followed by substitution therapy with oral methadone. Gradual withdrawal of methadone is performed.
○ Methadone is preferred for the substitution therapy because it is effective orally, has a prolonged duration of action, has slow development of tolerance and milder withdrawal signs and symptoms. Methadone also has a lower abuse potential than morphine.
○ Supportive management including psychological therapy, counseling etc. are important.

Administration of opioid antagonists such as naloxone in opioid dependent persons can lead to acute withdrawal syndrome.

Contraindications and Precautions

The key precautions and contraindications of morphine are mentioned below:
- Patients with bronchial asthma → can lead to bronchospasm due to release of histamine by morphine
- Head injury patients → morphine is contraindicated due to the reasons mentioned in Table 5.

TABLE 5	Morphine is contraindicated in head injury patients

- Morphine can produce effects such as nausea, vomiting, miosis and mental confusion, which can interfere with the assessment of neurological function/ clinical progress in patients of head injury.
- Morphine can cause respiratory depression which can lead to CO, retention. Increased CO, can cause cerebral vasodilatation leading to an increase in intracranial pressure.
- Increased sensitivity to respiratory depressant effects of morphine.

- Infants and elderly → increased risk of respiratory depression. Elderly are more prone for urinary retention
- Patients having impaired pulmonary function such as emphysema, pulmonary fibrosis
- Patients with undiagnosed acute abdominal pain
  - Administration of morphine in such patients may lead to aggravation of conditions such as diverticulitis, biliary colic etc.
- Patients with hypotensive conditions such as shock or those with decreased blood volume
- Patients with hepatic disease, renal disease and hypothyroidism exhibit increased sensitivity to the effects of morphine

Codeine

It is a naturally occurring opioid and is methyl-morphine. The analgesic potency and efficacy of codeine is lower than morphine. Codeine also has a low abuse potential.

The clinical uses of codeine include:
- Suppression of cough
- Analgesia (mild to moderate pain) → can lead to constipation.

SYNTHETIC OPIOID AGONISTS

Pethidine (Meperidine)

It is a synthetic opioid. The key features of pethidine and morphine are mentioned in Table 6.

TABLE 6	Morphine and pethidine	
	Morphine	Pethidine
Origin	Natural opium alkaloid	Synthetic opioid
Analgesic potency	More potent	Less potent (1/10th)
Antitussive effect	High	Not effective
Sedative, euphoric effects and abuse potential	Similar	Similar
Effects on smooth muscle (constipation, urinary retention, miosis)	More prominent	Less prominent

Contd...

	Morphine	Pethidine
Respiratory depression	Similar	Similar (If administered during labor, pethidine causes relatively less respiratory depression in the neonate)
Heart rate	Bradycardia	Tachycardia (antimuscarinic effect)
Histamine release	More	Less
Oral absorption	Slow and unreliable	Well absorbed

Pethidine is metabolized in the liver. The two metabolites are meperidinic acid (major metabolite) and norpethidine (minor metabolite). The metabolites are excreted in the urine.

Pethidine also has local anesthetic action.

Adverse Effects

The adverse effects of pethidine include the following:
- Pethidine has a similar adverse effect profile as that of morphine. Patients may have some antimuscarinic effects such as tachycardia, dry mouth and blurred vision.
- Overdose of pethidine may produce excitatory effects due to accumulation of norpethidine (which has excitatory effects). These include tremors, mydriasis, delirium and convulsions.
- Tolerance and dependence can also develop with pethidine.

Fentanyl

- It is a synthetic opioid and its potency is 80–100 times more than morphine.
- It has high lipid solubility and has a short duration of action.
- It is clinically used to provide analgesia during some surgical procedures. It is also available as transdermal patch and is used for cancer or other chronic painful conditions.

Methadone

- It is a synthetic opioid with similar actions as that of morphine.
- It is orally effective and has a long duration of action. It accumulates in tissues on repeated dosing.
- It is used as a substitution therapy for opioid dependence because it is effective orally, has a prolonged duration of action, has slow development of tolerance and milder and gradual withdrawal signs and symptoms. Methadone also has a lower abuse potential than morphine.
- It can also be used for analgesia.
- Rifampicin and phenytoin enhance the metabolism of methadone and hence, can precipitate withdrawal syndrome.

Tramadol

- Tramadol is a centrally acting synthetic opioid analgesic.
- It is a weak agonist at μ receptors. It also inhibits the reuptake of noradrenaline (NA) and 5-hydroxytryptamine (5-HT).
- It has a low abuse potential. It produces less respiratory depression, urinary retention, sedation and constipation as compared to morphine.
- Clinical uses include mild to moderate pain.

CLINICAL USES OF OPIOIDS

Some of the clinical uses of opioids are mentioned in Table 7.

TABLE 7	Clinical uses of opioids
Analgesia	• Useful in moderate to severe pain in conditions such as injury, trauma, burns, myocardial infarction, surgical and postsurgical patients, malignancies etc.
Preanesthetic medication	• Opioids such as morphine, pethidine can be used in some patients
Acute left ventricular failure	Morphine is useful in patients with acute left ventricular failure (cardiac asthma) due to the following effects: • Vasodilatation and peripheral pooling of blood → ↓ preload • Shifting of blood from the pulmonary to systemic circulation → ↓ pulmonary congestion • ↓ apprehension, ↓ anxiety, ↓ sympathetic stimulation and ↓ cardiac work Morphine can also reduce pulmonary edema due to causes such as infarction of lungs.
Cough (dry cough suppression)	• Drugs such as codeine and dextromethorphan are used
Diarrhea	• Drugs such as codeine, diphenoxylate and loperamide are used
Postanesthetic shivering	• Pethidine is useful

PARTIAL μ (MU) AGONIST AND κ (KAPPA) ANTAGONIST

BUPRENORPHINE

The analgesic potency of buprenorphine is 25 times more than morphine. Buprenorphine has a slower onset and a longer duration of action, as compared to morphine.

Compared to morphine, buprenorphine:
- Has higher analgesic potency
- Onset of action is slow, and duration of action is longer
- Produces less constipation
- Produces less dependence (physical, psychological) and tolerance
- Has lower abuse liability

The clinical uses of buprenorphine include chronic painful conditions such as pain associated with malignancies. Other uses include premedication, postoperative analgesia and morphine dependence.

AGONISTS-ANTAGONISTS

PENTAZOCINE

It has agonist action on κ (kappa) receptors and weak antagonist action on μ (mu) receptors.
- Acts on κ (kappa) receptors leading to analgesia
- Sympathetic stimulation can lead to tachycardia and rise in BP. Hence, pentazocine should be avoided in patients with coronary artery disease and MI.
- Sedation and respiratory depression are less as compared to morphine
- Compared to morphine, pentazocine has a lower severity of constipation and biliary spasm, lower incidence of vomiting
- Tolerance and dependence (physical and psychological) can develop on prolonged use
- It can also lead to dysphoric effects and hallucinations

Clinical uses of pentazocine include moderate to severe pain in conditions such as malignancies, trauma and burns. It can also be used for postoperative pain.

PURE ANTAGONISTS

NALOXONE

It is a competitive antagonist at opioid receptors and is the drug of choice in morphine poisoning.

Naloxone does not have any agonist activity and does not cause dependence (physical or psychological).

It can reverse all the effects of morphine including analgesic and respiratory depressant effects. It can block analgesia induced by placebo and acupuncture. Naloxone can precipitate withdrawal in morphine dependent patients.

Naloxone is inactive orally and is administered intravenously.

Clinical uses include the following:

- Morphine poisoning—it has a short duration of action which should be considered during treatment of morphine overdose. Repeated administration is required.
- Treatment of neonatal asphyxia due to opioid administration to the mother during labor.
- Overdose with other opioids except buprenorphine. Effects of buprenorphine are only partially reversed by naloxone because buprenorphine is very tightly bound to opioid receptors.

NALTREXONE

- It is orally active, more potent and has a longer duration of action, as compared to naloxone.
- Clinical uses include opioid blockade therapy in opioid dependent persons as well as treatment of alcoholics.
- The adverse effects include nausea and hepatotoxicity.

NALMEFENE

- Longer acting as compared to naloxone.

ASSESS YOURSELF (Examination Questions of Various Universities)

1. Classify opioid analgesics. Discuss the pharmacological effects, adverse effects and clinical uses of morphine.
2. Discuss the treatment of morphine poisoning giving relevant pharmacology of naloxone.
3. List important differences between morphine and pethidine.
4. Write short notes on:
   a. Methadone
   b. Tramadol
   c. Buprenorphine
   d. Pentazocine

e. Naloxone
f. Opioid antagonists
g. Orally effective pure morphine antagonist
5. Explain why:
   a. Morphine is contraindicated (i.e. not given) in patients with head injury
   b. Morphine is useful in acute left ventricular failure
   c. Methadone is used for maintenance therapy in chronic opioid dependence

MULTIPLE CHOICE QUESTIONS

1. Which of the following is seen due to opioid withdrawal? *(Recent Question Dec 2016)*
   a. Pupil dilation
   b. Constipation
   c. Sedation
   d. Respiratory depression
2. Opioid receptor which is responsible for dysphoria: *(AIIMS May 2013)*
   a. Mu
   b. Kappa
   c. Delta
   d. Sigma
3. Which is the mechanism of action of Buprenorphine? *(Recent Question 2016)*
   a. Partial agonist at mu and antagonist at kappa
   b. Partial agonist at kappa and antagonist at mu and delta
   c. Partial agonist at mu and kappa and antagonist at delta
   d. Partial agonist at mu kappa and delta
4. Buprenorphine is: *(Recent Question 2016)*
   a. Partial agonist at μ receptor
   b. Partial agonist at κ receptor
   c. Full agonist at μ receptor
   d. Full agonist at κ receptor
5. Tolerance develops to all of the following actions of opioids except: *(Recent Question 2016)*
   a. Miosis
   b. Analgesia
   c. Euphoria
   d. Nausea and vomiting
6. A newborn developed respiratory depression in a postoperative ward. It can result from the use of: *(Recent Question 2016)*
   a. Opioid
   b. Propofol
   c. Furosemide
   d. Heparin

7. Long-term use of pethidine is avoided because a metabolite of pethidine is associated with:
   a. Constipation *(Recent Question 2016)*
   b. Dependence
   c. Seizures
   d. Respiratory depression
8. In acute morphine poisoning, the drug of choice is: *(Recent Question 2016)*
   a. Atropine
   b. Methadone
   c. Naloxone
   d. Alcohol
9. Naltrexone is used for poisoning of: *(Recent Question 2016)*
   a. Heroin
   b. Atropine
   c. Cannabis
   d. Diazepam
10. Tramadol is: *(Recent Question 2016)*
    a. Antiflatulent
    b. Antireflux drug
    c. Beta-blocker
    d. Opioid analgesic
11. The effect of morphine which has least tolerance is: *(Recent Question 2016)*
    a. Analgesia
    b. Respiratory depression
    c. Constipation
    d. Bradycardia
12. Opioid with monoamine action is: *(Recent Question 2016)*
    a. Tramadol
    b. Pentazocine
    c. Pethidine
    d. Meperidine
13. Drug with agonist action to any opioid receptors are all except: *(Recent Question 2016)*
    a. Pentazocine
    b. Buprenorphine
    c. Levonorphan
    d. Naloxone
14. Opioid withdrawal is characterized by all except: *(Recent Question 2016)*
    a. Miosis
    b. Salivation
    c. Diarrhea
    d. Lacrimation

Ans.

1. (a)	2. (b)	3. (a)	4. (a)	5. (a)	6. (a)
7. (c)	8. (c)	9. (a)	10. (d)	11. (c)	12. (a)
13. (d)	14. (a)				

Antiparkinsonian Drugs

DRUGS USED FOR PARKINSON'S DISEASE

Parkinson's disease (PD), also known as 'paralysis agitans' or 'shaking palsy', was first described by Sir James Parkinson in 1817. It is one of the most common neurodegenerative disorders.

It affects approximately 1% of individuals over the age of 65 years.

CLINICAL FEATURES

Parkinson's disease is a chronic and progressive neurodegenerative disorder.

There are two main neuropathological features in PD: loss of pigmented dopaminergic neurons in the substantia nigra pars compacta (SNpc) and the presence of Lewy bodies (Figure 1).

Loss of dopaminergic neurons in substantia nigra pars compacta (SNpc)	Lewy bodies
• Approximately 60–80% of the dopaminergic neurons are lost before the motor signs of PD are observed.	• Lewy bodies are abnormal protein aggregates (eosinophilic inclusions) that develop inside residual dopaminergic neurons. • The primary structural component of Lewy bodies is **alpha-synuclein**.

Figure 1: Neuropathological features in Parkinson's disease

Parkinson's disease is mainly a clinical diagnosis. The clinical features of PD are mentioned in Figure 2.

Cardinal features			
Bradykinesia • Slowness of voluntary movement • Commonly observed as: ◆ *Micrographia*—small handwriting ◆ *Decreased movements* as walking, eating etc. ◆ *Hypomimia*—decreased facial expression ◆ *Hypophonia*—decreased vocal volume	**Rigidity** • Involuntary increase in muscle tone; present throughout the range of movement. • Two types are identified: ◆ *Cogwheel rigidity*: Jerky, ratchet-like resistance to passive movement, in which the muscles alternatively become tensed and relaxed. ◆ *Lead-pipe rigidity*: Smooth and consistent rigidity. More sustained resistance to passive movement.	**Resting tremors** • Rhythmic oscillatory movements around a joint. • Known as resting tremors because they are maximum at rest and disappear upon voluntary movements and sleep. • Occur at a frequency of 4–6 Hz. Commonly manifests as: ◆ *Pill-rolling tremor*: Back-and-forth rubbing of the thumb and forefinger.	**Postural imbalance*** • Leads to stooped posture and reduced arm swing. • The Parkinsonian gait is characteristic and is mentioned below: ◆ *Shuffling gait* which is characterized by short steps, with feet barely leaving the ground ◆ *Festination* is a combination of stooped posture, imbalance, and short steps. The gait progressively gets faster and faster, often resulting in a fall.
Note: * Postural imbalance (leading to disturbances of gait and falling) is a late feature and is sometimes considered as a 4th cardinal feature. * Prominent postural imbalance in the initial few years may suggest that PD may not be the correct diagnosis.			

Contd...

Noncardinal features

Some of the noncardinal features (observed in PD) are:
- **Cognitive decline:** Such as memory difficulties, slowed thinking, confusion and in some cases, dementia
- **Affective disorders:** Such as depression and anxiety
- **Abnormality of autonomic functions:** Such as bladder function abnormalities, orthostatic hypotension, sexual problems, excessive sweating and salivation etc.
- **REM behavior sleep disorder**
- **Weight loss, weight gain, fatigue**

Figure 2: Clinical features of Parkinson's disease

Without adequate treatment, PD progresses to a rigid akinetic state in 5–10 years, wherein the patients are unable to care for themselves. Death commonly results from complications of immobility, such as pulmonary embolism or aspiration pneumonia.

PATHOGENESIS

Parkinson's disease is primarily a disorder of the basal ganglia. Basal ganglia is mainly involved in body movement. The basal ganglia comprise of 5 interactive structures located on each side of the brain (Figure 3).

- Globus pallidus is divided into external and internal segments called globus pallidus externa (GPe) and globus pallidus interna (GPi)
- Substantia nigra is divided into substantia nigra pars compact (SNpc) and substantia nigra pars reticularis (SNpr)

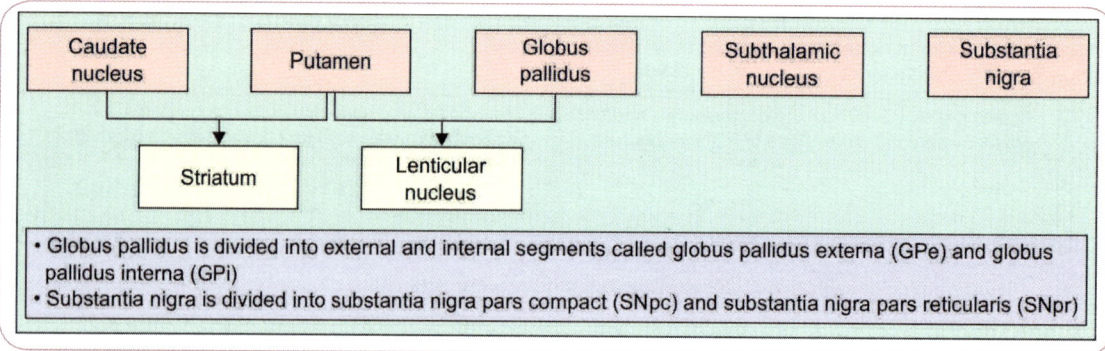

Figure 3: Components of basal ganglia

There are four neurotransmitters involved in the functioning of basal ganglia. These are mentioned in Figure 4.

Excitatory	Inhibitory
• Glutamate • Acetylcholine	• Dopamine • Gamma aminobutyric acid (GABA)

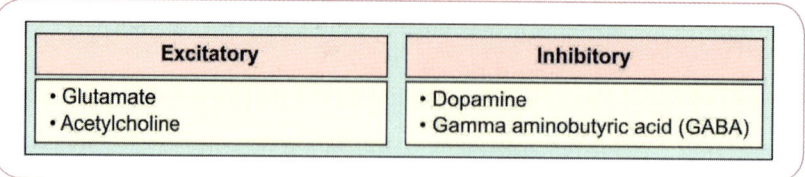

Figure 4: Neurotransmitters involved in basal ganglia

CLASSIFICATION

The classification of antiparkinsonian drugs is mentioned in Table 1.

TABLE 1	Classification of antiparkinsonian drugs
Drugs acting on brain dopaminergic system	**Dopamine precursor** • Levodopa (L-DOPA)
	Peripheral decarboxylase inhibitors • Carbidopa • Benserazide
	Dopamine receptor agonists • Bromocriptine • Pergolide • Apomorphine • Ropinirole • Pramipexole • Rotigotine
	COMT inhibitors • Entacapone • Tolcapone
	MAO B inhibitors • Selegiline (Deprenyl) • Rasagiline
Drugs acting on brain cholinergic system	**Centrally acting anticholinergics** • Trihexyphenidyl • Procyclidine • Benztropine
	Antihistaminics with anticholinergic activity • Promethazine • Orphenadrine

MECHANISM OF ACTION

Blood-brain barrier (BBB) plays an important role in the mechanism of action of various antiparkinsonian drugs. The BBB is a semipermeable membrane that separates the brain from the circulatory system.

In PD, there is a loss of the dopaminergic neurons leading to a deficiency of dopamine in the brain. This results in an imbalance between the dopaminergic and cholinergic system in the striatum that results in motor defects.

Pharmacotherapy of PD therefore, focuses on increasing dopamine availability or dopamine action in the brain. This is achieved by external supplementation of dopamine, decrease in metabolism of dopamine, direct dopamine receptor agonistic action and anticholinergic action.

There are 3 main enzymes that play an important role in therapeutics of PD:
○ DOPA decarboxylase—present both centrally and peripherally
○ Catechol-O-methyltransferase (COMT)—present both centrally and peripherally
○ Monoamine oxidase B (MAO-B)—present centrally

DOPA Decarboxylase

Dopamine does not cross the BBB, and therefore, does not have any therapeutic effect in PD when given in the peripheral circulation. However, levodopa which is a metabolic precursor of dopamine do cross the BBB and gets converted to dopamine in the brain via the enzyme DOPA decarboxylase.

An important aspect is that DOPA decarboxylase also exists in the peripheral circulation wherein it also converts levodopa to dopamine. This peripherally produced dopamine does not exert any therapeutic effect in PD (as it does not cross the BBB), but leads to several adverse effects such as nausea, vomiting, tachycardia, hypotension etc.

Peripheral decarboxylase inhibitors (carbidopa/benserazide) inhibit the enzyme DOPA decarboxylase; thereby preventing the peripheral conversion of levodopa to dopamine. This results in an increase in the amount of levodopa available to cross the BBB. Hence, co-administration of levodopa + carbidopa leads to an increase in the therapeutic benefit of levodopa and a decrease in its adverse effects.

The mechanism of action of various drugs used in the treatment of Parkinson's disease is mentioned in Figure 5.

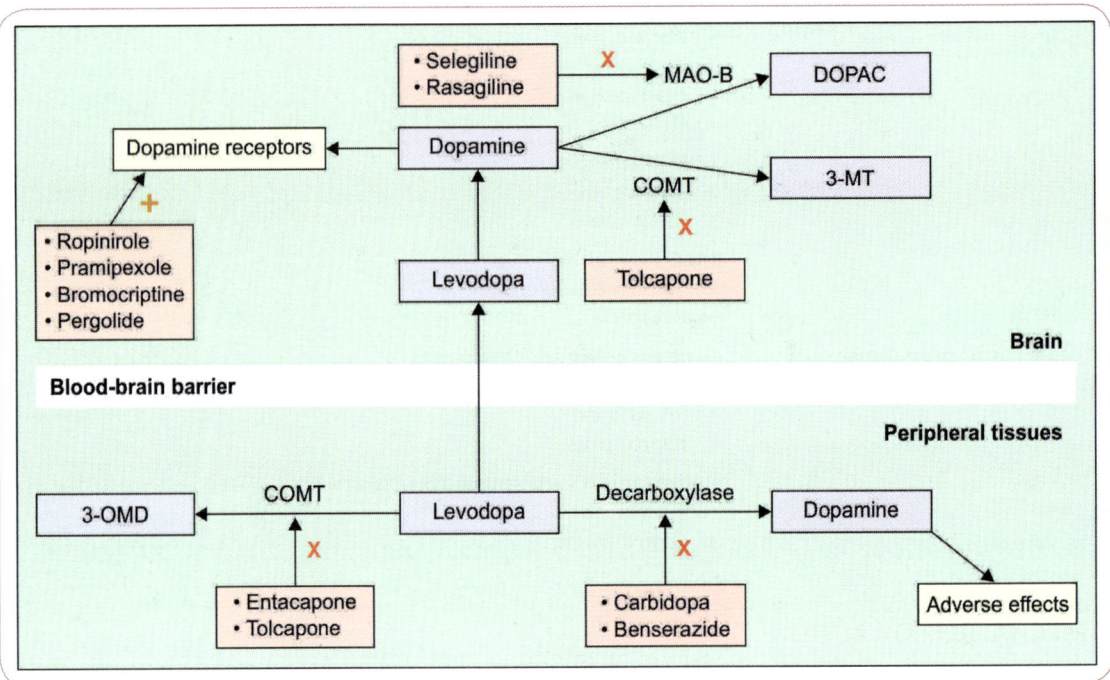

Figure 5: Pharmacological mechanisms for dopaminergic therapy in Parkinson's disease

Abbreviation: COMT: catechol-O-methyltransferase; MAO monoamine oxidase; 3-OMD: 3-O-methyl DOPA; 3-MT: 3-methoxytyramine; DOPAC; 3,4-dihydroxyphenylacetic acid

DRUGS ACTING ON BRAIN DOPAMINERGIC SYSTEM

LEVODOPA

Levodopa is the most effective drug for the treatment of Parkinson's disease. It is the metabolic precursor of dopamine. Levodopa is mostly inert and exerts therapeutic effects as well as adverse effects, by conversion to the neurotransmitter dopamine.

Levodopa when administered alone or when administered with a peripheral decarboxylase inhibitor, produce different results (Figure 6).

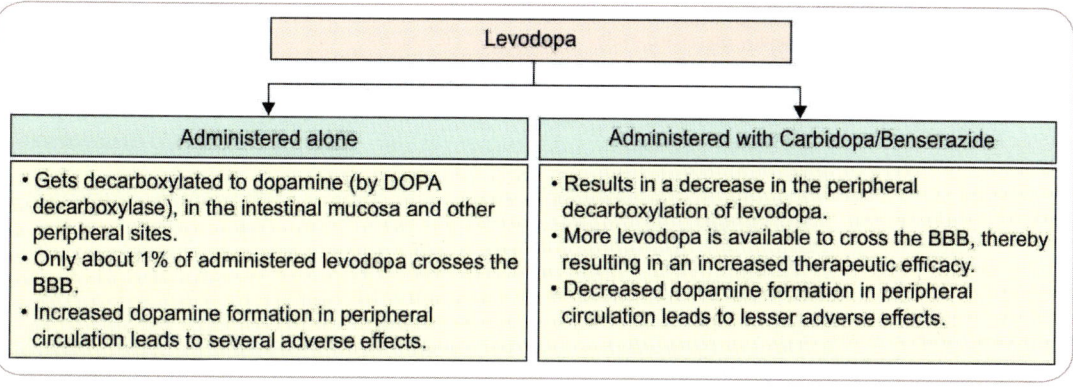

Figure 6: Fate of levodopa when administered alone or with a peripheral decarboxylase inhibitor

Carbidopa is a peripherally acting DOPA decarboxylase inhibitor that does not cross the BBB. Therefore, it does not have any effect on the central DOPA decarboxylase enzyme that is required for the conversion of levodopa to dopamine in the brain.

Levodopa significantly improves the symptoms of PD (i.e. bradykinesia, rigidity, tremors etc.) in the initial few years of treatment.

However, levodopa does not arrest the progression of the disease. The benefits of levodopa therapy start decreasing from 3rd to 5th year of therapy, regardless of the initial therapeutic response.

Pharmacokinetics

Levodopa is rapidly absorbed from the small intestine by an amino acid transport mechanism. The same transport mechanism is utilized during passage of levodopa across the BBB. Hence, dietary protein interferes with levodopa absorption from small intestine as well as levodopa entry into the brain.

The rate of absorption from small intestine also depends upon the pH of stomach and the rate of gastric emptying. Ingestion of food delays levodopa absorption. Therefore, levodopa should be taken on an empty stomach, usually 30 minutes before a meal.

The half-life is usually around 1–3 hours. The main metabolites are homovanillic acid (HVA) and 3,4-dihydrophenylacetic acid (DOPAC). The metabolites are mainly excreted in the urine.

Adverse Effects

The adverse effects of levodopa are mentioned in Figure 7.

Drug Interactions

The key drug interactions of levodopa are mentioned below:

- **Pyridoxine (Vitamin B$_6$):** Pyridoxine is a cofactor for the enzyme DOPA decarboxylase. Pyridoxine leads to an increase in extracerebral (peripheral) breakdown of levodopa. This results in a decrease in levodopa efficacy.

  If carbidopa is given along with levodopa, pyridoxine's action will be decreased. This is because carbidopa will inhibit DOPA decarboxylase, and hence, prevent pyridoxine from increasing peripheral breakdown of levodopa.

- **Nonselective monoamine oxidase (MAO) inhibitors and selective MAO-A inhibitors** prevents breakdown of peripherally synthesized catecholamines (can lead to hypertensive crisis)—hence, they should not be used along with levodopa.

- **Antipsychotics:** Dopamine D$_2$ receptor antagonists (e.g. phenothiazines, butyrophenones, risperidone) can reduce the therapeutic effect of levodopa.

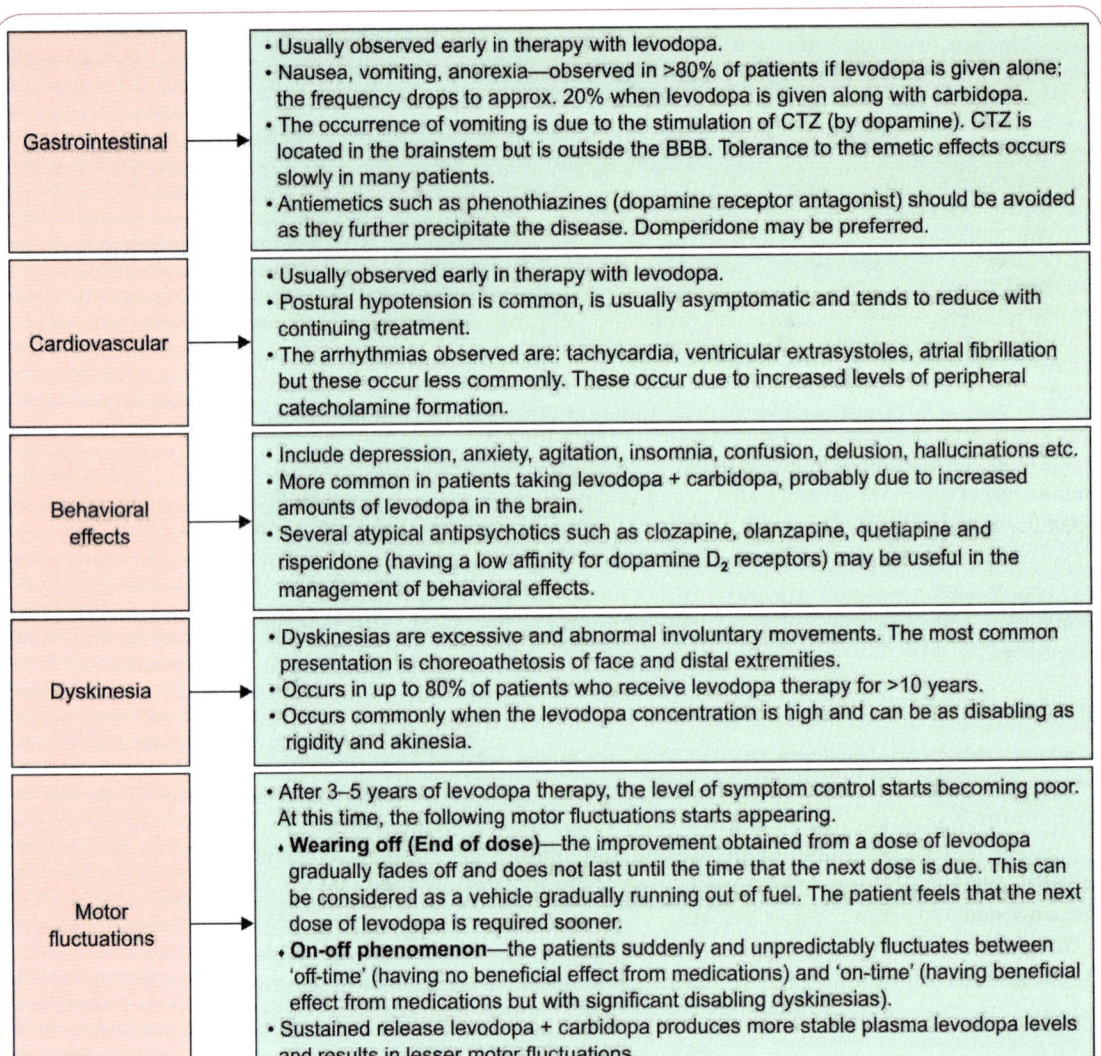

Gastrointestinal
- Usually observed early in therapy with levodopa.
- Nausea, vomiting, anorexia—observed in >80% of patients if levodopa is given alone; the frequency drops to approx. 20% when levodopa is given along with carbidopa.
- The occurrence of vomiting is due to the stimulation of CTZ (by dopamine). CTZ is located in the brainstem but is outside the BBB. Tolerance to the emetic effects occurs slowly in many patients.
- Antiemetics such as phenothiazines (dopamine receptor antagonist) should be avoided as they further precipitate the disease. Domperidone may be preferred.

Cardiovascular
- Usually observed early in therapy with levodopa.
- Postural hypotension is common, is usually asymptomatic and tends to reduce with continuing treatment.
- The arrhythmias observed are: tachycardia, ventricular extrasystoles, atrial fibrillation but these occur less commonly. These occur due to increased levels of peripheral catecholamine formation.

Behavioral effects
- Include depression, anxiety, agitation, insomnia, confusion, delusion, hallucinations etc.
- More common in patients taking levodopa + carbidopa, probably due to increased amounts of levodopa in the brain.
- Several atypical antipsychotics such as clozapine, olanzapine, quetiapine and risperidone (having a low affinity for dopamine D_2 receptors) may be useful in the management of behavioral effects.

Dyskinesia
- Dyskinesias are excessive and abnormal involuntary movements. The most common presentation is choreoathetosis of face and distal extremities.
- Occurs in up to 80% of patients who receive levodopa therapy for >10 years.
- Occurs commonly when the levodopa concentration is high and can be as disabling as rigidity and akinesia.

Motor fluctuations
- After 3–5 years of levodopa therapy, the level of symptom control starts becoming poor. At this time, the following motor fluctuations starts appearing.
  - **Wearing off (End of dose)**—the improvement obtained from a dose of levodopa gradually fades off and does not last until the time that the next dose is due. This can be considered as a vehicle gradually running out of fuel. The patient feels that the next dose of levodopa is required sooner.
  - **On-off phenomenon**—the patients suddenly and unpredictably fluctuates between 'off-time' (having no beneficial effect from medications) and 'on-time' (having beneficial effect from medications but with significant disabling dyskinesias).
- Sustained release levodopa + carbidopa produces more stable plasma levodopa levels and results in lesser motor fluctuations.

Figure 7: Adverse effects of levodopa

PERIPHERAL DECARBOXYLASE INHIBITORS

Carbidopa and benserazide are peripheral (extracerebral) DOPA decarboxylase inhibitors. They do not cross the BBB. Therefore, they inhibit the conversion of levodopa to dopamine only peripherally and not in the brain.

Levodopa is almost always given along with carbidopa or benserazide. Some of these combinations are mentioned in Table 2.

TABLE 2	Combinations of levodopa with peripheral decarboxylase inhibitors	
Combination	**Ratio**	**Strength**
Levodopa + carbidopa	10:1 or 4:1	L (100 mg) + C (10 mg) L (250 mg) + C (25 mg) L (100 mg) + C (25 mg)
Levodopa + benserazide	4:1	L (100 mg) + B (25 mg)

The therapy is usually started in a dose of levodopa (100 mg) + carbidopa (25 mg) to be taken three times a day.

As the disease progresses, the dose can be increased to levodopa (250 mg) + carbidopa (25 mg) to be taken three times a day. A dopamine receptor agonist can also be added.

The advantages of the combination therapy are mentioned in Table 3.

TABLE 3	Advantages of combination therapy with levodopa and carbidopa/benserazide

- Reduction in dose requirement of levodopa (by up to 75%). This is due to prolongation of plasma half-life of levodopa.
- Reduction in adverse effects (nausea, vomiting, cardiac effects etc.). This is due to decreased peripheral conversion of levodopa to dopamine.
- Reduction in motor fluctuations. This is due to stable cerebral dopamine levels.
- Reversal of levodopa effect by pyridoxine does not occur.

DOPAMINE RECEPTOR AGONISTS

The dopamine receptor agonists (DA agonists) clinically used are bromocriptine, pergolide, ropinirole and pramipexole. The older drugs (bromocriptine and pergolide) are ergot derivatives. The newer drugs (ropinirole and pramipexole) are nonergot derivatives.

These drugs act directly on the postsynaptic dopamine receptors in the corpus striatum.

The DA agonists are longer acting than levodopa (duration of action 8–24 hours for DA agonists versus 6–8 hours for levodopa). They are particularly useful in managing dose-related fluctuations and motor complications (i.e. on-off phenomenon).

The advantages of DA agonists include the following:
- Do not require enzymatic conversion to active dopamine as required for levodopa
- Do not have toxic metabolites
- Do not compete with other substances (for active transport) across intestinal wall and BBB

Bromocriptine and Pergolide

These are ergot derivatives. These are older drugs and have mostly been replaced by the newer nonergot drugs ropinirole and pramipexole (which have a better adverse effect profile).

Bromocriptine is a strong D_2 agonist and a partial D_1 agonist. Pergolide is a strong agonist of both D_1 and D_2 receptors.

Both have similar actions and adverse effect profile.

Adverse Effects

The adverse effects include nausea, vomiting, constipation, headache, postural hypotension, digital vasospasm, nasal congestion, cardiac arrhythmias and pleural or retroperitoneal fibrosis.

Pergolide has been associated with cardiac valvulopathy for which it has been withdrawn in many countries.

Pramipexole and Ropinirole

These are nonergot derivatives. Ropinirole is a pure D_2 agonist. Pramipexole has a selective affinity towards D_3 receptors. Both these drugs are used as monotherapy for mild parkinsonism.

They are also used as an adjunct to levodopa in advanced PD, particularly for smoothening out the response fluctuations due to levodopa ('on-off phenomenon').

Adverse Effects

These drugs are better tolerated than the ergot derivatives; hence, they have mostly replaced the ergot derivatives in the management of PD.

The adverse effects include nausea, vomiting, dizziness, somnolence (sometimes excessive irresistible urge to fall asleep), postural hypotension, confusion, delusions and hallucinations.

Impulse control disorders: Pathological gambling, compulsive spending or buying, binge eating, compulsive eating, increased libido and hypersexuality. These usually resolve with drug withdrawal or with dose reduction.

Rotigotine

Rotigotine is available only in a *transdermal patch formulation*. It is used mainly in the treatment of early Parkinson's disease. It provides more continuous dopaminergic receptor stimulation than the orally used drugs. The therapeutic effects and adverse effects are similar to other DA agonists.

■ CATECHOL-O-METHYL TRANSFERASE (COMT) INHIBITORS

Entacapone and tolcapone are reversible COMT inhibitors.

Normally, degradation of levodopa by DOPA decarboxylase is a major pathway of metabolism. Degradation by COMT is a minor pathway of peripheral levodopa metabolism.

When decarboxylation of levodopa is inhibited by giving carbidopa/benserazide, there is a compensatory activation of the other metabolic pathway (via COMT). This results in an increased production of 3-OMD (3-O methyl DOPA) and decreased half-life and efficacy of levodopa.

COMT inhibitors, therefore result in the following actions:

○ Prolongs bioavailability and action of levodopa by diminishing its peripheral metabolism
○ Prevents formation of 3-OMD which is beneficial, as 3-OMD competes with levodopa for transport across the intestinal wall and BBB

The key differences between entacapone and tolcapone are mentioned in Figure 8.

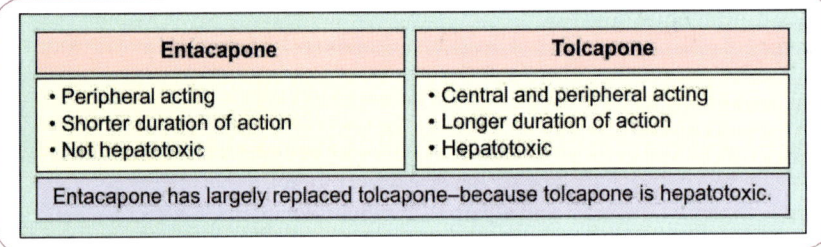

Entacapone	Tolcapone
• Peripheral acting • Shorter duration of action • Not hepatotoxic	• Central and peripheral acting • Longer duration of action • Hepatotoxic
Entacapone has largely replaced tolcapone–because tolcapone is hepatotoxic.	

Figure 8: Differences between entacapone and tolcapone

Adverse Effects

The adverse effects include nausea, diarrhea, abdominal pain, dyskinesia, orthostatic hypotension, confusion and hallucinations.

Tolcapone is *hepatotoxic*, can cause elevated liver enzymes; fatal cases of hepatic failure have rarely been reported. Entacapone does not cause hepatotoxicity and is preferred.

Clinical Uses

Both these drugs are used in patients with advanced PD (as an adjunct to levodopa + carbidopa/benserazide) who have developed motor fluctuations. Addition of COMT inhibitors results in smoother response and more prolonged 'on state.'

Entacapone is available in a fixed-dose combination with levodopa and carbidopa.

MONOAMINE OXIDASE (MAO) INHIBITORS

Monoamine oxidases are enzymes that catalyze the oxidation of monoamines.

There are two types of MAO enzymes:
- MAO-A—metabolize norepinephrine, serotonin and dopamine
- MAO-B—metabolize dopamine

Large amount of MAO-B (with very little MAO-A) is present in the striatum and globus pallidus.

Selegiline

Selegiline is a selective and irreversible inhibitor of MAO-B in the brain. It prevents the breakdown of dopamine in the brain; thereby prolongs the effect of levodopa.

If used alone, it has mild antiparkinsonian effect in early PD cases. However, when used along with levodopa, it reduces motor fluctuations and 'wearing off' and 'on-off' effect. This allows for a decrease in the dose of levodopa.

It is not used in advanced cases (or those with cognitive impairment) because it may aggravate the motor and cognitive adverse effects of levodopa.

It is metabolized to amphetamine and methamphetamine. Hence, it may cause insomnia, anxiety and other adverse effects.

Rasagiline

The mechanism of action and indications of rasagiline are similar to selegiline.

However, rasagiline is 5 times more potent than selegiline, and rasagiline is not metabolized to amphetamine like substances and does not cause insomnia, anxiety etc.

DRUGS ACTING ON THE CENTRAL CHOLINERGIC SYSTEM

CENTRAL ANTICHOLINERGICS

The centrally acting anticholinergics used are trihexyphenidyl (benzhexol) and benztropine.

Centrally acting anticholinergics are used in idiopathic parkinsonism. However, they are the treatment of choice and the only medications useful in drug (phenothiazine)-induced parkinsonism.

Levodopa is usually *not effective* in drug (phenothiazine)-induced parkinsonism because:
- The dopamine receptors are already blocked by phenothiazines
- Dopamine is not deficient, instead the receptors are blocked

In PD, there is a deficiency of dopamine, due to which the activity of cholinergic interneurons become dominant. Blockade of cholinergic transmission aids in the correction of imbalance in the dopamine : acetylcholine ratio.

These drugs are less efficacious than levodopa and have an adjunctive role in antiparkinsonian therapy. They relieve tremor and rigidity but have little effect on bradykinesia.

The adverse effect profile is similar to atropine and include dry mouth, constipation, urinary retention, blurring of vision, mood changes, confusion etc.

ANTIHISTAMINICS WITH ANTICHOLINERGIC ACTIVITY

Some antihistaminics such as promethazine and orphenadrine have anticholinergic activity and are occasionally used in the reduction of cholinergic overactivity in the basal ganglia.

MISCELLANEOUS DRUGS

APOMORPHINE

Apomorphine is a nonergot dopamine agonist that interacts with postsynaptic D_2 receptors. It is available as a subcutaneous injection.

It is used mainly for the temporary relief (rescue) in 'off-period' of akinesia, in patients on therapy with dopaminergic medications.

It is highly emetogenic. The other potentially serious adverse effects include dyskinesia, hallucinations, QT prolongation etc.

It is used only when the other drugs such as dopamine agonists or COMT inhibitors have not been able to control the 'off-periods' of akinesia.

AMANTADINE

Amantadine is an antiviral drug used to treat influenza. It was accidentally found to have weak antiparkinsonian effects.

The mode of action is unclear; however, it may potentiate dopaminergic action by increasing dopamine release, blocking cholinergic receptors and inhibiting N-methyl-D-aspartate (NMDA) type of glutamate receptors.

It has various undesirable adverse effects such as depression, hallucinations, confusion, dizziness, sleep disturbance, livedo reticularis, peripheral edema etc. Overdosage may lead to acute toxic psychosis.

It is used in mild PD as an initial therapy. It may also be used as an adjunct to levodopa for managing motor fluctuations and dyskinesias.

DRUGS USED FOR ALZHEIMER'S DISEASE

Alzheimer's disease (AD) is a progressive, irreversible, neurodegenerative brain disease that diminishes memory (dementia) and cognitive skills such as thinking, remembering and reasoning. *The most prominent neurochemical abnormality is acetylcholine deficiency.*

It is the most common neurodegenerative disorder followed by Parkinson's disease. It is the most common cause of dementia accounting for 60–70% cases among older adults.

NEUROPATHOLOGICAL FEATURES

The following neuropathological features are observed in the brain of AD patients: senile plaques and neurofibrillary tangles (Figure 9). This eventually leads to a loss of cortical neurons (mainly cholinergic neurons) and atrophy of brain tissue.

Senile plaques	Neurofibrillary tangles
• Main component is β_2 amyloid protein • Extracellular deposition • Neurotoxic effect in hippocampus, entorhinal cortex, but spares the cerebellum	• Main component is Protein Tau • Intracellular deposition • First appear in the entorhinal cortex, then hippocampus and then the cortex

Figure 9: Neuropathological features in Alzheimer's disease

The aim of drug therapy in AD is to improve cholinergic transmission in the brain and prevent excitotoxic effects due to overstimulation of NMDA receptors (Table 4).

TABLE 4	Drug therapy in Alzheimer's disease
Improve cholinergic transmission within the brain	Acetylcholinesterase inhibitors • Donepezil • Rivastigmine • Galantamine • Tacrine
Prevent excitotoxic effects resulting from overstimulation of NMDA glutamate receptors in the brain	NMDA receptor antagonist • Memantine

ACETYLCHOLINESTERASE INHIBITORS

The acetylcholinesterase inhibitors used in AD are donepezil, rivastigmine, galantamine and tacrine. These drugs are used in mild to moderate AD. They have a modest beneficial effect.

These drugs act by inhibiting acetylcholinesterase, the enzyme that catalyzes the breakdown of acetylcholine. Hence, both the level and duration of action of acetylcholine is increased.

Tacrine was the 1st cholinesterase inhibitor used in AD, but now rarely used because of hepatotoxicity and other adverse effects. It has been replaced with donepezil, rivastigmine and galantamine, which are orally active and adequately enter the CNS. All have some degree of selectivity for CNS compared to the periphery.

Rivastigmine is the only approved medication for dementia in PD. It is the only cholinesterase inhibitor available as a transdermal patch.

Rivastigmine (unlike donepezil and galantamine) is metabolized by esterases and not by CYP enzymes; therefore, it has no interactions with drugs that alter the CYP enzymes.

The key adverse effects include gastrointestinal disturbance (nausea, vomiting, anorexia), muscle cramps and abnormal dreams.

NMDA RECEPTOR ANTAGONIST

Memantine is the drug used in AD. It noncompetitively blocks the NMDA receptors and limits calcium influx in the neuron, thereby preventing toxic intracellular levels of calcium.

It is used in moderate to severe AD. It is often given in combination with cholinesterase inhibitors. It significantly reduces the rate of clinical worsening.

It is well tolerated; the adverse effects are mild and reversible and include headache, dizziness and confusion.

Drugs Acting on the Central Nervous System

SECTION D

ASSESS YOURSELF (Examination Questions of Various Universities)

1. Classify drugs used in the treatment of parkinsonism. Discuss the mechanism of action, drug interactions and adverse effects of levodopa.
2. What is the rationale (advantages) of combining carbidopa with levodopa?
3. Why is levodopa not effective in drug-induced parkinsonism.
4. Discuss the pharmacological role of:
   a. Ropinirole in parkinsonism
   b. COMT inhibitors in parkinsonism
   c. Trihexyphenidyl in parkinsonism
   d. Selegiline in parkinsonism
5. Write short notes on:
   a. Management of drug-induced parkinsonism
   b. Ropinirole and pramipexole
6. Name 2 drugs used in the treatment of Alzheimer's disease and mention their mechanism of action.

MULTIPLE CHOICE QUESTIONS

1. Drug used for Alzheimer's disease acting on NMDA receptor is: *(Recent Question Dec 2016)*
   a. Donepezil
   b. Memantine
   c. Tacrine
   d. Galantamine
2. Which of the following statement regarding Selegiline is false?
   (Recent Question Dec 2016)
   a. May be used in on-off phenomenon
   b. Does not cause cheese reaction
   c. It is used in parkinsonism
   d. It is a MAO-A inhibitor
3. Tolcapone is: *(Recent Question Dec 2016)*
   a. Hepatotoxic
   b. Nephrotoxic
   c. Ototoxic
   d. Neurotoxic
4. Peripheral vasospasm is observed with which of the following anti-Parkinsonian drugs?
   (AIIMS May 2014)
   a. Ropinirole
   b. Levodopa
   c. Bromocriptine
   d. Entacapone
5. Rotigotine is: *(Recent Question 2016)*
   a. Dopamine agonist
   b. Dopamine antagonist
   c. GABA agonist
   d. GABA antagonist
6. Anti–Parkinsonism drug that is a selective COMT inhibitor: *(Recent Question 2016)*
   a. Entacapone
   b. Ropinirole
   c. Pergolide
   d. Pramipexole
7. All are dopaminergic agonists used for parkinsonism except: *(Recent Question 2016)*
   a. Bromocriptine
   b. Ropinirole
   c. Pramipexole
   d. Selegiline
8. Antiparkinson drug known to cause cardiac valvular fibrosis is: *(Recent Question 2016)*
   a. Bromocriptine
   b. Ropinirole
   c. Pramiprexole
   d. Pergolide and cabergoline
9. Galantamine is used in: *(Recent Question 2016)*
   a. Alzheimer's disease
   b. Parkinson's disease
   c. Emesis
   d. Chorea
10. All are ergot derivatives used in parkinsonism except: *(Recent Question 2016)*
    a. Bromocriptine
    b. Pergolide
    c. Trihexyphenidyl
    d. Cabergoline
11. Ropinirole is a: *(NIMHANS 2011, 2008, 2007)*
    a. MAO inhibitor
    b. Dopamine agonist
    c. COMT inhibitor
    d. GABA inhibitor

Ans.

1. (b)	2. (d)	3. (a)	4. (c)	5. (a)	6. (a)
7. (d)	8. (d)	9. (a)	10. (c)	11. (b)	

23 Antipsychotic Drugs

Psychosis is a symptom of mental disease where the sense of reality is lost. The patient also has distorted perception (delusions and hallucinations), thought and behavior.

The common psychotic disorder includes the following:
- ○ Schizophrenia
- ○ Mood disorders (major depression or mania) with psychosis
- ○ Dementia with psychosis
- ○ Delirium with psychosis
- ○ Drug-induced psychosis

Schizophrenia occurs in about 1% of population worldwide and is considered as the prototypic disorder for psychosis. The antipsychotic drugs are effective against schizophrenia and other psychotic disorders.

SCHIZOPHRENIA

Schizophrenia is a chronic brain disorder characterized by delusions, hallucinations and thinking or speech disturbances.

The manifestations of schizophrenia include positive symptoms, negative symptoms and cognitive defects (Figure 1):

Positive symptoms	Negative symptoms	Cognitive defects
• Delusions • Hallucinations (usually auditory) • Disorganized speech and behavior	• Poverty of speech • Loss of interest and drive • Reduction in emotional range	• Deficits in working memory • Deficits in attention

- **Delusions:** False, firm, fixed beliefs that cannot be corrected by any amount of reasoning. For example, person believes that a rope present in the room is a snake.
- **Hallucinations:** Perception in the absence of an external stimulus. For example, person believes that there is a snake in the room in the absence of either a snake or a rope.

Figure 1: Manifestations of schizophrenia

Schizophrenia is thought to be due to an increased activity of dopamine in mesolimbic and mesocortical neuronal pathways (Figure 2). Other neurotransmitters such as serotonin and norepinephrine are also thought to be involved in the pathogenesis.

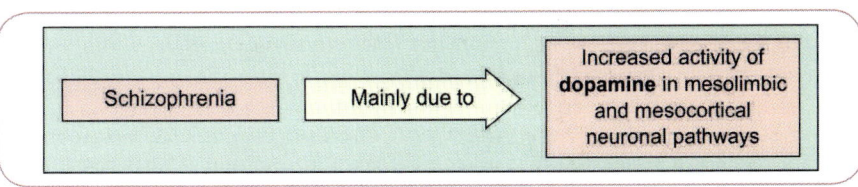

Figure 2: Pathophysiology of schizophrenia

ANTIPSYCHOTIC DRUGS

The antipsychotic drugs (also called neuroleptics or major tranquilizers) are mainly used to treat schizophrenia; however, they are also used in other psychotic and manic illnesses.

The classification of antipsychotic drugs based on the chemical structure as well as based on the sequence of their discovery is mentioned in Table 1 and Figure 3.

TABLE 1	Classification based on the chemical structure
Structure	**Examples**
Phenothiazines	Chlorpromazine, triflupromazine, trifluoperazine, thioridazine, fluphenazine
Butyrophenones	Haloperidol, droperidol, trifluperidol
Thioxanthenes	Thiothixene, flupenthixol
Others	Pimozide, loxapine
Atypical	Clozapine, olanzapine, quetiapine, risperidone, paliperidone, aripiprazole, ziprasidone

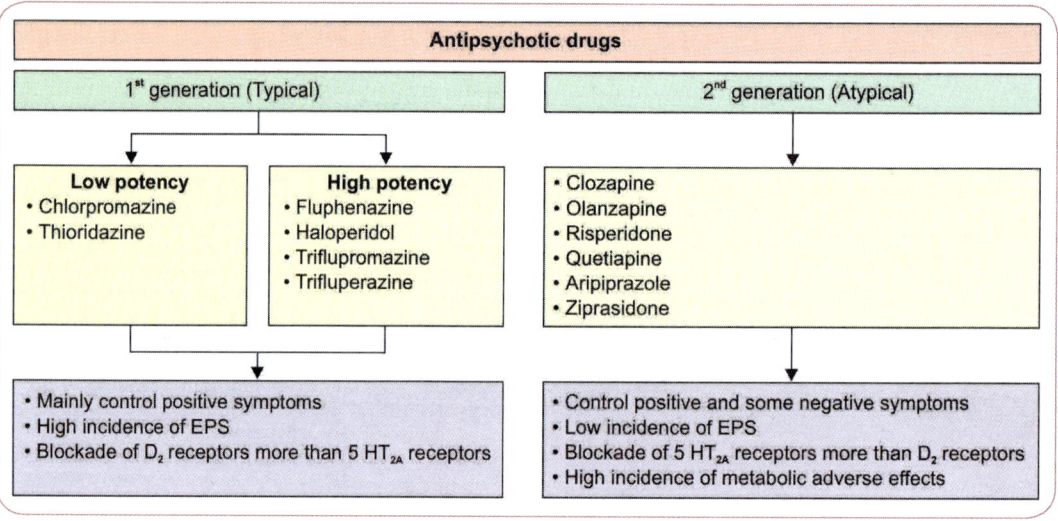

Figure 3: Classification based on the sequence of discovery

■ MECHANISM OF ACTION

Antipsychotic drugs exert beneficial effects by the following mechanisms (Figure 4):

Antipsychotic drugs	
Typical	**Atypical**
Mainly decrease dopaminergic neurotransmission Mainly block (Dopamine) D_2 receptors	**Mainly decrease serotonergic neurotransmission** Mainly block (Serotonin) $5\text{-}HT_{2A}$ receptors

- All antipsychotics are D_2 antagonists except **Aripiprazole** which is a partial D_2 agonist.
- Aripiprazole has D_2 receptor affinity slightly less than dopamine, but intrinsic activity of only 25% that of dopamine.
  Hence, in the presence of dopamine, if aripiprazole is given, it blocks D_2 receptors but only produces 25% of the response. This leads to a decrease in dopaminergic transmission, compared to when dopamine was functioning maximally.

Figure 4: Mechanism of action of antipsychotic drugs

TYPICAL ANTIPSYCHOTICS

CHLORPROMAZINE

Chlorpromazine is the prototype drug.

All typical antipsychotics reduce the positive symptoms of schizophrenia but have minimal effect on the negative symptoms and cognitive effects. The atypical antipsychotics decrease the negative symptoms and cognitive effects to some extent.

Pharmacological Actions

Chlorpromazine produces the following effects in schizophrenia patients:

Central Nervous System

Chlorpromazine produces the following CNS effects:
- Reduce irrational behavior, agitation and aggressiveness
- Suppress delusions, hallucinations and hyperactivity
- Reduce spontaneous movements
- Reduce anxiety
- Controls disturbed thought and behavior

Endocrine System

Dopamine is the prolactin inhibitory factor in the anterior pituitary. Chlorpromazine functions as a D_2 antagonist.

Therefore, chlorpromazine, by blocking D_2 receptors in the anterior pituitary, leads to loss of dopamine's inhibition on prolactin synthesis and release. This in turn results in hyperprolactinemia.

Hyperprolactinemia is manifested as galactorrhea, amenorrhea and infertility in females and gynecomastia in males.

Other Actions

- Chlorpromazine causes antiemetic effect by blocking D_2 receptors in the chemoreceptor trigger zone (CTZ).
- It causes extrapyramidal symptoms by blocking D_2 receptors in the basal ganglia.
- It causes anticholinergic (atropine-like) effects by blocking M_1 (muscarinic) receptors.
- It causes antihistaminic effects by blocking H_1 (histaminic) receptors.
- It causes anti α-adrenergic effects by blocking α_1-adrenergic receptors.

Chlorpromazine does not result in addiction. Tolerance develops to antihistaminic and anticholinergic effects over days to weeks. Tolerance does not develop to the antipsychotic effects.

The pharmacological actions of chlorpromazine are mentioned in Figure 5.

Beneficial effects	Adverse effects	Adverse effects	Adverse effects	Adverse effects
Inhibition of D_2/5-HT$_2$ receptors (in limbic and cortical system) • Antipsychotic effects • Reduction of hallucinations, delusions, hyperactivity, agitation etc. **Inhibition of D_2 receptors in CTZ** • Antiemetic effect	**Inhibition of D_2 receptors in basal ganglia/pituitary** • Extrapyramidal symptoms • Hyperprolactinemia	**Inhibition of M_1 (Muscarinic) receptors** • Anticholinergic effects • Dry mouth • Constipation • Urinary retention • Blurred vision • Tachycardia	**Inhibition of H_1 (Histaminic) receptors** • Antihistaminic effects • Sedation • Weight gain	**Inhibition of α_1-adrenergic receptors** • Anti α_1-adrenergic effects • Postural hypotension • Tachycardia

Figure 5: Pharmacological actions of chlorpromazine

Pharmacokinetics

Chlorpromazine is effective orally and parenterally. It undergoes high first-pass metabolism (systemic bioavailability ~30%). It is highly lipid soluble and highly plasma protein bound.

It accumulates in the brain and other tissues. The clinical duration of action is much longer as compared to its half-life. The volume of distribution is large (>7 L/kg). It is metabolized in the liver. It is excreted by the kidneys for a long duration of time (usually months) after discontinuation.

Other typical antipsychotics have broadly similar pharmacokinetic features.

The adverse effects and clinical uses of typical as well as atypical antipsychotics are discussed at the end.

THIORIDAZINE

Thioridazine is a low potency antipsychotic which has marked central anticholinergic action. The key distinguishing features of thioridazine are:

- Very low incidence of extrapyramidal adverse effects (due to central anticholinergic action).
- Causes retinal deposits. These may look like retinitis pigmentosa. These may be associated with 'browning of vision'.
- Causes cardiac abnormalities. Overdoses may result in ventricular arrhythmias and sudden cardiac death.

FLUPHENAZINE

Fluphenazine is a high potency antipsychotic. It has a high incidence of extrapyramidal adverse effects and tardive dyskinesia.

A depot injectable form of fluphenazine is available for rapid treatment initiation and maintenance in noncooperative patients.

HALOPERIDOL

Haloperidol is a high potency antipsychotic and is one of the most widely used typical antipsychotic drug. The other features of haloperidol are:

- It has a very high incidence of extrapyramidal adverse effects and tardive dyskinesia.
- It does not cause weight gain.
- It has a low incidence of autonomic adverse effects.
- It is the preferred drug for acute schizophrenia, Huntington's disease and Tourette's syndrome.

A depot injectable form of haloperidol is available for rapid treatment initiation and maintenance in noncooperative patients.

ATYPICAL ANTIPSYCHOTICS

The atypical antipsychotics commonly used are clozapine, olanzapine, quetiapine, risperidone, paliperidone, aripiprazole and ziprasidone.

These drugs are more potent $5HT_{2A}$ blockers and weak D_2 blockers. Hence, they have a lower incidence of extrapyramidal adverse effects.

The key features of atypical antipsychotics are mentioned in Table 2.

TABLE 2	Features of atypical antipsychotics
• Blockade of 5HT2A receptors is more than the blockade of D2 receptors	
• Controls positive symptoms and some negative symptoms	
• Lower incidence of extrapyramidal (neurological) adverse effects (as compared to typical antipsychotics)	
• Higher incidence of metabolic adverse effects (as compared to typical antipsychotics)	

CLOZAPINE AND OLANZAPINE

The key distinguishing features of clozapine and olanzapine are:
- High $5HT_{2A}/D_2$ ratio, i.e. selectively block $5HT_{2A}$ receptors with weak D_2 blocking action
- *Very low* incidence of extrapyramidal adverse effects
- *Very high* incidence of metabolic adverse effects
- Also block M_1, H_1 and α_1-adrenergic receptors; hence, they cause sedation and postural hypotension.

Adverse Effects

The key adverse effects include the following:

Agranulocytosis

Clozapine (but not olanzapine) causes agranulocytosis in 1–2% of patients.
- This serious, potentially fatal adverse effect usually occurs between 6 and 18 weeks of therapy.
- Patients receiving clozapine should have weekly monitoring of blood counts for the first 6 months and thrice weekly thereafter.

Seizure Risk

- Clozapine (and to a lesser extent olanzapine) have a dose-dependent risk of inducing seizures.

Other Adverse Effects

Both clozapine and olanzapine are associated with sedation, postural hypotension, weight gain and other metabolic effects. Clozapine causes increased salivation while olanzapine causes dry mouth and constipation.

Clinical Uses

Clozapine is the only drug effective in cases of refractory schizophrenia.

Clozapine is used only as a reserve drug due to a high incidence of adverse effects (mainly agranulocytosis).

Olanzapine is used for the treatment of schizophrenia and for the treatment of mania associated with bipolar disorder.

QUETIAPINE

Quetiapine has a shorter half-life and requires twice daily dosing (unlike other atypical drugs which require once daily dosing). It is highly sedating.

It is effective in schizophrenia and can be used as monotherapy in bipolar disorder.

RISPERIDONE

Risperidone is unique in the sense that it has a very low tendency to cause extrapyramidal adverse effects at lower doses (<8 mg/day). However, it has a high tendency of causing extrapyramidal adverse effects at higher doses.

Risperidone (like other atypical antipsychotics) has a weak D_2 blocking action. However, risperidone (unlike other atypical antipsychotics) leads to an increased prolactin secretion.

It is effective in schizophrenia and can be used for mania episodes in bipolar disorder.

ARIPIPRAZOLE

Aripiprazole is the only atypical antipsychotic that is a partial agonist of D_2 receptor. It has a long half-life (~3 days) and causes minimal weight gain and metabolic effects. It has a very low tendency of causing extrapyramidal adverse effects.

It is effective in schizophrenia and can be used in mania and bipolar disorder.

ZIPRASIDONE

It is a newer atypical antipsychotic drug with some anxiolytic and antidepressant properties.

It causes minimal weight gain and metabolic effects. It has a very low tendency of causing extrapyramidal adverse effects. However, it causes QTc prolongation—may lead to serious arrhythmias.

It is effective in schizophrenia and can be used in mania and bipolar disorder.

ADVERSE EFFECTS OF ANTIPSYCHOTIC DRUGS

The adverse effects of antipsychotic drugs are mostly an extension of their known pharmacological effects. However, some of them are allergic or idiosyncratic.

The various adverse effects are mentioned as per the individual body systems/organs:

Neurological

Extrapyramidal symptoms (EPS) are the main neurological effects that occur with the use of antipsychotic drugs. These reactions occur more frequently with drugs having a strong D_2 blocking action. The following are noteworthy regarding the development of EPS:

- ❍ EPS are the major dose limiting adverse effects.
- ❍ High-potency typical drugs are more likely to cause EPS (most with haloperidol).
- ❍ Low-potency typical drugs are less likely to cause EPS (least with thioridazine).
- ❍ Atypical drugs are less likely to cause EPS because they are strong $5HT_{2A}$ blockers and weak D_2 blockers.

Extrapyramidal symptoms may manifest in the form of acute dystonia, parkinsonism, akathesia, neuroleptic malignant syndrome and tardive dyskinesia (Figure 6).

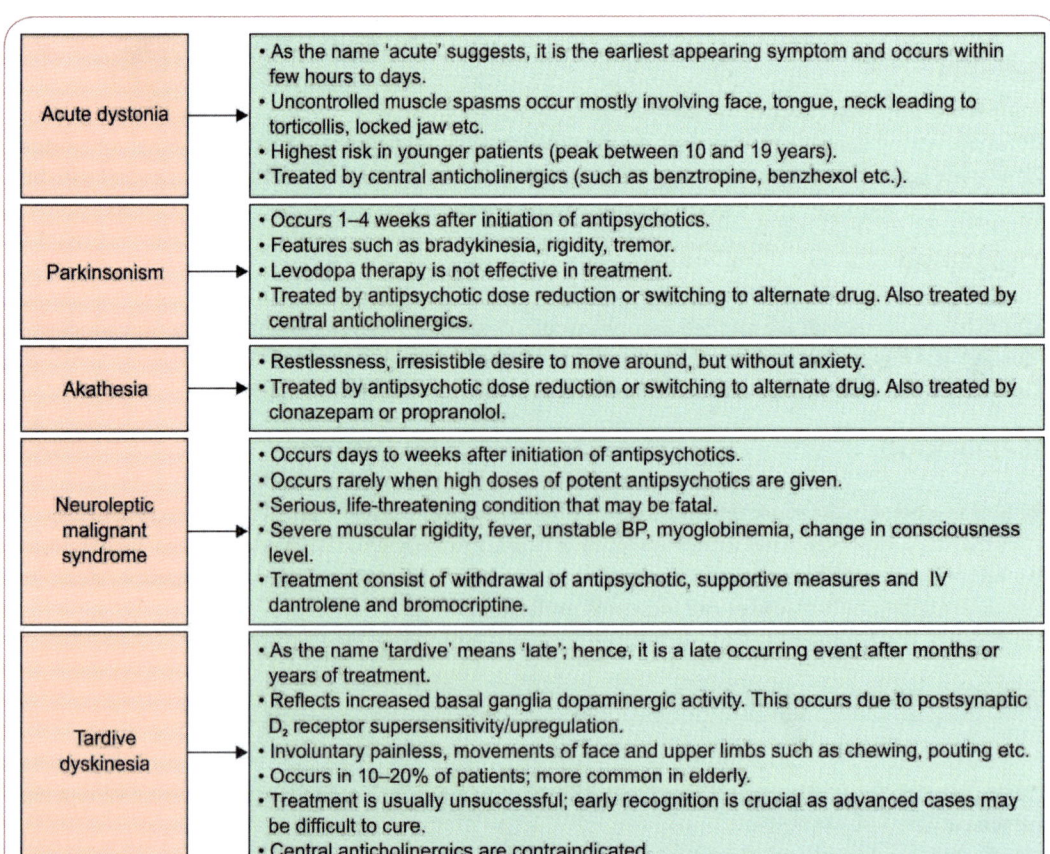

Acute dystonia	• As the name 'acute' suggests, it is the earliest appearing symptom and occurs within few hours to days. • Uncontrolled muscle spasms occur mostly involving face, tongue, neck leading to torticollis, locked jaw etc. • Highest risk in younger patients (peak between 10 and 19 years). • Treated by central anticholinergics (such as benztropine, benzhexol etc.).
Parkinsonism	• Occurs 1–4 weeks after initiation of antipsychotics. • Features such as bradykinesia, rigidity, tremor. • Levodopa therapy is not effective in treatment. • Treated by antipsychotic dose reduction or switching to alternate drug. Also treated by central anticholinergics.
Akathesia	• Restlessness, irresistible desire to move around, but without anxiety. • Treated by antipsychotic dose reduction or switching to alternate drug. Also treated by clonazepam or propranolol.
Neuroleptic malignant syndrome	• Occurs days to weeks after initiation of antipsychotics. • Occurs rarely when high doses of potent antipsychotics are given. • Serious, life-threatening condition that may be fatal. • Severe muscular rigidity, fever, unstable BP, myoglobinemia, change in consciousness level. • Treatment consist of withdrawal of antipsychotic, supportive measures and IV dantrolene and bromocriptine.
Tardive dyskinesia	• As the name 'tardive' means 'late'; hence, it is a late occurring event after months or years of treatment. • Reflects increased basal ganglia dopaminergic activity. This occurs due to postsynaptic D_2 receptor supersensitivity/upregulation. • Involuntary painless, movements of face and upper limbs such as chewing, pouting etc. • Occurs in 10–20% of patients; more common in elderly. • Treatment is usually unsuccessful; early recognition is crucial as advanced cases may be difficult to cure. • Central anticholinergics are contraindicated.

Figure 6: Extrapyramidal (neurological) adverse effects of antipsychotic drugs

Autonomic Nervous System and Histaminic

These may manifest as the following:
- *Anticholinergic (Atropine like) effects* (due to blockade of M_1 muscarinic receptors)
  - Dry mouth, constipation, urinary retention, blurred vision, tachycardia
- *Anti α-adrenergic effects* (due to blockade of α_1-adrenergic receptors)
  - Orthostatic (postural) hypotension, tachycardia
- *Antihistaminic effects* (due to blockade of H_1 histaminic receptors)
  - Sedation, weight gain.

Endocrine

Antipsychotics function as D_2 antagonists, thereby resulting in hyperprolactinemia.

Hyperprolactinemia is manifested as galactorrhea, amenorrhea and infertility in females and gynecomastia in males.

Hyperprolactinemia is more common with strong D_2 receptor blockers (e.g. typical antipsychotics). It is less likely with atypical antipsychotics (the exceptions are risperidone and paliperidone which cause dose dependent increase in prolactin levels).

Metabolic

These include weight gain, hypertriglyceridemia, hyperglycemia and new onset type 2 diabetes mellitus.

The metabolic effects are much more common with atypical antipsychotics. Of these, clozapine and olanzapine have the highest risk of causing metabolic effects.

Cardiac

The cardiac adverse effects can occur with the following drugs:
- Thioridazine mostly causes reversible minor abnormalities of T-wave in doses up to 300 mg/day. However, in overdoses, it may result in ventricular arrhythmias and sudden cardiac death.
- Ziprasidone has a high incidence of causing QT_C prolongation and should not be given along with other drugs with same effect (e.g. thioridazine, class 1A or 3 antiarrhythmics).

Ocular

The ocular adverse effects can occur with the following drugs:
- Chlorpromazine can cause deposits in the anterior part of the eye (i.e. in lens and cornea). The normal process of aging of the lens can be accentuated.
- Thioridazine may cause retinal deposits, which in advanced cases may mimic retinitis pigmentosa. This may result in browning of vision. To avoid this complication, thioridazine is not used in doses above 800 mg/day.

Allergic or Idiosyncratic

These are not dose-related adverse effects. They may occur in the following forms with specific antipsychotic drugs:
- Agranulocytosis with clozapine
- Cholestatic jaundice with chlorpromazine
- Skin reactions with chlorpromazine

CLINICAL USES OF ANTIPSYCHOTIC DRUGS

The antipsychotics are frequently used in the following clinical conditions:

Schizophrenia

Antipsychotic drugs are the mainstay of therapy in the treatment of schizophrenia.

They provide symptomatic relief but do not remove the cause of disease. Prolonged (lifelong) therapy may be required. The following are some of the key features for the use of these drugs:

- ○ *The atypical antipsychotics are more commonly used.* This is because they have a much lower risk of causing EPS.
- ○ *Clozapine is the only effective drug in resistant schizophrenia.* It is also the reserve drug because it has a high incidence of causing agranulocytosis and weight gain.
- ○ Of the typical antipsychotics, haloperidol is the most commonly used drug, although it has the highest incidence of causing EPS.

Mania

Antipsychotic drugs are needed for rapid control of symptoms in acute mania. This is because it takes 1–2 weeks for the effects of lithium to manifest.

Once the acute attack is controlled by antipsychotic drugs, lithium is then used for maintenance treatment.

The antipsychotic drugs commonly used in acute mania include chlorpromazine, haloperidol, olanzapine, risperidone, aripiprazole and quetiapine.

Depression

Antipsychotic drugs are now being used in depression in the following conditions:
- ○ **Acute bipolar depression:** Quetiapine is being used as a monotherapy, while olanzapine is used in combination with fluoxetine for the treatment of bipolar depression.
- ○ **Unipolar depression:** Quetiapine, olanzapine and aripiprazole are being used as adjunctive therapies to antidepressants, for the treatment of unipolar depression.

Antiemetic

The antiemetic effect of antipsychotic drugs is due to their D_2 receptor blocking action in the CTZ. However, they are not routinely used for this purpose due to adverse effects.

Prochlorperazine is an antipsychotic employed for treating drug-induced emesis, such as that with anticancer therapy.

Intractable Hiccoughs

Intractable hiccough can respond to parenteral chlorpromazine.

ASSESS YOURSELF (Examination Questions of Various Universities)

1. Classify antipsychotic drugs. Discuss the mechanism of action, adverse effects and clinical uses of chlorpromazine.
2. Discuss the pharmacotherapy of acute schizophrenia.

3. Write short notes on:
   a. Clozapine and Olanzapine
   b. Risperidone
   c. Haloperidol
   d. Atypical antipsychotics
   e. Adverse effects of chlorpromazine

MULTIPLE CHOICE QUESTIONS

1. Which of the following is true regarding typical antipsychotics?   *(Recent Question Dec 2016)*
   a. Increases seizure threshold
   b. Antiemetic property
   c. Pruritic effect
   d. Diarrhea
2. A patient, Hari has been diagnosed to have schizophrenia, which of the following acts as a limiting factor in the use of clozapine as an antipsychotic drug in this patient?
   (Recent Question 2016)
   a. Its potential to cause agranulocytosis
   b. Its inability to benefit negative symptoms of schizophrenia
   c. High incidence of extrapyramidal side effects
   d. Production of hyperprolactinemia
3. Most common receptor for typical antipsychotics is: *(Recent Question 2016)*
   a. D1   b. D2
   c. D3   d. D4
4. Drug causing agranulocytosis:
   (Recent Question 2016)
   a. Pimozide   b. Clozapine
   c. Risperidone   d. Olanzapine
5. Which of the following has highest potential to cause metabolic syndrome?
   (Recent Question 2016)
   a. Clozapine   b. Risperidone
   c. Quetiapine   d. Aripiprazole

6. Which of the following drug causes sedation but no extrapyramidal side effect?
   (Recent Question 2016)
   a. Clozapine   b. Pimozide
   c. Fluphenazine   d. Haloperidol
7. Antipsychotic drug with least extrapyramidal side effects is: *(Recent Question 2016)*
   a. Triflupromazine   b. Thioridazine
   c. Pimozide   d. Trifluoperazine
8. Antipsychotic drug is: *(Recent Question 2016)*
   a. Doxepin   b. Fluoxetine
   c. Clozapine   d. All
9. Clozapine   *(Recent Question 2016)*
   a. Has D2 agonist activity
   b. Cause agranulocytosis
   c. Cause hyperprolactinemia
   d. Anti-seizure property
10. A patient on antipsychotic treatment has an inability to sit at a place. He has to keep on moving to relieve his discomfort:
    (Recent Question 2016)
    a. Akathisia
    b. Tardive dyskinesia
    c. Malignant hyperthermia
    d. Neuroleptic malignant syndrome

Ans.

| 1. (b) | 2. (a) | 3. (b) | 4. (b) | 5. (a) | 6. (a) |
| 7. (b) | 8. (c) | 9. (b) | 10. (a) | | |

24

Antimanic Drugs

Mania is characterized by elevated or irritable mood, increased activity or energy, increased self-esteem, increased thought and speech and decreased need for sleep.

Bipolar disorder (manic-depressive psychosis, MDP) is a cyclical condition where mania alternates with depression.

The drugs effective in acute mania and/or MDP are lithium, anticonvulsants (valproate, carbamazepine, lamotrigine) and atypical antipsychotics (risperidone, aripiprazole, olanzapine).

■ LITHIUM

Lithium is a monovalent cation and is handled by the kidneys similarly as sodium. Lithium is mostly reabsorbed in the proximal convoluted tubule of the kidney.

Mechanism of Action

Inositol triphosphate (IP_3) and diacylglycerol (DAG) function as secondary messengers for muscarinic and α-adrenergic transmission.

The activity of these secondary messengers is postulated to be significantly increased in mania. Lithium selectively inhibits the generation of these messengers and has a beneficial effect in mania.

Lithium blocks the conversion of IP_2 to IP_1 and of IP_1 to inositol. This leads to decreased generation of phosphatidylinositol and phosphatidylinositol bisphosphate (PIP_2), which are the membrane precursors of IP_3 and DAG (Figure 1).

Lithium also decreases the release of dopamine and norepinephrine in the brain.

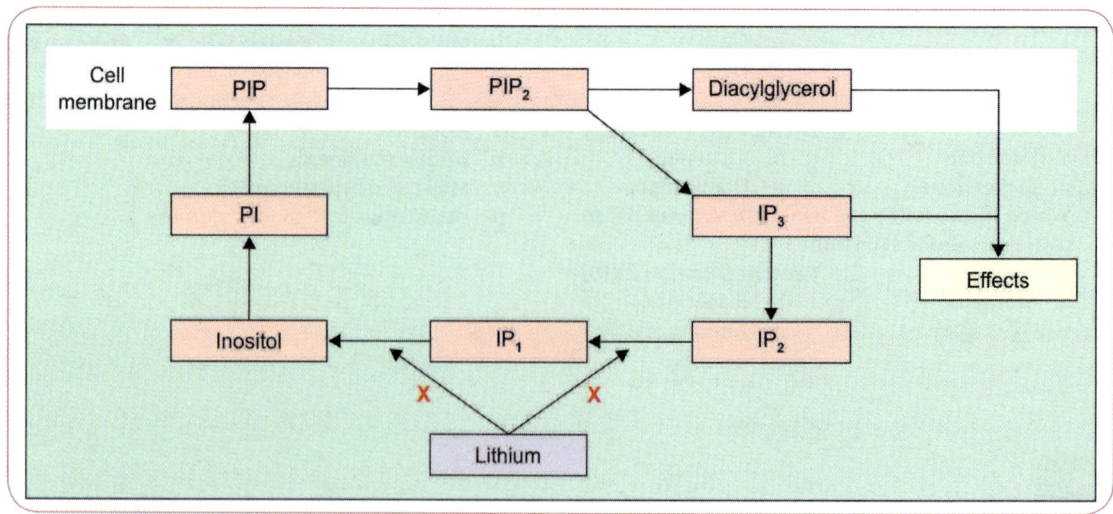

Figure 1: Mechanism of action of lithium

Abbreviation: PI, phosphatidylinositol; PIP, phosphatidylinositol monophosphate; PIP2, phosphatidylinositol biphosphate; IP_3, inositol triphosphate; IP_2, inositol biphosphate; IP_1, inositol monophosphate

Pharmacokinetics

Lithium is rapidly absorbed from the gastrointestinal tract. Complete absorption takes place in ~8 hours. The steady state is achieved after 5–7 days of daily lithium administration.

The distribution of lithium occurs in total body water. There is no plasma protein binding. Hence, the volume of distribution is equal to that of total body water, i.e. 0.7–0.9 L/kg. Passage through the blood brain barrier is slow. Lithium is not metabolized and gets excreted in urine, sweat, saliva etc.

Lithium is completely filtered at the glomerulus and 80% is reabsorbed in the proximal tubules. Lithium competes with sodium for reabsorption. The absorption of lithium is increased in conditions of sodium loss (diuretic use, diarrheal illness, etc.).

Lithium has a narrow safety margin (narrow therapeutic window); hence, it is an important candidate for therapeutic drug monitoring.

The concentration of lithium generally considered effective and safe is 0.5-1.5 mEq/L. Toxicity occurs at concentration >1.5 mEq/L (Figure 2).

However, there is marked individual variation in the pharmacokinetics of lithium.

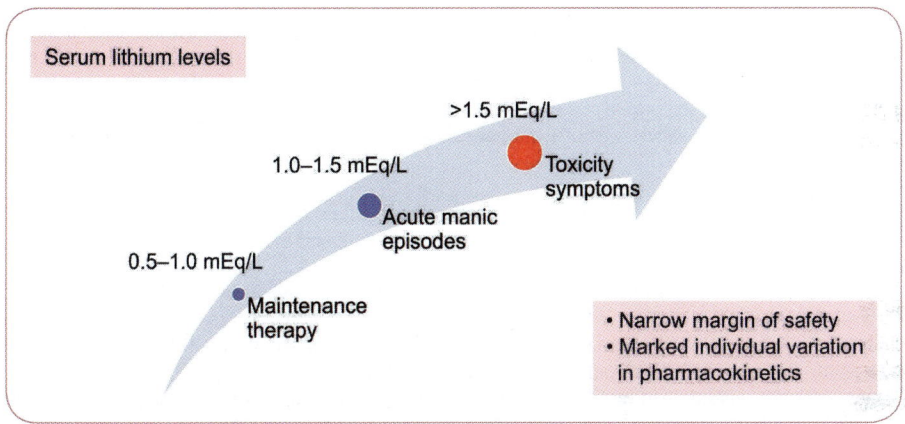

Figure 2: Serum lithium concentrations

Pharmacological Actions

Central Nervous System

- Lithium, when given in acute mania, gradually suppresses the excitatory CNS effects in 1–2 weeks
- Lithium, when given as prophylactic therapy in bipolar disorder, acts as a mood stabilizer and prevents cyclic mood changes
- It does not have any sedative or euphoriant effects

Other Body Tissues

- It inhibits ADH action on distal tubules, which may result in a diabetes insipidus like state
- It has an insulin like action on glucose metabolism
- It increases leukocyte count
- It decreases thyroxine synthesis

Adverse Effects and Overdose

The adverse effects of lithium are mentioned in Figure 3.

Neurologic and psychiatric	Renal	Cardiac	Thyroid	Others
Tremor • Most common adverse effect • Occurs at therapeutic doses • Propranolol and atenolol are effective as treatment **Choreoathetosis, aphasia, dysarthria (slurred speech), ataxia, mental confusion**	**Polyuria and polydipsia** • Occurs because lithium inhibits the action of ADH on kidney's distal tubule • Resistant to vasopressin • May respond to amiloride • Reversible on discontinuation	**Depression of the SA node** • Lithium is contraindicated in sick sinus (bradycardia – tachycardia) syndrome	**Decreased thyroid function** • Benign, nontender thyroid enlargement in few patients • Reversible and non-progressive	**Edema** • Occurs possibly due to sodium retention **Folliculitis, dermatitis, alopecia, worsening of acne or psoriasis**

Lithium overdose/toxicity
- Therapeutic overdoses are more common as compared to accidental or deliberate ingestion of lithium.
- Toxicity is usually due to modifications in the patient's status such as use of diuretics, decreased sodium levels or changes in the renal function.
- Toxicity symptoms are usually seen at levels >2 mEq/L.
- Symptoms include vomiting, diarrhea, tremors, giddiness, ataxia, confusion, convulsions, coma, cardiac arrhythmias.
- Management
  - No specific antidote for lithium. Discontinue lithium and monitor serum levels.
  - Supportive treatment should be initiated, including correction of fluid and electrolyte imbalance. Sodium restoration promotes lithium excretion.
  - Hemodialysis is the preferred treatment in severe toxicity (i.e. very high lithium levels >4 mEq/L).

Use during pregnancy
- *Ebstein's anomaly*—Lithium use increases the chances of cardiovascular anomalies in the newborn, especially Ebstein's anomaly. It usually can be surgically corrected after birth.
- *Floppy baby syndrome*—Lithium use may lead to CNS depression, hypotonia, neonatal goiter and cardiac murmur.

Figure 3: Adverse effects of lithium

Drug Interactions

- **Lithium × diuretics (such as thiazides/furosemide):** Diuretics cause Na^+ excretion leading to hyponatremia. This results in a compensatory increase in Na^+ and Li^+ reabsorption from the proximal tubule, leading to Li^+ toxicity.
- **Lithium × newer NSAIDs (such as indomethacin):** Indomethacin decreases the renal clearance of Li^+, leading to Li^+ toxicity.
- **Lithium × antipsychotics (such as haloperidol):** Lithium when given for prolonged periods may aggravate tremor, rigidity, confusion, and extrapyramidal symptoms due to haloperidol. Coadministration may also increase the risk of neuroleptic malignant syndrome.
- **Lithium × neuromuscular blockers:** Lithium may cause prolongation of neuromuscular blockade induced by both depolarizing (succinylcholine) and nondepolarizing (pancuronium) neuromuscular blockers.

Clinical Uses

The clinical uses of lithium are mentioned in Figure 4.

Treatment of acute mania	Prophylaxis of bipolar disorder	Treatment of unipolar depression
• Lithium has a slow onset of action (1–2 weeks are required for clinical effect). • Hence, lithium is always given along with atypical antipsychotics (e.g. olanzapine, ziprasidone, aripiprazole etc.). • Antipsychotics provide cover for the initial 1–2 weeks till lithium effects are visible. • Benzodiazepines are also used as adjunctive therapy.	• Prophylaxis of bipolar disorder is the most common indication for lithium. • Prophylactic use of lithium prevents both the depressive and manic phase (unlike anti-psychotics or antidepressants). • Lithium discontinuation results in a high risk of early recurrence.	• Lithium is used in the treatment of resistant recurrent cyclical depression. • Lithium is used (as an adjunct) in the treatment of resistant acute major depression. • The dosage required for the treatment of depression (0.4–0.8 mEq/L) is lower than that required for bipolar disorder (0.6–1.0 mEq/L).

Figure 4: Clinical uses of lithium

OTHER DRUGS USED IN MANIA AND BIPOLAR DISORDERS

There are certain other drugs such as anticonvulsants, atypical antipsychotics and benzodiazepines which are also used in the management of mania and bipolar disorders.

The specific drugs and the situations where these drugs are used are mentioned in Table 1.

TABLE 1	Other drugs used in mania and bipolar disorders

Sodium valproate	• It is being considered as the first line therapy of acute mania. As compared to lithium, it has:
	  ▪ Rapid onset of action
	  ▪ Favorable safety profile
	• It is also used in the prophylaxis of bipolar disorder

Carbamazepine	• Used in the treatment of acute mania and in the prophylaxis of bipolar disorder • It is an alternative drug to lithium when the latter is less effective • Induces CYP3A4 isoenzyme; hence, drug interactions remain a concern
Lamotrigine	• Used in the prophylaxis of bipolar disorder • Not effective in acute mania
Atypical antipsychotics	• Olanzapine, aripiprazole and ziprasidone are commonly used • These drugs are used in the treatment of acute mania (for rapid control of symptoms)
Benzodiazepines	• Diazepam and lorazepam are used as adjunctive therapies in agitated patients

SECTION D ■ Drugs Acting on the Central Nervous System

ASSESS YOURSELF (Examination Questions of Various Universities)

1. Discuss the mechanism of action and adverse effects of lithium.

2. Write short notes on:
   a. Lithium
   b. Lithium toxicity
   c. Therapeutic status of lithium in manic depressive psychosis

MULTIPLE CHOICE QUESTIONS

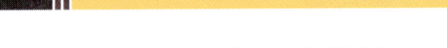 

1. Most common renal sequel of lithium toxicity is:
   (Recent Question 2016)
   a. Nephrogenic DI
   b. Renal tubular acidosis
   c. Glycosuria
   d. MPGN

2. Lithium use in pregnancy may result in fetal:
   (Recent Question 2016)
   a. Cardiac malformation
   b. Cranial abnormality
   c. Cleft lip and cleft palate

3. Coarse tremors, dysarthria and ataxia are side effects of: *(Recent Question 2016)*
   a. Lithium   b. Haloperidol
   c. Imipramine   d. None

4. Lithium causes all except:
   (Recent Question 2016)
   a. Exaggeration of psoriasis
   b. Nephropathy
   c. Ebstein's anomaly
   d. Hyperthyroidism

5. Toxic levels of serum lithium more than:
   (Recent Question 2016)
   a. 2 mEq   b. 4 mEq
   c. 6 mEq   d. 8 mEq

6. Lithium use in pregnancy leads to which effect on baby? *(AIIMS Nov 2018)*
   a. CVS defect   b. Urogenital defect
   c. Neural tube defect   d. Facial defects

Ans.

| 1. (a) | 2. (a) | 3. (a) | 4. (d) | 5. (a) | 6. (a) |

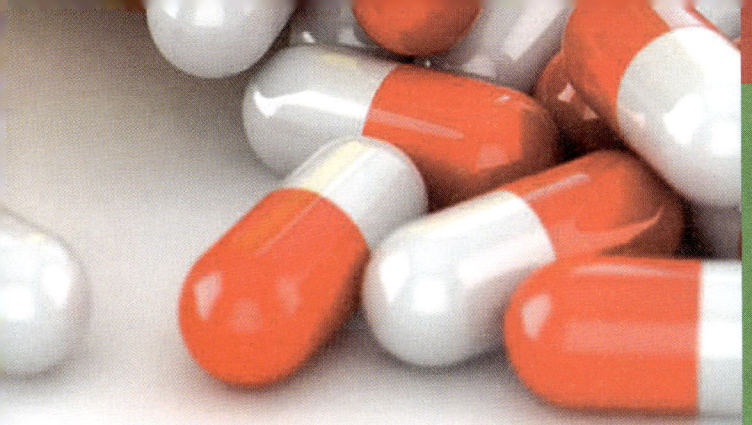

Drugs Used for Anesthesia

25

General Anesthetics

ANESTHESIA

The word anesthesia is derived from two Greek words: "an" which means "without" and "aesthesis" which means "sensation" (Figure 1).

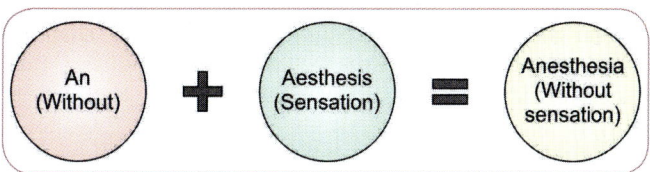

Figure 1: Anesthesia

GENERAL ANESTHESIA (GA)

General anesthesia is a state of controlled and reversible loss of consciousness.

General anesthetics are drugs that produce a reversible state of CNS depression resulting in unconsciousness and loss of all sensations.

The features of general anesthesia are mentioned in Figure 2.

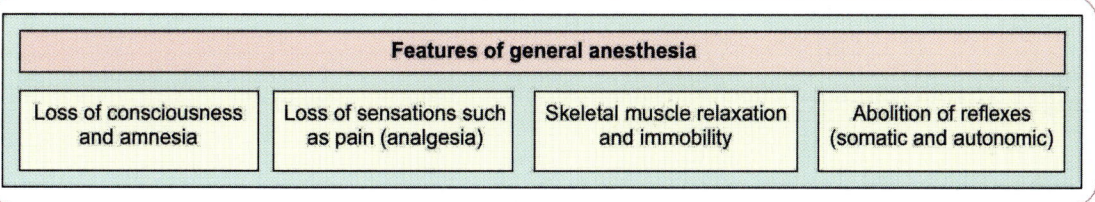

Figure 2: General anesthesia

The practice of balanced anesthesia depends upon utilizing various combinations of drugs (intravenous and inhaled) to achieve the above effects. This is because there is no single drug that can reversibly induce the features of general anesthesia.

Some examples of drugs that may be used in the conduct of anesthesia are mentioned in Figure 3.

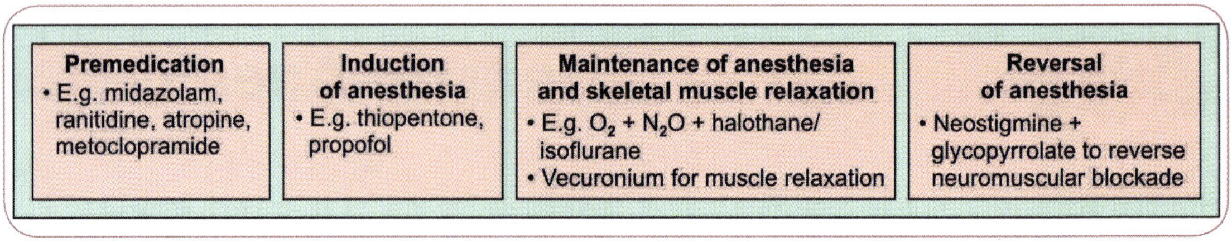

Premedication	Induction of anesthesia	Maintenance of anesthesia and skeletal muscle relaxation	Reversal of anesthesia
• E.g. midazolam, ranitidine, atropine, metoclopramide	• E.g. thiopentone, propofol	• E.g. O_2 + N_2O + halothane/ isoflurane • Vecuronium for muscle relaxation	• Neostigmine + glycopyrrolate to reverse neuromuscular blockade

Figure 3: Anesthesia

MECHANISM AND STAGES OF GA

The mechanism of action of general anesthetics is not clearly understood. These drugs may exert their effects at the cellular and the molecular level.

○ Cellular level → by affecting the synaptic transmission
○ Molecular level → affect the GABA receptors, NMDA receptors, two-pore K^+ channels

The stages of anesthesia were described by Guedel in 1920 with ether anesthesia. These stages are not seen in modern anesthesia due to premedication and concurrent use of many other anesthetic agents (Table 1).

TABLE 1	Stages of anesthesia	
Stage	**Start of stage**	**End of stage**
Stage 1 **(Stage of analgesia)**	Induction of general anesthesia	Loss of consciousness
Key features • Progressively diminished pain sensation • Consciousness and respiration are present		
Stage 2 **(Stage of excitement and delirium)**	Loss of consciousness	Start of regular respiration
Key features • Patient exhibits excitement → rise in BP and HR may be seen • Pupillary dilatation is observed		
Stage 3 **(Stage of surgical anesthesia)**	Start of regular respiration	Cessation of spontaneous breathing
Key features		
Plane 1	• Roving eyeballs	
Plane 2	• Corneal and laryngeal reflexes are lost	
Plane 3	• Start of pupillary dilatation and loss of light reflex	
Plane 4	• Pupillary dilatation, paralysis of intercostal muscles, shallow abdominal respiration	
Stage 4 **(Stage of medullary paralysis)**	Cessation of spontaneous breathing	Failure of circulation and death
Key features • Complete pupillary dilatation and flaccid muscular paralysis • Depression of respiratory and vasomotor center		

CLASSIFICATION OF DRUGS USED FOR GA

A classification of drugs used in GA is mentioned in Figure 4.

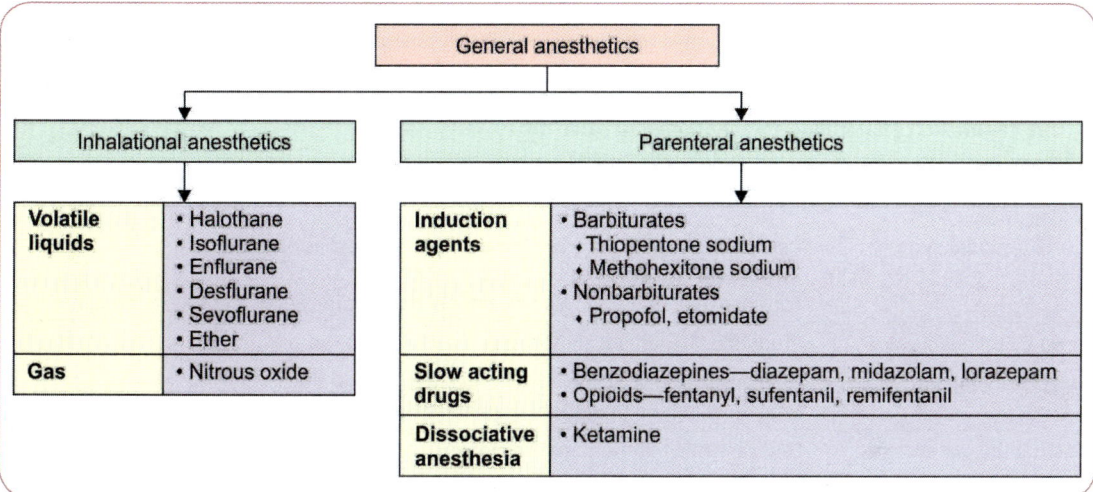

Figure 4: General anesthetics

INHALATIONAL ANESTHETIC DRUGS

Pharmacokinetics of Inhalational Anesthetics

The factors affecting the depth of anesthesia and induction and recovery from anesthesia are as follows:
- Depth of anesthesia
  - Potency (Minimal alveolar concentration [MAC]) of the anesthetic drug
  - Partial pressure of the anesthetic drug in the brain
- Induction and recovery from anesthesia
  - Rate of change of partial pressure in the brain

Minimal Alveolar Concentration (MAC)

It is lowest concentration of the anesthetic present in the alveoli that is required to produce immobility in response to a painful stimulus (surgical skin incision) in 50% of the patients.

It is a measure of potency of the anesthetic.

Partial Pressure

The anesthetic drug moves across a series of partial pressure gradients from the alveoli to blood to tissues (brain).

The factors affecting the partial pressure of the inhaled anesthetic drug achieved in the brain are mentioned in Table 2.

TABLE 2	Factors affecting the partial pressure of anesthetic in brain
Partial pressure of the drug in the inspired air	• Faster anesthetic induction can be obtained by a higher concentration of the drug in the inspired air
Pulmonary ventilation	• Increased ventilation can increase the delivery of the drug to the alveoli
Alveolar exchange	• Conditions such as emphysema can impair the alveolar exchange
Solubility of the drug in blood	• Induction of anesthesia is faster with drugs that have a lower blood solubility
Solubility of the drug tissues	• Drugs with a higher lipid solubility can enter the adipose tissue for a long time and also exit it gradually (e.g. halothane)
Blood flow to the brain	• Increased cerebral blood flow can increase the delivery of the drug to the brain

Halothane

It is a halogenated hydrocarbon having a sweet smell. It is nonirritant and noninflammable.

The MAC of halothane is 0.75% and the blood gas partition coefficient is 2.3. The delivery of halothane requires a special vaporizer.

It is a potent anesthetic and induction is relatively smooth and pleasant. It is neither a good muscle relaxant nor a good analgesic.

It is used for the induction and maintenance of general anesthesia.

The key effects of halothane are mentioned in Table 3.

TABLE 3	Effects of halothane
Cardiovascular system	• Decrease in cardiac contractility with reduced cardiac output • Decrease HR and BP • Sensitize the heart to arrhythmogenic action of catecholamines (e.g. adrenaline)
Central nervous system	• Production of general anesthesia
Respiratory system	• Depression of respiration • Bronchodilatation (beneficial in asthmatic patients)
Gastrointestinal system	• Decrease salivation and gastric motility
Genitourinary system	• Decrease renal blood flow and GFR • Reduce tone of pregnant uterus

Adverse Effects

The adverse effects include:
- Risk of arrhythmias (especially in the presence of hypoxia, hypercapnia or increased catecholamines)
- Hepatotoxicity
- Malignant hyperthermia

Halothane Hepatotoxicity

The administration of halothane is associated with two types of hepatotoxicity. The characteristic features of these two types are mentioned in Figure 5.

Halothane hepatotoxicity	
Type I (mild)	**Type 2 (fulminant)** Halothane hepatitis
• Relatively common and self-limiting • Elevation of serum transaminases is mild and transient. Jaundice is not seen clinically • Possibly due to reductive metabolism of halothane in the body as compared to the usual oxidative metabolism • Does not occur with other volatile anesthetics	• Massive centrilobular hepatic cell necrosis • Jaundice, fever and gross elevations of hepatic enzymes. Can lead to fulminant liver failure • Possible mechanism involves immune mediated damage to the liver cells following oxidative metabolism of halothane • Can occur with other volatile anesthetics (e.g. isoflurane, enflurane), but the incidence of hepatitis is higher with halothane • Has a genetic predisposition

Figure 5: Halothane hepatotoxicity

Isoflurane

It is halogenated methyl ether and is slightly irritant. The delivery of isoflurane requires a special vaporizer.
It has the following effects on the body:
- Cardiovascular system → ↓ BP, ↑ HR

○ Respiratory system → Irritant, depression of respiration, bronchodilatation
○ Does not sensitize the heart to arrhythmogenic action of catecholamines

Adverse effects include triggering of malignant hyperthermia and rare incidence of hepatotoxicity.

It is used for induction and maintenance of general anesthesia. It is a useful anesthetic for neurosurgery as it does not provoke seizures.

Enflurane

It is halogenated methyl-ethyl ether.

It can precipitate seizure activity and is not recommended in epileptic patients.

Desflurane

It is fluorinated methyl isopropyl ether. It is a highly volatile agent. It requires a specific pressurized and heated vaporizer for delivery.

Desflurane has very low blood solubility; hence the induction and recovery are very fast. It can be used for outpatient surgery.

It has a pungent odor; hence is not preferred for induction of anesthesia.

Like isoflurane, it does not invoke seizures and does not sensitize the heart to arrhythmogenic action of catecholamines.

Sevoflurane

It is halogenated ether. It is not pungent and induction is smooth and pleasant. The delivery of sevoflurane requires a special vaporizer.

Induction and recovery are fast; hence, it can be used for both inpatient and outpatient surgery.

It is unstable in the presence of moist soda lime.

Ether

It is a volatile liquid and produces vapors that are inflammable and explosive. It has the following properties:
○ Good analgesia
○ Potent anesthesia
○ Good muscle relaxation

Ether is highly soluble in blood. Induction with ether is prolonged and unpleasant (struggling, salivation, secretions etc.). Premedication with atropine is given.

Ether is not used in modern anesthesia because of its inflammable and unpleasant properties.

It should not be used along with electrocautery as it is inflammable.

Ether is supplied in amber colored bottles that are covered with black paper, as it can form ether peroxide (irritant) upon exposure to sunlight.

A comparison of some of the features of inhaled volatile anesthetic drugs is shown in Table 4.

TABLE 4	Comparison of inhaled anesthetics				
	Ether	Halothane	Isoflurane	Desflurane	Sevoflurane
Chemical composition	Diethyl ether	Halogenated hydrocarbon	Halogenated methyl ether	Fluorinated methyl isopropyl ether	Halogenated ether
Inflammable	Yes	No	No	No	No
MAC (%)	1.9	0.75	1.2	6.0	2.0
Blood: Gas partition coefficient	12.1	2.3	1.4	0.42	0.68
Induction	Slow	Intermediate	Fast	Fast	Fast
Risk of hepatotoxicity	Not hepatotoxic	Some risk	Low risk	Low risk	Low risk

Nitrous Oxide

Nitrous oxide (N_2O) (also called laughing gas) is a colorless, nonirritant, odorless gas that is supplied in steel cylinders.

It has a low potency (MAC: 105%). Hence, loss of consciousness cannot be produced in a patient without the risk of associated hypoxia.

It has good analgesic effect but is a poor muscle relaxant.

Nitrous oxide is often administered in combination with oxygen and other inhaled anesthetic gases such as halothane or isoflurane.

One such combination is N_2O (70%) + O_2 (25–30%) + other anesthetic gas (halothane/isoflurane/sevoflurane in smaller concentrations).

The rationale of combining N_2O with inhaled anesthetic gases such as halothane/isoflurane/sevoflurane is as follows:

- Second gas effect (Figure 6)
  - Second gas effect is observed when N_2O is used in high concentrations along with low concentrations of inhaled anesthetic agents such as halothane/isoflurane/sevoflurane.
  - It occurs due to low solubility of N_2O in the blood that results in rapid absorption of N_2O from the alveoli.
  - This leads to a sharp increase in concentration of other inhaled anesthetic agent (e.g. halothane/isoflurane) in the alveoli.
  - Hence, a reduced concentration of the other inhaled anesthetic (e.g. halothane/isoflurane) is required to produce anesthesia.
  - Reduced concentration of the other inhaled anaesthetic (e.g. halothane/isoflurane) leads to a decreased incidence of adverse effects associated with these drugs.
- Reduction in concentration of the other inhaled anesthetic gas (halothane/isoflurane) leads to a faster recovery from anesthesia.
- N_2O has a low potency but good analgesic properties. Inhaled anesthetic agents such as halothane/isoflurane have high potency, but poor analgesic properties. Hence, combination of N_2O with these agents allows a better administration of anesthesia.

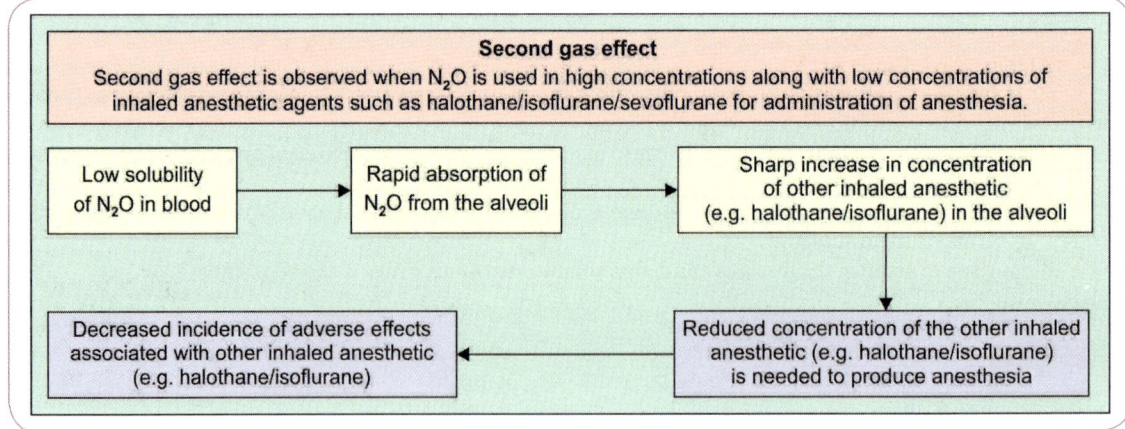

Figure 6: Second gas effect

Diffusion Hypoxia

Diffusion hypoxia is practically the reverse of second gas effect. It is observed following discontinuation of N_2O after prolonged anesthesia (Figure 7).

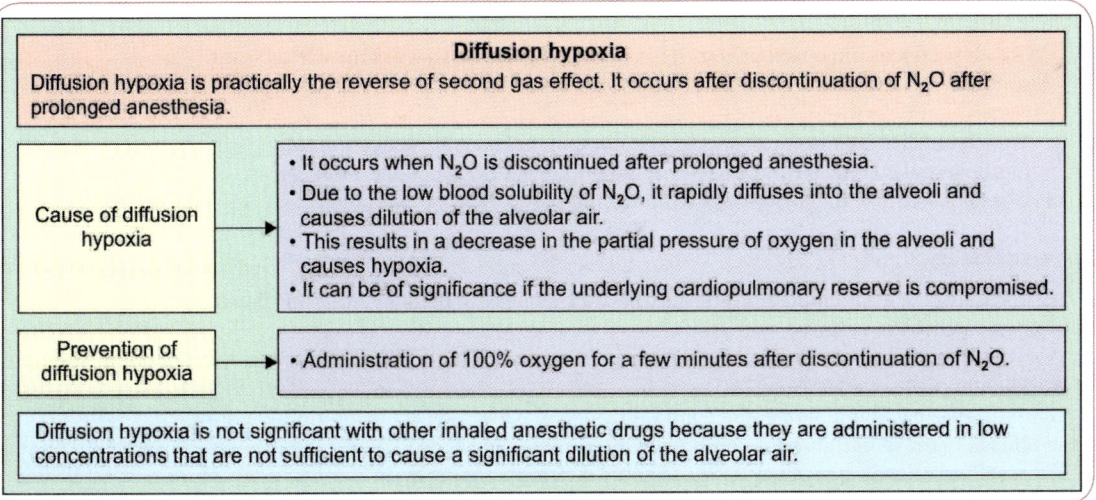

Figure 7: Diffusion hypoxia

Entonox

Entonox is a mixture of N_2O and O_2 in the ratio of 50:50. It can be used for obstetric analgesia with maintenance of consciousness. It can also be used for minor procedures that require transient analgesia.

Nitrous oxide should not be used in patients with bowel obstruction, pneumothorax or sinus disease. This is because N_2O can replace nitrogen in the air spaces faster than nitrogen can leave those spaces. This can result in an increase in pressure (sinuses) or an increase in the volume (pneumothorax) of closed body compartments.

PARENTERAL ANESTHETIC DRUGS—INDUCTION AGENTS

Induction agents are drugs that rapidly produce unconsciousness in one arm-brain circulation time which is approximately 11 seconds.

Thiopentone Sodium

Thiopentone sodium is an ultrashort acting thiobarbiturate that is used as an intravenous induction agent.

Pharmacokinetics

It is a highly lipid soluble drug. It has a rapid onset with short duration of action.

Following intravenous injection, thiopentone rapidly enters the brain and produces anesthesia, resulting in a decline in blood levels of thiopentone.

This leads to diffusion of the drug back from the brain into the blood. This is followed by redistribution of thiopentone into other less vascular tissue. The patient soon regains consciousness (Figure 8).

Repeated injections can lead to gradual accumulation of the drug in the extracerebral sites that can prolong the duration of action and delay the recovery.

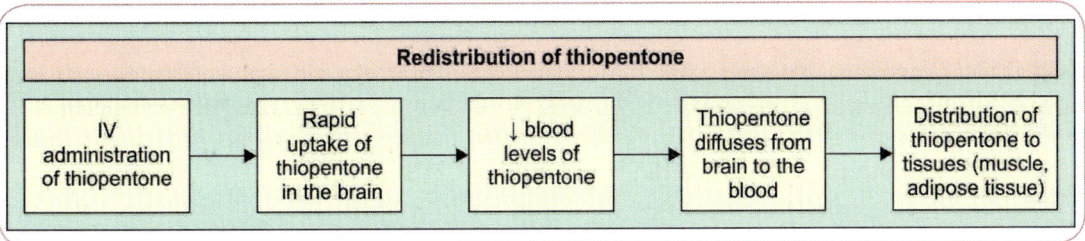

Figure 8: Redistribution of thiopentone

Physiological Effects

- CNS → It produces unconsciousness. It is a poor analgesic and a weak muscle relaxant.
- Respiration → Respiratory depression may be observed.
- CVS →
  - Transient fall in BP may be observed at induction that usually recovers rapidly.
  - Cardiovascular collapse may be seen in patients of shock, hypovolemia or sepsis.
  - Does not sensitize the heart to arrhythmogenic action of catecholamines.

Adverse Effects

- Extravasation or accidental intra-arterial injection can lead to pain, necrosis and gangrene
- Hypersensitivity reactions
- Laryngospasm can occur especially in the presence of respiratory secretions or when intubation is attempted in a lighter plane of anesthesia
- Barbiturates (e.g. thiopentone) are contraindicated in patients of acute intermittent porphyria:
  - This is because barbiturates can induce microsomal enzymes (ALA synthetase) and cause an increase in porphyrins, leading to precipitation of acute intermittent porphyria
- Suxamethonium and thiopentone should not be mixed in the same syringe as they react chemically.

Clinical Uses

The clinical uses of thiopentone include:

- Induction of general anesthesia—commonly used drug for this purpose
- Adjunct to provide hypnosis during balanced anesthesia with other anesthetic agents such as analgesics and muscle relaxants
- Control of convulsions
- Narcoanalysis.

Propofol

Propofol is a short acting intravenous induction agent. It is available as 1% emulsion for intravenous injection or for infusion.

The mechanism of action is unclear but is believed to be due to an inhibitory effect on $GABA_A$ receptors leading to CNS depression.

It does not cause airway irritation and has a rapid onset of action with quick recovery. It also has decreased residual impairment. It does not have analgesic effects.

Propofol has a low incidence of postoperative nausea and vomiting.

Clinical uses include the following:

- Induction and maintenance of general anesthesia in adults and children (age >1 month)
- Sedation for diagnostic and surgical procedures in adults and children (age >1 month)
- Sedation of ventilated patients (age >16 years) in the intensive care unit
- Propofol is particularly useful for outpatient (daycare) surgery

It can cause local pain during injection which is reduced by co-administration with lidocaine and by injection in the larger veins of the forearm/antecubital fossa.

It is one of the commonly used anesthetic induction agents.

Etomidate

It is short acting intravenous induction agent. The incidence of cardiovascular and respiratory depression is low.

It has a higher incidence of restlessness, rigidity, pain on injection and postoperative nausea and vomiting.

■ PARENTERAL ANESTHETIC DRUGS—SLOWER ACTING DRUGS

Benzodiazepines

Drugs such as diazepam, midazolam and lorazepam are used in anesthesia practice.

They produce sedation, amnesia and loss of consciousness. They are poor analgesics; hence, can be administered along with opioids. However, co-administration with opioids can significantly compromise the respiratory and cardiac function.

They do not lead to postoperative nausea and vomiting.

Benzodiazepines are used for procedures such as angiographies, endoscopies, cardiac catheterizations, electroconvulsive therapy, etc. They are also used for conscious sedation along with local or regional anesthesia.

Opioids

Opioids such as fentanyl, alfentanil and sufentanil are used in balanced anesthesia. Opioids are potent analgesics. The administration of opioids allows the use of lower concentrations of other anesthetics agents.

Dexmedetomidine

It is a centrally acting selective α_2 adrenergic receptor agonist.

It is used for the sedation of adult patients in the intensive care unit. It produces analgesia and sedation. The contraindications include uncontrolled hypotension and acute cerebrovascular conditions.

PARENTERAL ANESTHETIC DRUGS—DISSOCIATIVE ANESTHESIA (KETAMINE)

Ketamine

Ketamine is general anesthetic that is used intravenously or intramuscularly. It is a NMDA receptor antagonist.

Ketamine causes dissociative anesthesia. The key features of dissociative anesthesia are mentioned in Figure 9.

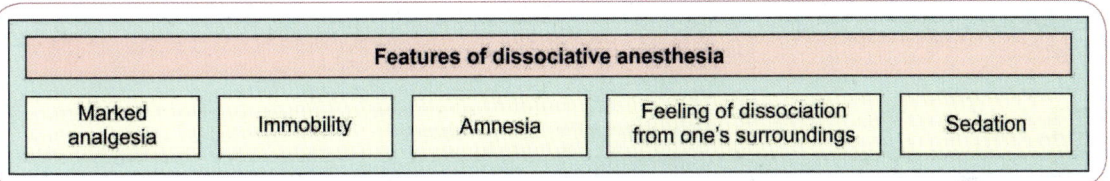

Figure 9: Dissociative anesthesia

The airway reflexes are intact and respiratory depression is not present. There is an increase in the muscle tone.

Ketamine causes sympathetic stimulation that leads to an increase in heart rate, cardiac output and blood pressure; hence it may be useful in patients with hypovolemia or shock.

Ketamine causes bronchodilatation; hence, can be used in asthmatic patients.

Contraindications and Adverse Effects

Emergence delirium, abnormal motor movements and hallucinations may be observed in patients during recovery.

It can cause an increase in the intracranial pressure.

Ketamine is contraindicated in patients in whom an increase in the blood pressure would result in a significant hazard. Hence, it should not be used in patients with severe coronary or cardiac disease, cerebral trauma or cerebrovascular accident.

It should not be used in women with eclampsia or preeclampsia.

Clinical Uses

The clinical uses of ketamine include:
- Head, neck or face surgeries
- Short procedures such as burn dressings, wound debridement, skin grafting
- Surgical procedures in an asthmatic patient.

COMPLICATIONS OF GA

Some of the complications of general anesthesia are mentioned in Table 5.

TABLE 5	Complications of general anesthesia
Cardiovascular	• Cardiac depression, hypotension • Cardiac arrhythmias • Cardiac arrest
Respiratory	• Laryngospasm, bronchospasm, hypoxia • Respiratory depression, apnea • Aspiration pneumonitis
Gastrointestinal	• Nausea and vomiting
Central nervous system	• Seizures, delirium • Prolonged sedation and impaired psychomotor function • Increased intracranial pressure • Awareness
Others	• Hepatotoxicity • Nephrotoxicity • Malignant hyperthermia • Precipitation of porphyria

PREANESTHETIC MEDICATION

Preanesthetic medications are used prior to the use of anesthetic drugs, to make anesthesia safer and pleasant (Table 6).

TABLE 6	Preanesthetic medications
Objectives	**Preanesthetic medications**
Antianxiety, amnesia	• Benzodiazepines (e.g. midazolam, diazepam)
Antiemetic	• Metoclopramide, domperidone • Ondansetron
Pre- and postoperative analgesia	• Opioids (e.g. pethidine, fentanyl)
Reduction of acid secretion	• H_2 blockers (e.g. ranitidine) • Proton pump inhibitors (e.g. omeprazole)
Increase gastric emptying	• Prokinetics (e.g. metoclopramide or domperidone) These drugs are often used prior to emergency surgery to increase gastric emptying and reduce the incidence of aspiration pneumonitis
Reduction of salivary and bronchial secretions Prevent vagal bradycardia	• Anticholinergics (e.g. atropine, glycopyrrolate) Glycopyrrolate is often preferred because it is less likely to cause CNS effects. It also causes relatively less tachycardia

CONSCIOUS SEDATION

The key features of conscious sedation are:
- ○ Patient is conscious, but sedated
- ○ Analgesia is present
- ○ Verbal communication can be done with the patient
- ○ Preservation of protective airway reflexes

Conscious sedation is used for dental procedures, endoscopies, liver, breast and kidney biopsies, etc. It is often useful in uncooperative and anxious patients.

The following agents can be used for conscious sedation:
- ○ Benzodiazepines → Diazepam, midazolam
- ○ Propofol
- ○ Nitrous oxide and oxygen
- ○ Fentanyl

Careful monitoring (heart rate, blood pressure, respiration, oxygen level, alertness, etc.) of the patient is extremely important during and after conscious sedation.

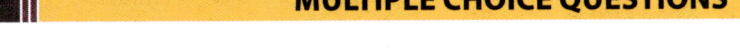

ASSESS YOURSELF (Examination Questions of Various Universities)

1. Pre-anaesthetic medication
2. Dissociative anaesthesia
3. I.V. general anaesthetics
4. Inhalational anaesthetic agents

MULTIPLE CHOICE QUESTIONS

1. **Which of the following intravenous induction agent is the most suitable for day care surgery?**
    (Recent Question Dec 2016)
    a. Morphine
    b. Ketamine
    c. Propofol
    d. Diazepam

2. **Which of the following anesthetic agent is a potent bronchodilator?**
    (Recent Question Dec 2016)
    a. Propofol
    b. Ketamine
    c. Thiopentone
    d. Methoxytone

3. **Which of the following drugs produces dissociative anesthesia?**
    (Recent Question Dec 2016)
    a. Ketamine
    b. Propofol
    c. Thiopentone
    d. Enflurane

4. **Thiopentone is contraindicated in:**
    (Recent Question Dec 2016)
    a. Acute intermittent porphyria
    b. Electro convulsive therapy
    c. Sarcoidosis
    d. Diabetic patients

5. **Inducing agent of choice in shock:**
    (Recent Question Dec 2016)
    a. Isoflurane
    b. Desflurane
    c. Ketamine
    d. Thiopentone

6. **Anesthetic agent used for maintenance in ICU is:** *(Recent Question Dec 2016)*
    a. Thiopentone
    b. Propofol
    c. Ketamine
    d. None of the above

7. **Hallucinations are seen with:**
    (Recent Question Dec 2016)
    a. Propofol
    b. Sevoflurane
    c. Ketamine
    d. Isoflurane

8. **Anesthetic of choice for status asthmaticus:**
    (Recent Question Dec 2016)
    a. Ketamine
    b. Thiopentone
    c. Ether
    d. Propofol

9. **Intracranial pressure is increased by:**
    (Recent Question Dec 2016)
    a. Barbiturate
    b. Ketamine
    c. Etomidate
    d. Propofol

10. **Ketamine is the preferred anesthetic in the following cases except:**
    (Recent Question Dec 2016)
    a. Hypertension
    b. Trauma cases that have bled significantly
    c. Burn dressing
    d. Short operations on asthmatics

11. **Most potent analgesic agent among following:**
    (AIIMS Nov 2012)
    a. Nitrous oxide
    b. Nitric oxide
    c. CO_2
    d. Oxygen

12. **Potency of inhalational anesthetic agent is measured by:**
    (Recent Question Dec 2016)
    a. Minimum alveolar concentration
    b. Diffusion coefficient
    c. Dead space concentration
    d. Alveolar blood concentration

13. **Following is the most severe adverse effect of halothane:** *(Recent Question Dec 2016)*
    a. Asthma
    b. Hepatitis
    c. Tachycardia
    d. Hypertension

Ans.

1.	(c)	2.	(b)	3.	(a)	4.	(a)	5.	(c)	6.	(b)
7.	(c)	8.	(a)	9.	(b)	10.	(a)	11.	(a)	12.	(a)
13.	(b)										

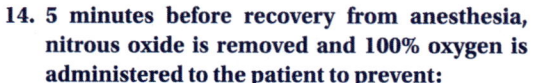

14. **5 minutes before recovery from anesthesia, nitrous oxide is removed and 100% oxygen is administered to the patient to prevent:**
(Recent Question Dec 2016)
   a. Diffusion hypoxia
   b. Second gas effect
   c. Hyperoxia
   d. Bronchospasm

15. **Second gas effect is seen with:**
(Recent Question Dec 2016)
   a. Ether
   b. Nitrous oxide
   c. Desflurane
   d. Sevoflurane

16. **Malignant hyperthermia is caused by:**
(Recent Question Dec 2016)
   a. Succinylcholine + halothane
   b. Propranolol
   c. Lidocaine
   d. Bupivacaine

17. **MAC of desflurane is:**
(Recent Question Dec 2016)
   a. 1.15
   b. 2
   c. 4
   d. 6

18. **Diffusion hypoxia seen during:**
(Recent Question Dec 2016)
   a. Induction of anesthesia
   b. Reversal of anesthesia
   c. Postoperative period
   d. None of the above

19. **Laughing gas is** *(Recent Question Dec 2016)*
   a. Nitrous oxide
   b. Halothane
   c. Chloroform
   d. Diethyl ether

20. **Ratio of O_2 : N_2O in entonox is:**
(Recent Question Dec 2016)
   a. 50:50
   b. 60:40
   c. 40:60
   d. 25:75

21. **MAC is:** *(Recent Question Dec 2016)*
   a. Minimum arterial concentration
   b. Maximum arterial concentration
   c. Minimum alveolar concentration
   d. Maximum alveolar concentration

22. **Second gas effect is exerted by which of the following gas when co-administered with halothane:** *(Recent Question Dec 2016)*
   a. Nitrous oxide
   b. Cyclopropane
   c. Nitrogen
   d. Helium

23. **Anesthetic agent which is explosive in the presence of cautery:**
(Recent Question Dec 2016)
   a. Nitrous oxide
   b. Ether
   c. Trilene
   d. Halothane

24. **Ketamine acts on:** *(NIMHANS 2008)*
   a. NMDA receptor
   b. Glycine receptor
   c. GABAa receptor
   d. Ach receptor

Ans.											
14.	(a)	15.	(b)	16.	(a)	17.	(d)	18.	(b)	19.	(a)
20.	(a)	21.	(c)	22.	(a)	23.	(b)	24.	(a)		

26

Skeletal Muscle Relaxants

Skeletal muscle relaxants reduce the muscle tone and/or cause muscular paralysis.

Based on the site and mechanism of action, they can be classified into peripherally acting and centrally acting muscle relaxants (Figure 1).

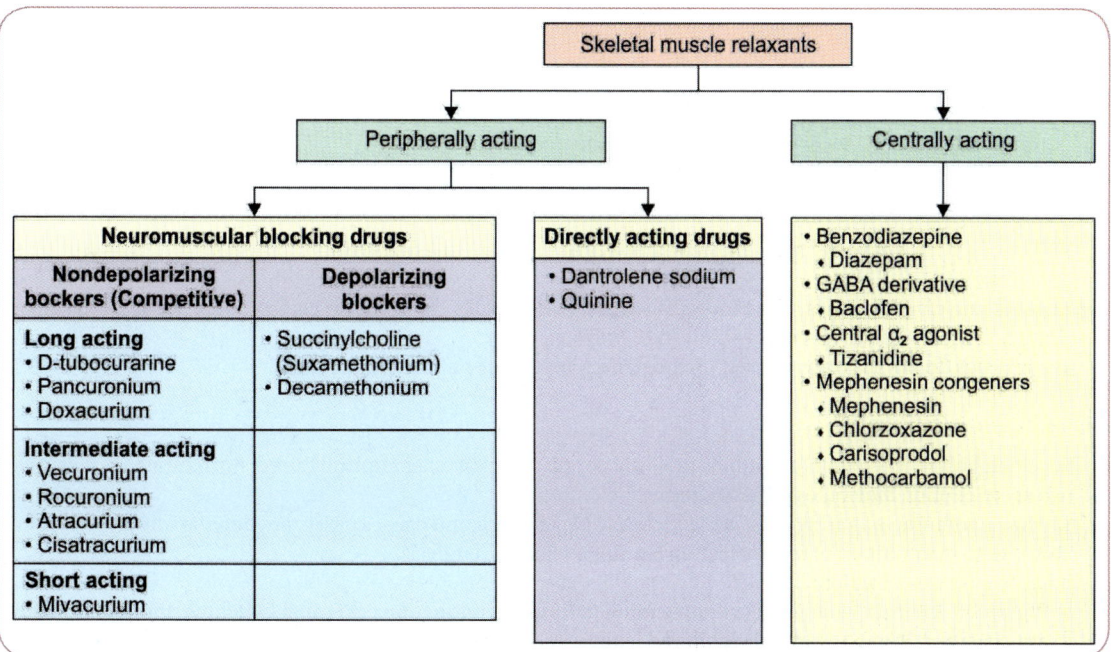

Figure 1: Skeletal muscle relaxants

NEUROMUSCULAR BLOCKING DRUGS (PERIPHERALLY ACTING MUSCLE RELAXANTS)

These drugs block neuromuscular transmission at the neuromuscular junction (at the nicotinic receptors). This results in a reduction in skeletal muscle tone and muscle paralysis.

Physiology of Neuromuscular Transmission

The neuromuscular junction (NMJ) is vital in the production of skeletal muscle contraction and consists of:
○ Motor neurone
○ Motor endplate
○ Synaptic cleft or junctional gap between the motor neurone and motor endplate
The neurotransmitter at the NMJ is acetylcholine (ACh) (Figure 2).

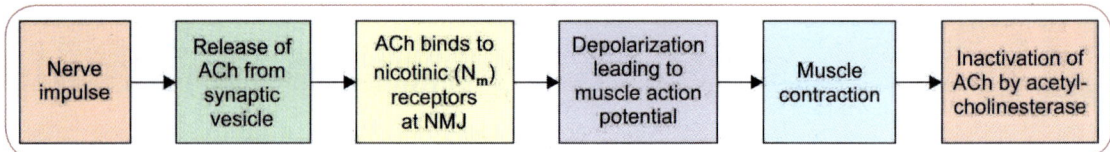

Figure 2: Neuromuscular transmission

Mechanism of Action of Neuromuscular Blockers

Nondepolarizing Blockers (Competitive)

- They are competitive antagonists of acetylcholine at the N_M receptors and prevent acetylcholine from stimulating the N_M receptors. This results in paralysis of muscles.
- The antagonism is competitive; hence, can be reversed by increasing the concentration of acetylcholine at the receptor sites (Figure 3).

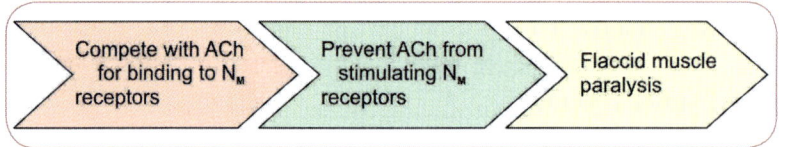

Figure 3: Mechanism of action of nondepolarizing (Competitive) blockers

The onset of muscle paralysis is in the following order: Eye muscles → Hands → Feet → Neck → Face → Trunk → Respiratory muscles. The recovery is usually in the reverse order.

These drugs do not have any impact on the consciousness or on pain perception.

Depolarizing Blockers

- Succinylcholine or suxamethonium is the only depolarizing blocker clinically used. Structurally, it resembles two acetylcholine molecules joined together.
- Succinylcholine acts as an agonist at the nicotinic N_M receptor and causes persistent depolarization of the NMJ. This results in inhibition of repolarization leading to flaccid paralysis.
- It has two phases of action:
  - Phase I → Initial brief depolarization leading to muscle contractions → initial twitching and fasciculations are observed. Repolarization is inhibited leading to flaccid paralysis. This type of block cannot be reversed by neostigmine (acetylcholinesterase inhibitor).
  - Phase II → Desensitization blockade in which the motor end plate loses its sensitivity after prolonged exposure to succinylcholine. This leads to a nondepolarizing type of block that can be reversed by neostigmine.

Pharmacokinetics of Neuromuscular Blockers

All neuromuscular blockers are quaternary polar compounds that have the following features:
- Not absorbed orally; hence, administered parenterally (usually IV)
- Do not cross cell membranes
- Do not cross placental or the blood brain barrier
- Have low volumes of distribution

Succinylcholine (Suxamethonium)

Succinylcholine has a very short duration of action (3–5 minutes). This is because it undergoes rapid hydrolysis (inactivation) by plasma cholinesterase (pseudocholinesterase) enzyme (Figure 4).

SECTION E ■ Drugs Used for Anesthesia

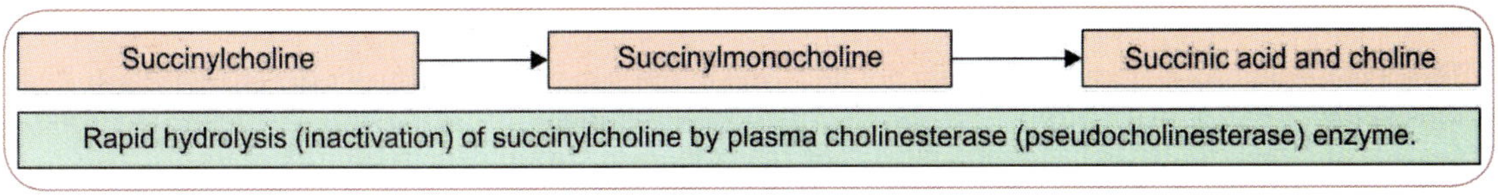

Figure 4: Succinylcholine—hydrolysis

Some patients may demonstrate a prolonged neuromuscular block (succinylcholine apnea) with succinylcholine. This may be due to the following:

o Congenital causes such as genetic deficiency of pseudocholinesterase that may result in ineffective succinylcholine inactivation
o Acquired causes such as severe hepatic failure or patients of severe burns

Prolonged neuromuscular blockade results in prolonged muscle paralysis and apnea. It is vital to maintain the airway and adequate ventilation until spontaneous respiration returns. Fresh frozen plasma to increase the patient's plasma cholinesterase levels may be considered.

Pharmacological Actions

o Skeletal muscles
  □ Flaccid paralysis
  □ Apnea
o Histamine release
  □ Among the nondepolarizing blockers, d-tubocurarine has a higher potential to cause histamine release from mast cells
  □ Succinylcholine and atracurium can also cause histamine release
  □ Histamine release may cause symptoms such as hypotension, flushing, bronchospasm and increased respiratory secretions
o Ganglion blockade
o CVS
  □ Hypotension may result from histamine release and ganglion blockade
  □ Pancuronium may also cause tachycardia.

Adverse Effects

Succinylcholine (Suxamethonium)

o Bradycardia → resulting from stimulation of muscarinic receptors in the SA node
o Rise in intraocular pressure
o Rise in intragastric pressure that may lead to aspiration of gastric contents
o Muscle pain → due to initial fasciculations
o Hyperkalemia
  □ Succinylcholine can lead to an increase in the serum potassium levels
  □ Cardiac arrhythmias and death may result in patients with pre-existing hyperkalemia
  □ Patients with burns, muscular dystrophies and paraplegics can develop fatal hyperkalemia
o Prolonged apnea (Succinylcholine apnea) and respiratory paralysis → due to congenital or acquired deficiency of pseudocholinesterase enzyme
o Malignant hyperthermia
o Hypersensitivity reactions.

Nondepolarizing Blockers

o Increased heart rate
o Hypersensitivity reactions
o Histamine release may lead to hypotension, bronchospasm and increased secretions.

Drug Interactions

- Thiopentone and succinylcholine should not be mixed in the same syringe as they react chemically and can precipitate
- General anesthetics such as halothane, isoflurane can potentiate the nondepolarizing blockers
- Antibiotics can potentiate the neuromuscular blockade
  - Aminoglycosides (e.g. gentamicin, streptomycin) can potentiate the effects of nondepolarizing NMBs by reducing the release of acetylcholine from nerve endings
  - Tetracyclines can potentiate the effects of NMBs by chelating calcium
- Calcium channel blockers (verapamil) can potentiate both nondepolarizing and depolarizing NMBs
- Diuretics (thiazides, furosemide) can cause hypokalemia that can potentiate the effects of nondepolarizing NMBs.

Clinical Uses

- These drugs are used as adjuvants to general anesthetics. They produce muscle relaxation to facilitate endotracheal intubation, mechanical ventilation and multiple surgical and obstetric procedures.
- Suxamethonium is used for rapid sequence induction/emergency endotracheal intubation in anesthesia because of its fast, predictable and short duration of action. Rapid sequence induction is done in patients who have an increased risk of gastric aspiration.
- Suxamethonium is used to decrease the incidence of convulsions and trauma resulting from electroconvulsive therapy.
- Nondepolarizing NMBs are used in intensive care for the management of status asthmaticus and tetanus. They are also used for assisted ventilation in critically ill patients.

Factors Affecting the Actions of Neuromuscular Blockers

- Acidosis and hypothermia can potentiate the neuromuscular block.
- Drugs such as general anesthetics (inhalational), calcium channel blockers, antibiotics (aminoglycosides, tetracyclines) can potentiate the neuromuscular block.
- Myasthenia gravis: It is an autoimmune condition in which there is development of autoantibodies against acetylcholine (ACh) nicotinic postsynaptic receptors. There is also a reduction in the numbers of postsynaptic acetylcholine receptors at the NMJ. Patients with myasthenia gravis are very sensitive to the effects of neuromuscular blockers.

Reversal of Neuromuscular Blockade

Anticholinesterases such as neostigmine or edrophonium may be used for the reversal of neuromuscular blockade.

Anticholinesterases inhibit the true cholinesterase enzyme in the synaptic cleft. This results in prolongation and intensification of the muscarinic and nicotinic effects of acetylcholine.

Anticholinergics such as atropine or glycopyrrolate are given along with anticholinesterases to block the muscarinic effects (bradycardia, increased secretions etc.) of acetylcholine.

Other indications of neostigmine include myasthenia gravis, paralytic ileus and postoperative urinary retention.

Sugammadex

It is used for the reversal of neuromuscular blockade induced by rocuronium or vecuronium in adults.

It is a selective relaxant binding agent that forms a complex with the neuromuscular blockers (rocuronium or vecuronium) in plasma.

Hence, it decreases the amount of neuromuscular blocker available to bind to nicotinic receptors in the neuromuscular junction.

This leads to the reversal of neuromuscular blockade induced by rocuronium or vecuronium.

INDIVIDUAL NEUROMUSCULAR BLOCKERS

Depolarizing

Succinylcholine (Suxamethonium)

- Depolarizing neuromuscular blocker
- Suxamethonium is used for rapid sequence induction/emergency endotracheal intubation in anesthesia because of its fast, predictable and short duration of action
- It is also used to decrease the incidence of convulsions and trauma resulting from electroconvulsive therapy
- Adverse effects include bradycardia, hyperkalemia and prolonged apnea (succinylcholine apnea)
- Patients with burns, muscular dystrophies and paraplegics can develop fatal hyperkalemia → cause is postulated to be an increase in the extrajunctional receptors.

Nondepolarizing

D-tubocurarine

- Not currently used due to its higher propensity to cause histamine release, ganglion blockade and cardiac effects.

Pancuronium

- Longer duration of action than newer agents; hence used only in prolonged operations
- Causes tachycardia due to vagolytic action
- Minimal release of histamine.

Vecuronium

- Intermediate duration of action
- Better cardiac stability
- Commonly used in anesthesia practice.

Atracurium

- Shorter acting
- Undergoes spontaneous inactivation in the plasma by nonenzymatic degradation (Hoffman elimination), in addition to inactivation by pseudocholinesterases
- It is preferred in patients with hepatic or renal disease
- Can cause histamine release and lead to hypotension.

Cisatracurium

- Undergoes inactivation by nonenzymatic degradation (Hoffman elimination)
- It is not inactivated by pseudocholinesterases
- Does not cause histamine release
- More potent than atracurium.

Rocuronium

- Rapid onset with intermediate duration of action
- It can be used to facilitate tracheal intubation during rapid sequence induction in adults.

Mivacurium

- Shortest acting nondepolarizing neuromuscular blocker
- Inactivated rapidly by plasma cholinesterase
- Prolonged apnea can occur in deficiency of pseudocholinesterase enzyme.

The salient pharmacological features of d-tubocurarine and succinylcholine are mentioned in Table 1.

TABLE 1	Difference between d-tubocurarine and succinylcholine	
Drug	**D-tubocurarine**	**Succinylcholine**
Type of block	• Nondepolarizing	• Depolarizing
Mechanism of action	• Competitive antagonism of ACh at N_M receptors	• Persistent depolarization of the N_M receptors leading to desensitization
Duration of action	• Long acting	• Short acting
Onset of action	• Slow	• Fast
Type of paralysis	• Flaccid paralysis	• Initial fasciculations → flaccid paralysis
Effect of anticholinesterases (neostigmine)	• Reversal (antagonism) of neuromuscular blockade	• Potentiation of phase I neuromuscular blockade

NEUROMUSCULAR BLOCKING DRUGS (DIRECTLY ACTING MUSCLE RELAXANTS)

Dantrolene is a directly acting muscle relaxant. It inhibits the release of calcium from the skeletal muscles by acting on the ryanodine receptors.

Oral dantrolene is used in chronic, severe spasticity of skeletal muscle in adults. It is used in conditions such as multiple sclerosis, cerebral palsy, paraplegia, upper motor neuron diseases, etc.

Intravenous dantrolene is the therapy of choice in malignant hyperthermia, which occurs due to persistent Ca^{++} release from sarcoplasmic reticulum. It also provides some benefit in neuroleptic malignant syndrome.

The adverse effects include muscular weakness, dizziness, somnolence, diarrhea and hepatic damage including fatal hepatic failure.

CENTRALLY ACTING MUSCLE RELAXANTS

Benzodiazepines—Diazepam

Diazepam enhances GABA transmission in the brain. It has antianxiety, anticonvulsant, sedative, amnesic and central muscle relaxant action. A reduction in the muscle tone is observed.

Clinical uses include:
- Control muscle spasms in tetanus
- Management of cerebral spasticity in some patients

The adverse effects include respiratory depression and dependence.

GABA Derivatives—Baclofen

Baclofen is a selective $GABA_B$ receptor agonist and has the following actions:
- Decreases synaptic reflex transmission in the spinal cord
- Antinociceptive action

Baclofen is used to reduce spasticity in neurological conditions such as multiple sclerosis, amyotrophic lateral sclerosis, spinal injuries and other spinal lesions.

The adverse effects include drowsiness, confusion, sedation, nausea and muscle weakness.

Central α_2 Agonist—Tizanidine

Tizanidine is a centrally acting skeletal muscle relaxant.

It is a α_2 receptor agonist and inhibits the release of excitatory amino acids in the spinal cord. Inhibition of polysynaptic reflexes is seen that reduces the muscle tone.

Clinical uses include:
- Spasticity associated with neurological disorders
- Painful muscle spasms of spinal origin

The adverse effects include hallucinations, somnolence, insomnia, dizziness and dry mouth.

Clinical Uses of Centrally Acting Muscle Relaxants

The clinical uses include the following:
- Acute muscle spasms
- Torticollis, neuralgias
- Spastic neurological diseases
- Tetanus
- Electroconvulsive therapy

The key difference between centrally acting and peripherally acting muscle relaxants is mentioned in Table 2.

TABLE 2	Centrally acting versus peripherally acting muscle relaxants
Centrally acting muscle relaxants	**Peripherally acting muscle relaxants**
• Cause reduction in muscle tone	• Cause muscle paralysis
• Inhibit polysynaptic reflexes	• Block transmission at neuromuscular junction
• Propensity to cause CNS depression	• Do not cross the blood brain barrier—no effect on the CNS
• Oral and parenteral administration	• Parenteral administration (usually IV)
• Clinically used in spastic conditions	• Used as muscle relaxants in anesthesia to facilitate endotracheal intubation, mechanical ventilation and multiple obstetric and surgical procedures
• Examples—diazepam, baclofen	• Examples—vecuronium, succinylcholine

BOTULINUM TOXIN TYPE B AND BOTULINUM TOXIN TYPE A

These are neurotoxins derived from *Clostridium botulinum.*

Botulinum Toxin Type A

It is a neurotoxin that blocks the release of acetylcholine at presynaptic cholinergic nerve terminals. This causes chemical denervation leading to muscle relaxation.

Clinical uses of botulinum toxin type A include:
- Treatment of focal spasticity
- Blepharospasm, idiopathic cervical dystonia
- Bladder dysfunction such as overactive bladder
- Temporary improvements in the facial lines in adults

The adverse effects include viral infections, paresthesia, exaggerated muscle weakness, distant spread of toxin, dysphagia, dyspnea, aspiration pneumonia (some with fatal outcome).

Botulinum Toxin Type B

It inhibits the release of acetylcholine from nerve terminals at the neuromuscular junction.

Clinical indication of botulinum toxin type B includes the treatment of cervical dystonia (torticollis) in adults.

The adverse effects include injection site pain, dry mouth, dysphagia, exaggerated muscle weakness, distant spread of toxin, dyspnea, aspiration pneumonia (some with fatal outcome).

ASSESS YOURSELF (Examination Questions of Various Universities)

1. **Classify skeletal muscle relaxants. State the mechanism of action, adverse effects and therapeutic uses of succinylcholine.**
2. **Centrally acting muscle relaxants**
3. **Depolarizing neuromuscular blocking agents**

MULTIPLE CHOICE QUESTIONS

1. **All of the following act on neuromuscular junction except:** *(AIIMS May 2016)*
   a. Pipercurium
   b. Dantrolene sodium
   c. Succinylcholine
   d. Mivacurium

2. **A drug that undergoes Hoffmann elimination is:** *(AIIMS May 2016)*
   a. Atracurium
   b. Vecuronium
   c. Pancuronium
   d. Mivacurium

3. **Cisatracurium is preferred over atracurium due to advantage of:** *(AIIMS Nov 2011)*
   a. Rapid onset
   b. Short duration of action
   c. No histamine release
   d. Less cardiodepressant

4. **Which drug can be eliminated by nonenzymatic degradation?** *(Recent Question Dec 2016)*
   a. Atracurium
   b. Pancuronium
   c. Mivacurium
   d. Doxacurium

5. **Only available depolarizing muscle relaxant is:** *(Recent Question Dec 2016)*
   a. Decamethonium
   b. Suxamethonium
   c. Mivacurium
   d. None

6. **Nondepolarizing blocking agent among the following is:** *(Recent Question Dec 2016)*
   a. Suxamethonium
   b. Decamethonium
   c. Pancuronium
   d. Baclofen

7. **Which of the following is directly acting skeletal muscle relaxant?** *(Recent Question Dec 2016)*
   a. Dantrolene
   b. Suxamethonium
   c. Pancuronium
   d. Atracurium

8. **Shortest acting muscle relaxant:** *(Recent Question Dec 2016)*
   a. Pancuronium
   b. Atracurium
   c. Mivacurium
   d. Vecuronium

9. **Drug used for d-TC reveral is:** *(Recent Question Dec 2016)*
   a. Atropine
   b. Atracurium
   c. Diazepam
   d. Neostigmine

10. **Receptor responsible for malignant hyperthermia:** *(Recent Question Dec 2016)*
    a. Nicotinic receptor
    b. Muscarinic receptor
    c. Ryanodine receptor
    d. NMDA receptor

11. **Dantrolene acts by:** *(Recent Question Dec 2016)*
    a. Inhibiting calcium release from smooth muscle cells
    b. Inhibiting sodium release from smooth muscle cells
    c. Inhibiting potassium release from smooth muscle cells
    d. Increase calcium release from smooth muscle cells

12. **Baclofen is a:** *(Recent Question Dec 2016)*
    a. Peripherally acting muscle relaxant
    b. Both centrally and peripherally acting muscle relaxant
    c. Directly acting muscle relaxant
    d. Centrally acting muscle relaxant

13. **Which of the following is a skeletal muscle relaxant that acts as a central a_2 adrenergic agonist?** *(Recent Question Dec 2016)*
    a. Tizanidine
    b. Brimonidine
    c. Chlormezanone
    d. Quinine

Ans.

1.	(b)	2.	(a)	3.	(c)	4.	(a)	5.	(b)	6.	(c)
7.	(a)	8.	(c)	9.	(d)	10.	(c)	11.	(a)	12.	(d)
13.	(a)										

27

Local Anesthetics

Local anesthetics (LA) are drugs which when applied topically or injected locally, reversibly prevent the transmission of nerve impulse in the region to which they are applied.

This results in loss of sensory perception in the area supplied by the nerve. They can also block the motor impulses and may result in motor paralysis.

They do not impair consciousness.

The important feature of LA is that the effects are reversible and complete recovery of nerve function results with no evidence of nerve damage.

Different neural fibers have varying degrees of sensitivity to local anesthetics (Figure 1).

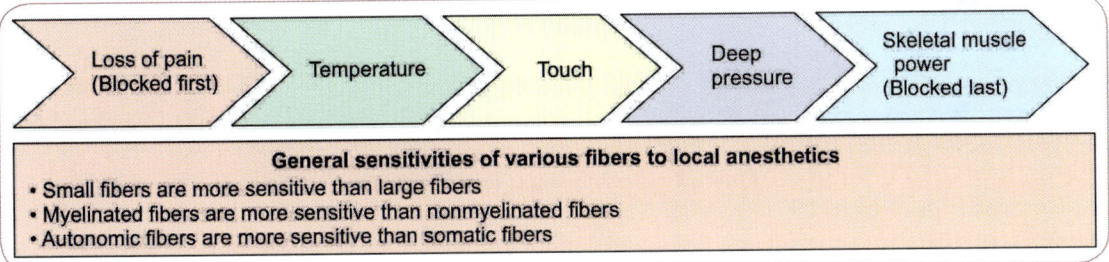

> Loss of pain (Blocked first) → Temperature → Touch → Deep pressure → Skeletal muscle power (Blocked last)
>
> **General sensitivities of various fibers to local anesthetics**
> - Small fibers are more sensitive than large fibers
> - Myelinated fibers are more sensitive than nonmyelinated fibers
> - Autonomic fibers are more sensitive than somatic fibers

Figure 1: Sensitivity to local anesthetics

CHEMICAL STRUCTURE OF LOCAL ANESTHETICS

Local anesthetics usually have a lipophilic aromatic group and a hydrophilic amino group. These two groups are linked together by either an ester bond or an amide bond (Figure 2).

Depending upon the linkage, the anesthetics can be classified as:
○ Ester anesthetics—e.g. cocaine, procaine, chloroprocaine, tetracaine, benzocaine
○ Amide anesthetics—e.g. lignocaine, bupivacaine, mepivacaine, ropivacaine, prilocaine

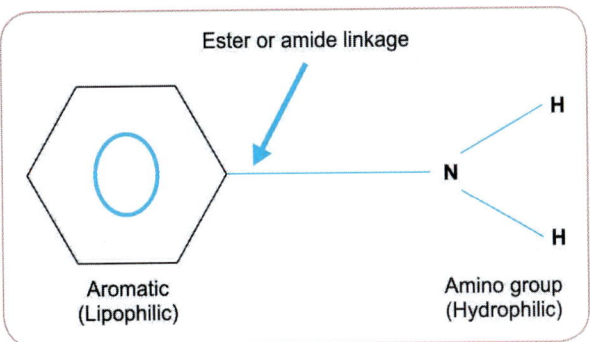

Ester or amide linkage

Aromatic (Lipophilic) — N — H, H

Amino group (Hydrophilic)

Figure 2: Structure of local anesthetics

CLASSIFICATION

Local anesthetics can be classified according to their clinical use or as per their chemical structure (Figure 3).

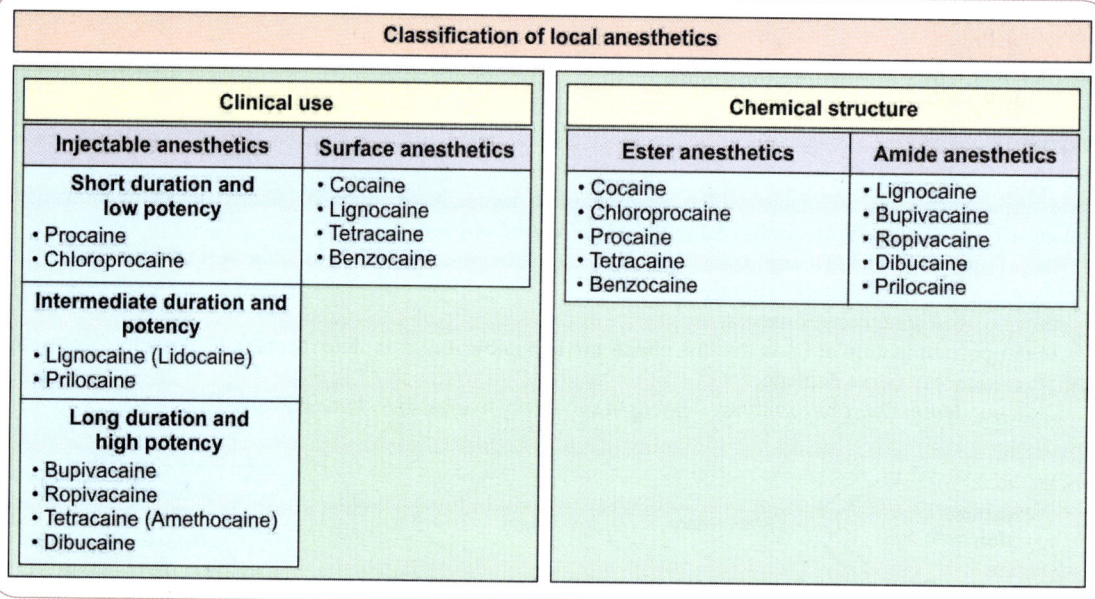

Classification of local anesthetics			
Clinical use		**Chemical structure**	
Injectable anesthetics	**Surface anesthetics**	**Ester anesthetics**	**Amide anesthetics**
Short duration and low potency • Procaine • Chloroprocaine	• Cocaine • Lignocaine • Tetracaine • Benzocaine	• Cocaine • Chloroprocaine • Procaine • Tetracaine • Benzocaine	• Lignocaine • Bupivacaine • Ropivacaine • Dibucaine • Prilocaine
Intermediate duration and potency • Lignocaine (Lidocaine) • Prilocaine			
Long duration and high potency • Bupivacaine • Ropivacaine • Tetracaine (Amethocaine) • Dibucaine			

Figure 3: Classification of local anesthetics

MECHANISM OF ACTION

The action of local anesthetics is based upon blockade of the voltage-gated Na^+ channels. Blockade of Na^+ channels prevent the generation of action potential. This interrupts the nerve conduction and results in local anesthesia (Figure 4).

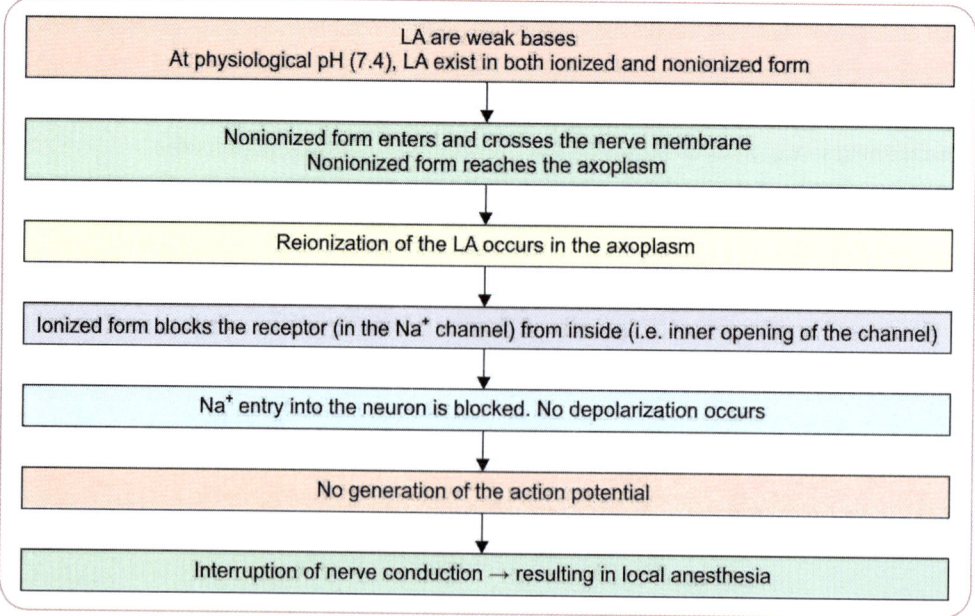

LA are weak bases
At physiological pH (7.4), LA exist in both ionized and nonionized form

↓

Nonionized form enters and crosses the nerve membrane
Nonionized form reaches the axoplasm

↓

Reionization of the LA occurs in the axoplasm

↓

Ionized form blocks the receptor (in the Na^+ channel) from inside (i.e. inner opening of the channel)

↓

Na^+ entry into the neuron is blocked. No depolarization occurs

↓

No generation of the action potential

↓

Interruption of nerve conduction → resulting in local anesthesia

Figure 4: Mechanism of action of local anesthetics

FACTORS AFFECTING THE ACTIONS OF LOCAL ANESTHETICS

The factors affecting the actions of LAs are mentioned below:

- Lipid solubility
  - High lipid soluble drugs can penetrate the nerve membrane easily as compared to less lipid soluble drugs
  - Lipid solubility correlates with the potency of the drug
  - Bupivacaine is more lipid soluble than lignocaine and is a more potent local anesthetic
- Protein binding
  - High plasma protein bound drugs have a longer duration of action
  - Bupivacaine is more plasma protein bound than lignocaine and has a longer duration of action
- pKa (Dissociation constant)
  - pKa (of a LA) determines the proportion of LA that exists in the ionized state
  - Nonionized form of LA enters the nerve membrane more easily and is converted to ionized form in the axoplasm, that blocks the Na^+ channels
  - Hence, the LA which is *more* nonionized at physiological pH will penetrate the nerve membrane faster as compared to the LA which is *less* nonionized at physiological pH
  - Lignocaine (pKa-7.8) has a faster onset of action than bupivacaine (pKa-8.1) because lignocaine is more nonionized at physiological pH
- External substances such as addition of vasoconstrictors (e.g. adrenaline), bicarbonate, glucose to local anesthetics
  - Vasoconstrictors (e.g. adrenaline)

  The rationale, advantages and disadvantages of adding vasoconstrictors (e.g. adrenaline) to LA is mentioned in Figure 5.

Use of vasoconstrictors (e.g. adrenaline) with local anesthetics

Rationale
- Vasoconstrictors (e.g. adrenaline) reduce the vasodilator effect of LAs and decrease blood flow to the site of action.
- This reduces the rate of absorption of LA into the systemic circulation, and hence, prolongs the duration of action of the LA.

Advantages
- Prolongs the duration of action of the LA.
- Reduces the systemic toxicity of LA by decreasing its absorption in the systemic circulation.
- Reduces bleeding at the site of surgery.

Disadvantages and contraindications
- Can lead to vasospasm and gangrene of the tissues. Hence, vasoconstrictors are contraindicated for use in fingers, toes, penis, tip of nose, ear lobule etc.
- Systemic toxicity can result from the absorption of adrenaline. This may result in cardiac complications such as hypertension, angina, myocardial infarction, arrhythmias, etc. Hence, vasoconstrictors should be avoided in patients with cardiac disorders such as hypertension, ischemic heart disease, arrhythmias, etc.
- Reduction of blood flow to the affected site may delay wound healing.

Figure 5: Addition of vasoconstrictors with local anesthetics

---

- Bicarbonate
  - Addition of bicarbonate to the LA solution increases the pH. This results in more nonionized form of LA and hence an increase in the onset of anesthesia.
- Glucose
  - Addition of glucose to the LA increases the baricity of the solution and makes it hyperbaric (as compared to CSF). This is used in spinal anesthesia to more effectively control the intrathecal spread of the LA solution.
- **Presence of infection**: Presence of infection can reduce the effectiveness of local anesthetics. The reasons for reduced effectiveness are mentioned in Figure 6.

Reduced effectiveness of LA at the infection site
Reasons   • Reduced pH at the site of inflammation causes an increase in the proportion of ionized form of LA. The ionized form is less able to penetrate the nerve cell resulting in decreased effect.   • Increased blood flow to the inflamed area enhances the absorption of the LA into the systemic circulation. Less LA is available at the site of action.   • Inflammatory mediators can also oppose the action of the LA.

Figure 6: Effectiveness of LA at infection site

SYSTEMIC ACTIONS

Local anesthetics can have systemic effects as they are absorbed into systemic circulation from the site of action. Some of the key systemic effects are as follows:

Cardiovascular System

Heart

○ LAs have depressant action on the heart that can manifest at higher doses or on inadvertent IV injection.
  ❑ LAs block cardiac Na^+ channels and reduce contractility, conductivity and automaticity. They also increase the effective refractory period (ERP). They can lead to cardiac arrhythmias.
  ❑ Bupivacaine is relatively more cardiotoxic than other LAs.
  ❑ The cardiotoxic effects of bupivacaine are difficult to treat as it is strongly bound to cardiac Na^+ channels. Hence the displacement of bupivacaine from myocardium is difficult.
○ Lignocaine is also used as an antiarrhythmic drug.

Blood Vessels

○ Vasodilatation induced by LA may result in hypotension.

Central Nervous System

○ LAs can initially cause CNS stimulation followed by CNS depression.
○ Toxicity of LAs can manifest as euphoria, confusion, tremors, muscle twitching, seizures, respiratory depression, loss of consciousness and death.

PHARMACOKINETICS

The metabolism of ester local anesthetics is different from that of amide local anesthetics.
○ Ester anesthetics (except cocaine)
  ❑ Rapidly metabolized by plasma (pseudo) cholinesterase to inactive metabolites
  ❑ Para-aminobenzoate is one of the key metabolites that has been associated with hypersensitivity reactions
  ❑ Cocaine is metabolized in the liver
○ Amide anesthetics
  ❑ Metabolized in the liver
  ❑ Hepatic disease can decrease the metabolism of amides
The salient differences between an ester and amide local anesthetic are shown in Table 1.

TABLE 1	Ester versus amide local anesthetics	
	Ester local anesthetics	**Amide local anesthetics**
Chemical bond	Ester	Amide

Contd...

	Ester local anesthetics	Amide local anesthetics
Metabolism	Fast metabolism by plasma (pseudo) cholinesterase	Slow metabolism by hepatic enzymes
Allergic reaction	High incidence	Low incidence
Stability	Low	High
Onset of action	Slow	Relatively fast
Examples	Procaine, chloroprocaine	Lignocaine, bupivacaine

ADVERSE EFFECTS

The adverse effects of local anesthetics are mentioned in Table 2.

TABLE 2	Adverse effects of local anesthetics
Allergic reactions	• Hypersensitivity reactions including rashes, urticaria, bronchospasm, anaphylaxis • Incidence is higher with ester LAs, possibly due to para-aminobenzoate which is a metabolite of ester LAs • Methylparaben (preservative used in LAs) can also cause allergic reactions
Central nervous system	• CNS stimulation followed by CNS depression • Tingling of lips, euphoria, confusion, tremors, muscle twitching, seizures, respiratory depression, loss of consciousness and death
Cardiovascular system	• Cardiac depression • Bradycardia, hypotension, arrhythmias including ventricular fibrillation, cardiac collapse (including fatalities) • Bupivacaine is more cardiotoxic than other LAs
Others	• Cocaine → mucosal irritation • Prilocaine → methemoglobinemia in susceptible individuals. It is due to a metabolite (o-toluidine) of prilocaine.

SALIENT FEATURES OF INDIVIDUAL LOCAL ANESTHETICS

Lignocaine (Lidocaine)

- Most commonly used amide LA. It is the prototypic amide LA
- Blocks nerve conduction within 3 minutes when injected around a nerve
- Causes vasodilatation in the injected area
- Used for surface, infiltration anesthesia, nerve blocks, neuraxial blocks, etc.
- Also has antiarrhythmic properties

Bupivacaine

- Potent and long acting amide LA
- Causes more sensory than motor block
- Based on the above features, it is a commonly used drug for prolonged analgesia during labor and postoperative period
- Used for infiltration anesthesia, nerve blocks, neuraxial blocks, etc.
- Highly cardiotoxic and may cause ventricular arrhythmias. Hence it should not be used in intravenous regional anesthesia (Bier's block).

Ropivacaine

- Less cardiotoxic and slightly less potent than bupivacaine
- Duration of action similar as bupivacaine
- Used for epidural and regional anesthesia

Tetracaine

- Long acting ester LA
- More potent and more slowly metabolized than procaine
- Used for surface and spinal anesthesia

Prilocaine

- Intermediate acting amide LA
- Pharmacological actions similar to lignocaine, except that it causes minimal vasodilatation; hence, can be used without a vasoconstrictor
- Tendency to cause methemoglobinemia (due to formation of o-toluidine); hence it should be avoided in obstetric anesthesia
- Used for intravenous regional anesthesia (Bier's block)

Dibucaine (Cinchocaine)

- Has the highest potency and longest duration of action
- Most toxic local anesthetic

Oxethazaine

- Potent local anesthetic that is used to anesthetize gastric mucosa
- Used in gastritis

EMLA Cream (Lignocaine and Prilocaine)

EMLA – (Eutectic Mixture of Local Anesthetics) → A eutectic mixture has a melting point that is lower than that of any of its individual components.

EMLA cream contains:
- Lignocaine 2.5% w/w (25 mg/g)
- Prilocaine 2.5% w/w (25 mg/g)

EMLA can penetrate intact skin and produce anesthesia up to a maximum depth of 5 mm. EMLA cream is applied on intact skin under an occlusive dressing for 1 hour prior to the procedure (e.g. venipuncture and intravenous catheter insertion).

The clinical uses of EMLA cream include the following:
- Topical anesthesia of the skin → for insertion of intravenous catheters
- Topical anesthesia of the genital mucosa
- Topical anesthesia of leg ulcers → to allow cleaning

CLINICAL USES AND TECHNIQUES OF LOCAL ANESTHESIA

Surface Anesthesia (Topical Anesthesia)

Topical application of local anesthetics on mucous membranes and abraded skin can result in surface/topical anesthesia.

The drugs used include tetracaine, lignocaine, oxethazaine and benzocaine.

The addition of adrenaline does not prolong the duration of LA action (in surface anesthesia) because of the poor absorption of adrenaline.

Some of the sites and uses of surface anesthesia are mentioned in Table 3.

TABLE 3	Surface anesthesia
Eye	• **Formulations:** Eyedrops, ointments • For minor surgery, tonometry • E.g. tetracaine
Pharynx, larynx, trachea, bronchi	• **Formulation:** Spray • For intubation, endoscopy • E.g. lignocaine
Stomach and esophagus	• **Formulation:** Suspension • For gastritis, esophagitis • E.g. oxethazaine
Urethra	• **Formulation:** Jelly • For catheterization • E.g. lignocaine
Intact skin	• **Formulation:** Cream • For insertion of IV catheters • E.g. EMLA cream (lignocaine and prilocaine)

Infiltration Anesthesia

Infiltration of a dilute solution of anesthetic is done beneath the skin at the site of surgery. It results in the block of sensory nerve endings leading to anesthesia of the affected area.

It is used for minor surgeries such as excision, hydrocele, abscess drainage, etc.

This technique is only suitable for anesthetizing a smaller area. A disadvantage is that relatively large amounts of anesthetic drugs are required to anesthetize a smaller area.

Drugs used include lignocaine and bupivacaine.

Conduction Block

Conduction block is of two types:

Field Block

- LA is injected subcutaneously so that all the nerves coming to a specific field are blocked
- Clinically used for stitching of scalp, herniorrhaphy
- Anesthesia of a larger area can be done with relatively lesser amount of drug
- Drugs used are lignocaine and bupivacaine.

Nerve Block

- LA is injected around specific nerve trunks or neural plexus. This allows anesthesia of the area supplied by that neural plexus and also causes paralysis of the skeletal muscles.
- Clinically used for upper limb surgeries (brachial plexus block), lower limb surgeries (femoral or sciatic plexus block), neck surgeries (cervical plexus block) etc.
- Anesthesia of a larger area can be done with relatively lesser amounts of drug.
- Drugs used are lignocaine and bupivacaine.

Neuraxial Anesthesia

Neuraxial anesthesia is a type of regional anesthesia in which the local anesthetic is placed around the nerves of the central nervous system.

Neuraxial anesthesia is of two types—spinal anesthesia and epidural anesthesia (Figure 7).

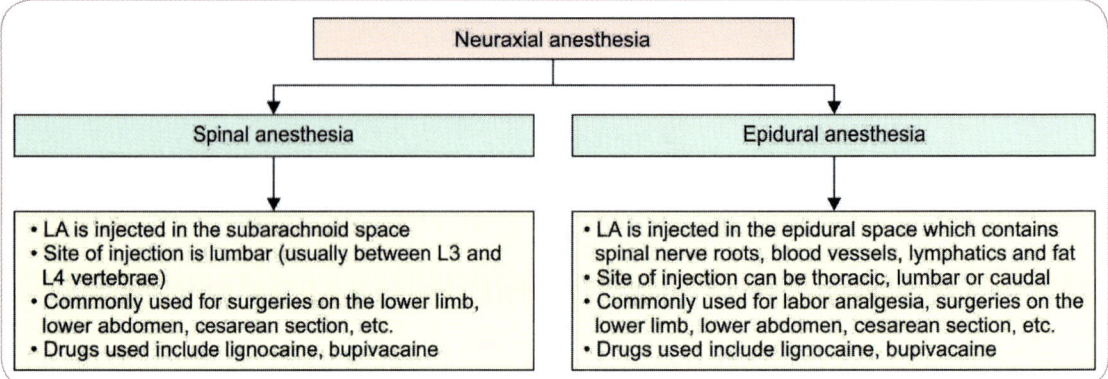

Figure 7: Neuraxial anesthesia

Spinal Anesthesia

The LA is injected in the cerebrospinal fluid (CSF) in subarachnoid space and the main site of action are the nerve roots in the cauda equina.

The injection of the spinal anesthetic is done with a very fine needle in the lumbar region, usually between the L3 and L4 vertebrae.

Spinal anesthesia leads to anesthesia of the lower abdomen and lower limbs.

It is used for surgeries such as hernia, prostatectomy, cesarean section, appendicectomy, etc.

The advantages of spinal anesthesia include preservation of consciousness, good analgesia with good muscle relaxation.

Complications of spinal anesthesia include the following:
- Headache due to leakage of CSF → can be reduced by using a smaller bore needle
- Hypotension → Due to blockade of sympathetic nerves, peripheral venous pooling, and reduced venous return to the heart. Management includes administration of oxygen, fluid infusion (preload), manipulation of patient's position, sympathomimetic drugs such as ephedrine or mephentermine.
- Respiratory paralysis
- Infection including septic meningitis
- Cauda equina syndrome.

Some of the contraindications of spinal anesthesia are mentioned below:
- Absolute contraindications → lack of consent from the patient, allergy to local anesthetic, active infection at the site of injection, insurmountable technical issues
- Relative contraindications → Uncorrected hypovolemia, bleeding diathesis, thrombophilia, raised intracranial pressure, severe cardiac stenotic disease.

Intravenous Regional Anesthesia (Bier's Block)

Intravenous regional anesthesia is produced by injection of a local anesthetic in the vein of a limb whose blood circulation is occluded by using a tourniquet.

It is used for short operative procedures on the hand, forearm or elbow.

Lignocaine or prilocaine are commonly used in this technique.

There are chances of premature failure of tourniquet resulting in toxic systemic levels of the LA. Bupivacaine being a cardiotoxic LA, therefore should not be used for this technique.

ASSESS YOURSELF (Examination Questions of Various Universities)

1. Classify local anaesthetics, Explain the mechanism of action, adverse effects and uses of lignocaine
2. Merits and demerits of using adrenaline along with local anaesthetic
3. Bupivacaine
4. Eutectic lidocaine/prilocaine
5. Spinal anaesthesia

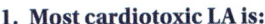

MULTIPLE CHOICE QUESTIONS

1. **Most cardiotoxic LA is:**
   (Recent Question Dec 2016)
   a. Bupivacaine
   b. Ropivacaine
   c. Prilocaine
   d. Etidocaine

2. **Intravenous regional anesthesia is used in:**
   (Recent Question Dec 2016)
   a. PPS surgeries
   b. Upper limb surgeries
   c. Lower limb surgeries
   d. Neurosurgeries

3. **Local anesthetic act by:**
   (Recent Question Dec 2016)
   a. Na^+ channel inhibition
   b. Ca^{++} channel inhibition
   c. Mg^{++} channel inhibition
   d. K^+ channel inhibition

4. **Not included in neuraxial block:**
   (Recent Question Dec 2016)
   a. Spinal block
   b. Epidural block
   c. Bier's block
   d. Caudal block

5. **Which of the following is *not* an amide?**
   (Recent Question Dec 2016)
   a. Lignocaine
   b. Procaine
   c. Mepivacaine
   d. Dibucaine

6. **Drug contraindicated for Bier's block:**
   (Recent Question Dec 2016)
   a. Lidocaine
   b. Prilocaine
   c. Dibucaine
   d. Bupivacaine

7. **Local anesthetic causing methemoglobinemia:**
   (Recent Question Dec 2016)
   a. Procaine
   b. Prilocaine
   c. Etidocaine
   d. Ropivacaine

8. **Agent added to local anesthetics to speed the onset of action is:** *(Recent Question Dec 2016)*
   a. Methylparaben
   b. Bicarbonate
   c. EDTA
   d. Adrenaline

9. **Local anesthetics:** *(Recent Question Dec 2016)*
   a. Block the release of neurotransmitters
   b. Increase the release of inhibitory neurotransmitters
   c. Inhibit the efflux of sodium from neurons
   d. Block the influx of sodium into the cell

10. **First sensation to be lost in local anesthetic use:**
    (Recent Question Dec 2016)
    a. Touch
    b. Pain
    c. Temperature
    d. Pressure

11. **EMLA contains:** *(Recent Question Dec 2016)*
    a. 2.5% lignocaine and 5% prilocaine
    b. 2.5% lignocaine and 2.5% prilocaine
    c. 5% lignocaine and 2.5% prilocaine
    d. 5% lignocaine and 5% prilocaine

Ans.											
1.	(a)	2.	(b)	3.	(a)	4.	(c)	5.	(b)	6.	(d)
7.	(b)	8.	(b)	9.	(d)	10.	(b)	11.	(b)		

NOTES

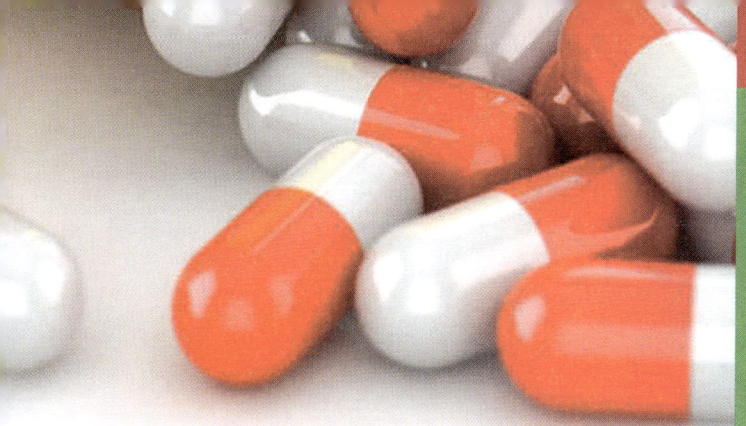

Autacoids and Associated Drugs

SECTION OUTLINE

28 Histamine and Antihistamines

HISTAMINE

Histamine is a biogenic amine that belongs to the group called autacoids which are biological factors that have a local site of action. Other autacoids include serotonin, prostaglandins, leukotrienes, kinins, angiotensin and platelet activating factor.

Histamine is synthesized locally by the decarboxylation of amino acid histidine. It is mainly present in the storage granules of mast cells and basophils.

Histamine is involved in multiple cellular responses including:
- Immune and inflammatory responses including hypersensitivity
- Gastric acid secretion
- Central nervous system (CNS) neurotransmission

Histamine exerts its actions by binding to various histamine receptors. All the 4 types of histamine receptors are G protein coupled receptors (Figure 1 and Table 1).

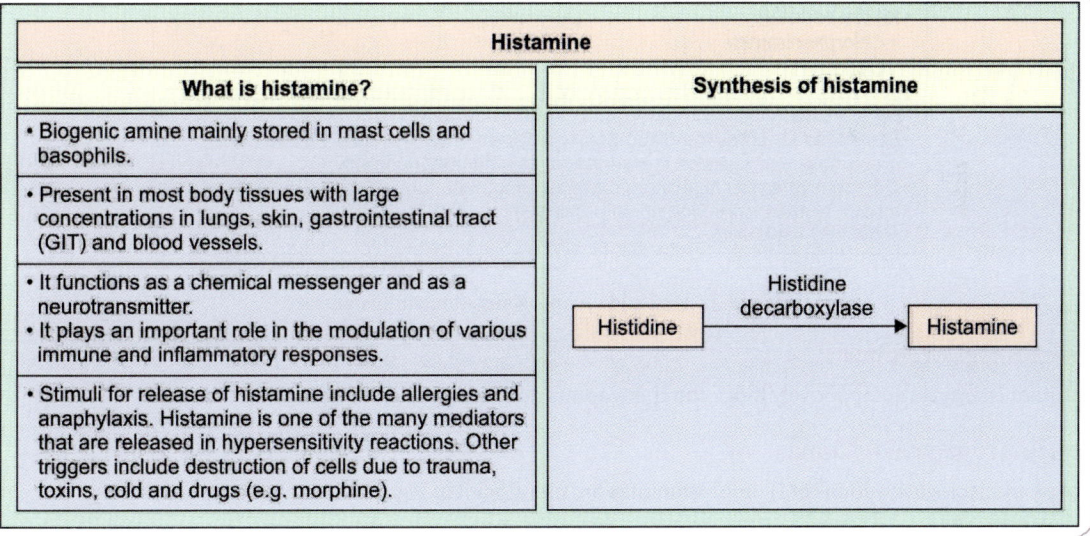

Figure 1: Histamine

TABLE 1	Histamine receptors			
Type	Location	Mechanism	Key actions	Clinically used antagonists
H_1	Smooth muscle, brain, endothelium	↑ IP_3, DAG	Smooth muscle contraction, increase capillary permeability	Chlorpheniramine, cetirizine
H_2	Gastric mucosa, heart, brain, mast cells	↑ cAMP	Increase gastric acid secretion	Cimetidine, ranitidine
H_3	Brain, myenteric plexus	↓ cAMP	Reduce histamine release	Limited clinical application
H_4	Neutrophils, eosinophils, T cells	↓ cAMP	Cytokine secretion, chemotaxis	Limited clinical application

Histamine currently has no clinical use.

BETAHISTINE

It is an H_1 selective histamine analogue used orally. It acts possibly by causing vasodilatation in the internal ear.

It is used for the control of vertigo in Meniere's disease. It should not be used in patients with bronchial asthma and peptic ulcer.

H_1 RECEPTOR ANTAGONISTS (ANTIHISTAMINES)

H_1 receptor antagonists are also commonly known as antihistamines. They can be divided into first-generation and second-generation antihistamines (Figure 2).

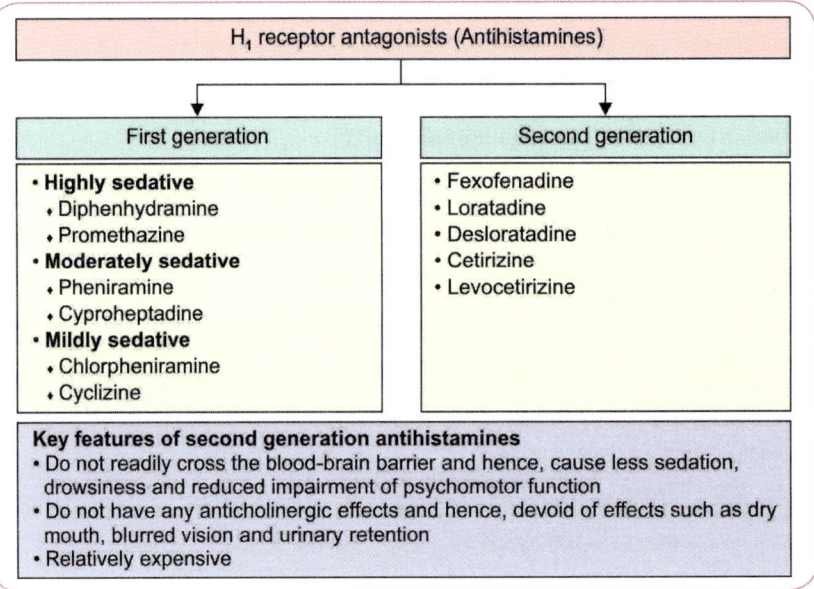

Figure 2: First and second-generation antihistamines

Mechanism of Action

The antihistamines competitively block the H_1 receptors and antagonize the effects of histamine.

Pharmacological Actions

The pharmacological actions of H_1 antihistamines are mentioned in Figure 3.

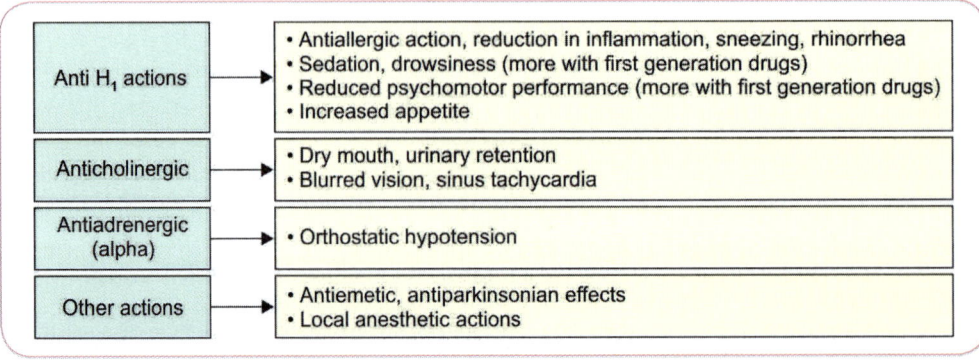

Figure 3: Pharmacological actions of H_1 antihistamines

Autacoids and Associated Drugs

SECTION F

Pharmacokinetics

The H_1 antihistamines are well absorbed following oral administration and are widely distributed in the body tissues. They are metabolized in the liver and excreted in the urine.

Adverse Effects

The first-generation antihistamines not only interact with H_1 receptors, but also interact with other receptors such as cholinergic, α-adrenergic and serotoninergic receptors. They can therefore cause several adverse effects:

- Sedation, drowsiness, lack of coordination, dizziness and impaired psychomotor performance. Hence, these drugs should be avoided while driving or operating machinery. The incidence of these adverse reactions is reduced with second-generation antihistamines as they do not readily cross the blood-brain barrier.
- Anticholinergic effects such as dry mouth, blurred vision and urinary retention. The second-generation antihistamines do not have any anticholinergic effects.
- Nausea, vomiting, gastrointestinal (GI) discomfort
- Cardiac adverse effects such as tachycardia and palpitations
- Hypersensitivity reactions (including angioedema and anaphylaxis)

Clinical Uses

- **Allergic and inflammatory conditions**
  - Including hay fever, allergic rhinitis, perennial rhinitis, urticaria, angioneurotic edema, drug and serum reactions, food allergy, insect bites etc.
  - H_1 antihistamines are not used in treating bronchial asthma. This is because other mediators such as leukotrienes (e.g. LTC_4 and LTD_4) play a much more important role (than histamine) in the pathogenesis of bronchial asthma.
- **Motion sickness and nausea**
  - Drugs such as diphenhydramine, promethazine are used
  - These drugs should be taken prior to the start of travel as they are generally not effective after the occurrence of symptoms
  - These drugs exert antiemetic effect possibly due to blockade of central H_1 and M_1 (muscarinic) receptors
  - They also reduce or prevent nausea by both vestibular and chemoreceptor pathway
- **Parkinsonism**
  - Promethazine may be useful in parkinsonism due to its sedative and anticholinergic effects to control tremor, rigidity and sialorrhea
  - Useful in drug-induced parkinsonism
- **Vertigo**
  - Cinnarizine is useful in patients of vertigo as it has anticholinergic, antiserotonergic, vasodilator and sedative properties
- **Preanesthetic medication**
  - Promethazine may be used due to its sedative and anticholinergic properties.

SECOND GENERATION H_1 RECEPTOR ANTAGONISTS (ANTIHISTAMINES)

The key features of second-generation H_1 receptor antagonists (antihistamines) are as follows:
- Highly selective for H_1 receptors
- Do not readily cross the blood-brain barrier and hence, cause less sedation, drowsiness and reduction in psychomotor impairment
- Do not have any anticholinergic effects and hence, are devoid of effects such as dry mouth, blurred vision and urinary retention
- Relatively expensive

Fexofenadine

It is an active metabolite of terfenadine and is a nonsedating H_1 antihistamine. It does not cause anticholinergic adverse effects.

Loratadine

It is a long-acting H_1 antihistamine. It does not have clinically significant sedative or anticholinergic properties in majority of the population. Convulsions have been reported as an adverse effect.

Cetirizine

Apart from having a H_1 antihistaminic effect, cetirizine also demonstrates other antiallergic activities such as inhibition of the late phase recruitment of eosinophils and prevent the release of histamine and other cytotoxic mediators from platelets.

Levocetirizine

It is an enantiomer of cetirizine and is more potent than cetirizine with comparatively lesser adverse effects.

Azelastine

It has good topical activity and is available for nasal application and as eye drops. It is indicated for symptomatic management of seasonal and perennial allergic conjunctivitis.

Rupatadine

It is a H_1 antihistamine with additional antiplatelet activating factor (anti-PAF) activity.

The main clinical uses of second-generation H_1 receptor antagonists are as follows:
○   Allergic conjunctivitis and rhinitis
○   Chronic idiopathic urticaria

▌DRUGS USED IN VERTIGO

Vertigo is a feeling that either one's self or one's surrounding are spinning or rotating. The key drugs used for treating vertigo include the following (Table 2).

TABLE 2	Drugs used for vertigo treatment
H_1 receptor antagonists (antihistamines)	• Cyclizine • Cinnarizine • Diphenhydramine, dimenhydrinate • Promethazine
Anticholinergics	• Hyoscine
Phenothiazine	• Prochlorperazine
H_1 analogue	• Betahistine
Diuretics	• Thiazide • Furosemide • Acetazolamide
Benzodiazepines	• Diazepam
Tricyclic antidepressants	• Amitriptyline

1. Enumerate second-generation antihistamines. Discuss their advantages over first-generation antihistamines.

2. Write short notes on:
   a. Cetirizine
   b. Uses of H_1 antihistamines
   c. H_1 receptor antagonists
   d. Second-generation antihistamines

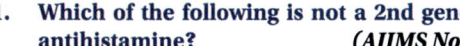

MULTIPLE CHOICE QUESTIONS

1. Which of the following is not a 2nd generation antihistamine? *(AIIMS Nov 2012)*
   a. Cetirizine
   b. Cyclizine
   c. Loratadine
   d. Fexofenadine

2. Which of the following is not a second generation antihistaminic? *(AIIMS May 2008, Nov 2006)*
   a. Cyclizine
   b. Fexofenadine
   c. Loratadine
   d. Acrivastine

3. Which antihistaminic can be used in day times? *(Recent Question Dec 2016)*
   a. Diphenhydramine
   b. Dimenhydrinate
   c. Chlorpheniramine maleate
   d. Promethazine

4. Fexofenadine is metabolic product of: *(Recent Question 2016)*
   a. Loratadine
   b. Astemizole
   c. Cetirizine
   d. Terfenadine

5. Least sedative antihistaminic is: *(JIPMER 2006)*
   a. Cetirizine
   b. Hydroxyzine
   c. Chlorpheniramine
   d. Carbinoxamine

6. Antihistaminic used in motion sickness is: *(WBPG 2008)*
   a. Cetirizine
   b. Meclizine
   c. Diphenhydramine
   d. Fexofenadine

Ans.

| 1. (b) | 2. (a) | 3. (c) | 4. (d) | 5. (a) | 6. (c) |

29

Serotonin Agonists and Antagonists and Drugs Used for Migraine

Serotonin (5-hydroxytryptamine, 5-HT) is an important neurotransmitter, and has diverse physiological roles in the body. It is widely distributed in plants, animals, stings and venoms. In humans, 90% of serotonin is found in intestine (enterochromaffin cells); most of the remainder is found in platelets and brain.

Serotonin is synthesized from the essential amino acid tryptophan, by the action of enzymes tryptophan hydroxylase followed by aromatic L-amino acid decarboxylase. Degradation occurs by monoamine oxidase (MAO) followed by oxidation, to form 5-hydroxyindole acetic acid (5-HIAA) which is excreted in the urine (Figure 1).

In the pineal gland, serotonin is converted to melatonin.

The urinary excretion of 5-HIAA during 24 hours can be used as a diagnostic test for tumors that synthesize excess amounts of serotonin, e.g. carcinoid tumors.

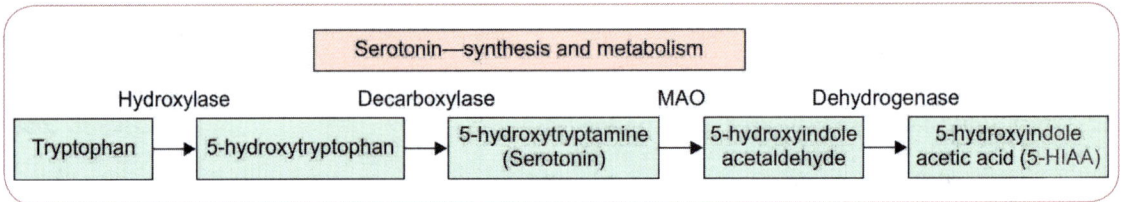

Figure 1: Biosynthesis and metabolism of serotonin

Serotonin is involved in numerous pathological conditions such as migraine, depression, anxiety, gastrointestinal disorders etc.

SEROTONIN RECEPTORS

There are 7 types of serotonin receptors (5-HT$_1$ to 5-HT$_7$). All of these are G-protein coupled receptors, except 5-HT$_3$ which is a ligand gated ion channel.

The various serotonin receptors along with their features are mentioned in Table 1.

TABLE 1	Serotonin receptors		
Receptor	Location	Mechanism	Key actions
5-HT$_1$	• Brain • Cranial blood vessels	GPCR ($\downarrow$ cAMP)	• Autoreceptors • Constriction of cranial blood vessels • Decreased norepinephrine release from sympathetic nerve endings
5-HT$_2$	5-HT$_{2A}$ • Platelets • Smooth muscles • Cerebral cortex 5-HT$_{2B}$ • Stomach fundus 5-HT$_{2C}$ • Choroid plexus	GPCR ($\uparrow$ IP$_3$, DAG)	• Platelet aggregation • Smooth muscle contraction • Excitation of neurons • Stomach contraction • CSF production

Contd...

Receptor	Location	Mechanism	Key actions
5-HT$_3$	• Area postrema and nucleus tract solitarius (NTS) in brainstem • Parasympathetic nerves in GIT	Ion channel	• Vomiting • Increased peristalsis
5-HT$_4$	• Hippocampus • GIT	GPCR ($\uparrow$ cAMP)	• CNS excitation • Increased peristalsis
5-HT$_{5-7}$	• CNS	GPCR ($\downarrow$ cAMP: 5-HT$_5$) ($\uparrow$ cAMP: 5-HT$_{6/7}$)	• Not clearly known

The drugs acting at various types of serotonin receptors and their specific indications are mentioned in Figure 2.

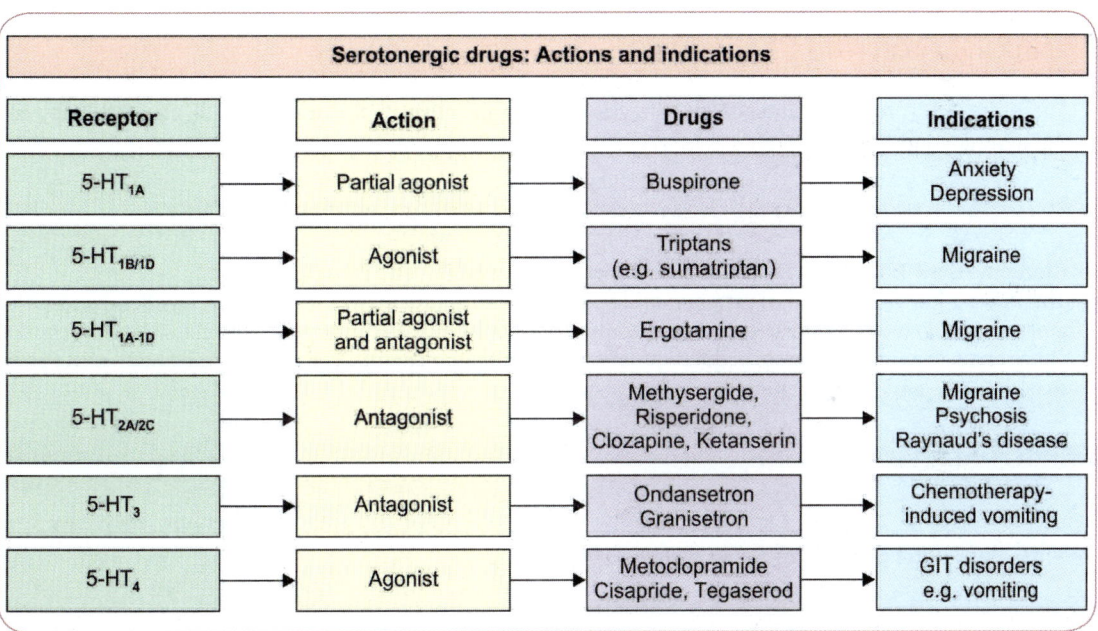

Figure 2: Serotonergic drugs: Actions and indications

SEROTONIN ANTAGONISTS

The salient features of clinically used serotonin receptor antagonists are mentioned below:

CYPROHEPTADINE

o It is a 5-HT$_{2A}$ and H$_1$ receptor blocker. It also has weak anticholinergic and mild CNS depressant activity.
o It is used in allergic conditions due to H$_1$ receptor antagonism; 5-HT$_{2A}$ receptors have no role in allergic responses.
o It is useful in migraine prophylaxis and in controlling GIT symptoms in carcinoid syndrome and postgastrectomy dumping syndrome.
o The adverse effects include drowsiness, dry mouth and weight gain.

METHYSERGIDE

- It is a 5-HT$_{2A/2C}$ antagonist.
- It belongs to the ergot group; has effect on vascular smooth muscle but does not have other ergot effects.
- It was previously used for migraine prophylaxis.

  Prolonged use causes **inflammatory fibrosis** (e.g. retroperitoneal fibrosis, pulmonary and endocardial fibrosis) which is a serious complication. Because of this risk, other drugs are now preferred for migraine prophylaxis.

KETANSERIN

- It is a 5-HT$_{2A/2C}$ antagonist. It potently blocks 5-HT$_{2A}$ receptors but weakly blocks 5-HT$_{2C}$ receptors. It also has weak α_1 and H$_1$ blocking action.
- It is an effective antihypertensive drug, but this effect is due to α_1 blocking action and not due to 5-HT$_{2A}$ receptor blocking action.

ONDANSETRON AND GRANISETRON

- These are 5-HT$_3$ receptor antagonists. They are highly effective in the treatment of chemotherapy and radiotherapy-induced vomiting.

ATYPICAL ANTIPSYCHOTICS (CLOZAPINE, RISPERIDONE, QUETIAPINE)

- Clozapine is a 5-HT$_{2A/2C}$ and D$_2$ antagonist. Risperidone is a 5-HT$_{2A}$ and D$_2$ antagonist.
- They have a lower incidence of extrapyramidal adverse effects (due to weaker D$_2$ blocking effect) and have a greater effect in reducing the negative symptoms of schizophrenia, as compared to the classic antipsychotics.
- Other atypical antipsychotics (e.g. quetiapine) act on multiple receptors, but their antipsychotic effect is due to both 5-HT$_{2A}$ and D$_2$ antagonism.

ERGOT ALKALOIDS

Ergot is produced by a fungus *Claviceps purpurea* that grows on rye and some other grains. They have been classified into natural and semisynthetic alkaloids (Figure 3).

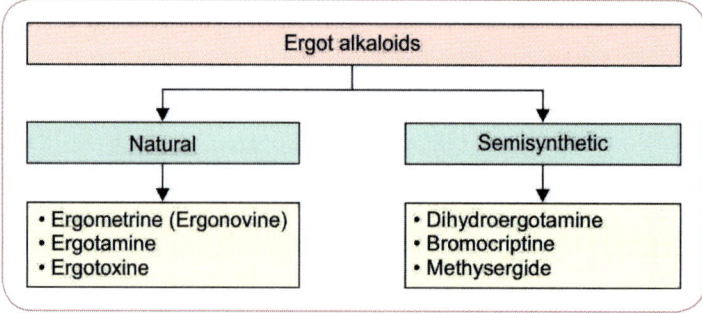

Figure 3: Ergot alkaloids

The pharmacological effects of ergot alkaloids are diverse and varied; they usually result from actions (as agonists or antagonists) on serotonergic, dopaminergic and α-adrenergic receptors.

The pharmacological properties of various ergot alkaloids are mentioned in Figure 4.

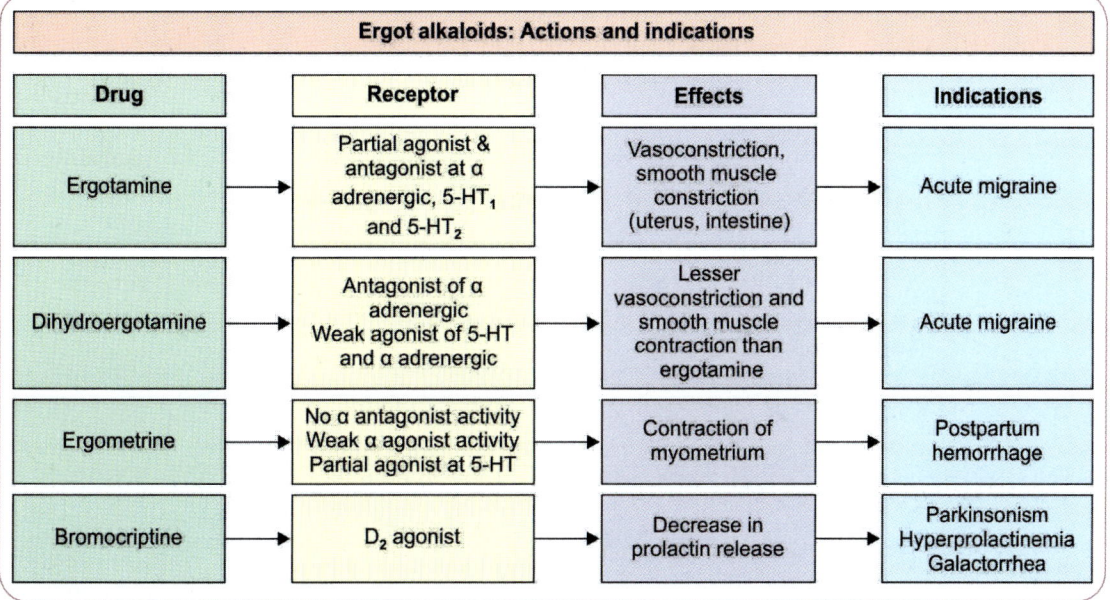

Figure 4: Ergot alkaloids: Actions and indications

DRUG THERAPY OF MIGRAINE

Migraine is a common, potentially debilitating and recurring disorder characterized by pulsatile, throbbing headache usually lasting for 4–72 hours. The pain is usually unilateral and is often associated with symptoms such as nausea, vomiting, sensitivity to light and sound etc.

It is the 2nd most common cause of headache (most common being tension headache). Migraine affects around 15% of population. It is 3 times more common in females.

There are 2 types of migraine headaches: classic migraine and common migraine (Figure 5).

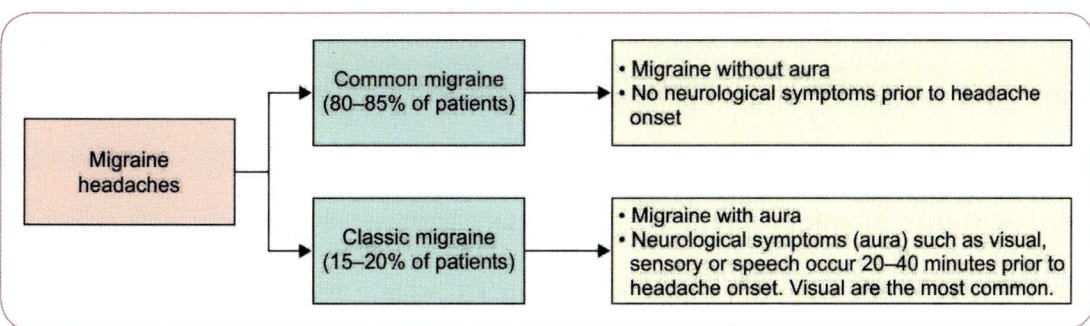

Figure 5: Migraine headaches

The main cause of pain in migraine is dilatation of large intracranial blood vessels.

There is a strong evidence to suggest that serotonin plays a critical role in the pathogenesis of migraine. Hence, most of drugs used in the treatment of migraine are either agonists or antagonists of 5-HT receptors.

The drugs used for the treatment of migraine are classified into those used in acute migraine and those used for migraine prophylaxis. The drugs used in acute migraine are further subdivided into those used in mild, moderate or severe migraine (Figure 6).

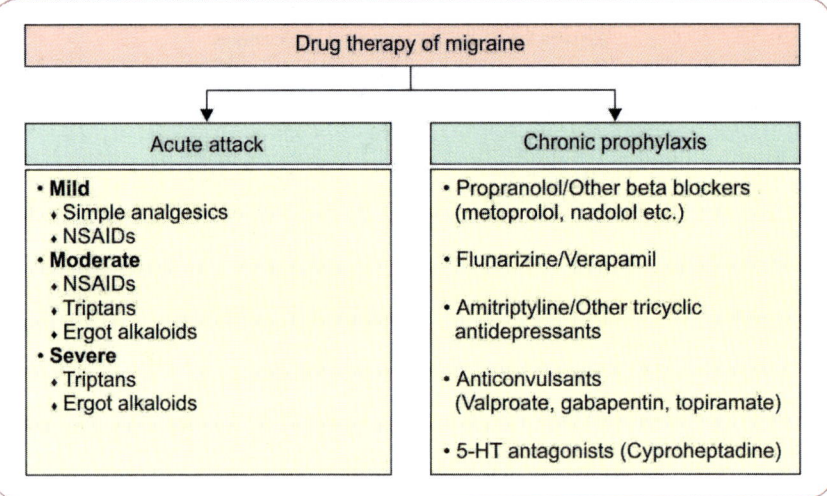

Figure 6: Drug therapy in migraine

ACUTE ATTACK OF MIGRAINE

NONSTEROIDAL ANTI-INFLAMMATORY DRUGS (NSAIDs)

The NSAIDs (such as ibuprofen, naproxen, indomethacin, mefenamic acid etc.) are either used alone or in combination with paracetamol, diazepam, antihistaminic, caffeine etc. They are used only during an acute attack of migraine for the relief of symptoms. They should not be taken for prolonged periods.

ANTIEMETICS

Antiemetics (such as metoclopramide, domperidone, prochlorperazine etc.) are used to treat nausea and vomiting associated with migraine headache.

Gastric stasis occurs during migraine which decreases drug absorption. Metoclopramide and domperidone promote gastric emptying and hence, increase the absorption of other drugs simultaneously being used to treat migraine.

ERGOT ALKALOIDS

Ergotamine is the effective ergot alkaloid used in acute attack of migraine.

It produces dramatic relief when given early during the attack. However, if given later, higher doses are required and the time to obtain relief is also prolonged.

It is administered by oral or sublingual route, or as a suppository. It is not safe to be used parenterally.

Dihydroergotamine is also as effective as ergotamine in acute attack of migraine. However, it can be given parenterally (IV, SC, or IM).

Ergotamine is marketed in combination with caffeine. Ergot alkaloids have a very low bioavailability due to slow and incomplete absorption. Caffeine increases the absorption of ergot alkaloids and also potentiate their cranial vasoconstricting effect.

Mechanism of Action

They are partial agonist in 5-$HT_{1B/1D}$ receptors in the cranial blood vessels. This leads to constriction of the dilated cranial blood vessels and decrease in neurogenic inflammation.

Adverse Effects and Contraindications

The adverse effects include nausea, vomiting, leg weakness, muscle cramps, paresthesia, coronary vasospasm and other vascular spasm.

Ergots are contraindicated in peripheral vascular disease, coronary artery disease, liver and kidney disease, hypertension, pregnancy and sepsis.

TRIPTANS

Triptans (such as sumatriptan, rizatriptan, zolmitriptan, naratriptan, frovatriptan etc.) are selective agonist of 5-$HT_{1B/1D}$ receptors. Sumatriptan was the first to be introduced and is the prototype of this class.

Triptans are now the preferred drugs for the treatment of acute attacks of migraine in patients who do not respond to initial analgesic therapy.

Triptans are preferred over ergots because of their ability to decrease nausea and vomiting (*Note:* Ergots increase nausea and vomiting). Ergots are nowadays used only in few patients.

Mechanism of Action

The triptans are selective agonist of 5-$HT_{1B/1D}$ receptors with little or no activity on any other type of receptors. They cause constriction of the dilated cranial blood vessels and specifically of the arterio-venous shunts of carotid artery.

Other actions include a decrease in the release of serotonin and other inflammatory neuropeptides (around affected blood vessels) as well as a decrease in neurogenic inflammation.

Pharmacokinetics

Sumatriptan has a bioavailability of ~15% after oral administration and ~97% after subcutaneous administration. It is metabolized mainly by MAO-A and the metabolites are excreted in urine. The elimination half-life is 1-2 hours.

The oral bioavailability of other triptans is higher than sumatriptan. Naratriptan and frovatriptan have longer half-lives than sumatriptan.

The key pharmacokinetic features of various triptans are mentioned in Table 2.

TABLE 2	Key pharmacokinetic features of triptans				
	Sumatriptan	Rizatriptan	Zolmitriptan	Naratriptan	Frovatriptan
Oral bioavailability	15%	45%	40%	70%	25%
Plasma $t_{1/2}$ (hours)	1–2	2–3	2–3	6	26

Adverse Effects and Contraindications

The common adverse effects include paresthesia, fatigue, tightness of chest, neck and jaw, dizziness, nausea and sweating.

The rare serious adverse effects include coronary artery vasospasm, bradycardia, ventricular arrhythmias and myocardial infarction. These occur mostly in patients having risk factors for coronary artery disease.

Triptans are contraindicated in patients with history of ischemic or coronary artery disease, cerebrovascular or peripheral vascular disease, hypertension, severe liver or kidney disease and pregnancy.

Triptans are contraindicated in patients who have taken MAO inhibitors within the last 2 weeks. Triptans should not be given within 24 hours of ergot administration.

Clinical Uses

Triptans are effective in acute attacks of migraine (both common and classical migraine). The treatment should be started as soon as possible after a migraine attack.

Triptans rapidly abort or markedly reduce the severity of migraine headache in around 70% of patients.

PROPHYLAXIS OF MIGRAINE

Prophylactic treatment is considered when 2–3 or more migraine attacks occur per month. It is required if during the attacks, the patient has significant functional impairment. The drugs commonly used in prophylactic treatment of migraine are mentioned in Table 3.

TABLE 3	Migraine prophylaxis
Beta blockers	• Propranolol is the most commonly used drug • Other drugs used are metoprolol, atenolol and nadolol
Calcium channel blockers	• Flunarizine and verapamil are used • Flunarizine is a cerebroselective calcium channel blocker • They decrease the frequency of attacks
Antidepressants	• Tricyclic antidepressants such as amitriptyline are used • It reduces migraine attacks but produce many adverse effects
Anticonvulsants	• Valproate, gabapentin and topiramate are used • These are used when the other drugs such as propranolol are not effective or are contraindicated
5-HT antagonists	• Cyproheptadine and methysergide are not commonly used

ASSESS YOURSELF (Examination Questions of Various Universities)

1. Mention drugs used in the prophylaxis of migraine.
2. Write short notes on:
   a. 5-HT antagonists
   b. Sumatriptan
   c. Ergotamine in acute migraine
3. Discuss the pharmacotherapy of migraine.

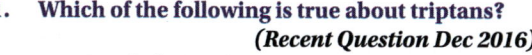

MULTIPLE CHOICE QUESTIONS

1. Which of the following is true about triptans?
   (Recent Question Dec 2016)
   a. Prophylaxis migraine
   b. Indicated in heart disease
   c. Variable pharmacokinetics
   d. Variable pharmacodynamics
2. Methysergide used as drug of choice in migraine but not now because *(Recent Question Dec 2016)*
   a. Peptic ulcer
   b. Arrhythmias
   c. Pulmonary fibrosis
   d. MI
3. Sumatriptan acts as an agonist at this receptor:
   (Recent Question Dec 2016)
   a. $5HT_{-1}$
   b. $5HT_{-2A/2C}$
   c. $5HT_{1B/1D}$
   d. $5HT_{2A/2C}$
4. Drug used in treatment of migraine
   (Recent Question 2016)
   a. $5HT_1$ agonist
   b. $5HT_1$ antagonist
   c. D_1 agonist
   d. D_1 antagonist
5. Drug of choice for acute migraine is
   (Recent Question 2016)
   a. Sumatriptan
   b. Ergot alkaloids
   c. Ondansetron
   d. Ketanserin

6. Drugs used in prophylaxis of migraine are all except: *(Recent Question 2016)*
   a. Propranolol
   b. Flunarizine
   c. Topiramate
   d. Levetiracetam
7. Which of the following serotonergic receptors is an autoreceptor? *(Recent Question 2016)*
   a. $5\text{-}HT_{1A}$
   b. $5\text{-}HT_4$
   c. $5\text{-}HT_{2A}$
   d. $5\text{-}HT_3$
8. One of the following is not a 5-HT receptor antagonist: *(Recent Question 2016)*
   a. Ketanserin
   b. Lanreotide
   c. Methysergide
   d. Tropisetron
9. $5HT_{2A}$ antagonist is: *(Recent Question 2016)*
   a. Cisapride
   b. Clozapine
   c. Ketanserin
   d. Sumatriptan
10. Sumatriptan is contraindicated in:
    (JIPMER 2009)
    a. Asthma
    b. DM
    c. Sepsis
    d. Peripheral vascular disease
11. Longest acting triptan: *(JIPMER 2006)*
    a. Rizatriptan
    b. Zolmitriptan
    c. Naratriptan
    d. Frovatriptan

Ans.

1. (c)	2. (c)	3. (c)	4. (a)	5. (a)	6. (d)
7. (a)	8. (b)	9. (c)	10. (d)	11. (d)	

30

Eicosanoids—Prostaglandins and Leukotrienes

Prostaglandins and leukotrienes are collectively called eicosanoids because they are all derived from eicosa (20 carbon atoms) tri/tetra/penta enoic acids.

Arachidonic acid (eicosatetraenoic acid) is the fatty acid that is released in the largest amount from membrane phospholipids.

Eicosanoids are widely distributed in the body. The metabolites of arachidonic acid (prostaglandins and leukotrienes) can be synthesized in virtually all cells of the body.

Prostaglandins and leukotrienes are synthesized locally and there are no preformed stores of these substances.

The key steps in the synthesis of prostaglandins and leukotrienes along with some of their salient actions are shown in Figure 1.

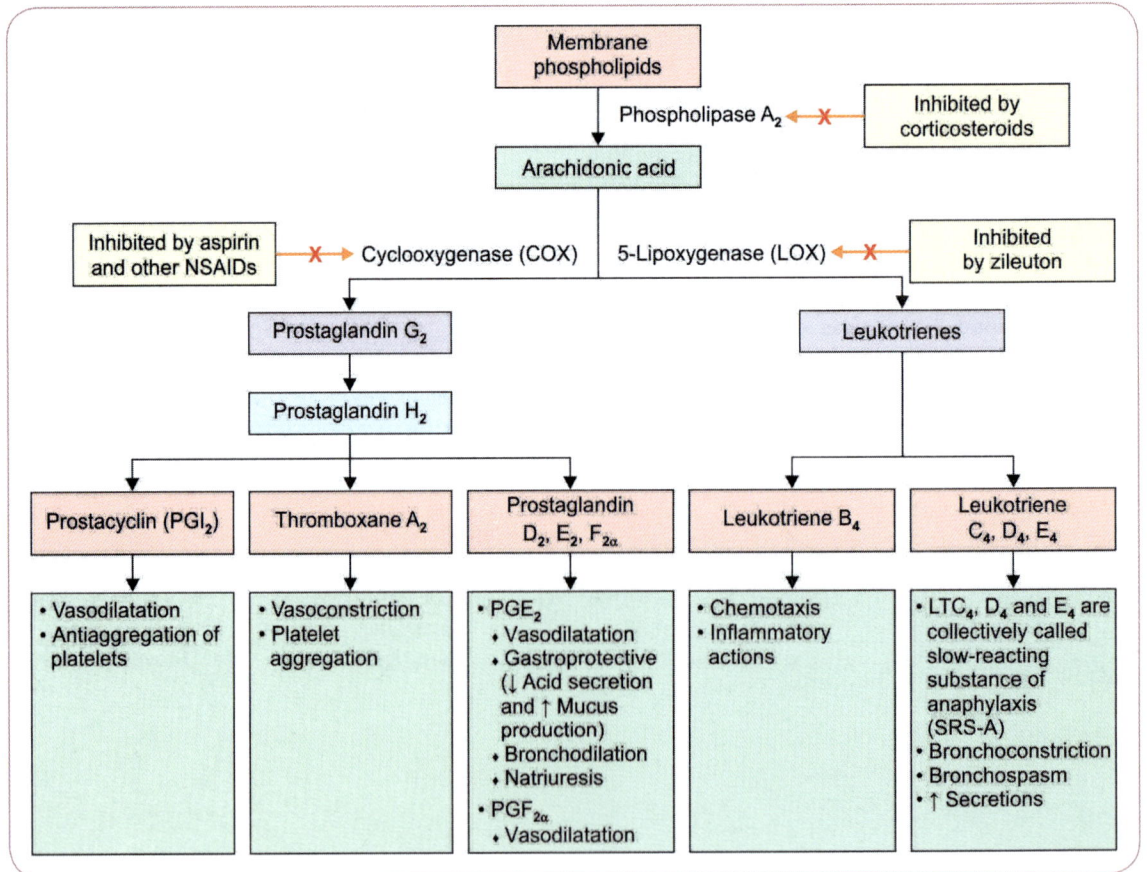

Figure 1: Prostaglandins and leukotrienes

The cyclooxygenase enzyme play a vital role in the biosynthesis of prostaglandins. The key differences between the two isoforms of cyclooxygenase enzyme are shown in Table 1.

TABLE 1	Cyclooxygenase-1 (COX-1) and cyclooxygenase-2 (COX-2)	
	Cyclooxygenase-1 (COX-1)	Cyclooxygenase-2 (COX-2)
Type of enzyme	• **Constitutional enzyme** → produced in the body under all physiological conditions	• **Inducible enzyme** → produced in the body under specific conditions such as inflammation • Also present as a constitutive enzyme in brain and juxtaglomerular cells
Key location(s)	• Gastrointestinal tract (stomach, intestine), renal tissue, platelets	• Predominantly at the site of inflammation
Key function(s)/ Action(s)	• Physiological (housekeeping) • Gastroprotective actions • Regulation of vascular function/ hemostasis • Preservation of renal function	• Involved in inflammatory response • Pain • Pyrexia
Inhibited by	• Aspirin • Nonselective NSAIDs such as ibuprofen, diclofenac etc.	• COX-2 selective drugs such as celecoxib, etoricoxib etc. • Aspirin and other NSAIDs also inhibit COX-2

PROSTAGLANDINS

Prostaglandins are synthesized locally from arachidonic acid.

Pharmacological Actions

The key pharmacological actions of prostaglandins on various body tissues are mentioned in Table 2.

TABLE 2	Prostaglandins: Pharmacological actions
Cardiovascular system	• PGE_2 and PGI_2 cause vasodilatation • TXA_2 cause vasoconstriction • $PGF_{2\alpha}$ generally cause vasodilatation; however, vasoconstriction occurs in pulmonary artery and vein *Significance* • PGE_2 and PGI_2 are continuously produced in ductus arteriosus during fetal life—keeps it patent. • Aspirin and indomethacin inhibit PGs and are used to induce closure of ductus arteriosus at birth, when it fails to close spontaneously. • PGE_1 (alprostadil) is used to maintain the patency of ductus arteriosus in neonates (with congenital heart disease) till surgery is performed. • PGI_2 (epoprostenol and treprostinil) is one of the preferred drug for pulmonary arterial hypertension. ▪ It provides benefit by vasodilatation of pulmonary and systemic arteries and inhibition of platelet aggregation.

Contd...

Gastrointestinal system	• PGE_2 and PGI_2 decrease acid secretion in stomach • PGE_2 and PGI_2 increase mucus secretion in stomach • PGE_2 and PGI_2 have cytoprotective effect—antiulcerogenic *Significance* • Aspirin and other NSAIDs decrease PG synthesis resulting in a loss of cytoprotective effect – leads to gastric erosion/ulcers. • PGE_1 analogue (misoprostol) is used for healing NSAID-induced peptic ulcers.
Uterus	• PGE_2 and $PGF_{2\alpha}$ contract pregnant uterus • PGE_2 and $PGF_{2\alpha}$ induce labor at term • PGE_2 and $PGF_{2\alpha}$ produce cervical ripening, making it favorable for induction of labor *Significance* • PGE_1 analogue (misoprostol) is used to induce early abortion (in the 1st few weeks). It is given in combination with mifepristone (antiprogestin). • PGE_2 (dinoprostone) is used to induce midterm abortion (in the 2nd trimester). It is also used for missed abortion and for benign hydatidiform mole. • $PGF_{2\alpha}$ analogue (carboprost) is used to induce 2nd trimester abortion and to control postpartum hemorrhage.
Platelet	• TXA_2 (produced by platelets) induce platelet aggregation • PGI_2 (produced by endothelium) inhibit platelet aggregation *Significance* • Aspirin inhibits COX enzyme—inhibits generation of TXA_2 in platelets and PGI_2 in endothelium. ▪ Platelets cannot regenerate COX while endothelium can. Thus, aspirin selectively inhibits the generation of TXA_2. The effect of PGI_2 predominates. This is the basis of antithrombotic effect of aspirin. • PGI_2 (epoprostenol) is used during hemodialysis to prevent platelet aggregation.
Eye	• $PGF_{2\alpha}$ decrease intraocular tension by increasing aqueous humor outflow via the uveoscleral tract *Significance* • $PGF_{2\alpha}$ analogues (latanoprost, bimatoprost, travoprost, unoprostone) are used in open-angle glaucoma.
Kidney	• PGE_2 and PGI_2 have diuretic effect: Salt and water excretion • PGE_2 and PGI_2 cause renal vasodilatation • PGE_2 antagonize ADH action: Diuretic effect *Significance* • NSAIDs inhibit PG synthesis and tend to retain salt and water. Hence, the diuretic effect of furosemide is decreased when NSAIDs (e.g. indomethacin) are given along with it.
Male reproductive system	• PGs have a smooth muscle relaxant effect *Significance* • PGE_1 (alprostadil) is a 2nd line treatment of erectile dysfunction. The treatment of choice is PDE5 inhibitors such as sildenafil, tadalafil etc.

Adverse Effects

The key adverse effects of prostaglandins include nausea, vomiting, fever, diarrhea, hypotension, flushing, tachycardia and uterine cramps.

Clinical Uses

The use of prostaglandins and its analogues is limited because of short duration of action, adverse effects and cost. However, despite these limitations, several prostaglandins and its analogues are of utility in certain clinical situations. The prostaglandins and their clinical uses are mentioned in Figure 2.

Prostaglandin (PG) and its analogues: Clinical uses		
PGE$_1$/PGE$_2$ and its analogues	**PGF$_{2\alpha}$ and its analogues**	**PGI$_2$ and its analogues**
Alprostadil (PGE$_1$) • Maintenance of patency of ductus arteriosus (in congenital heart disease) • Erectile dysfunction	**Carboprost (PGF$_{2\alpha}$ analogue)** • Midterm abortion • Postpartum hemorrhage	**Epoprostenol & treprostinil (PGI$_2$)** • Pulmonary arterial hypertension
Misoprostol (PGE$_1$ analogue) • Peptic ulcer—NSAID induced • Abortion—in early pregnancy	**Latanoprost, travoprost (PGF$_{2\alpha}$ analogue)** • Open-angle glaucoma	
Dinoprostone (PGE$_2$) • Midterm abortion • Cervical softening		

Figure 2: Clinical uses of prostaglandins

Prostaglandins in Obstetrics

The prostaglandins and its analogues find its highest utility in obstetric conditions. Some of the clinical situations where these drugs are used are mentioned below:

Abortion

○ Misoprostol and gemeprost (PGE$_1$ analogue)— is used for termination of early pregnancy (given in combination with mifepristone [antiprogestin] or methotrexate).
○ Dinoprostone (PGE$_2$)—is used for midterm abortion, for missed abortion and for benign hydatidiform mole.
○ Carboprost (PGF$_{2\alpha}$ analogue)—is used for 2nd trimester abortion and to control postpartum hemorrhage.

Postpartum Hemorrhage

○ Carboprost or misoprostol can be used to control bleeding in postpartum hemorrhage.

LEUKOTRIENES

The leukotrienes are formed from arachidonic acid by the enzyme lipoxygenase.

The important leukotrienes are leukotrienes B$_4$, C$_4$, D$_4$ and E$_4$.

Leukotrienes C$_4$, D$_4$ and E$_4$ are known as 'cysteinyl leukotrienes' or the 'slow reacting substance of anaphylaxis (SRS-A)'. These are produced in bronchial asthma and anaphylaxis.

The leukotrienes (C$_4$ and D$_4$) are potent bronchoconstrictors and play a significant role in pathogenesis of bronchial asthma.

The leukotriene antagonists e.g. montelukast, zafirlukast and zileuton are discussed along with the treatment for bronchial asthma.

ASSESS YOURSELF (Examination Questions of Various Universities)

1. Mention the preparations and uses of prostaglandins.
2. Discuss briefly the obstetrical uses of prostaglandins.
3. Discuss the therapeutic uses of prostaglandin analogues.

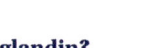

MULTIPLE CHOICE QUESTIONS

1. **Misoprostol is a:** *(Recent Question 2016)*
   a. Prostaglandin E_1 analog
   b. Prostaglandin E_2 analog
   c. Prostaglandin antagonist
   d. Antiprogestin

2. **Which of the following drugs inhibit an enzyme in the prostaglandin synthesis?**
   (Recent Question 2016)
   a. Aminocaproic acid   b. Aspirin
   c. Aprotinin   d. Alteplase

3. **Which prostaglandin helps in cervical ripening?**
   (Recent Question 2016)
   a. PGI_2 b. PGF_2
   c. PGF_2 d. PGD_2

4. **Inhibitor of platelet aggregation includes:**
   (Recent Question 2016)
   a. TXA_2 b. PGI_2
   c. PGG_2 d. All of the above

5. **Which is not a side effect of prostaglandin?**
   (Recent Question 2016)
   a. Vomiting   b. Fever
   c. Convulsion   d. Diarrhea

6. **Alprostadil is used in all except:**
   (Recent Question 2016)
   a. Congenital heart disease
   b. Maintain PDA
   c. Erectile dysfunction
   d. Closure of PDA

7. **Drug causing patency of ductus:**
   (Recent Question 2016)
   a. Alprostadil   b. Apraclonidine
   c. Aripiprazole   d. Aspirin

Ans.

1. (a)	2. (b)	3. (c)	4. (b)	5. (c)	6. (d)
7. (a)					

31

Nonsteroidal Anti-inflammatory Drugs

The nonsteroidal anti-inflammatory drugs (NSAIDs) are a group of drugs that have analgesic, antipyretic and anti-inflammatory actions.

CLASSIFICATION OF NSAIDs

Classification of nonsteroidal anti-inflammatory drugs (NSAIDs) has been depicted below in Figure 1.

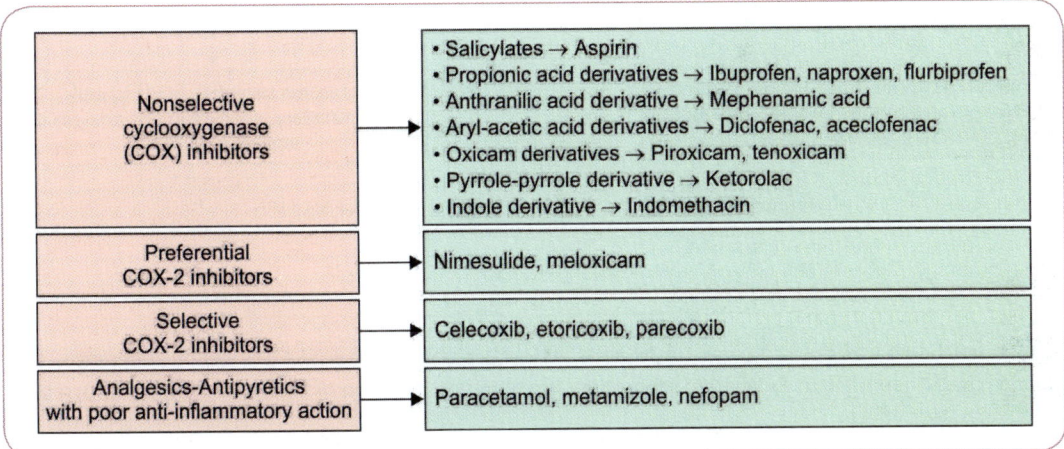

Figure 1: Classification of NSAIDs

ASPIRIN AND OTHER NSAIDs

MECHANISM OF ACTION

The NSAIDs inhibits the enzyme cyclooxygenase (COX) that has a vital role in the biosynthesis of prostaglandins. Inhibition of cyclooxygenase leads to reduced synthesis of prostaglandins.

Cyclooxygenase has at least two isoforms: COX-1 and COX-2.

Aspirin and other nonselective NSAIDs inhibit both COX-1 and COX-2. However, aspirin irreversibly inhibit the COX enzymes, whereas other NSAIDs reversibly inhibit the COX enzymes.

Preferential COX-2 inhibitors have a higher COX-2/COX-1 selectivity ratio whereas selective COX-2 inhibitors mainly inhibit COX-2 isoform (Figure 2).

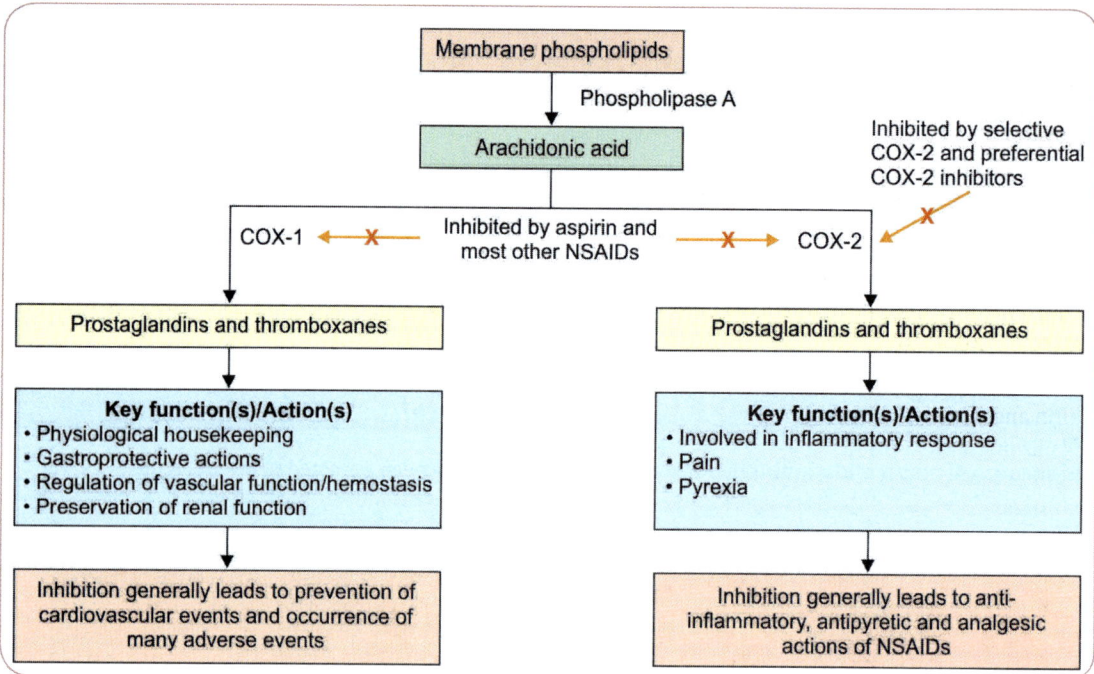

Figure 2: Mechanism of action of aspirin and other NSAIDs

PHARMACOLOGICAL ACTIONS

Aspirin is considered as the prototype for NSAIDs. The other nonselective NSAIDs exhibit differences in the pharmacokinetic and pharmacodynamic properties—e.g. potency, duration of action, analgesic, antipyretic and anti-inflammatory effects.

Analgesic Effect

The NSAIDs produce analgesia by inhibiting the synthesis of prostaglandins. They block the sensitization to pain (induced by various mediators of inflammation). NSAIDs are effective in inflammation induced pain, tissue injury related pain and musculoskeletal pain. They are comparatively ineffective in visceral, ischemic pain. They are ineffective in neuropathic pain.

Compared to opioids (morphine), they are less effective analgesics and they do not depress the CNS or produce physical dependence.

The NSAIDs are also called non-narcotic or non-opioid analgesics.

Antipyretic Effect

The antipyretic effect results mainly due to inhibition of prostaglandin synthesis.

The NSAIDs also reset the hypothalamic thermostat and promote heat loss by causing vasodilatation and sweating.

Anti-inflammatory Effect

The anti-inflammatory effect is mainly due to inhibition of prostaglandin synthesis at the site of inflammation. Suppression of signs of inflammation such as pain, swelling, tenderness, erythema and infiltration of leukocytes is observed.

The anti-inflammatory effect of aspirin is observed at high doses (3–6 g/day in divided doses).

Antiplatelet Effect (Inhibition of Platelet Aggregation)

Low dose aspirin irreversibly inactivates (acetylates) the COX-1 enzyme and therefore, reduces the production of thromboxane A_2 (TXA_2). Low dose aspirin has a clinically useful antiplatelet action (inhibition of platelet aggregation) due to the following factors:

- Irreversible inactivation of the COX enzyme
- Lack of nucleus in the platelets → platelets cannot synthesize new COX enzymes
- Antiplatelet action of aspirin lasts for the lifetime of the platelets (~7–10 days)

Aspirin at higher doses reduces the synthesis of both TXA_2 and prostaglandin I_2 (PGI_2) leading to reduced antiplatelet effect.

The dose of aspirin ranges from 75 mg to 325 mg daily.

Gastrointestinal

Aspirin and other NSAIDs can cause gastric pain, mucosal ulceration and GI blood loss. The mechanism includes the following (Figure 3):

- Inhibition of COX-1 enzyme leading to inhibition of prostaglandin-mediated gastric protection
- Ion trapping of acidic NSAIDs in the ionized form inside the mucosal cell

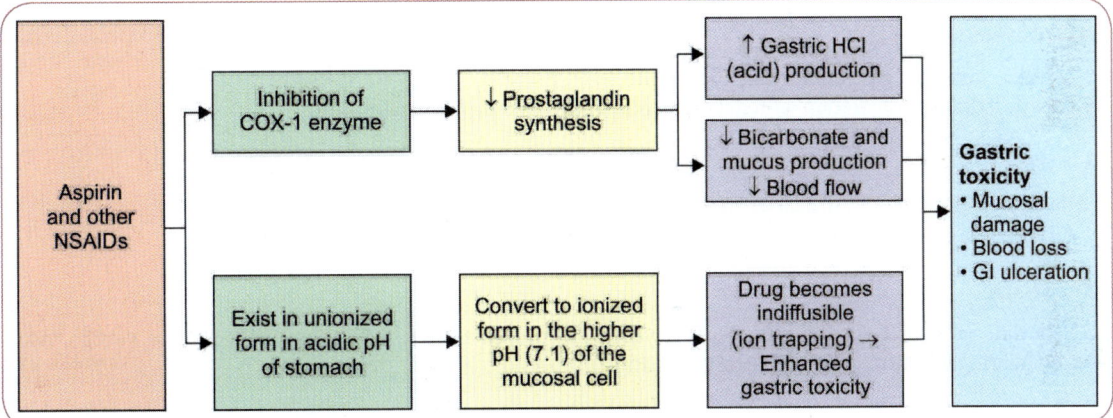

Figure 3: Gastric toxicity of aspirin and other NSAIDs

They also cause nausea and vomiting by stimulation of the CTZ.

Renal

The NSAIDs have the following effects on the renal system:

- Reduction in renal blood flow and decrease in GFR. It can lead to worsening of renal insufficiency.
- Salt and water retention
- Chronic intake can lead to renal papillary necrosis (known as analgesic nephropathy)

The effects of NSAIDs on the renal system are not significant in normal persons, but can be of significance in patients with hypovolemia, cirrhosis, underlying renal insufficiency, heart failure or those on antihypertensive or diuretic therapy.

Acid Base and Electrolyte Balance

The NSAIDs can cause initial respiratory stimulation leading to respiratory alkalosis. Toxic doses may lead to depression of the respiratory center resulting in respiratory acidosis. Subsequently, uncompensated metabolic acidosis may result.

Urate Excretion

Aspirin can cause a dose related effect on the uric acid.

- Low doses → decreases uric acid excretion; causes a rise in uric acid level
- High doses → increases uric acid excretion; causes a fall in uric acid level (uricosuric effect)

Cardiovascular System

The NSAIDs may precipitate heart failure in patients with decreased cardiac reserve.

PHARMACOKINETICS

Aspirin is rapidly absorbed from the GIT (stomach and small intestine).

It undergoes glycine and glucuronide conjugation in the liver and is excreted in the urine.

The kinetics of aspirin change from first order (low dose) to zero order (high dose) as the metabolic processes get saturated.

ADVERSE EFFECTS

Gastrointestinal (GIT)

- Nausea, vomiting, gastrointestinal discomfort
- Gastric irritation, ulceration with occult bleeding, GIT hemorrhage, perforation

Hypersensitivity

- Rashes, drug eruptions, urticaria, angioedema, bronchospasm
- Allergic reactions, including anaphylactic/anaphylactoid reactions

Salicylism

- Salicylates at higher doses can lead to salicylism. The presentation includes tinnitus, dizziness, vertigo, visual and hearing impairment and mental confusion.

Reye's Syndrome

- Administration of salicylates in children having viral infection (e.g. influenza, chickenpox) has been associated with liver damage and encephalopathy. It can be fatal, and survivors may also develop permanent brain damage. Treatment usually requires hospitalization and intensive care management. Salicylates are contraindicated in children with viral infections.

Renal

- Salt and water retention
- Interstitial nephritis, papillary necrosis, nephropathy
- Chronic renal failure

Hematological

- Bleeding, thrombocytopenia, leucopenia, anemia (including hemolytic and aplastic anemia), agranulocytosis

Liver

- Elevated liver enzymes, hepatitis
- Liver failure (rare)

CNS

- Headache, vertigo, mental confusion, memory impairment
- Convulsion, anxiety

CVS

○ Cardiac failure, myocardial infarction, stroke, thrombosis
  ❑ Low dose aspirin however, has an antiplatelet effect (inhibition of platelet aggregation) and is used in acute coronary syndrome including acute myocardial infarction, unstable angina, coronary artery disease, transient ischemic attack, prosthetic cardiac valves, coronary angioplasty, stents and peripheral vascular disease.

Acute Salicylate Poisoning

The clinical features of acute salicylate poisoning include:
○ Vomiting, dehydration, tinnitus, hearing impairment, sweating, warm extremities, hyperventilation
○ Acid base abnormalities such as metabolic acidosis
○ Coagulation abnormalities, bleeding, hypoglycemia, thrombocytopenia, hypokalemia
○ Pulmonary edema, convulsions, coma

Acute salicylate poisoning is more common in children as compared to adults.

The treatment of acute salicylate poisoning is as follows:
○ There is no specific antidote for salicylate toxicity. Treatment requires hospitalization and includes supportive and symptomatic management such as:
  ❑ Gastric lavage and activated charcoal
  ❑ External cooling
  ❑ Urine alkalinization → hastens renal excretion of salicylates because salicylates are ionized in alkaline pH
  ❑ Hemodialysis
  ❑ Fluid and electrolyte management including administration of sodium bicarbonate
  ❑ Correction of blood sugar levels
  ❑ Correction of coagulation abnormalities with vitamin K, blood transfusions

PRECAUTIONS AND CONTRAINDICATIONS (TABLE 1)

The key contraindications of NSAIDs include the following:
○ Hypersensitivity to the active substance or any of the excipients
○ Gastric, peptic or intestinal ulcer, GI bleeding or perforation
○ Coagulation abnormalities including bleeding
○ Children with viral infections
○ Patients with hepatic or renal failure
○ Patients with heart failure or those with reduced cardiac reserve
○ Patients with ischemic heart disease, peripheral arterial disease or cerebrovascular disease (→ *low dose aspirin is used in some of these patients due to its antiplatelet effect i.e. inhibition of platelet aggregation*)
○ Pregnancy
  ❑ Inhibition of prostaglandin synthesis can adversely affect the pregnancy and/or development of the fetus
  ❑ There is an increased risk of miscarriage and/or congenital anomalies including cardiac malformations
  ❑ When used during the third trimester of pregnancy, there is an increased risk of the following:
    • Cardiopulmonary toxicity (premature closure of ductus arteriosus and pulmonary hypertension)
    • Kidney dysfunction that can progress to renal failure
    • Coagulation abnormalities including prolongation of bleeding time → may lead to postpartum bleeding
    • Delayed or prolonged labor due to inhibition of prostaglandin synthesis
○ Aspirin prolong bleeding time due to irreversible inactivation of COX-1 enzyme in the platelets, and therefore, reduce the production of TXA_2. Reduced levels of TXA_2 leads to an inhibition of platelet aggregation. Aspirin at higher doses reduce the synthesis of both TXA_2 and prostaglandin I_2 (PGI_2) leading to reduced antiplatelet efficacy. Aspirin should be stopped one week prior to elective surgery.
○ High doses of aspirin can lead to hemolytic anemia in patients with glucose 6-phosphate dehydrogenase (G6-PD) deficiency.

TABLE 1	Contraindications of NSAIDs	
• Hypersensitivity		• Hepatic or renal failure
• Gastric, peptic or intestinal ulcer, GI bleeding or perforation		• Heart failure or those with reduced cardiac reserve
• Coagulation abnormalities		• Ischemic heart disease, peripheral arterial disease or cerebrovascular disease
• Children with viral infections		• Pregnancy

CLINICAL USES OF NSAIDs

Analgesic

Aspirin is used for pain relief in headache, toothache, backache, dysmenorrhea, myalgia, neuralgia, joint pain etc. The effective analgesic dose is 300–600 mg every 6–8 hourly.

Antipyretic

At the analgesic doses, aspirin is effective in reducing fever of any origin. However, paracetamol is preferred for antipyretic action because of the following:
- Less adverse effects, safer for use
- Does not cause Reye's syndrome in children

Acute Rheumatic Fever

Aspirin is the preferred drug for the treatment of acute rheumatic fever. It is to be given in high doses (4-8 g/day in divided doses). This brings about marked symptomatic relief in 1–3 days.

Fever, joint pain and swelling are reduced, but the underlying disease progression is not altered.

Osteoarthritis

Paracetamol is used in mild cases of osteoarthritis. In severe cases when paracetamol is not effective, other NSAIDs are preferred because aspirin causes adverse effects when given for prolonged periods. They give symptomatic relief, but the underlying disease continues to progress.

Rheumatoid Arthritis

The NSAIDs have anti-inflammatory action and provide symptomatic relief in pain, swelling and stiffness of the joints. Aspirin is not preferred as it causes adverse effects when given for prolonged periods. The underlying disease continues to progress.

Cardiovascular Uses

Aspirin in low doses (75–162 mg daily) inhibits TXA_2 generation and platelet aggregation, and therefore, decreases subsequent risk of cardiovascular complications.

Low dose aspirin is used for:
- Acute coronary syndrome including:
  - Acute myocardial infarction—ST elevation myocardial infarction (STEMI) and non-ST elevation myocardial infarction (NSTEMI)
  - Unstable angina
- Coronary artery disease
- Transient ischemic attack

- Prosthetic cardiac valves, coronary angioplasty, stents
- Peripheral vascular disease

Other Uses

- Closure of patent ductus arteriosus (indomethacin is the drug of choice)
- Familial colonic polyposis—aspirin and other NSAIDs suppress polyp formation
- Prevention of colon cancer
- Prevention of flushing associated with nicotinic acid (niacin) ingestion
- Preeclampsia—low dose of aspirin is useful
- Alzheimer' disease—aspirin reduces the risk and retards progression

---

Note:

Aspirin is rarely used nowadays because of the following disadvantages:
- High incidence of adverse effects, especially gastrointestinal toxicity
- Risk of Reye's syndrome in children
- Short duration of action

Paracetamol and other NSAIDs are preferred for most of the clinical situations.

DRUG INTERACTIONS

The key drug interactions of NSAIDs are mentioned in Figure 4.

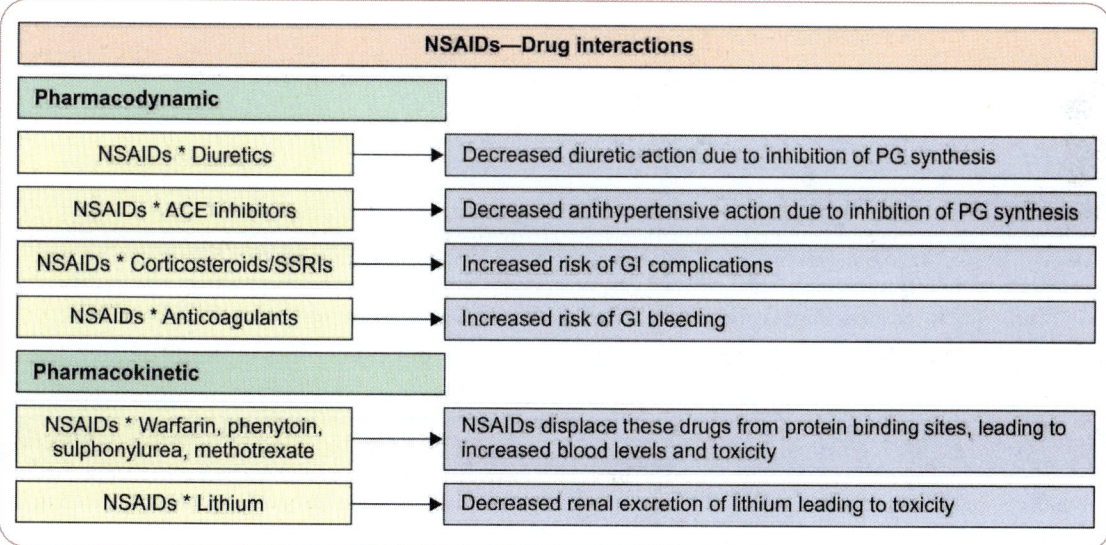

Figure 4: Drug interactions of NSAIDs

OTHER NSAIDs

Other NSAIDs have similar mechanism of action, pharmacological actions, adverse effects and therapeutic effects, as compared to aspirin. The individual drugs differ primarily in analgesic and anti-inflammatory effects, and pharmacokinetic parameters such as potency, half-lives and duration of action.

The salient features of key NSAIDs are mentioned in Table 2.

TABLE 2	Salient features of NSAIDs
Ibuprofen	• Better tolerated than aspirin • One of the safest and most commonly used NSAID • Lesser anti-inflammatory efficacy (at therapeutic doses) • Half-life of 2 hours (*Note:* Naproxen is more potent and longer acting than ibuprofen, with a half-life of 14 hours)
Diclofenac	• One of the most commonly used NSAID • It is highly potent • Gets concentrated in synovial fluid in the joints; hence, preferred in inflammatory arthritis • Hepatotoxicity occurs more commonly • It is also available in combination with misoprostol. This combination reduces the incidence of gastric ulcers.

Indomethacin	• It is ~20 times more potent than aspirin
	• High toxicity:
	  ▪ Gastrointestinal (GI) adverse effects—vomiting, diarrhea, bleeding
	  ▪ CNS adverse effects—frontal headache, dizziness, confusion
	• It is commonly used in neonates for medial closure of patent ductus arteriosus
	• It is a reserve drug for malignancy associated fevers and severe refractory inflammatory conditions (e.g. ankylosing spondylitis, acute gout)
	• It is contraindicated in psychiatric and epilepsy patients, machinery operators and pregnancy

Piroxicam	• It is long acting (half-life 2 days) • It is highly potent • Increased frequency of GI adverse effects
Ketorolac	• Potent analgesic effect; analgesic efficacy equal to morphine • Moderate anti-inflammatory effect • Used in postoperative pain, renal colic and metastatic pain • Adverse effects include GI effects and CNS effects • Not to be given continuously for >5 days
Mefenamic acid	• Analgesic, antipyretic and weak anti-inflammatory effect • Used in dysmenorrhea as well as muscle and joint pain where anti-inflammatory effect is not required • Adverse effects commonly include diarrhea and epigastric distress; rarely causes hemolytic anemia

SELECTIVE COX-2 INHIBITORS (COXIBs)

These drugs selectively inhibit the COX-2 isoenzyme (induced at the site of inflammation) without affecting the function of COX-1 isoenzyme (present in GIT and platelets).

Some of the COX-2 inhibitors clinically used are celecoxib, parecoxib and etoricoxib. Parecoxib is the only COX-2 inhibitor given parenterally. It is a prodrug of valdecoxib.

Although there are lesser GI adverse effects with selective COX-2 inhibitors; there is a higher incidence of cardiovascular thrombotic episodes.

○ This occurs because COX-2 inhibitors decrease endothelial PGI_2 production but have no effect on platelet TXA_2 production.

○ Selective COX-2 inhibitors should be avoided in patients susceptible to cardiovascular or cerebrovascular disease e.g. hypertension, diabetes, history of ischemic heart disease etc.

Note: Rofecoxib and valdecoxib have been withdrawn due to significantly increased risk of cardiovascular complications.

The key differences between nonselective COX inhibitors and selective COX-2 inhibitors are mentioned in Figure 5.

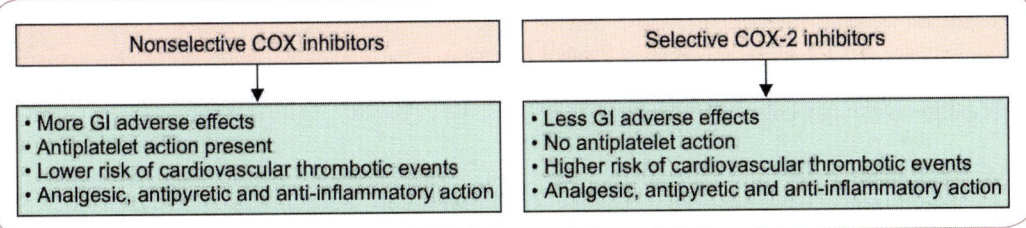

Nonselective COX inhibitors	Selective COX-2 inhibitors
• More GI adverse effects • Antiplatelet action present • Lower risk of cardiovascular thrombotic events • Analgesic, antipyretic and anti-inflammatory action	• Less GI adverse effects • No antiplatelet action • Higher risk of cardiovascular thrombotic events • Analgesic, antipyretic and anti-inflammatory action

Figure 5: Differences between nonselective COX and selective COX-2 inhibitors

CELECOXIB

It is about 10–20 times more selective for COX-2 than COX-1. It causes less GI irritation than most other NSAIDs. It does not affect platelet aggregation.

It is metabolized mainly by CYP2C9. The plasma half-life is around 10 hours. It is a sulfonamide, hence may occasionally cause rashes; other adverse effects may include dyspepsia, edema and mild hypertension.

It is primarily used in osteoarthritis, rheumatoid arthritis and dysmenorrhea.

PARACETAMOL (ACETAMINOPHEN)

Paracetamol is one of the most commonly used analgesic and antipyretic drug. It however has weak anti-inflammatory effect.

PHARMACOLOGICAL ACTIONS

The analgesic effect of paracetamol is like aspirin i.e. it raises pain threshold. The antipyretic effect is also similar to that of aspirin. However, in contrast to aspirin, it has much weaker anti-inflammatory effect.

Unlike aspirin, paracetamol does not stimulate respiration, does not affect acid-base balance and does not affect platelet aggregation. It usually does not cause gastric mucosal injury. It does not have uricosuric action. The key differences between aspirin and paracetamol are mentioned in Figure 6.

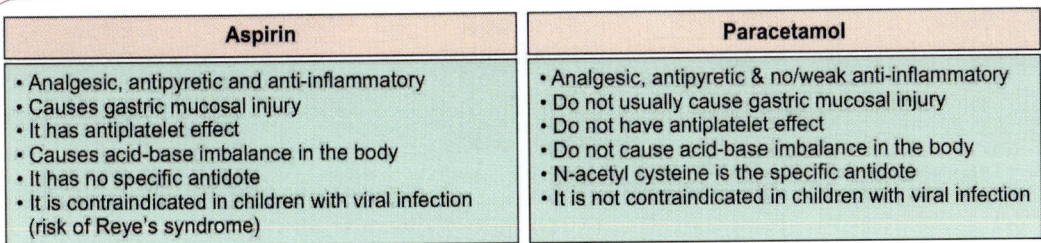

Aspirin	Paracetamol
• Analgesic, antipyretic and anti-inflammatory • Causes gastric mucosal injury • It has antiplatelet effect • Causes acid-base imbalance in the body • It has no specific antidote • It is contraindicated in children with viral infection (risk of Reye's syndrome)	• Analgesic, antipyretic & no/weak anti-inflammatory • Do not usually cause gastric mucosal injury • Do not have antiplatelet effect • Do not cause acid-base imbalance in the body • N-acetyl cysteine is the specific antidote • It is not contraindicated in children with viral infection

Figure 6: Differences between aspirin and paracetamol

PHARMACOKINETICS

Paracetamol is well-absorbed orally and has high bioavailability. Peak plasma concentration occurs in 30–60 minutes and the plasma half-life is around 2 hours. The effect of an oral dose lasts for 3–6 hours. The metabolism occurs in the liver mainly by glucuronide conjugation (~60%) and sulfate conjugation (~35%).

A small portion (5–10%) undergoes CYP dependent hydroxylation to form a toxic metabolite N-acetyl P-benzoquinone (NAPQI). NAPQI then reacts in the following ways:

- At normal doses of paracetamol, NAPQI reacts with the sulfhydryl groups of glutathione (present in liver) and nontoxic metabolites are formed.
- At toxic doses of paracetamol, NAPQI is formed in excess. The liver's glutathione stores gets depleted. The excess NAPQI then reacts with the sulfhydryl groups of liver and kidney cells causing hepatic and renal damage.

The metabolites are finally excreted in the urine.

ADVERSE EFFECTS

At recommended therapeutic doses, paracetamol is very well tolerated.

- The occasional adverse effects may include nausea, rashes and other allergic reactions.
- Hepatic toxicity occurs in both acute overdose and on long-term use.
- Renal toxicity occurs usually on long-term use.

ACUTE PARACETAMOL POISONING

It usually occurs in adults when >10 gm of paracetamol is ingested in a single dose.

The initial symptoms (in the first 24 hours) reflect gastric distress and include nausea, vomiting, abdominal pain and anorexia.

The clinical indications of liver damage become apparent 2–4 days after ingestion and the symptoms include tender hepatomegaly, right subcostal pain and jaundice. In severe poisoning, hepatic failure may progress to encephalopathy, hypoglycemia, cerebral edema and death.

Acute renal failure (due to renal tubular necrosis) manifests as loin pain, hematuria and proteinuria.

Mechanism of Toxicity and Treatment

Paracetamol is mainly metabolized in the liver by glucuronide and sulfate conjugation to nontoxic metabolites. However, a minor toxic metabolite NAPQI is also formed (by CYP mediated hydroxylation).

The toxic metabolite NAPQI is normally detoxified by conjugation with glutathione, followed by its elimination.

When toxic doses of paracetamol are taken, glucuronide conjugation gets saturated and increasing amount of paracetamol undergo CYP mediated hydroxylation, to generate more NAPQI.

Increased NAPQI depletes glutathione stores in the liver. The highly reactive NAPQI then binds to liver and kidney cells leading to cell damage (Figure 7).

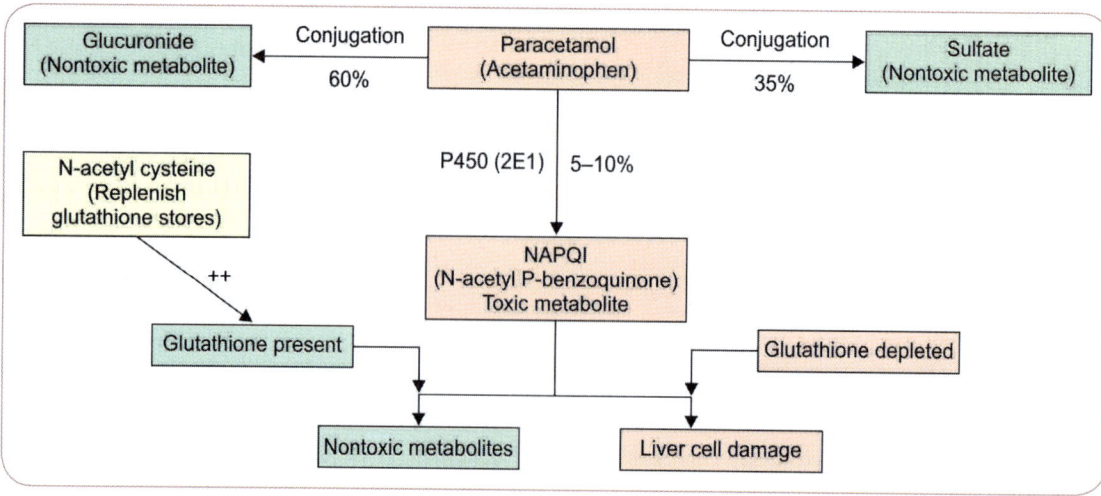

Figure 7: Paracetamol toxicity

Management of Paracetamol Toxicity

○ Paracetamol toxicity requires immediate management in a hospital setting. Patients with significant liver damage may require management in a specialized hepatic unit.

○ Initial symptoms may include nausea and vomiting, and may not reflect the severity of toxicity or the risk of organ damage.

○ N-acetylcysteine is the antidote for paracetamol toxicity which should be promptly administered. Treatment with N-acetylcysteine may be used up to 24 hours after ingestion of paracetamol; however, the maximum benefit is obtained up to 8 hours following ingestion.

○ N-acetylcysteine replenishes the stores of glutathione in the liver and inhibits the binding of NAPQI to hepatic cells.

○ Activated charcoal may be considered if the patient presents within 1 hour of overdose.

○ Supportive and symptomatic management should be done.

SECTION F ■ Autacoids and Associated Drugs

ASSESS YOURSELF (Examination Questions of Various Universities)

1. Classify nonsteroidal anti-inflammatory drugs. Discuss the mechanism of action, therapeutically useful actions and adverse effects of aspirin.
2. List important differences between aspirin and paracetamol.
3. Why aspirin use is contraindicated during pregnancy.

4. Explain the rationale of using:
   a. Low dose aspirin in myocardial infarction
   b. N-acetyl cysteine in paracetamol poisoning
5. Write short notes on:
   a. Ibuprofen
   b. Selective COX-2 inhibitors
   c. Therapeutic uses and adverse effects of aspirin

MULTIPLE CHOICE QUESTIONS

1. False about NSAIDs: *(AIIMS Nov 2014)*
   a. Used in neuropathic pain
   b. Decreases efficacy of antihypertensives
   c. Cause renal failure
   d. Can be used topically

2. Anti-inflammatory dose of aspirin:
   (Recent Question 2016)
   a. 500 g/day   b. 1–2 g/day
   c. 3–6 g/day   d. 6–12 g/day

3. NSAID given as a single daily dose is:
   (Recent Question 2016)
   a. Naproxen   b. Ketorolac
   c. Piroxicam   d. Paracetamol

4. Mechanism of action of aspirin is:
   (Recent Question 2016)
   a. Inhibits COX-2 preferentially
   b. Inhibits COX-1 preferentially
   c. Inhibits COX 1 and COX2 reversibly
   d. Inhibits COX 1 and COX2 irreversibly

5. Which of the following drug is associated with highest cardiac mortality?
   (Recent Question 2016)
   a. Rofecoxib   b. Nicorandil
   c. Losartan   d. Metoprolol

6. Aspirin inhibits: *(Recent Question 2016)*
   a. Lipoprotein lipase   b. Lipoxygenase
   c. Cyclooxygenase   d. Phospholipase

7. Which of the following drugs inhibit platelet cyclooxygenase reversibly?
   (Recent Question 2016)
   a. Alprostadil   b. Aspirin
   c. Ibuprofen   d. Prednisolone

8. All are reversible inhibitors of COX except:
   (Recent Question 2016)
   a. Diclofenac   b. Ibuprofen
   c. Aspirin   d. Indomethacin

9. Drug of choice for paracetamol poisoning:
   (Recent Question 2016)
   a. Adrenaline   b. Atropine
   c. Acetyl-cysteine d. Insulin

10. False about NSAIDs: *(Recent Question 2016)*
    a. Cause addiction
    b. Cause gastric irritation
    c. Used in acute gout
    d. NAPQI COX

11. NAPQI inhibitor used in acute acetaminophen poisoning is: *(Recent Question 2016)*
    a. Parabenzol   b. Rotenone
    c. N-acetylcysteine d. Thermogenin

12. Renal papillary necrosis is caused by:
    (Recent Question 2016)
    a. NSAIDs   b. Cocaine
    c. Heroin   d. Morphine

Ans.

| 1. (a) | 2. (c) | 3. (c) | 4. (d) | 5. (a) | 6. (c) |
| 7. (c) | 8. (c) | 9. (c) | 10. (a) | 11. (c) | 12. (a) |

32 Drugs Used for Gout

Gout is a disorder of purine metabolism characterized by increased uric acid levels in the blood (hyperuricemia). Hyperuricemia can be due to reduced excretion of uric acid, increased production of uric acid or increased intake of purine rich foods (Figure 1).

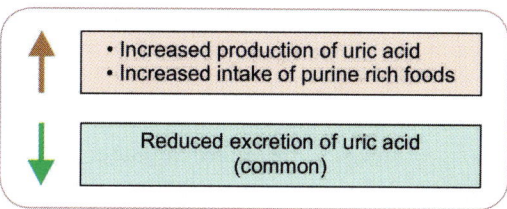

Figure 1: Hyperuricemia

Hyperuricemia can be either primary or secondary (Figure 2).

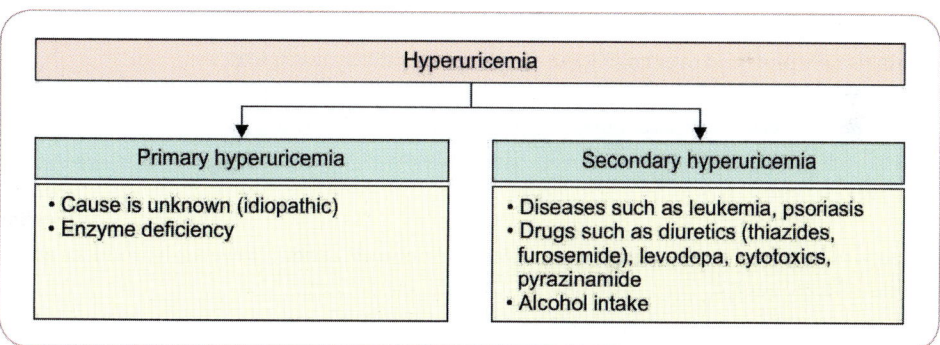

Figure 2: Hyperuricemia

In gout, there is a deposition of monosodium urate crystals in and around joints leading to recurrent acute or chronic arthritis.

In patients with severe chronic hyperuricemia, urate crystals may be deposited in larger joints and in organs such as kidneys.

CLASSIFICATION OF DRUGS USED FOR GOUT

The drugs used in the treatment of acute and chronic gout are mentioned in Figure 3.

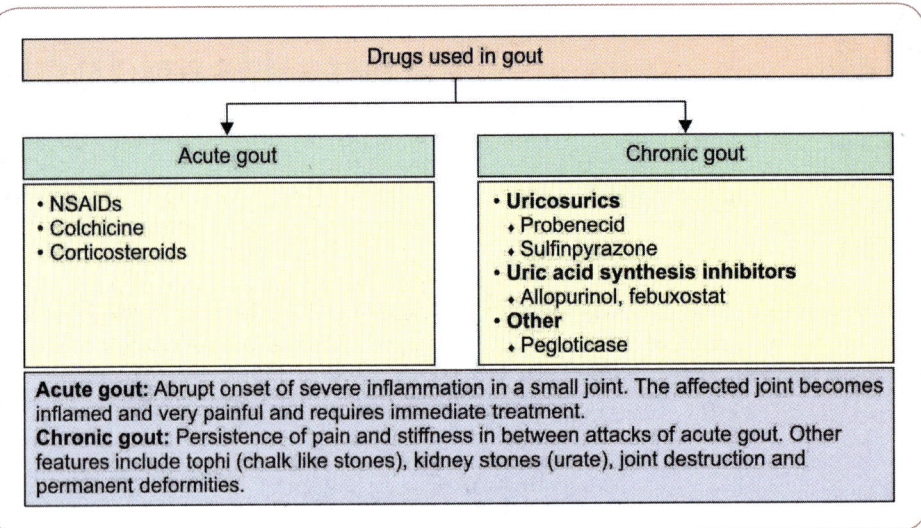

Figure 3: Drugs used for gout

DRUGS USED FOR ACUTE GOUT

NONSTEROIDAL ANTI-INFLAMMATORY DRUGS (NSAIDs)

The NSAIDs are used in acute gout as they have potent anti-inflammatory actions. They do not have any uricosuric action. They are usually preferred over colchicine due to comparatively lesser toxicity.

Some of the NSAIDs used for acute gout include—indomethacin, naproxen, diclofenac and piroxicam. Prolonged use of NSAIDs is not recommended due to risk of toxicity.

COLCHICINE

Colchicine is an alkaloid that does not have any analgesic or uricosuric action. However, it produces dramatic relief in the symptoms of acute gout.

Mechanism of Action

Colchicine has a selective anti-inflammatory effect in acute gout. It binds to tubulin and causes its depolymerization. This inhibits the migration of granulocytes to the site of inflammation (Figure 4). Colchicine also has an antimitotic effect. It causes metaphase arrest by binding to microtubules and interfere with spindle formation.

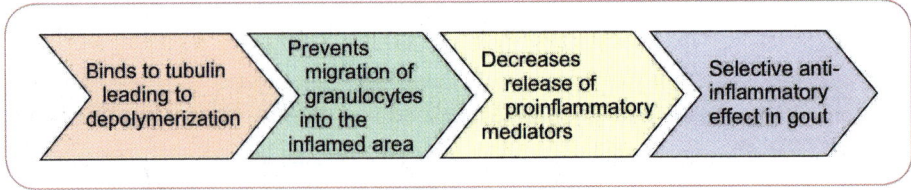

Figure 4: Selective anti-inflammatory effect of colchicine in acute gout

Adverse Effects

Colchicine has high toxicity and is poorly tolerated.

The most common adverse effects include gastrointestinal toxicity manifesting as nausea, vomiting, diarrhea and abdominal pain. These are dose-limiting and colchicine should be discontinued once these adverse effects appear.

Chronic therapy can lead to severe bone marrow depression (agranulocytosis and aplastic anemia), myopathy and alopecia.

Overdose can result in multisystem organ dysfunction including CNS depression, renal damage and GIT bleeding. Death can occur due to cardiovascular collapse and respiratory depression.

Clinical Uses

- Treatment of acute gout—produces rapid response, but not generally preferred due to toxicity. NSAIDs are usually preferred for acute therapy.
- Prophylaxis of acute gout during initiation of therapy with allopurinol and uricosuric drugs.

CORTICOSTEROIDS

They are used in situations that are nonresponsive to NSAIDs and colchicine. They can also be considered in situations where the patients are unable to receive NSAIDs due to toxicity.

Systemic steroids such as prednisolone and methylprednisolone can be used. Intra-articular injection of steroids such as triamcinolone can be considered for monoarticular or single joint involvement.

DRUGS USED FOR CHRONIC GOUT

URICOSURIC DRUGS—PROBENECID, SULFINPYRAZONE

Probenecid

It is a uricosuric drug used in the management of chronic gout.

Mechanism of Action

Probenecid competitively inhibits the anion transporter in the renal tubules and hence, blocks the transport of organic acids.

Uric acid which is mainly reabsorbed from the renal tubules is prevented from being reabsorbed, and is therefore excreted in the urine.

Antibiotics such as penicillins, cephalosporins and sulfonamides are mainly secreted in the renal tubules. Hence, probenecid can enhance and prolong the action of such antibiotics because their tubular secretion is decreased by probenecid (Figure 5).

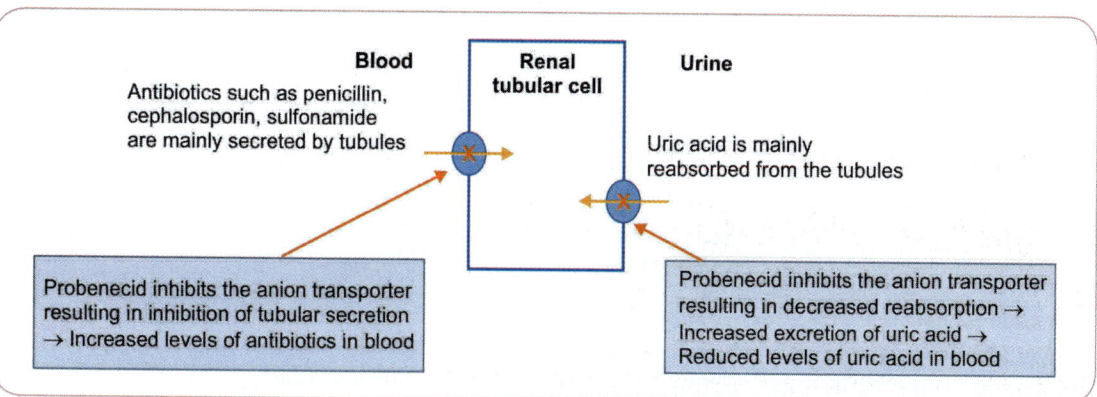

Figure 5: Probenecid

Adverse Effects

It is usually well tolerated and adverse effects include dyspepsia, skin rashes etc.

Drug Interactions

o Probenecid inhibits the excretion of drugs such as penicillins, cephalosporins and sulfonamides causing a rise in their blood levels. Hence, probenecid can enhance and prolong the action of such antibiotics.
o Probenecid can inhibit the tubular secretion of methotrexate and indomethacin.
o Probenecid can inhibit the tubular secretion of nitrofurantoin leading to a failure of nitrofurantoin to attain antibacterial concentration in the urine.
o Aspirin can block the uricosuric action of probenecid.

Clinical Uses

o Chronic gout
  ❑ Probenecid should not be given in acute gout because it can precipitate an attack.
  ❑ As probenecid increases the renal excretion of uric acid, liberal fluid intake is advised to decrease the risk of uric acid stones in urinary tract.
  ❑ It is ineffective in the presence of renal insufficiency and should be avoided in patients with creatinine clearance <50 mL/min.
o Enhance and prolong the action of antibiotics such as penicillin.

Sulfinpyrazone

It is a uricosuric drug used in the management of chronic gout. It inhibits the tubular reabsorption of uric acid and has an additive action with probenecid.

Adverse effects include gastric irritation and must be avoided in patients of peptic ulcer.

URIC ACID SYNTHESIS INHIBITOR—ALLOPURINOL, FEBUXOSTAT

ALLOPURINOL

It is a purine antimetabolite used in the management of chronic gout.

Mechanism of Action

Allopurinol is an inhibitor of xanthine oxidase enzyme and decreases the synthesis of uric acid (Figure 6).

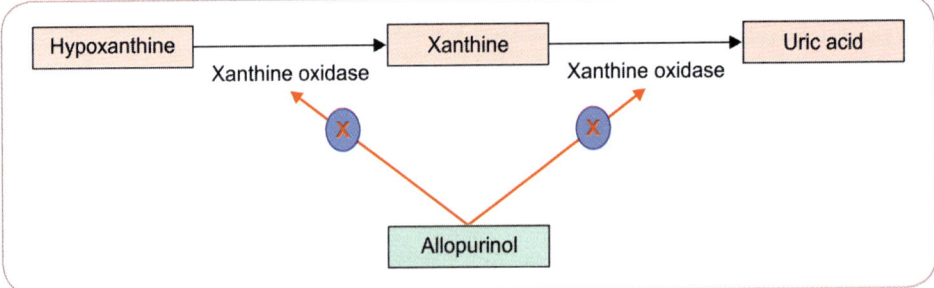

Figure 6: Mechanism of action of allopurinol

Allopurinol inhibits xanthine oxidase competitively, but its major metabolite alloxanthine is a noncompetitive inhibitor of xanthine oxidase. Administration of allopurinol leads to reduction in the levels of uric acid, but there is an increase in the levels of hypoxanthine and xanthine, which are more soluble and are excreted in the urine.

It can also cause some feedback inhibition of *de novo* purine synthesis.

Pharmacokinetics

Allopurinol is well absorbed orally and is not bound to plasma proteins.

Adverse Effects

- ○ Hypersensitivity reaction
- ○ Stevens Johnson syndrome
- ○ GIT: Nausea, vomiting

It is contraindicated in pregnancy and lactation.

Allopurinol should be used cautiously in elderly, children, and in patients with hepatic or renal disease.

Drug Interactions

- ○ Allopurinol and 6-Mercaptopurine
  - ❑ Allopurinol prevents the degradation of 6-mercaptopurine and azathioprine by inhibition of the enzyme xanthine oxidase. Hence, if allopurinol is administered along with 6-mercaptopurine or azathioprine, then the dosage of 6-mercaptopurine or azathioprine should be reduced to around 1/3rd of the normal dose.
- ○ Allopurinol can inhibit the metabolism of warfarin and theophylline and potentiate their action.

Clinical Uses

- ○ It is the preferred drug for chronic gout
  - ❑ Therapy with allopurinol and uricosuric drugs should not be initiated during acute gout due to the risk of precipitation of an acute attack. The chances of precipitation of an acute attack are higher during initial 1–2 months of therapy.
- ○ It is used in secondary hyperuricemia resulting from drugs such as thiazides, anticancer medications and radiation therapy.
- ○ It can be used to potentiate the effects of 6-mercaptopurine and azathioprine in patients receiving anticancer and immunosuppressant therapy.
- ○ It can be used in resistant cases of Kala-azar, as it inhibits *Leishmania* by modifying its purine metabolism.

FEBUXOSTAT

- ○ It is a nonpurine inhibitor of xanthine oxidase and hence, reduces the formation of uric acid.
- ○ It is used in chronic hyperuricemia in patients of gout. It can be used in patients who are intolerant to allopurinol.
- ○ Adverse effects include hepatic dysfunction, headache and diarrhea.

PEGLOTICASE

It is a recombinant uricase that converts uric acid to allantoin. Allantoin, being an inert and water soluble compound is excreted primarily in the urine. This leads to a decrease in the uric acid levels (Figure 7).

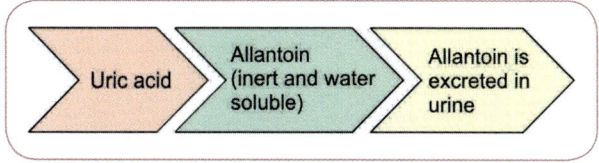

Figure 7: Mechanism of action of pegloticase

Pegloticase is indicated for the treatment of chronic gout in adult patients refractory to conventional therapy.

Flaring of gout can occur during initiation of antihyperuricemic therapy. Hence, prophylaxis for gout flare is recommended with an NSAID or colchicine starting at least 1 week before initiation of therapy with pegloticase and lasting for at least 6 months.

Autacoids and Associated Drugs

SECTION F

1. Discuss the pharmacotherapy of chronic gout.
2. Why allopurinol should not be used in acute gout.
3. Write short notes on:
   a. Allopurinol
   b. Colchicine
   c. Uricosuric drugs
   d. Febuxostat
4. Discuss 2 drugs used in acute gout with different mechanism of action.
5. Explain the drug interaction between:
   a. Probenecid and penicillin G
   b. Allopurinol and 6-mercaptopurine

MULTIPLE CHOICE QUESTIONS

1. Mechanism of action of colchicine is:
   (Recent Question 2016)
   a. Inhibits gouty inflammation
   b. Inhibits the release of chemotactic factors
   c. Inhibits granulocyte migration
   d. All the above

2. Uricosuric drug not used in acute gout is:
   (Recent Question 2016)
   a. NSAIDs
   b. Colchicine
   c. Corticosteroids
   d. Sulfinpyrazone

3. Febuxostat is used for: *(Recent Question 2016)*
   a. Hyperkalemia
   b. Hyperuricemia
   c. Hypernatremia
   d. Hypercalcemia

4. Allopurinol inhibits which enzyme:
   (Recent Question 2016)
   a. Xanthine oxidase
   b. Carbonic anhydrase
   c. Pyrimidine synthase
   d. Dihydroorotate dehydrogenase

5. The most common effect of colchicines which is dose limiting is: *(Recent Question 2016)*
   a. Diarrhea
   b. Dyspepsia
   c. Retinal damage
   d. Loss of taste sensation

6. Drug used in acute gout: *(Recent Question 2016)*
   a. Allopurinol
   b. Febuxostat
   c. Steroids
   d. All of the above

7. Which of the following is not a uricosuric drug?
   (JIPMER 2010)
   a. Probenecid
   b. Benzbromarone
   c. Sulfinpyrazone
   d. Febuxostat

8. Which one of the following is the mechanism of action of rasburicase? *(APPG 2009)*
   a. Increases the excretion of uric acid
   b. Increases the formation of uric acid
   c. Catalyzes the conversion of uric acid to allantoin
   d. Catalyzes the conversion of urea to ammonia

9. Colchicine is: *(MHCET 2011)*
   a. Analgesic
   b. Anti-inflammatory
   c. Uricosuric
   d. None of the above

10. Drug not causing hyperuricemia: *(WBPG 2008)*
    a. Probenecid
    b. Thiazide
    c. Pyrazinamide
    d. Ethambutol

Ans.

1.	(d)	2.	(d)	3.	(b)	4.	(a)	5.	(a)	6.	(c)
7.	(d)	8.	(c)	9.	(b)	10.	(a)				

Drugs Used for Rheumatoid Arthritis

Rheumatoid arthritis is a chronic, systemic autoimmune disorder. It is characterized by:
○ Inflammation of the joints
○ Synovial infiltration
○ Destruction of the articular cartilage

Patients with rheumatoid arthritis present with systemic symptoms such as early morning stiffness of affected joints, fatigue, malaise, anorexia, generalized weakness and low-grade pyrexia.

The affected joints are painful, warm and swollen with limitation of movement. Gradually joint deformities such as Boutonnière and swan-neck deformities may be present.

CLASSIFICATION OF ANTIRHEUMATOID DRUGS

The drugs used in the management of rheumatoid arthritis are mentioned in Figure 1.

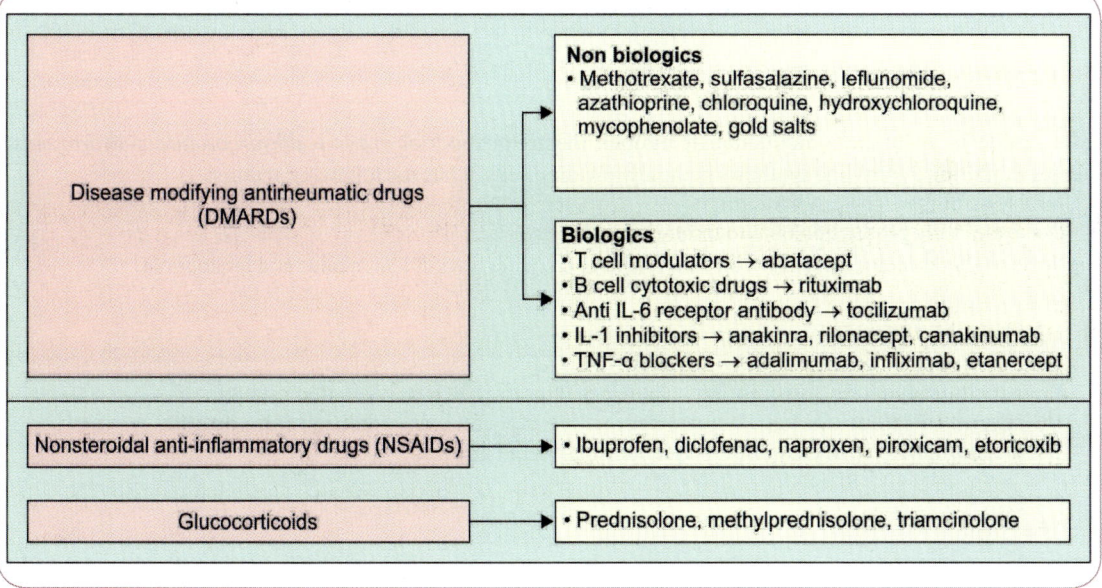

Figure 1: Drugs used for rheumatoid arthritis

An integrated approach consisting of both nonpharmacologic and pharmacologic therapies is considered for the management of rheumatoid arthritis.
○ Nonpharmacologic therapy includes exercise, dietary management, counseling, physiotherapy, stress management and surgery.
○ Pharmacologic therapy consists of multiple classes of drugs used as per the requirement of patient and the disease condition. Early therapy with DMARDs is considered the standard of care, because it can retard disease progression more efficiently than treatment at a later stage and potentially induce more remissions.

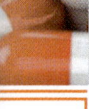

DISEASE MODIFYING ANTIRHEUMATIC DRUGS (DMARDs)—NONBIOLOGICS

METHOTREXATE

It is a first line DMARD for the management of rheumatoid arthritis.

It is a folate antagonist and inhibits the production of cytokines. This results in anti-inflammatory and immunosuppressive effects. The dose of methotrexate required for rheumatoid arthritis is much lower than that required for cancer chemotherapy.

The toxicity of methotrexate can be reduced by the use of folinic acid.

The adverse effects include nausea, mucosal ulceration, intestinal ulceration, hematological abnormalities (such as neutropenia) and liver damage including cirrhosis.

It is contraindicated in severe renal or hepatic impairment, serious acute or chronic infections and blood dyscrasias (such as significant anemia, leucopenia or thrombocytopenia). It is also contraindicated in active gastrointestinal ulcer disease.

It is teratogenic and is contraindicated in pregnancy and breastfeeding.

CHLOROQUINE AND HYDROXYCHLOROQUINE

These are drugs used for the treatment of malaria. The exact mechanism of action in rheumatoid arthritis is unclear. The onset of action is slow; takes 6 weeks to 6 months. They have low efficacy and are generally used in mild disease. They are used either alone or along with sulfasalazine and/or methotrexate.

Prolonged therapy can lead to ocular toxicity such as retinal damage and corneal deposits.

LEFLUNOMIDE

Leflunomide is an immunomodulator. It inhibits the mitochondrial enzyme *dihydroorotate dehydrogenase*, thereby inhibiting pyrimidine synthesis in rapidly dividing cells. It has the following actions:
○ Inhibition of the T cell proliferation
○ Decrease in the production of autoantibodies by B cells
The adverse effects include diarrhea, elevation of liver enzymes, loss of hair, rashes and leukopenia.

GOLD COMPOUNDS

○ These include auranofin and aurothiomalate and suppress the cell mediated immunity.
○ The adverse effects include bone marrow depression, liver and kidney damage and stomatitis.
○ These compounds are not commonly used for rheumatoid arthritis.

SULFASALAZINE

Sulfasalazine is split by the colonic bacteria to 5-aminosalicylic acid (5-ASA) and sulfapyridine. The sulfapyridine gets absorbed and acts systemically in rheumatoid arthritis. In contrast, 5-ASA acts locally in the colon in ulcerative colitis.

The exact mechanism is unclear but it is postulated that sulfapyridine exerts an anti-inflammatory effect that may be beneficial in rheumatoid arthritis.

The adverse effects include nausea, vomiting, hematological abnormalities (leukopenia, agranulocytosis, aplastic anemia, hemolytic anemia) and pulmonary toxicity.

DISEASE MODIFYING ANTIRHEUMATIC DRUGS (DMARDs)—BIOLOGICS

These drugs are usually produced by recombinant DNA technology.

T CELL MODULATORS → ABATACEPT

It inhibits the activation of T cells and is administered via IV infusion.

The adverse effects include infections (mainly respiratory). Patients should be screened for latent tuberculosis and hepatitis prior to therapy initiation.

Concomitant administration of abatacept with TNF-α inhibitors can lead to severe infections and hence, is not recommended.

B CELL CYTOTOXIC DRUGS → RITUXIMAB

Rituximab causes depletion of B lymphocytes and hence, reduces inflammation.

It is indicated for use in combination with methotrexate for the treatment of adult patients with severe active rheumatoid arthritis who have had an inadequate response or intolerance to other DMARDs (including one or more TNF-α inhibitors).

The adverse effects include rashes, serious and sometimes fatal infections.

ANTI IL-6 RECEPTOR ANTIBODY → TOCILIZUMAB

Tocilizumab is a monoclonal antibody that blocks the IL-6 receptor and inhibits the actions of IL-6.

The adverse effects include serious and sometimes fatal infections and an increased risk of malignancy.

IL-1 INHIBITORS → ANAKINRA, RILONACEPT, CANAKINUMAB

These drugs block the effects of IL-1. The adverse effects include injection site reactions and serious infections.

TNF-α BLOCKERS → ADALIMUMAB, INFLIXIMAB, ETANERCEPT

These drugs block the effects of TNF-α. The adverse effects include risk of infections, risk of malignancies, hematologic reactions (e.g. pancytopenia, leukopenia) and congestive heart failure.

NONSTEROIDAL ANTI-INFLAMMATORY DRUGS (NSAIDs)

These drugs have anti-inflammatory action and hence, can produce rapid symptomatic relief.

They have limited effect on the disease progression. Some of the NSAIDs used in patients of rheumatoid arthritis include ibuprofen, diclofenac, naproxen, piroxicam and etoricoxib.

GLUCOCORTICOIDS

They are used to rapidly suppress inflammation and can be administered systemically or topically (intra-articular).

Some of the glucocorticoids used in patients of rheumatoid arthritis include prednisolone, methylprednisolone and triamcinolone.

SECTION F ■ Autacoids and Associated Drugs

ASSESS YOURSELF (Examination Questions of Various Universities)

1. Discuss the pharmacotherapy of rheumatoid arthritis.
2. Enumerate the disease modifying antirheumatic drugs (DMARDs) used in rheumatoid arthritis.
3. Write short notes on:
   a. Methotrexate
   b. Leflunomide

MULTIPLE CHOICE QUESTIONS

1. Which of the following is not a TNF alpha inhibitor? *(Recent Question Dec 2016)*
   a. Mycophenolate mofetil b. Etanercept
   c. Adalimumab   d. Infliximab
2. Not a DMARD in RA *(Recent Question Dec 2016)*
   a. BAL
   b. Gold
   c. Methotrexate
   d. Hydroxychloroquine
3. Abatacept is used in: *(AIIMS Nov 2014)*
   a. Osteoarthritis
   b. Rheumatoid arthritis
   c. Multiple sclerosis
   d. Sarcoidosis
4. Which among the following is an IL-1 antagonist?
   (Recent Question 2016)
   a. Anakinra   b. Adalimumab
   c. Etanercept   d. Infliximab
5. First choice DMARD in RA:
   (Recent Question 2016)
   a. Gold salts   b. Infliximab
   c. Methotrexate   d. Steroids
6. Leflunomide is used in the treatment of:
   (Recent Question 2016)
   a. Rheumatoid arthritis
   b. Dermatomyositis
   c. Bony metastasis
   d. Postmenopausal osteoporosis
7. Which of the following drugs is not used in Rheumatoid arthritis? *(AIIMS May 2018)*
   a. Etanercept
   b. Leflunomide
   c. Febuxostat
   d. Methotrexate

Ans.

1. (a)	2. (a)	3. (b)	4. (a)	5. (c)	6. (a)
7. (c)					

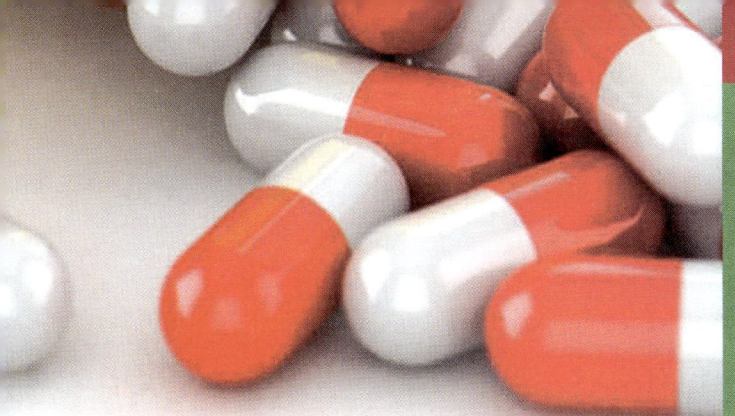

Drugs Acting on the Respiratory System

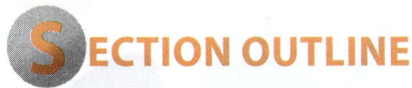 **ECTION OUTLINE**

○ Drugs Used for Bronchial Asthma and Cough

34 Drugs Used for Bronchial Asthma and Cough

Bronchial asthma is a respiratory disease characterized by airway hyperresponsiveness and chronic airway inflammation.

Patients of bronchial asthma experience episodes of acute bronchoconstriction that can cause symptoms such as dyspnea (shortness of breath), cough, wheeze and chest tightness. These symptoms are often accompanied with variable expiratory airflow limitation (Figure 1).

There is a considerable variation in the intensity and timing of the symptoms and expiratory airflow limitation. Triggering factors for episodes of bronchoconstriction are multiple and can include exercise, irritants, allergens, respiratory infections, aspirin, climatic changes etc.

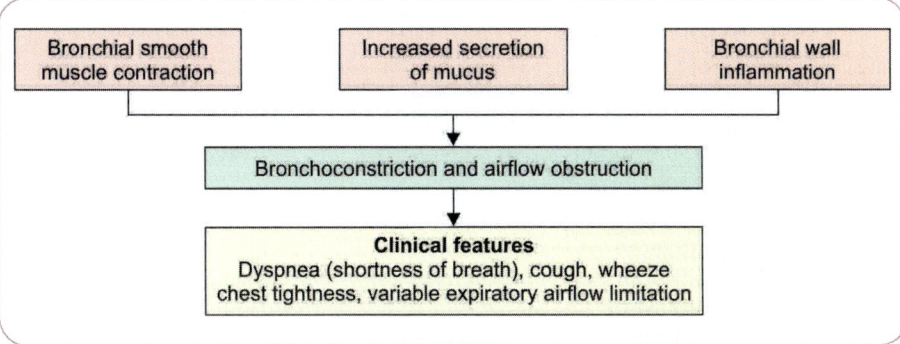

Figure 1: Bronchial asthma

CLASSIFICATION OF DRUGS FOR BRONCHIAL ASTHMA (TABLE 1)

TABLE 1	Drugs used for bronchial asthma
Bronchodilators	

Sympathomimetics	• *Selective* short-acting β_2 agonists (SABAs)
	  ▪ Salbutamol, terbutaline
	• *Selective* long-acting β_2 agonists (LABAs)
	  ▪ Salmeterol, formoterol
	• Nonselective
	  ▪ Adrenaline

Anticholinergics	Ipratropium bromide, tiotropium bromide
Methylxanthines	Theophylline, aminophylline
Mast cell stabilizers	Sodium cromoglycate, ketotifen
Leukotriene antagonists	Montelukast, zafirlukast, zileuton

Corticosteroids	• Inhaled corticosteroids
	  ▪ Beclomethasone, budesonide, fluticasone, ciclesonide, triamcinolone
	• Systemic corticosteroids
	  ▪ Prednisolone, methylprednisolone, hydrocortisone

Monoclonal antibody	• Omalizumab (Anti IgE) • Reslizumab (Anti IL-5)

SYMPATHOMIMETICS

Sympathomimetics cause bronchodilation by stimulation of β_2 adrenergic receptors, decrease in mast cell degranulation, inhibition of histamine release and promotion of mucociliary clearance.

SELECTIVE SHORT-ACTING β_2 AGONISTS (SABAs)

The drugs in this category include salbutamol (albuterol) and terbutaline.

These drugs provide rapid relief in acute exacerbations of asthma and hence are called 'reliever or rescue' medications.

They have a rapid (within minutes) onset and a short duration of action.

Inhaled route is commonly used as it reduces the adverse effects typically associated with the systemic use of β_2 agonists.

The adverse effects include tremors, tachycardia, palpitations, hypokalemia, hyperglycemia and ankle edema. Prolonged, regular use of β_2 agonists is not advisable as it can worsen bronchial hyperreactivity. Regular use also downregulates the beta receptors that may further lead to diminished responsiveness. They should not be used alone for long-term maintenance of persistent asthma.

SELECTIVE LONG-ACTING β_2 AGONISTS (LABAs)

The drugs in this category include salmeterol and formoterol.

Salmeterol

- First *selective* long-acting β_2 agonist
- Slow and prolonged onset of action
- Clinically used in moderate to severe persistent asthma
- Salmeterol is not used to manage an acute attack as it has a slow onset of action
- Not used as monotherapy because of:
  - Increased risk of asthma-related death when used as monotherapy. Hence, these drugs should be used only in combination with an inhaled corticosteroid.

Formoterol

- It has a faster onset of action as compared to salmeterol
- Clinically used in moderate to severe persistent asthma.

NONSELECTIVE SYMPATHOMIMETIC

Adrenaline (Epinephrine) is a nonselective sympathomimetic drug. It has a powerful bronchodilator effect by directly acting on β_2 receptors. It can be used in acute severe attack of asthma; however, it is not frequently used due to dangerous cardiac adverse effects.

ANTICHOLINERGICS

They cause bronchodilation by anticholinergic action, i.e. by blockade of the effects of acetylcholine. The main effect is on the larger airways.

Anticholinergic drugs are less efficacious than sympathomimetic drugs. They are not preferred as a single agent for acute attack of asthma because they have a slower response.

Combination of inhaled ipratropium + β_2 agonist drugs leads to significant and prolonged bronchodilation. Hence, they can be used in patients of acute severe asthma.

Anticholinergic drugs are the preferred bronchodilators in patients of COPD. They are also utilized in patients of bronchial asthma.

METHYLXANTHINES

Methylxanthines are not currently considered as first line therapy in bronchial asthma due to the availability of drugs that are more effective and have a better safety profile. Methylxanthines have a narrow margin of safety.

MECHANISM OF ACTION

Methylxanthines inhibit the phosphodiesterase (PDE) enzyme leading to an increase in cAMP and cGMP levels. Methylxanthines are also adenosine receptor blockers (Figure 2).

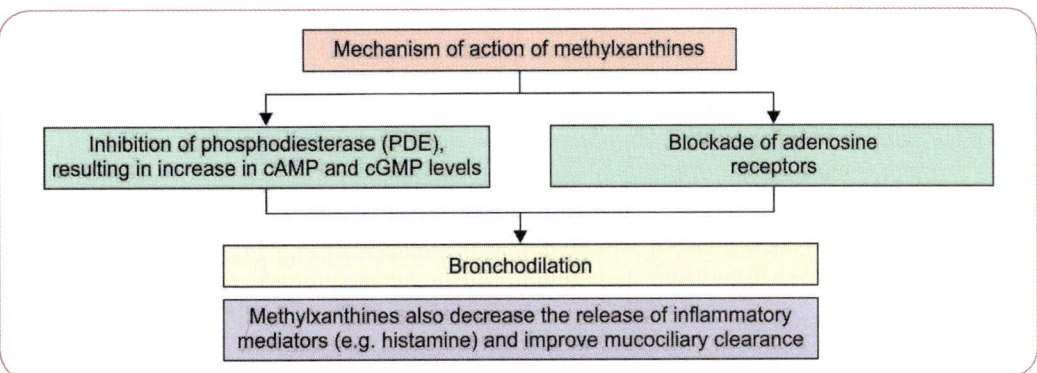

Figure 2: Mechanism of action of methylxanthines

PHARMACOKINETICS

Methylxanthines are well-absorbed orally.
Theophylline is metabolized in the liver and is eliminated via kidneys.

ADVERSE EFFECTS

The key adverse effects of methylxanthines are mentioned in Table 2.

TABLE 2	Adverse effects of methylxanthines
Central nervous system	• Tremors, delirium, vomiting, convulsions
Gastrointestinal system	• Gastric irritation (nausea, vomiting), dyspepsia
Cardiovascular system	• Tachycardia, palpitation, arrhythmia, hypotension, shock
Others	• Diuresis
Methylxanthines have a narrow margin of safety and fatalities can occur	

DRUG INTERACTIONS

The key drug interactions of methylxanthines are mentioned below:
- The effects of drugs such as sympathomimetics and furosemide can be potentiated by methylxanthines.
- Theophylline reduces the effects of phenytoin, lithium.
- Metabolism of theophylline is induced by drugs such as phenytoin, rifampicin, phenobarbitone leading to a decrease in the plasma level of theophylline.
- Metabolism of theophylline is inhibited by drugs such as erythromycin, cimetidine, ciprofloxacin, oral contraceptives leading to an increase in the plasma level of theophylline.

CLINICAL USES

The clinical uses of methylxanthines include the following:
- Bronchial asthma and COPD
- Apnea in premature infants—theophylline can decrease the duration and frequency of apneic episodes.

MAST CELL STABILIZERS

Mast cell stabilizers have the following actions:
- Prevent degranulation of the mast cells and inhibit the release of inflammatory mediators such as histamine, leukotrienes, interleukins etc.
- Long-term use can lead to:
  - Reduced cellular inflammatory response
  - Decreased bronchial hyperreactivity
  - May prevent bronchospasm induced by allergens, cold air, irritant, exercise etc.

SODIUM CROMOGLYCATE

Sodium cromoglycate is not effective if administered during an acute attack of bronchial asthma because it is not a bronchodilator and it also does not oppose the bronchoconstrictor effects of mediators such as histamine, acetylcholine and leukotrienes.

Sodium cromoglycate inhibits the release of mediators (e.g. histamine and leukotrienes) from the mast cells.

Sodium cromoglycate is not absorbed orally and is administered via inhalation. The onset of action is slow.

Adverse Effects

- Sodium cromoglycate is minimally absorbed → systemic adverse effects are rare
- Local adverse effects include cough, bronchospasm, headache, etc.

Clinical Uses

The clinical uses include:
- Bronchial asthma → prophylactic agent in mild to moderate asthma. Can be useful in exercise induced asthma
- Allergic rhinitis and allergic conjunctivitis.

KETOTIFEN

- It has some sodium cromoglycate like effect along with additional antihistaminic (H_1) effect
- It is not a bronchodilator and has a slow onset of action
- Orally effective and can cause sedation.

LEUKOTRIENE ANTAGONISTS

MONTELUKAST, ZAFIRLUKAST

Leukotrienes (leukotrienes C_4, D_4) are potent bronchoconstrictors and play a significant role in pathogenesis of bronchial asthma.

The leukotrienes act on the $cysLT_1$ receptors to cause airway hyperresponsiveness, bronchoconstriction, plasma exudation etc.

Montelukast, zafirlukast are competitive antagonists at $cysLT_1$ receptors. They have the following effects:
- Bronchodilation
- Suppression of bronchial hyperactivity and inflammation

The adverse effects include rashes, headache and eosinophilia (rare).

The clinical uses include prophylactic treatment of mild to moderate bronchial asthma.

ZILEUTON

It inhibits the enzyme 5-lipoxygenase and blocks the synthesis of leukotrienes B_4, C_4 and D_4. Zileuton can cause hepatotoxicity and hence the clinical use is restricted.

CORTICOSTEROIDS

Corticosteroids have anti-inflammatory effects and are used in patients of bronchial asthma (Table 3).

TABLE 3	Corticosteroids in bronchial asthma
• Anti-inflammatory, antiallergic and immunosuppressant action	
• Decrease bronchial hyperreactivity	
• Decrease mucosal edema	
• Suppress inflammatory response to antigen-antibody reaction	
• Corticosteroids do *not* have a bronchodilator effect	

INHALED CORTICOSTEROIDS

The inhaled corticosteroids (ICS) used clinically include beclomethasone, budesonide, fluticasone and ciclesonide.

The ICS have a high topical and low systemic activity. ICS reduce the need for rescue medications, decrease asthma exacerbations and may influence airway modeling. They are used as prophylactic medications in patients of bronchial asthma.

Combination of ICS + long acting β_2 agonists (LABA) is advantageous because ICS potentiates the effect of β_2 agonists and may also prevent the development of tolerance to β_2 agonists.

They are not useful in acute exacerbation or in status asthmaticus.

Adverse Effects

○ Local effects of inhaled corticosteroids include dysphonia, hoarseness and oral candidiasis. These effects can be reduced or prevented by using a spacer device or by doing post inhalation gargle.
○ Use of inhaled corticosteroids avoids the adverse effects typically associated with the systemic use of corticosteroids.
○ Systemic adverse effects are dose related and can occur with oral or inhaled forms. They include suppression of the pituitary adrenal axis, osteoporosis, gastric irritation, hyperglycemia, bruising etc.

Ciclesonide

○ Prodrug that is converted to active form by esterases in bronchial epithelium.

SYSTEMIC CORTICOSTEROIDS—PREDNISOLONE, HYDROCORTISONE

Systemic steroids (prednisolone, hydrocortisone) are used in the management of severe chronic asthma, status asthmaticus and acute asthma exacerbation.

The incidence of systemic adverse effects is higher as compared to inhalational steroids.

MONOCLONAL ANTIBODY

OMALIZUMAB (ANTI IgE)

○ Omalizumab is a monoclonal antibody.

- Omalizumab prevents the binding of IgE to mast cells. This prevents the release of inflammatory mediators from mast cells.
- Clinical uses include allergic asthma and allergic rhinitis.
- Local adverse effects include injection site reactions and anaphylaxis.

DRUG THERAPY FOR STATUS ASTHMATICUS (ACUTE SEVERE ASTHMA)

It is a medical emergency and can be potentially life-threatening. The treatment measures are mentioned in Table 4.

TABLE 4	Status asthmaticus
1. High flow humidified oxygen therapy	
2. Inhaled *selective* short-acting β_2 agonists (SABAs) • Salbutamol (albuterol) administered via nebulization • Inhaled anticholinergics (ipratropium bromide) can be administered along with inhaled SABA	
3. Systemic corticosteroids • Prednisolone or hydrocortisone can be used	
4. Other measures to be considered • Treatment of chest infections with antibiotics • Intubation and mechanical ventilation • Supportive treatment to correct dehydration, electrolyte imbalance and acidosis	

DRUGS USED FOR COUGH

Cough is a protective reflex that helps to remove respiratory secretions or foreign matter from the respiratory tract.

It is important to identify and treat the underlying cause of cough.

Productive cough is helpful in clearing the respiratory passages. Suppression of productive cough is not recommended and may be harmful. Suppression is recommended in nonproductive cough.

The drugs used for the symptomatic treatment of cough are mentioned in Table 5.

TABLE 5	Drugs for symptomatic treatment of cough
Antitussives (Cough center suppressants)	• Codeine, pholcodine, dextromethorphan, noscapine • Antihistaminics → Chlorpheniramine, diphenhydramine, promethazine
Expectorants	• Mucolytics → Bromhexine, ambroxol, acetylcysteine, carbocisteine • Others → Sodium citrate, potassium citrate, guaiphenesin, potassium iodide
Pharyngeal demulcents	• Cough drops, lozenges, glycerine

ANTITUSSIVES (COUGH CENTER SUPPRESSANTS)

These drugs exert either one or both of the following actions to suppress cough:

- Central action → increase the threshold of cough center in the brain
- Peripheral action → decrease cough impulses from the respiratory tract

These drugs are used for dry, nonproductive cough. Salient features of antitussives are mentioned in Table 6.

TABLE 6	Antitussives
Codeine	• Suppresses the cough center in the brain • Can lead to constipation, drowsiness, respiratory depression • Has low abuse liability
Pholcodine	• Analgesic or addicting properties are practically nonexistent • Similar antitussive activity as codeine; has a longer duration of action
Noscapine	• Suppresses cough but does not have any analgesic, dependence producing or narcotic activities • Adverse effects include headache, nausea and bronchoconstriction in patients of asthma
Dextromethorphan	• Increase the threshold of cough center in the brain • Constipation or addicting properties are practically nonexistent
Antihistaminics	• Provide benefit in cough due to their anticholinergic and sedative effects • Examples inlcude chlorpheniramine, diphenhydramine, promethazine

EXPECTORANTS—MUCOLYTICS

BROMHEXINE

It has mucolytic and mucokinetic properties.

Bromhexine reduces the viscosity of the sputum by depolymerizing the mucopolysaccharides. Depolymerization of mucopolysaccharides is due to bromhexine-induced release of lysosomal enzymes and also due to direct action. The thick tenacious sputum is broken down into thin copious secretions that are relatively easy for the patient to cough out.

Adverse effects include gastric irritation, lacrimation and rhinorrhea.

AMBROXOL

○ It is a metabolite of bromhexine.
○ Clinical uses and adverse effects are similar to bromhexine.

ACETYLCYSTEINE

○ It makes the sputum thin and less viscid by opening the disulfide bonds in the mucoproteins in the sputum.
○ Clinical uses include mucolytic adjuvant in patients with thick, viscous mucus production.
○ Adverse effects include headache, vomiting and bronchospasm.

EXPECTORANTS—OTHERS

Expectorants (mucokinetics) increase the amount of bronchial secretions or decrease the viscosity of the sputum. This makes it relatively easy for the patient to cough out the secretions.

PHARYNGEAL DEMULCENTS

Pharyngeal demulcents are throat soothing agents. They are useful in dry irritating cough arising from the pharynx.

Drugs Acting on the Respiratory System

SECTION G

ASSESS YOURSELF (Examination Questions of Various Universities)

1. Enumerate second-generation antihistamines. Discuss their advantages over first-generation antihistamines.
2. Write short notes on:
   a. Cetirizine
   b. Uses of H₁ antihistamines
   c. H₁ receptor antagonists
   d. Second-generation antihistamines
3. Describe the pharmacotherapy of bronchial asthma

4. Role of corticosteroids in bronchial asthma
5. Long acting β2-agonists in asthma
6. Salbutamol in bronchial asthma
7. Drug treatment of status asthmaticus
8. Mast cell stabilizers
9. Montelukast in bronchial asthma
10. Drug management of cough
11. Enumerate and discuss the role of inhaled steroids in bronchial asthma

MULTIPLE CHOICE QUESTIONS

1. Omalizumab is: *(Recent Question 2016)*
   a. Anti-IgM antibody
   b. Anti-lgG antibody
   c. Anti-IgE antibody
   d. Anti-IgD antibody
2. Montelukast is: *(Recent Question 2016)*
   a. Leukotriene antagonist
   b. Potassium channel opener
   c. Smooth muscle relaxant
   d. Anti-inflammatory
3. Mechanism of action of theophylline in bronchial asthma is: *(Recent Question 2016)*
   a. Inhibition of phosphodiesterase-IV
   b. Beta 2 agonism
   c. Anticholinergic action
   d. Inhibition of mucociliary clearance
4. Inhibition of 5-lipoxygenase is useful in:
   a. Cardiac failure *(Recent Question 2016)*
   b. Bronchial asthma
   c. Hepatic failure
   d. Arthritis
5. Which of the following anti-asthma drugs is not a bronchodilator? *(Recent Question 2016)*
   a. Ipratropium bromide
   b. Theophylline
   c. Formoterol
   d. Sodium cromoglycate
6. Most common side effect of inhaled corticos-teroids: *(Recent Question 2016)*
   a. Pneumonia
   b. Oropharyngeal candidiasis
   c. Atrophic rhinitis
   d. Pituitary adrenal suppression

7. All of the following drugs useful in bronchial asthma are bronchodilators except:
   (Recent Question 2016)
   a. Theophylline   b. Salmeterol
   c. Beclomethasone   d. Ipratropium
8. Dextromethorphan is an:
   (Recent Question 2016)
   a. Antihistaminic   b. Antitussive
   c. Expectorant   d. Antiallergic
9. In theophylline metabolism, drug interactions occurs with all except: *(Recent Question 2016)*
   a. Cimetidine   b. Phenobarbitone
   c. Rifampin   d. Tetracyclines
10. Mechanism of action of zileuton is:
    (Recent Question 2016)
    a. Inhibits production of lgE
    b. Inhibits lipoxygenase
    c. Inhibits cyclooxygenase
    d. Inhibits activity of mast cells
11. All are inhalational steroids except:
    (Recent Question 2016)
    a. Sodium cromoglycate
    b. Triamcinolone
    c. Beclomethasone
    d. Budesonide
12. Corticosteroid which is given by inhalation route is: *(Recent Question 2016)*
    a. Prednisolone   b. Beclomethasone
    c. Dexamethasone   d. Hydrocortisone
13. Side effects of salbutamol are all except:
    (AIIMS Nov 2018)
    a. Hypokalemia   b. Hypoglycemia
    c. Tremor   d. Tachycardia

Ans.

1. (c)	2. (a)	3. (a)	4. (b)	5. (d)	6. (b)
7. (c)	8. (b)	9. (d)	10. (b)	11. (a)	12. (b)
13. (b)					

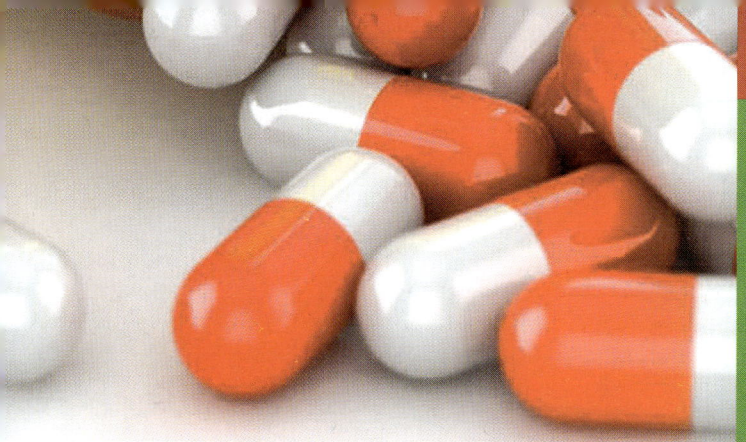

Drugs Acting on the Endocrine Physiology

35

Overview, Hypothalamic and Anterior Pituitary Hormones

Hormones are chemical substances that are produced by cells in the specific glands, and are directly released into the bloodstream.

They are transported in the circulation and act on target organs which are far away from the site of their production and release.

CLASSIFICATION OF HORMONES

As per the site of production (Figure 1):

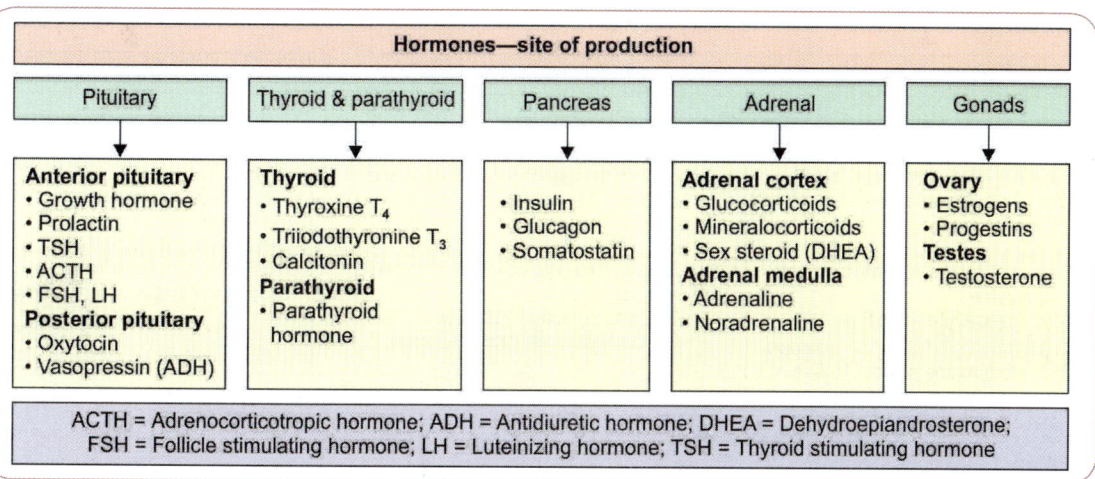

Figure 1: Hormones—site of production

As per the chemical structure (Table 1):

TABLE 1	Hormones—structural subtypes
Type of hormones	**Examples**
Peptide hormones	• Hypothalamic regulatory hormones • Pituitary hormones • Insulin, glucagon • Parathyroid hormone
Amino acid hormones	• Catecholamines (e.g. adrenaline, noradrenaline, dopamine) • Thyroid hormones (e.g. thyroxine T_4, triiodothyronine T_3) **Note:** All these end with 'ine' as they are derived from amino acid 'tyrosine'
Steroid hormones	• Glucocorticoids • Mineralocorticoids • Sex hormones (e.g. estrogens, progestins, androgens)

Drugs Acting on the Endocrine Physiology

SECTION H ■

As per the site and mechanism of action (Figure 2):

The hormones produce effects by acting on specific receptors in the target organs. The hormone receptors can be membrane, cytoplasmic or nuclear receptors.

> **Note:**
> ○ Peptide and amino acid hormones
>   □ are water soluble
>   □ cannot diffuse the lipid bilayer of the cell membrane
>   □ have their receptors at the cell membrane
> ○ Steroid hormones
>   □ are lipid soluble
>   □ can easily diffuse through the cell membrane
>   □ have their receptors inside the cell i.e. either in the cytoplasm or in the nucleus
> The only exception to the above is thyroid hormones which are amino acid hormones, but they are lipid soluble; diffuse through the cell membrane and act through the nuclear receptors.

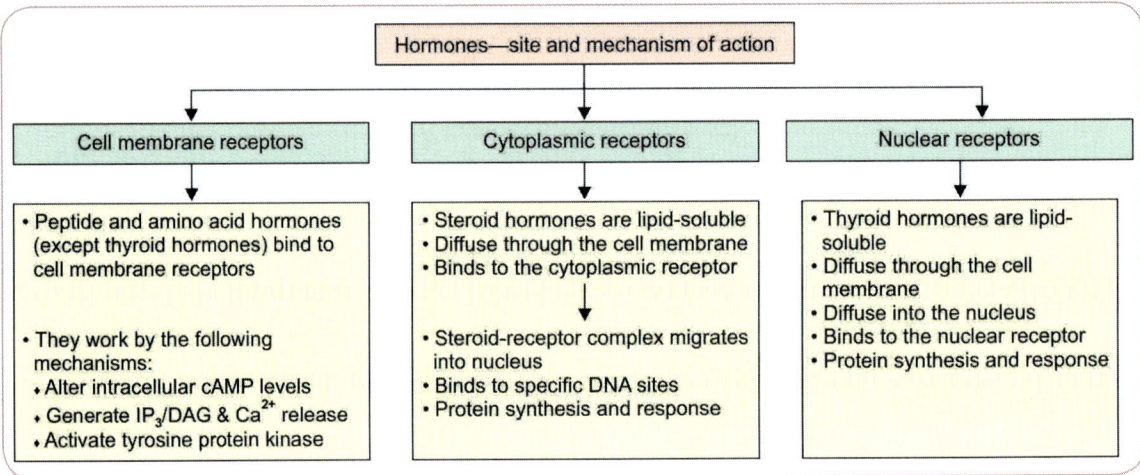

Figure 2: Hormones—site and mechanism of action

HYPOTHALAMIC HORMONES

The anterior pituitary hormones TSH, FSH, LH and ACTH are regulated by specific hormones from the hypothalamus. These specific hormones from the hypothalamus are mainly stimulating (releasing hormones).

○ TSH release is stimulated by thyrotropin releasing hormone (TRH)

○ FSH & LH release is stimulated by gonadotropin releasing hormone (GnRH)

○ ACTH release is stimulated by corticotropin releasing hormone (CRH)

The other anterior pituitary hormones growth hormone (GH) and prolactin differs from TSH, FSH, LH and ACTH in the following aspects:

○ GH is regulated by 2 hormones secreted by hypothalamus: GHRH (that stimulates GH secretion) and somatostatin that inhibits GH secretion.

○ Prolactin is regulated by 1 hormone secreted by hypothalamus: dopamine (that inhibits prolactin secretion). There is no releasing hormone for prolactin from the hypothalamus. The only exception is that TRH, if raised in hypothyroidism, can stimulate prolactin release.

The hypothalamic hormones TRH, CRH and GHRH, and the pituitary hormones TSH and ACTH are rarely used therapeutically. Hence, they are not further discussed.

The GnRH and its analogues are clinically used, and will be discussed along with the discussion on gonadotropins (FSH & LH).

Regulation of Anterior Pituitary Hormones by Hypothalamic Hormones

The secretion of various hormones is regulated by an interaction between hypothalamus, pituitary and the endocrine glands. This hypothalamo-pituitary-endocrine axis is depicted in Figure 3.

The hypothalamus produces various releasing and release-inhibitory hormones that are secreted into the anterior pituitary gland.

The anterior pituitary gland then produces various stimulating hormones which are transported to the respective endocrine glands, which then produces respective hormones.

The hormonal levels are regulated and maintained under precise control by the following regulatory mechanisms:

○ Feed-forward regulation (Positive)—the master signal hormones from hypothalamus & anterior pituitary **stimulate** the synthesis of hormones from target endocrine glands.

○ Feed-back regulation (Negative)—hormones released from target endocrine glands **inhibit** the synthesis of the following: releasing hormones from hypothalamus and stimulating hormones from the anterior pituitary.

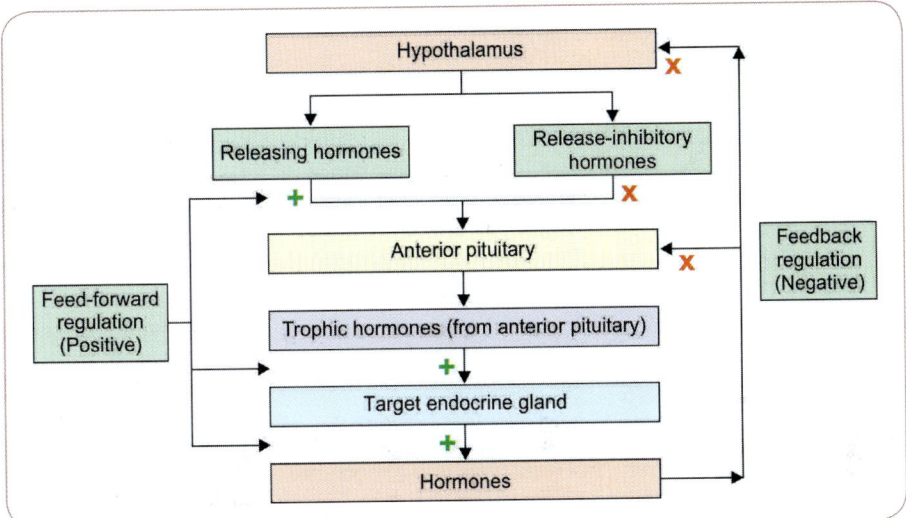

Figure 3: Regulation of anterior pituitary hormones

ANTERIOR PITUITARY HORMONES

The pituitary gland has 2 lobes: an anterior lobe and a posterior lobe. The hormones secreted by the 2 lobes of the pituitary are mentioned in Figure 1.

The anterior pituitary secretes the following hormones: Growth hormone, prolactin, TSH, FSH, LH and ACTH. The posterior pituitary secretes oxytocin and vasopressin (ADH).

Growth Hormone

Growth hormone (GH) is a peptide hormone secreted by the anterior pituitary.
The secretion of GH is regulated by the following hypothalamic hormones:
○ Growth hormone releasing hormone (GHRH) which stimulates GH secretion
○ Growth hormone inhibitory hormone (Somatostatin) which inhibits GH secretion
Somatostatin is also released by the D cells of islets of Langerhans in the pancreas.

Physiological Functions of GH

GH produces effects by direct and indirect actions (Table 2).

TABLE 2	Growth hormone—physiological actions	
Direct actions	**Indirect actions**
• No mediator is involved. GH acts directly to produce effects	• A mediator IGF-1, is involved. GH causes the release of IGF-1, which in turn produce effects

• Direct actions are:
   ▪ Increase lipolysis
   ▪ Increase gluconeogenesis
• This leads to an anti-insulin, diabetes-like state
	• Indirect actions (via IGF-1) are:
	   ▪ Positive nitrogen balance
	   ▪ Increase muscle mass
	   ▪ Increase longitudinal bone growth (if epiphyses have not fused)

Disorders Associated with Excess/Deficiency of GH

The disorders associated with excess or deficient secretion of GH are mentioned in Table 3.

TABLE 3	Growth hormone secretion disorders		
GH excess (In children)	**GH excess (In adults)**	**GH deficiency (In children)**
• Gigantism occurs	• Acromegaly occurs	• Pituitary dwarfism occurs
• As the bone epiphyses are open in children, the bones grow longitudinally resulting in increased height and body size. Other features of GH excess occur.	• As the bone epiphyses have already fused in adults, the longitudinal growth of bones cannot occur. Other features of GH excess occur.	• The body size remains small with stunted growth due to GH deficiency.
• Treatment consists of pituitary surgery, irradiation and drugs.	• Treatment consists of pituitary surgery, irradiation and drugs.	• Treatment consists of replacement therapy with drugs.
• The drugs used are somatostatin analogues (e.g. octreotide, lanreotide) and pegvisomant.	• The drugs used are somatostatin analogues (e.g. octreotide, lanreotide) and pegvisomant.	• The drugs used are human recombinant GH e.g. somatropin and somatrem.

Clinical Uses

The human recombinant GH (Somatropin & Somatrem) is used to treat the following conditions:

○ Growth failure in children (that may be associated with GH deficiency, chronic renal insufficiency, Turner syndrome, Prader Willi syndrome etc.)
○ GH deficiency in adults
○ AIDS related muscle wasting

Growth Hormone Antagonists

Somatostatin Analogues

Somatostatin is a peptide hormone that is secreted by the hypothalamus, parts of the CNS, pancreas and the GIT.

It mainly functions as an inhibitory hormone, and inhibits the release of GH & TSH (From anterior pituitary), insulin & glucagon (From pancreas) and gastrin (From GIT).

Somatostatin has very limited utility because, it has a very short half-life (1–3 minutes) and it has multiple effects in various secretory systems.

Therefore, long acting analogues of somatostatin (e.g. octreotide, lanreotide) have been developed for clinical use.

Octreotide

Octreotide is 40 times more potent than somatostatin in inhibiting GH secretion. It also has a longer duration of action ($t_{1/2}$~90 minutes).

Octreotide 50–200 µg (every 8 hourly) is given subcutaneously for the treatment of the following conditions:

○ *Hormone secreting tumors*—acromegaly, carcinoid syndrome, gastrinoma, insulinoma, glucagonoma etc.

○ *Diarrheas*—associated with diabetes, AIDS, chemotherapy, hormone secreting tumors etc.

○ *Acute control of bleeding from esophageal varices*—as it decreases mucosal blood flow

The adverse effects of octreotide include nausea, vomiting, abdominal cramps and flatulence. It may also cause biliary sludge and gallstones in around 20–30% of patients after more than 6 months of use.

Sandostatin

Sandostatin is a long-acting slow-release formulation of octreotide. It is given intramuscularly (into gluteal muscles) in a dose of 20–30 mg at 4-weekly intervals.

It is given only after a brief course of shorter-acting formulation of octreotide has been found safe and effective.

Lanreotide

It is a longer-acting analogue of octreotide. It is administered intramuscularly in a dose of 30 mg. As compared to sandostatin, its duration of action is shorter and is given at 10–14 day intervals.

Pegvisomant

Pegvisomant is a *GH receptor antagonist* that is approved for the treatment of acromegaly. It is used as an alternative in patients who do not respond to somatostatin analogues.

It is administered subcutaneously, and long-term therapy has been shown to reduce IGF-1 levels. It may cause an increase in liver enzymes.

Prolactin

Prolactin is a peptide hormone. It is secreted by the anterior pituitary. It is the main hormone responsible for lactation in females.

The control of prolactin secretion by the hypothalamus is mainly inhibitory. This is a unique phenomenon because the control of other anterior pituitary hormones is mainly stimulatory. Prolactin secretion is mainly regulated by prolactin release inhibitory hormone (PRIH). This PRIH is **dopamine** which acts on lactotrope D_2 receptors, to inhibit prolactin secretion.

The effect of dopamine agonists and antagonists on prolactin secretion is mentioned in Figure 4.

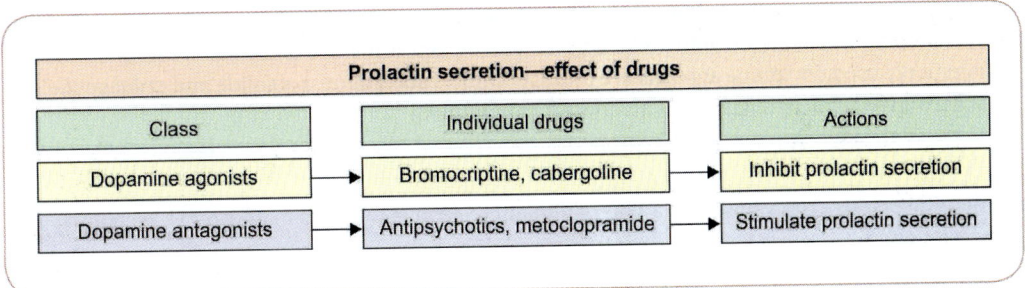

Figure 4: Prolactin secretion—effect of dopaminergic drugs

Physiological Functions of Prolactin

Prolactin stimulates growth and differentiation of ductal and alveolar epithelial cells in the breast and causes milk production.

Prolactin levels are low in nonpregnant females. During pregnancy, serum prolactin levels start increasing from 8th week of gestation and peaks at delivery. Thereafter, high levels are maintained by suckling during breast-feeding.

If breastfeeding is not initiated or is stopped, serum prolactin levels gradually decline to nonpregnant levels.

High prolactin levels during breast-feeding ensures natural contraception to the lactating mothers (Figure 5).

High prolactin levels (during lactation) causes natural contraception
• Suckling in lactating mothers leads to an increased prolactin secretion. • Prolactin inhibits GnRH release and causes an inhibition of hypothalamic-pituitary-gonadal axis. • Decreased GnRH leads to decreased levels of gonadotropins (FSH & LH). • Ovulation (Ovarian function) is inhibited, and this results in infertility. **Suckling therefore, provides natural contraception to the breast-feeding mothers. Once, breast-feeding is stopped, prolactin levels return to normal and fertility is restored.**

Figure 5: Effect of prolactin levels on fertility

Hyperprolactinemia

It is a relatively common endocrine disorder that may result from pituitary or hypothalamic disease. The common causes of hyperprolactinemia include:

○ **Pituitary tumors**
  ❑ Prolactin secreting adenomas are the most common
  ❑ Treated by pituitary surgery, irradiation and/or drugs (Somatostatin analogues e.g. (Octreotide & lanreotide) and pegvisomant.

○ **Dopamine antagonists**
  ❑ Common dopamine antagonist drugs include antipsychotics (Chlorpromazine, haloperidol etc.) and metoclopramide.

The clinical features of hyperprolactinemia include galactorrhea, amenorrhea and infertility in females. It may cause erectile dysfunction, loss of libido and infertility in males.

Hyperprolactinemia is commonly treated by dopamine agonists such as bromocriptine and cabergoline.

Dopamine Agonists

Dopamine agonists functionally behave as prolactin secretion inhibitors. Hence, they are used to treat hyperprolactinemia. They decrease both prolactin secretion as well as the size of the adenoma.

The commonly used dopamine agonists are bromocriptine, cabergoline, pergolide and quinagolide. The first 3 are ergot derivatives while quinagolide is a nonergot compound.

Bromocriptine

It is a semisynthetic ergot derivative. It is a potent dopamine agonist that acts mainly on D_2 receptors, to inhibit prolactin secretion.

Pharmacological Actions

The pharmacological actions of bromocriptine are mentioned in Table 4.

TABLE 4	Pharmacological actions of bromocriptine	
Endocrinal	**Neurological**	**Others**
Decrease in prolactin secretion • Dopamine inhibits prolactin secretion. Hence, bromocriptine (being a dopamine agonist) inhibits prolactin secretion. It is the 1st line treatment for hyperprolactinemia.	**Antiparkinsonian effect** • Bromocriptine, in higher doses (than used for endocrinal uses) is used in the treatment of Parkinson's disease. • It used in combination with levodopa therapy.	**CTZ stimulation** • Bromocriptine may cause nausea and vomiting because of stimulation of dopaminergic receptors in the chemoreceptor trigger zone (CTZ).
Decrease in GH levels • Bromocriptine decreases GH levels in patients with acromegaly.		**Weak α-blocking activity** • Hypotension may occur due to this effect.

Pharmacokinetics

Bromocriptine is well absorbed orally; however, the bioavailability is only ~7% due to high first-pass metabolism in the liver. It has a short half-life (3–6 hours); hence, it needs to be given multiple times in a day.

Adverse Effects

The key adverse effects include the following:
○ Gastrointestinal system—nausea, vomiting, constipation, abdominal pain
○ Cardiovascular system—postural hypotension, nasal blockade, digital vasospasm
○ Central nervous system—headache, hallucinations, insomnia, psychosis

Clinical Uses

Bromocriptine is mainly used in the treatment of hyperprolactinemia, acromegaly and Parkinson's disease.

Cabergoline

○ It is an ergot derivative. It has a longer half-life (~65 hours) with a higher affinity and greater selectivity for D_2 receptors, as compared to bromocriptine.
○ It causes less nausea, and leads to better patient compliance, due to twice weekly dosing requirement.
○ At higher doses required for Parkinson's disease, it may cause valvular heart disease.
○ It is being used in the treatment of hyperprolactinemia and acromegaly.

Gonadotropins (FSH & LH) & Human Chorionic Gonadotropin (HCG)

Follicle Stimulating Hormone (FSH) & Luteinizing Hormone (LH)

The anterior pituitary secretes 2 gonadotropins: Follicle stimulating hormone (FSH) and luteinizing hormone (LH).

The functions of FSH and LH are mentioned in Table 5.

TABLE 5	Functions of gonadotropins (FSH & LH)
Follicle stimulating hormone (FSH)	**Luteinizing hormone (LH)**
In females • Stimulate follicle development (in the ovaries). • Stimulate estrogen production (in the ovaries).	**In females** • Induce ovulation (in the ovaries). • Stimulate estrogen production (in the ovaries). • Stimulate progesterone production (by corpus luteum in the ovaries).

Contd...

Follicle stimulating hormone (FSH)	Luteinizing hormone (LH)
In males • Stimulate and maintain spermatogenesis in Sertoli cells (of testes). • Increase production of androgen binding protein (ABP) by the Sertoli cells. This maintains high concentration of testosterone near the sperm. • Convert testosterone to estrogen in Sertoli cells.	**In males** • Production of testosterone by the interstitial Leydig cells (of the testes).

The available preparations of FSH and LH are mentioned below:
- FSH
  - Urofollitropin
  - Follitropin alfa & Follitropin beta (recombinant forms)
- LH—Lutropin alfa (recombinant form)

Human Chorionic Gonadotropin (hCG)

Human chorionic gonadotropin is secreted by the placenta during pregnancy. Its main action is to maintain corpus luteum during initial phase of pregnancy. This allows corpus luteum to secrete progesterone which maintains the growing fetus.

The hCG initially was obtained from the urine of pregnant females. A recombinant form of hCG is now available i.e. choriogonadotropin alfa.

Adverse Effects of Gonadotropins

The adverse effects of gonadotropins in females include ovarian hyperstimulation syndrome and multiple pregnancies. The adverse effects in males include gynecomastia.

Clinical Uses of Gonadotropins

Gonadotropins are used to induce ovulation in females who are anovulatory secondary to hypogonadotropic hypogonadism or polycystic ovarian syndrome.

However, clomiphene is preferred, and gonadotropins are reserved for patients who do not respond to clomiphene therapy.

Gonadotropins are used in hypogonadal infertile males to stimulate sperm production.

Although the signs of hypogonadism (e.g. delayed puberty, decreased secondary sex characteristics) can be treated with testosterone provided from outside, however sperm production and infertility cannot be treated by testosterone. The sperm production and treatment of infertility requires the activity of both FSH and LH. This is achieved by injecting hCG in hypogonadal men.

Gonadorelin (Synthetic GnRH)

It is a synthetic human GnRH. It has a very short plasma half-life (~4 minutes) and is given IV or SC.

Pulsatile administration of gonadorelin results in an increased FSH & LH release from the anterior pituitary. This results in an increased synthesis of estrogen, progesterone and testosterone.

GnRH Agonist Analogues (Goserelin, Buserelin, Nafarelin, Leuprolide)

Several GnRH agonists have been developed. These GnRH agonists have the following advantages over gonadorelin:
- Longer duration of action
- Increased potency
- Can be given IM, SC or as a nasal spray (nafarelin)

Pharmacological Actions

The actions of gonadorelin and GnRH agonists vary when they are administered continuously vs. when they are administered in a pulsatile manner (Figure 6).

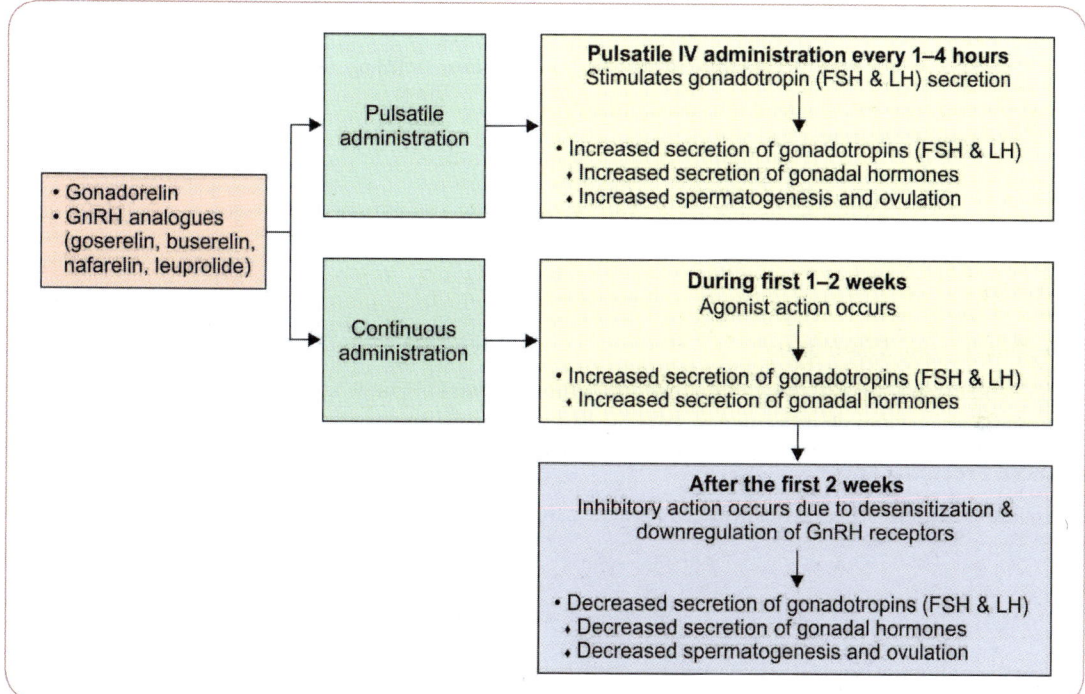

Figure 6: Pharmacological actions of gonadorelin and GnRH analogues

Clinical Uses

The GnRH agonist analogues are mostly used for suppression of gonadotropin release.

By decreasing gonadotropin levels and the levels of gonadal hormones in both males and females, the GnRH agonists brings about a state of reversible virtual orchiectomy or oophorectomy.

Hence, they are used in the following clinical conditions:

- **Prostate cancer:** Combined antiandrogen therapy with the following drugs is recommended:
  - Continuous GnRH agonist therapy + Androgen receptor blocker (e.g. flutamide, bicalutamide)

  The GnRH agonist used is one of the long-acting depot formulations.

  The GnRH agonist decrease the secretion of gonadotropins and hence, decrease testosterone levels. As prostate cancer is testosterone dependent, decrease in testosterone levels slows the growth and spread of cancer. Androgen receptor blocker is combined to block disease flare-up in the initial stages, as testosterone levels initially increases with GnRH therapy.

- **Precocious puberty:** Continuous GnRH agonist therapy is indicated for central precocious puberty. The treatment is continued up to the age of 11 years in females and 12 years in males.

  The advantage obtained is due to a decrease in gonadotropin (FSH & LH) levels in both males and females resulting in a decrease in the levels of gonadal hormones (estrogen, progesterone and testosterone).

- **Endometriosis and uterine fibroids**
- **Controlled ovarian stimulation in assisted reproductive techniques**
- **Breast and ovarian cancers**

GnRH Antagonist Analogues (Ganirelix, Cetrorelix, Abarelix, Degarelix)

The GnRH antagonists competitively block GnRH receptors in the anterior pituitary. This results in a decrease in gonadotropin (FSH & LH) levels and subsequently, a decrease in the level of gonadal hormones.

The advantages of GnRH antagonist over GnRH agonist analogues are mentioned in Figure 7.

Advantages of GnRH antagonists over GnRH agonists
• Initial increase in FSH/LH/Gonadal hormones do not occur
• Immediate onset of action
• More complete suppression of LH secretion is achieved

Figure 7: Advantages of GnRH antagonist over GnRH agonist analogues

Clinical Uses

Controlled Ovarian Stimulation

Ganirelix and cetrorelix are used for this indication as they suppress LH surge and estrogen production in females. Thus, premature ovulation is prevented.

Advanced Prostate Cancer

Degarelix and abarelix are used in advanced prostate cancer as they suppress testosterone production in males.

ASSESS YOURSELF (Examination Questions of Various Universities)

1. Mention three therapeutic uses and adverse effects of octreotide. Mention the advantages of octreotide over somatostatin.
2. Discuss the drugs used in the treatment of acromegaly.
3. Write short notes on:
   a. GnRH analogues
   b. Bromocriptine
   c. Somatostatin and its analogues
4. Explain why continuous GnRH agonists are used in the treatment of precocious puberty in both boys and girls.

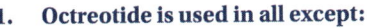

MULTIPLE CHOICE QUESTIONS

1. Octreotide is used in all except:
   (AIIMS May 2011)
   a. Glucagonoma
   b. Insulinoma
   c. Carcinoid syndrome
   d. Glioma
2. Which of the following statements about octreotide is true? *(AIIMS Nov 2011)*
   a. Stimulates growth hormone
   b. Used in secretory diarrhea
   c. Used orally
   d. Contraindicated in acromegaly
3. Cabergoline is used in *(Recent Question 2016)*
   a. Acromegaly
   b. Hyperprolactinoma
   c. Both a and b
   d. None of the above
4. Pegvisomant is a: *(Recent Question 2016)*
   a. Growth hormone receptor agonist
   b. Growth hormone receptor antagonist
   c. GnRH agonist
   d. GnRH analogue
5. Drug of choice for esophageal varices
   (Recent Question 2016)
   a. Demeclocycline
   b. Dopamine
   c. Octreotide
   d. Adrenaline

6. Treatment for acromegaly
   (Recent Question 2016)
   a. Octreotide
   b. Sermorelin
   c. Hexarelin
   d. Nafarelin
7. In hyperprolactinoma, which drug is used for controlling lactation *(APPG 2010)*
   a. Danazol
   b. Clomiphene citrate
   c. Stilbestrol
   d. Bromocriptine
8. GnRH analogue used in hormonal treatment of carcinoma prostate? *(MHCET 2007)*
   a. Goserelin
   b. Nilutamide
   c. Cyproterone acetate
   d. Finasteride
9. Which of the following is given at intervals as a pulsatile therapy? *(MHCET 2007)*
   a. GnRH
   b. GH
   c. PSH
   d. Estrogen

Ans.											
1.	(d)	2.	(b)	3.	(c)	4.	(c, d)	5.	(c)	6.	(a)
7.	(d)	8.	(a)	9.	(a)						

36

Corticosteroids

Corticosteroids are hormones that are released from the adrenal gland. The term corticosteroids refer to both glucocorticoids and mineralocorticoids.

The adrenal gland consists of an outer cortex and an inner medulla that secrete different hormones (Figure 1).

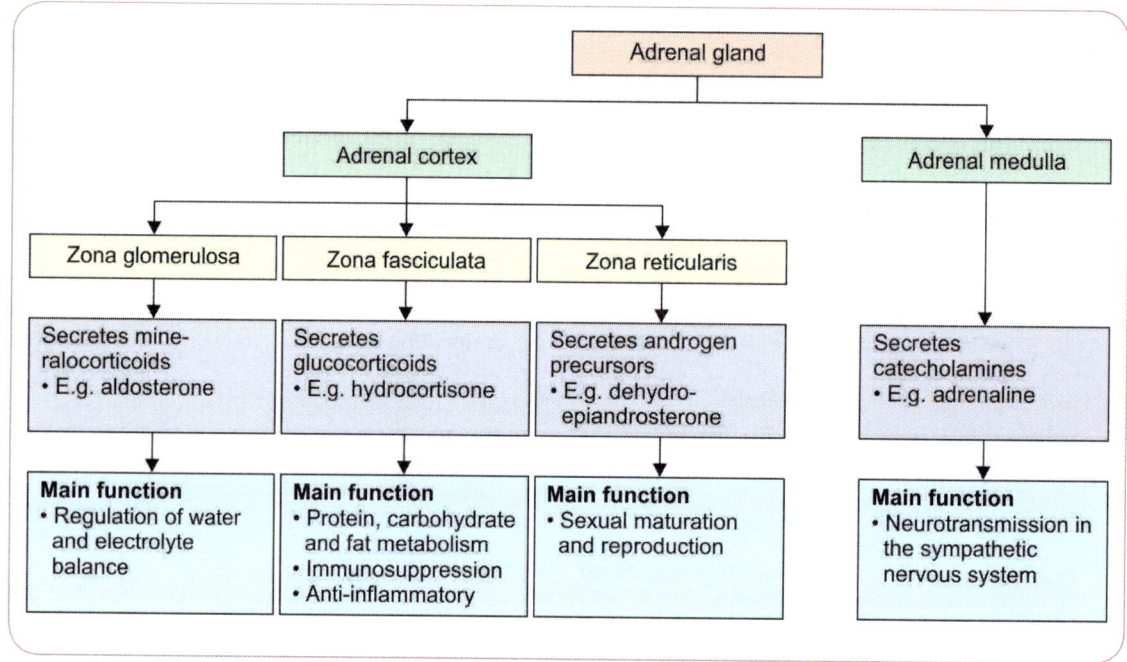

Figure 1: Adrenal gland hormones

The deficiency or excess of adrenocortical hormones can result in the following disease conditions:
- ○ Chronic deficiency of adrenocortical hormones → Addison's disease
- ○ Hypersecretion of mineralocorticoids → Conn's syndrome (Primary hyperaldosteronism)
- ○ Hypersecretion of glucocorticoids → Cushing's syndrome
- ○ Hypersecretion of androgens → Adrenogenital syndrome (Precocious puberty)

BIOSYNTHESIS OF ADRENOCORTICAL HORMONES

The adrenocortical hormones are synthesized from cholesterol in the adrenal cortex. The key steps are mentioned in Figure 2.

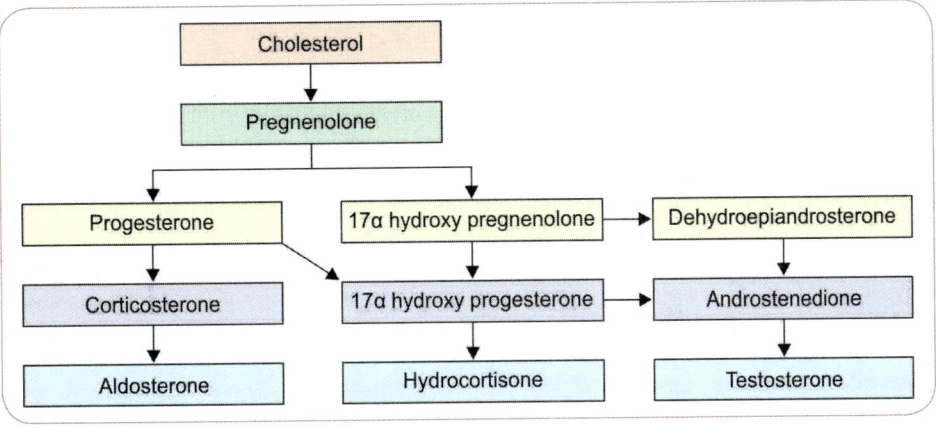

Figure 2: Key steps in biosynthesis of adrenocortical hormones

CLASSIFICATION AND COMPARATIVE EFFICACY OF CORTICOSTEROIDS

The comparison of the relative activity of various corticosteroids is presented in Figure 3.

Glucocorticoids		
Anti-inflammatory activity	Salt-retaining activity	Clinical features
Short acting (8–12 hours)		
Hydrocortisone (Cortisol) — 1	1	Rapid acting; short duration of action. Preferred drug for replacement therapy in adrenal insufficiency. Also used in status asthmaticus and shock
Cortisone — 0.8	0.8	Cortisone is inactive and gets converted to active hydrocortisone in the liver; rarely used now
Intermediate acting (12–36 hours)		
Prednisolone — 4	0.8	Commonly used in allergic, inflammatory & autoimmune disorders. Causes lesser HPA axis suppression by a single morning dose
Methylprednisolone — 5	0.5	Useful as a retention enema in ulcerative colitis. Useful as high dose pulse therapy in acute RA, renal transplant etc.
Triamcinolone — 5	0	Commonly used in skin conditions (eczema, psoriasis etc.), arthritis etc.

Contd...

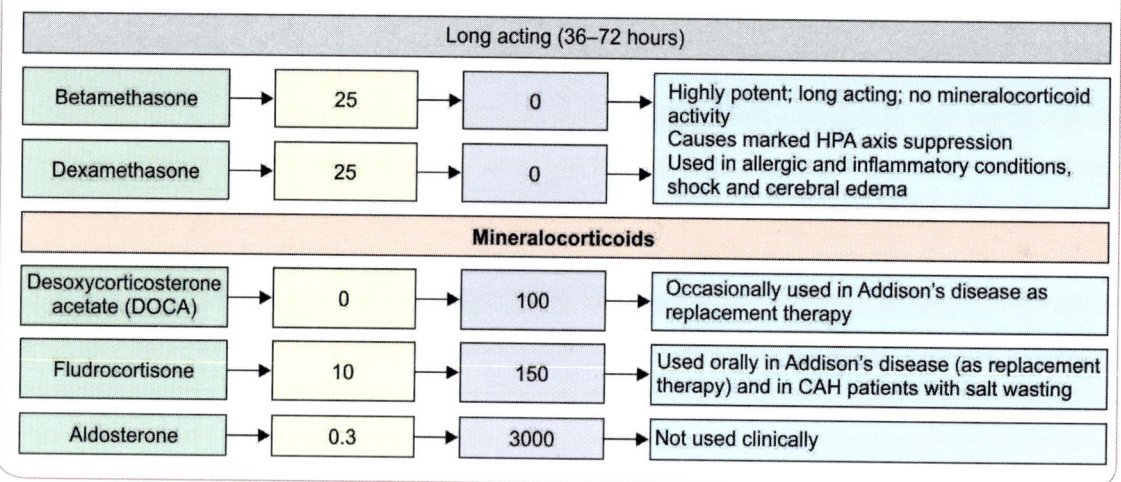

Long acting (36–72 hours)			
Betamethasone	25	0	Highly potent; long acting; no mineralocorticoid activity Causes marked HPA axis suppression Used in allergic and inflammatory conditions, shock and cerebral edema
Dexamethasone	25	0	
Mineralocorticoids			
Desoxycorticosterone acetate (DOCA)	0	100	Occasionally used in Addison's disease as replacement therapy
Fludrocortisone	10	150	Used orally in Addison's disease (as replacement therapy) and in CAH patients with salt wasting
Aldosterone	0.3	3000	Not used clinically

Figure 3: Comparative presentation of corticosteroids (Hydrocortisone taken as standard)

REGULATION OF BIOSYNTHESIS OF CORTICOSTEROIDS

The synthesis and release of glucocorticoids (by the adrenal cortex) is stimulated by ACTH (adrenocorticotropic hormone), which is produced by the anterior pituitary gland.

The synthesis and release of ACTH is stimulated by CRH (corticotropin releasing hormone), which is produced by the hypothalamus (Figure 4).

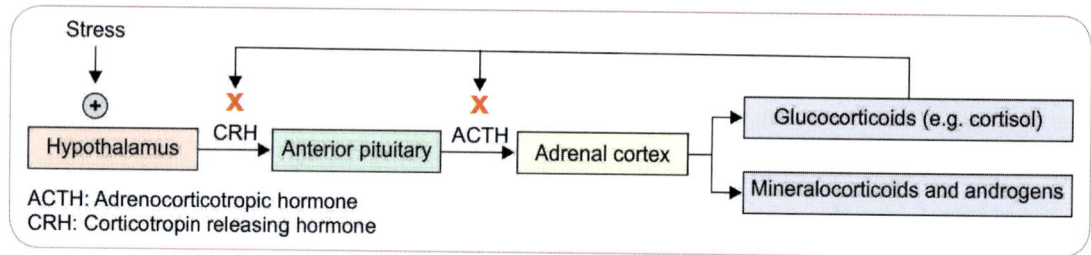

Figure 4: Regulation of glucocorticoid synthesis

The release of mineralocorticoids is controlled by the renin angiotensin system (Figure 5).

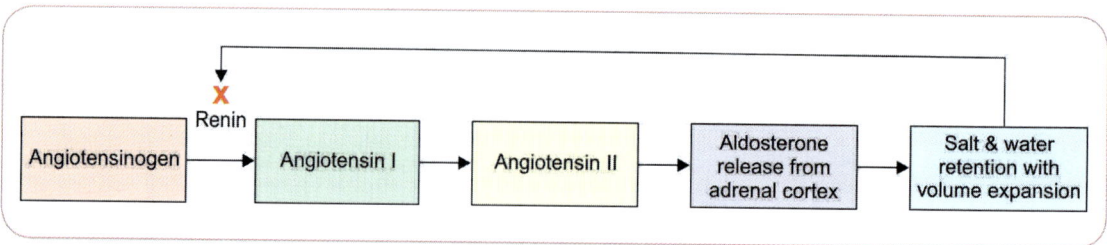

Figure 5: Regulation of mineralocorticoid synthesis

Mechanism of Action

Corticosteroids enter the cells and binds to the cytoplasmic glucocorticoid receptor.

The glucocorticoid-receptor complex then enters the nucleus and binds to the glucocorticoid response elements on the DNA. This leads to RNA transcription and regulation of protein synthesis resulting in manifestations of the physiological effects.

Pharmacological Actions

The actions of corticosteroids can be of two types:
- **Glucocorticoid** → Actions on carbohydrate, fat, and protein metabolism and other related activities
- **Mineralocorticoid** → Actions on Na^+, K^+ and water balance

The relative glucocorticoid and mineralocorticoid activities differ across various corticosteroids—e.g. hydrocortisone (cortisol) has both glucocorticoid and mineralocorticoid activities whereas dexamethasone has selective glucocorticoid effects.

The key actions of corticosteroids are mentioned in Table 1.

TABLE 1	Pharmacological actions of corticosteroids

Anti-inflammatory effects

Glucocorticoids suppress the inflammatory responses in the body.
The following factors contribute to the anti-inflammatory effects of glucocorticoids:
- Reduced production of prostaglandins and leukotrienes by inhibition of phospholipase A_2
- Reduced production of proinflammatory mediators such as IL-1, IL-6, TNF-α
- Reduced ability of macrophages and leukocytes to respond to antigens
- Decrease in the number of lymphocytes, eosinophils and basophils
- Stabilization of the basement membranes of mast cells and basophils → reduced release of inflammatory mediators such as histamine

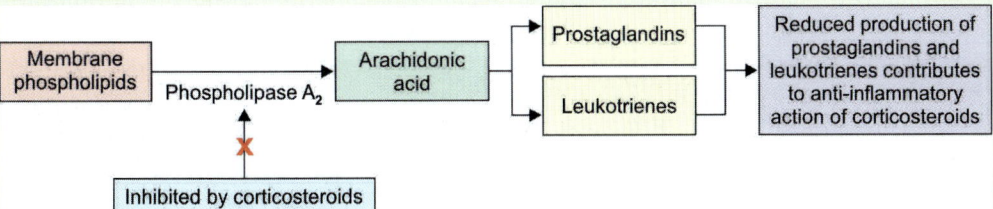

Immunosuppressant effects

Glucocorticoids have prominent immunosuppressant effects. The following factors contribute to the immunosuppressant effects of glucocorticoids:
- Suppression of T lymphocytes → impairment of cell mediated immunity
- Suppression of B lymphocytes → impairment of humoral immunity

They also inhibit the release of cytokines such as IL-1 and IL-2. All type of hypersensitivity and allergic reactions are suppressed by glucocorticoids.

Metabolic effects—Carbohydrate metabolism

- Promote glycogen deposition in liver
- Promote gluconeogenesis
- Decrease peripheral utilization of glucose

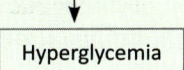

Hence, diabetes may be aggravated; hence, steroid use is considered a relative contraindication.

Contd...

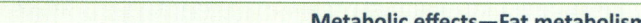

SECTION H ■ Drugs Acting on the Endocrine Physiology

Metabolic effects—Fat metabolism
• Permissive effect leading to lipolysis • Redistribution of body fat leading to increase fat over neck, shoulder, face (resulting in moon face or buffalo hump) and loss of fat in the limbs

Metabolic effects—Protein metabolism
• Catabolic action leading to protein breakdown • Muscle wasting, skin thinning, growth retardation, impaired wound healing

Effects on calcium and bones
• Decrease calcium absorption from the GIT • Increase calcium excretion in the urine • Increase activity of osteoclasts (cells involved in bone resorption) • Decrease activity of osteoblasts (cells involved in bone formation) ↓ Reduced calcium levels may lead to osteoporosis, bone fractures

Cardiovascular effects
• Retain sodium and water • Permissive effect on actions of adrenaline and angiotensin II • Results in hypertension and exacerbation of heart failure

Effects on skeletal muscles
• Steroids are required for normal skeletal muscle activity • Muscle weakness and fatigue are observed in both hyper- and hypocorticism

Hypercorticism	Hypocorticism
↑ Mineralocorticoids → Hypokalemia ↑ Glucocorticoids → Muscle wasting	Mainly due to hypodynamic circulation

Gastrointestinal effects
• Inhibition of prostaglandins results in increased secretion of gastric acid and pepsin → Aggravation of peptic ulcer can result

Hematologic and lymphoid effects
• Increase in RBC, neutrophils and platelets in the blood • Decrease in lymphocytes, eosinophils, monocytes and basophils

CNS effects
• Sense of wellbeing, mood elevation, euphoria, insomnia

Water and electrolyte metabolism
The mineralocorticoid actions include: • Retention of Na^+ and water • Excretion of K^+ and H^+ • Metabolic alkalosis

Adverse Effects of Corticosteroids

Corticosteroids are frequently used in life threatening conditions and hence, the benefit-risk balance of the drug should be carefully considered.

The incidence of the usual adverse effects including suppression of the hypothalamic-pituitary-adrenal (HPA) axis is generally related to factors such as relative strength of the drug, dosage, duration of therapy, time of administration etc.

A single dose of glucocorticoids is practically without significant adverse effects. A short course of therapy (up to 1 week) is unlikely to have significant adverse effects, if there are no specific contraindications.

An increase in duration of glucocorticoid therapy beyond 1 week can have time and dose dependent increases in the incidence of adverse effects that may be disabling and potentially fatal.

The key adverse effects of corticosteroids are mentioned in Figure 6.

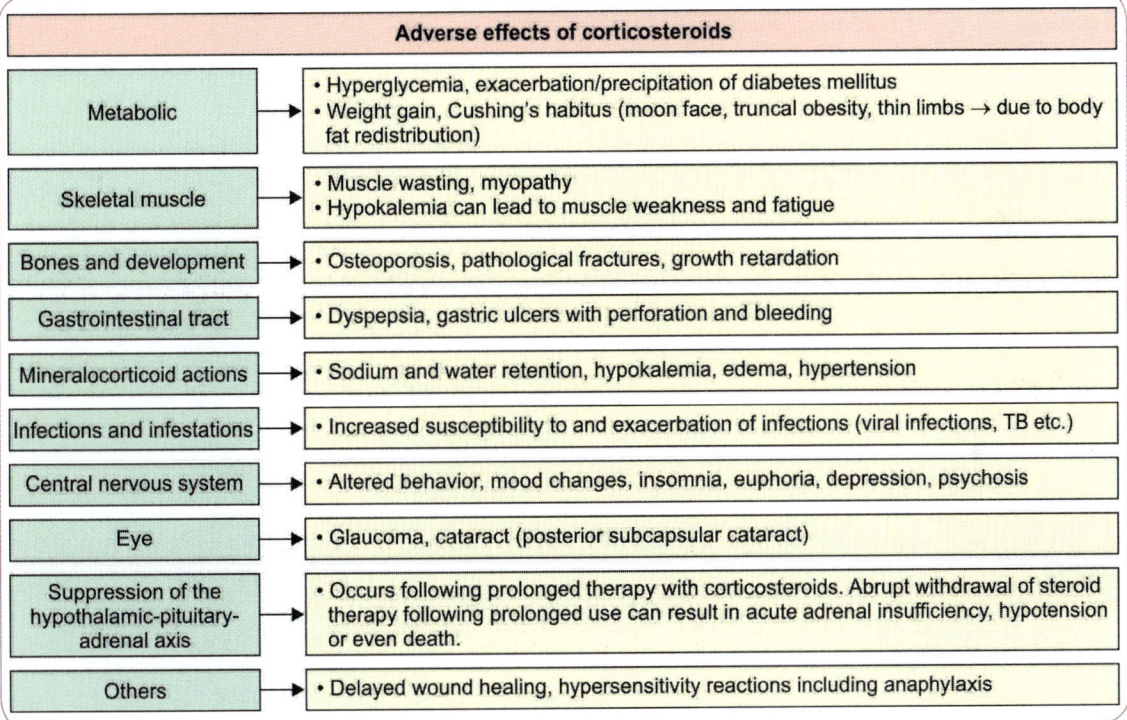

Figure 6: Adverse effects of corticosteroids

Suppression of the Hypothalamic-pituitary-adrenal (HPA) Axis

The suppression of HPA axis is observed following prolonged therapy with corticosteroids. Abrupt withdrawal of steroid therapy following prolonged use can result in steroid withdrawal syndrome and acute adrenal insufficiency (Figure 7).

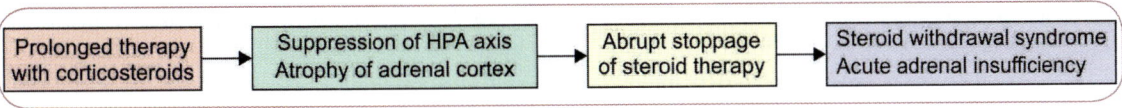

Figure 7: Suppression of hypothalamic-pituitary-adrenal (HPA) axis

Steroid withdrawal syndrome manifests with fever, malaise, postural hypotension and reactivation/flare up of the underlying disease.

Acute adrenal insufficiency is a potentially fatal condition and can be precipitated if such patients are subjected to stress. The clinical manifestations of acute adrenal insufficiency include nausea, vomiting, dehydration, hyponatremia, hyperkalemia and hypotension.

The following measures should be considered during long-term steroid therapy:
- If possible, topical therapy should be preferred over systemic therapy
- If possible, therapy with short-acting steroids should be administered
- Single morning dose therapy is preferable
- Gradual withdrawal or tapering of steroid therapy should be done in patients on prolonged therapy.

Clinical Uses

The corticosteroids are used either as replacement therapy in deficiency states (endocrine uses) or as pharmacotherapy in a variety of conditions (nonendocrine uses).

Replacement Therapy (Endocrine Uses)

The corticosteroids are used as replacement therapy in deficiency states such as acute adrenal deficiency, chronic adrenal insufficiency and congenital adrenal hyperplasia (Table 2).

TABLE 2 Glucocorticoids: Replacement therapy		
Acute adrenal insufficiency	**Chronic adrenal insufficiency (Addison's disease)**	**Congenital adrenal hyperplasia (Adrenogenital syndrome, CAH)**
• Is a medical emergency	• Hydrocortisone given orally is the most commonly used drug	• Due to genetic deficiency of steroidal enzyme (usually 21-hydroxylase)
• Treated with IV hydrocortisone + NaCl + 5% glucose	• 2/3 of hydrocortisone dose is given in the morning and 1/3 in the evening (mimics normal diurnal variation) along with adequate salt and water	• In CAH, steroid synthesis decreases, ACTH increases, leading to excess androgen production
• Precipitating cause e.g. trauma, infection, hemorrhage must be treated	• Fludrocortisone may be added, as required	• Steroids when given, suppress ACTH secretion and androgen production
• After stabilization, the patient is treated like chronic adrenal insufficiency		• Hydrocortisone is usually given, fludrocortisone may be added, as required

Pharmacotherapy (Nonendocrine Uses)

Glucocorticoids are used in a variety of clinical conditions. Their benefits are mainly due to anti-inflammatory and immunosuppressive actions.

They frequently produce a dramatic improvement in symptoms in many severe diseases. On the flip side, they have the potential of causing a large number of adverse effects; hence, steroids should be prescribed only after carefully considering the benefits and risks in each patient. The following principles should be considered:

- Short courses of steroids (up to 1 week) are not likely to be harmful in the absence of contraindications.
- When the duration of therapy is beyond 1 week, there is a significant increase in the incidence of severe and potentially lethal adverse effects.
- The dose is determined by severity of the disease:
  - Severe disease: Start with a high dose and then reduce gradually
  - Mild disease: Start with a low dose and then increase gradually
- Steroids should be given for the shortest duration and in the lowest dose possible.
- Abrupt withdrawal of steroids after prolonged therapy should not be done, as it may lead to adrenal insufficiency.
- Local therapy is to be administered wherever possible.

The glucocorticoids are frequently used in the following conditions:

Rheumatoid Arthritis

Although glucocorticoids produce marked symptomatic relief, they are not routinely used. Their use is considered only in the following scenarios:

- In severe disease which fails to respond to 1st line therapies such as NSAIDs and physiotherapy. Even in this situation, they are used only to provide temporary relief until the effect of other slower acting drugs (e.g. methotrexate) becomes evident.
- Intra-articular injections are administered if only 1 or 2 joints are involved.

Osteoarthritis

Osteoarthritis is a noninflammatory degenerative joint disease. It is mainly treated with NSAIDs.

Systemic glucocorticoids are not used. However, intra-articular steroid injections may be used in acute flare-up. The main problem with repeated intra-articular steroid injections is that there may be painless destruction of the joints.

Rheumatic Fever

Aspirin is the mainstay of therapy in rheumatic fever. Glucocorticoids are only used in severe cases (i.e. with CHF and carditis) because they produce more rapid symptomatic relief than aspirin. Prednisolone and aspirin are initiated together. After the control of symptoms, prednisolone is tapered off while aspirin is continued.

Gout

Glucocorticoids are the reserve drugs for acute gout. They are used only when the disease is not controlled by NSAIDs.

Collagen Disorders

Collagen diseases such as polyarteritis nodosa, systemic lupus erythematosus, dermatomyositis, glomerulonephritis etc. require large doses of glucocorticoids for their control. After remission is achieved, the dose is then tapered down to maintenance doses.

Allergic Disorders

Allergic diseases such as anaphylaxis and angioneurotic edema require drugs which act immediately. Hence, epinephrine is preferred, as glucocorticoids take 1-2 hours to act.

Glucocorticoids may be used in allergic diseases such as drug reactions, contact dermatitis, serum sickness, urticaria etc.

Bronchial Asthma

Glucocorticoids provide relief by their anti-inflammatory action on the hyperreactive airways in bronchial asthma.

In acute severe asthma, IV glucocorticoids are administered. In less severe asthma, oral glucocorticoids are administered.

In chronic asthma, inhalational steroids (such as beclomethasone, budesonide, fluticasone, triamcinolone etc.) are preferred because the systemic uptake and adverse effects are minimized.

Infectious Diseases

Although the use of immunosuppressive steroids in infectious diseases appear contradictory, there are a few situations where glucocorticoids are indicated.

One classic example is its use in *Pneumocystis carinii* pneumonia in AIDS patients. Adding a steroid to antibiotics increase oxygenation and decrease the chances of respiratory failure. In another example, steroids decrease the incidence of neurological damage in *Haemophilus influenzae* meningitis in infants.

Ocular Diseases

Glucocorticoids are used to suppress inflammation in the eye in inflammatory conditions such as keratitis, iridocyclitis etc. They help to preserve vision. They may be used topically, systemically or by intraocular injection.

Steroids are contraindicated in herpes simplex keratitis (may cause irreversible corneal opacity) and ocular injuries (may delay healing and promote development of infection).

Skin Diseases

Glucocorticoids are used in several inflammatory skin conditions. Topical steroids are used in many eczematous conditions. Systemic steroids are required in severe conditions such as pemphigus vulgaris, Stevens-Johnson syndrome, exfoliative dermatitis etc. Intralesional steroids are used in keloids, hypertrophic scars etc.

Intestinal Diseases

Glucocorticoids are used in inflammatory bowel diseases such as ulcerative colitis and Crohn's disease.

Steroids are used in acute flare-ups of the disease when it is not controlled by conservative treatment (diet and sulfasalazine). They may be given orally or by retention enemas.

Renal Diseases

Glucocorticoids are the first-line therapy in nephrotic syndrome (secondary to minimal change disease). They are used in both children and adults.

Cerebral Edema

Glucocorticoids are effective in treating or preventing cerebral edema associated with tumors, tubercular meningitis and neurocysticercosis.

Glucocorticoids are not effective in the treatment of cerebral edema associated with trauma or cerebrovascular accidents (poststroke).

The steroid which does not have salt and water retaining property is preferred (e.g. dexamethasone).

Autoimmune Diseases

Glucocorticoids are used in diseases such as autoimmune hemolytic anemia, idiopathic thrombocytopenia and chronic active hepatitis.

Organ Transplantation

Glucocorticoids in high doses are used to prevent graft rejection. They are used along with other immunosuppressive drugs. The doses are subsequently tapered to maintenance doses.

Malignancies

Glucocorticoids have antilympholytic effects. Hence, they are used (in combination with other chemotherapeutic drugs) for the treatment of acute lymphocytic leukemias, Hodgkin's and other lymphomas.

Hypercalcemia

Hypercalcemia of sarcoidosis, vitamin D intoxication and malignancy responds to prednisolone.

Shock

Glucocorticoids may be used in septic shock when blood pressure does not respond effectively to fluids and vasopressors.

Testing of adrenal-pituitary axis function

Relative Contraindications of Corticosteroids

The following conditions are worsened using steroids. In general, no contraindications are applicable in situations where steroids may be used for life-saving measures. Hence, these can be considered as relative contraindications (Table 3).

TABLE 3	Corticosteroids: Relative contraindications	
• Peptic ulcer	• Psychosis	
• Hypertension	• Epilepsy	
• Diabetes mellitus	• Renal failure	
• Osteoporosis	• Congestive heart failure	
• Tuberculosis	• Cataract	
• Herpes simplex keratitis		

INHALED CORTICOSTEROIDS

Asthma is an inflammatory disease and hence, corticosteroids are beneficial in asthma due to their anti-inflammatory action. Inhaled corticosteroids (ICS) do not have any bronchodilator action.

The ICS are indicated as a controller medication for regular, maintenance treatment of asthma.

The commonly used ICS are beclomethasone, budesonide, fluticasone, flunisolide and ciclesonide.

MECHANISM OF ACTION

The mechanism of action of corticosteroids in bronchial asthma is mentioned in Table 4.

TABLE 4	Mechanism of action of corticosteroids in bronchial asthma

Anti-inflammatory, anti-allergic action
- Suppress bronchial inflammation
- Reduce bronchial hyperreactivity
- Decrease mucosal edema
- Suppress inflammatory response to antigen-antibody reaction

- ICS have high topical activity and low systemic activity
- ICS decrease need for rescue medications, decrease asthma exacerbations and may influence airway modeling
- ICS have no role during acute exacerbation or in status asthmaticus
- Combination of ICS + LABA (long-acting β-adrenergic agonists) is advantageous because ICS potentiate the action of LABA and may also prevent the development of tolerance to LABA

Adverse Effects

- Local effects of ICS include dysphonia, hoarseness and oral candidiasis. These effects can be reduced or prevented by using a spacer or by doing post inhalation gargle with water.
- Use of ICS significantly decreases the incidence of adverse effects associated with systemic corticosteroids.
- Systemic adverse effects are dose related and can occur with oral or inhaled forms. Systemic adverse effects of inhaled corticosteroids are clinically relevant with doses >600 μg/day. They include mood changes, suppression of the adrenal-pituitary axis, osteoporosis, cataracts, skin atrophy, hyperphagia, hyperglycemia and bruising.

Fluticasone Propionate

- Negligible oral bioavailability—low propensity to cause systemic adverse effects.

Flunisolide

- Used for the prophylaxis and treatment of seasonal and perennial rhinitis.

Ciclesonide

- Prodrug that is converted to active form by esterases in bronchial epithelium.
- Improves topical: systemic activity ratio.

ASSESS YOURSELF (Examination Questions of Various Universities)

1. Classify glucocorticoids. Discuss the pharmacological actions of glucocorticoids.
2. Describe briefly with clinical significance pharmacological effects of glucocorticoids on cardiovascular and immune system.
3. Discuss the measures to minimize HPA axis suppression during chronic steroid therapy.
4. Why glucocorticoids should not be stopped abruptly after long-term administration.
5. Mention the management of acute and chronic adrenal insufficiency.
6. Write short notes on:
   a. Adverse effects of glucocorticoids
   b. Therapeutic uses of glucocorticoids
   c. Inhaled glucocorticoids

MULTIPLE CHOICE QUESTIONS

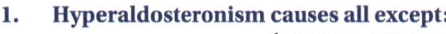

1. Hyperaldosteronism causes all except:
   (AI 2009, AIIMS May 2010)
   a. Hypernatremia
   b. Hypokalemia
   c. Hypertension
   d. Metabolic acidosis

2. Compared to hydrocortisone maximum glucocorticoid action is found in:
   (Recent Question 2016)
   a. Dexamethasone   b. Prednisolone
   c. Methyl prednisolone   d. Cortisone

3. Long-acting corticosteroid is:
   (Recent Question 2016)
   a. Triamcinolone   b. Betamethasone
   c. Hydrocortisone   d. Prednisolone

4. Drug of choice for acute adrenal insufficiency is:
   (Recent Question 2016)
   a. Oral prednisone   b. Hydrocortisone
   c. Betamethasone   d. Dexamethasone

5. Corticosteroid which is given by inhalation route:
   (Recent Question 2016)
   a. Prednisolone
   b. Beclomethasone
   c. Dexamethasone
   d. Hydrocortisone

6. Steroids are contraindicated in all except:
   (Recent Question 2016)
   a. Eczematous lesion
   b. Peptic ulcer
   c. Diabetes mellitus
   d. Herpes simplex keratitis

7. Glucocorticoids do not cause:
   (Recent Question 2016)
   a. Osteoporosis   b. Hypoglycemia
   c. Peptic ulceration   d. Cataracts

Ans.

| 1. | (d) | 2. | (a) | 3. | (b) | 4. | (b) | 5. | (b) | 6. | (a) |
| 7. | (b) | | | | | | | | | | |

37

Estrogens, Progesterones and Oral Contraceptives

ESTROGENS

Estrogen is the primary female sex hormone. It is produced by the ovary, adrenal gland and the placenta. The estrogens can be classified as natural and synthetic estrogens (Figure 1).

Natural estrogens comprise of estradiol or 17-β estradiol (E_2), estrone (E_1) and estriol (E_3).

Estradiol is the most potent estrogen.

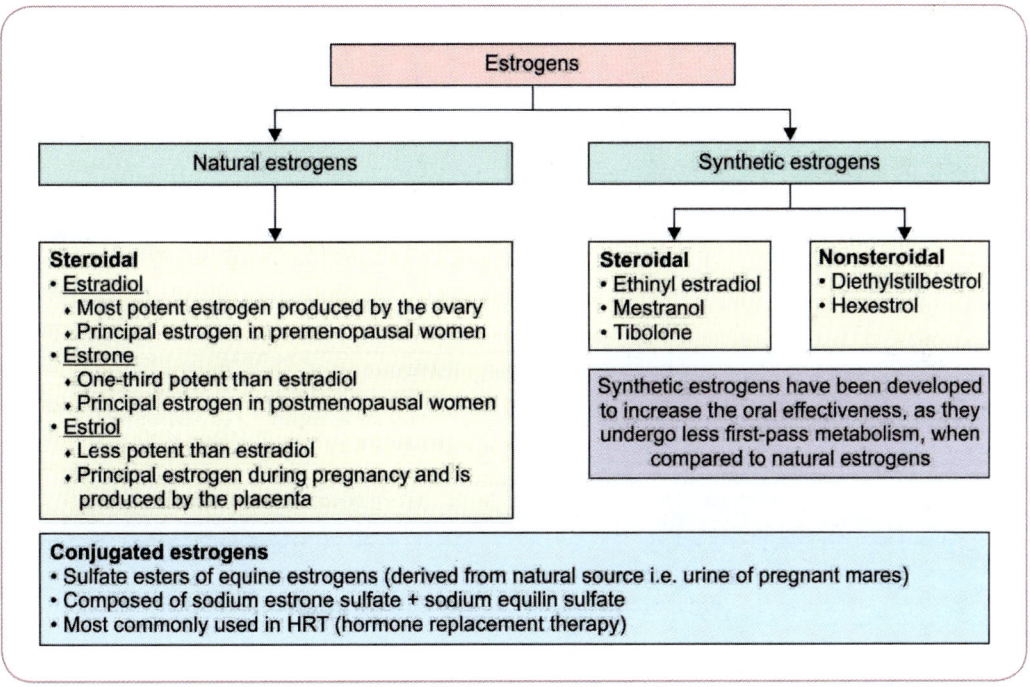

Figure 1: Classification of estrogens

Biosynthetic Pathway for Natural Estrogens

Steroidal estrogens are synthesized in the body from the precursors, androstenedione and/or testosterone (Figure 2).

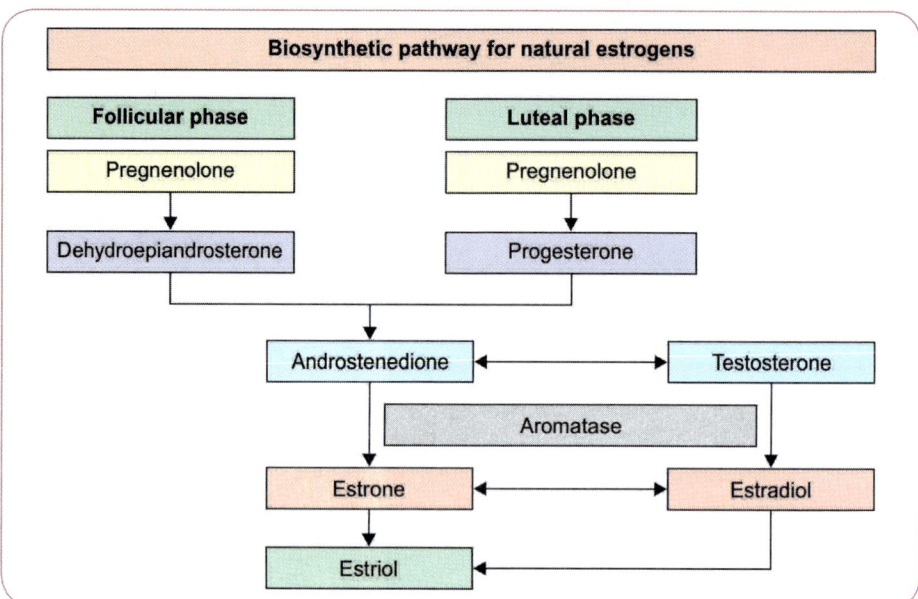

Figure 2: Biosynthetic pathway for natural estrogens

Mechanism of Action

Estrogens in the blood and interstitial fluid are bound to sex-hormone binding globulin (SHBG) and albumin.

They dissociate from their binding sites, cross the cell membrane, enter the nucleus and bind to their receptors known as estrogen receptors (ER) (Figure 3).

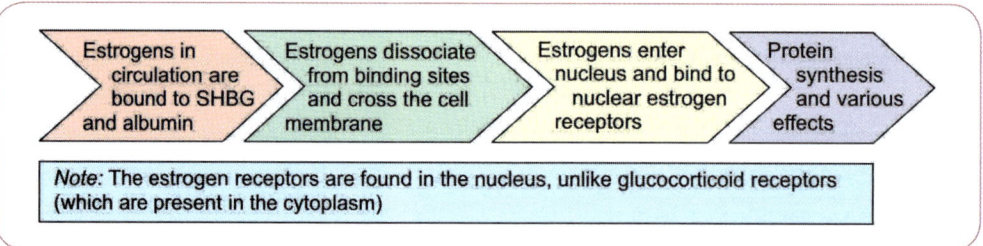

Figure 3: Mechanism of action of estrogens

There are 2 classes of nuclear estrogen receptors: ERα and ERβ.

Many tissues have both subtypes of estrogen receptors. However, the predominant location of individual subtype of receptors is mentioned in Figure 4.

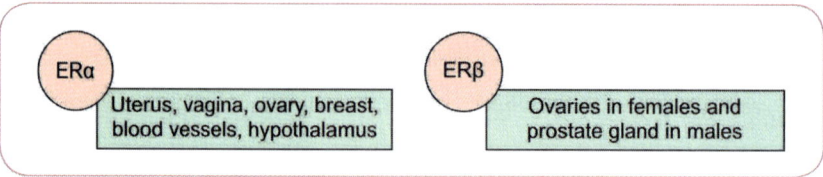

Figure 4: Types of estrogen receptors

Regulation of Secretion

The secretion of estrogen and progesterone from the ovary is regulated by:
o   Gonadotropins (FSH and LH) secreted by the anterior pituitary
o   Gonadotropin releasing hormone (GnRH) secreted by the hypothalamus

The estrogen and progesterone in turn regulates the secretion of FSH, LH and GnRH in a feedback mechanism as mentioned in Figure 5.

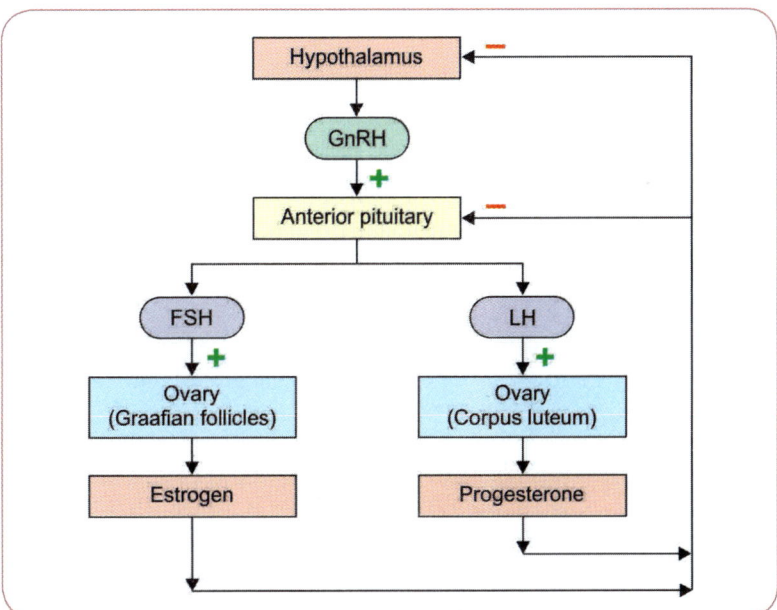

Figure 5: Regulation of secretion of estrogen and progesterone

Note:
o   The release of GnRH is intermittent; hence, the secretion of FSH and LH occurs in pulses.
o   The intermittent, pulsatile release of these hormones is necessary for the maintenance of a normal menstrual cycle. This is because a continuous external infusion of the GnRH leads to a stoppage of production of FSH/LH as well as estrogen/progesterone.
o   In the follicular (preovulatory) phase of the cycle, estrogen inhibits gonadotropin release from the pituitary (negative feedback).
o   In the mid-cycle, estrogen stimulates gonadotropin release from the pituitary (positive feedback) leading to the mid-cycle FSH/LH surge.

Pharmacokinetics

The estrogens are available as oral, parenteral, transdermal or topical formulations.

The estrogens are well absorbed orally, but natural estrogens are not active orally due to high first-pass metabolism in the liver.

Estradiol is converted into estrone which further changes to estriol.

The natural estrogens are metabolized by conjugation with glucuronic acid and sulfate. The metabolites are excreted in bile and urine.

In the intestine, the bacteria unconjugates (hydrolyzes) the conjugated estrogens; frees them so that they are again reabsorbed from the intestinal epithelium. This results in enterohepatic circulation of estrogens (Figure 6) and the final excretion occurs subsequently in urine.

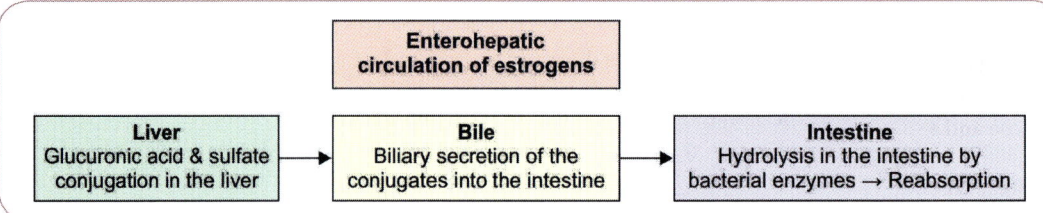

Figure 6: Enterohepatic circulation of estrogens

Pharmacological Actions

The pharmacological actions of estrogens are mentioned in Table 1.

TABLE 1	Pharmacological actions of estrogens
Sex organs	• **Growth and development of female sex organs** ▪ Vagina ▪ Uterus ▪ Fallopian tubes • **Development of secondary sexual characteristics** ▪ Growth of breasts (ductal and stromal growth) ▪ Axillary and pubic hair ▪ Body fat redistribution, leading to female body contour ▪ Increased bone growth and epiphyseal closure
Endometrium	• Growth/proliferation of uterine (endometrial) lining during 1st half (proliferative phase) of the menstrual cycle
Cervix	• Makes cervical secretions thin, watery and alkaline; hence, facilitates sperm penetration
Fallopian tubes and myometrium	• Induces rhythmic contractions of tubes and myometrium
Metabolic	• Decreases bone resorption by inhibiting osteoclasts • Increases HDL and triglyceride levels • Decreases LDL levels • Mild salt-water retention and edema
Coagulation	• Increases blood coagulation by an: ▪ Increase in clotting factors (II, VII, IX and X) ▪ Decrease in antithrombin III

Adverse Effects

The key adverse effects of estrogens are mentioned in Figure 7.

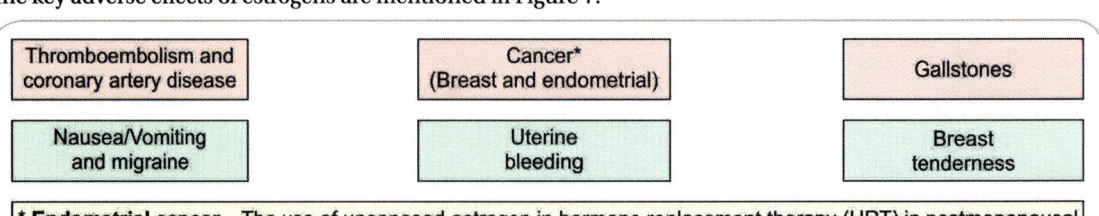

* **Endometrial cancer**—The use of unopposed estrogen in hormone replacement therapy (HRT) in postmenopausal women increases the risk of endometrial cancer by 5- to 15-fold. This risk is prevented if a progesterone is co-administered with estrogen. Hence, a progesterone is always given along with an estrogen for HRT.
* **Breast cancer**—Addition of progesterone to estrogen does not have a protective effect in breast cancer. Further studies are required to assess the association between progesterone use and breast cancer risk.
* **Adenocarcinoma of vagina and cervix**—This cancer has been reported with an increased incidence in young women whose mothers were treated with diethylstilbestrol during 1st trimester of pregnancy.

Figure 7: Adverse effects of estrogens

Clinical Uses

Estrogens are most commonly used as contraceptive therapy and postmenopausal hormone replacement therapy. The specific drugs and doses employed are different in each of these indications.

These and the other uses of estrogens are discussed below:

Contraceptive Therapy

- ○ Estrogens are used in combination with progestins for reversible suppression of fertility
- ○ Synthetic estrogens are most commonly used for this purpose
- ○ These are described later after the discussion on progestins

Postmenopausal Hormone Replacement Therapy (HRT)

At menopause, the ovarian function decreases. This leads to a decrease in the secretion of estrogen; hence, resulting in several medical problems in the female. Some of the key problems are mentioned in Table 2.

TABLE 2	Menopausal problems
Vasomotor instability	Hot flushes, night sweats, fainting
Urogenital atrophy	Vaginal atrophy, vaginal drying, vaginitis
Osteoporosis	Loss of osteoid and calcium, bone thinning, predisposition to fractures
Skin changes	Thinning, drying, loss of elasticity of skin
Cardiovascular changes	Increased risk of coronary artery disease, myocardial infarction and stroke
Cognitive changes	Depression, irritability, headache, anxiety

Postmenopausal HRT for women with an intact uterus should include a progestin along with an estrogen, to decrease the risk of estrogen related-endometrial cancer.

For hysterectomized women (i.e. where uterus has been removed), endometrial cancer is not a concern and estrogen alone is recommended (Figure 8).

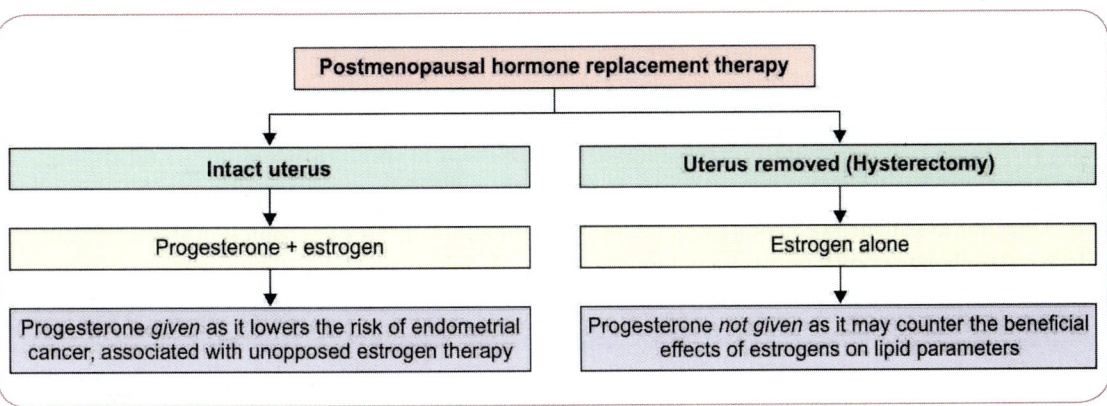

Figure 8: Postmenopausal hormone replacement therapy

Salient Features Regarding HRT

- ○ HRT is highly effective in relieving the menopausal symptoms.
- ○ The main indication of HRT is to relieve menopausal symptoms, rather than prevention of chronic disease.
- ○ The most common estrogens used are conjugated estrogens (0.625 mg/day).
- ○ The most common progestins used are medroxyprogesterone acetate (MPA) and norethindrone.

○ HRT should be used at the lowest effective dose for the shortest duration of time. This is due to the concern regarding the risks of using HRT (e.g. increased risk of cancer and cardiovascular events).

○ The dose of estrogen used in HRT is significantly less than the dose used in oral contraception therapy (OCT) (Table 3).

TABLE 3	Dose of estrogen	
Estrogen dose for HRT	**Estrogen dose for OCT**
• Conjugated estrogen 0.625 mg/day = Ethinyl estradiol 10 µg/day	• Ethinyl estradiol 20–35 µg/day

Hence, the adverse effects of estrogens are lesser when used as an HRT, as compared to OCT.

○ Women with intact uterus should receive estrogen + progestin; while hysterectomized women should receive estrogen alone.

○ HRT may be given by 'continuous' or 'cyclic' regimens. A common cyclic regimen is mentioned in Figure 9.

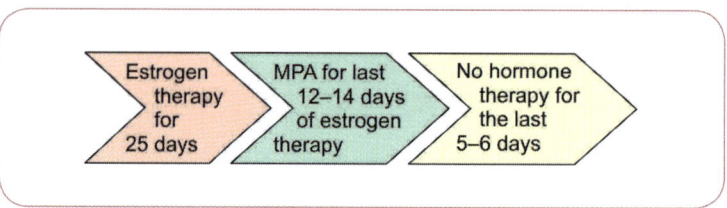

Figure 9: Cyclic regimen for HRT

Delayed Puberty in Females

Estrogens are used in the treatment of Turner's syndrome or hypopituitarism. The treatment is given to stimulate growth, secondary sexual characteristics and to prevent osteoporosis.

Senile Vaginitis

Topical estrogens are preferred. It may be combined with an antibiotic.

Dysmenorrhea

Estrogens with progestins suppress ovulation in patients with dysmenorrhea. Anovulatory cycles are painless.

Acne

Acne occurs due to an increased androgen secretion. Estrogens are helpful as they suppress ovarian production of androgens by inhibiting GnRH release from the pituitary.

SELECTIVE ESTROGEN RECEPTOR MODULATORS

Selective estrogen receptor modulators (SERMs) are nonsteroidal compounds with tissue selective actions.

By saying tissue selective, it is meant that SERMs show selective agonistic or antagonistic activity (on estrogen receptors) depending on the tissue type. In other words, they have estrogen-like actions in some tissues and estrogen-antagonistic actions in some other tissues.

The aim of using these drugs is to:

○ produce beneficial estrogenic actions in some tissues (e.g. bone, brain, liver)

○ prevent deleterious estrogenic actions in some other tissues (e.g. breast and endometrium)

The commonly used SERMs are mentioned in Figure 10.

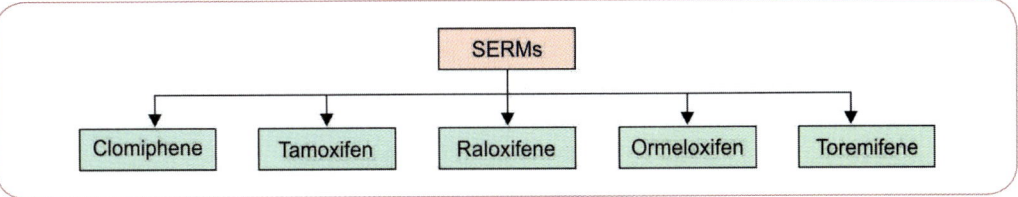

Figure 10: Commonly used SERMs

Previously, clomiphene was classified as a pure estrogen antagonist. Later on, it was observed that its actions differs in various tissues, i.e. agonist in some and antagonist in others. Hence, clomiphene has recently been classified as a SERM.

CLOMIPHENE CITRATE

Clomiphene has both agonistic and antagonistic effects at estrogen receptors.

The agonistic effects are best demonstrated in animals, when the endogenous estrogen levels are extremely low in situations of marked gonadal deficiency. Overall, in humans, the antagonistic effects prevail.

Mechanism of Action

The mechanism of action of clomiphene is mentioned in Figure 11.

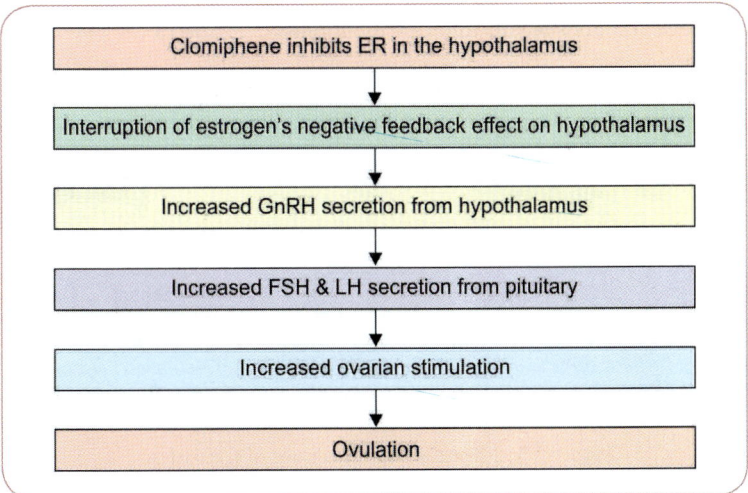

Figure 11: Mechanism of action of clomiphene

Pharmacokinetics

Clomiphene is well absorbed orally. It has a long plasma half-life of 5–7 days due to high plasma protein binding, enterohepatic circulation and accumulation in fatty tissues.

Adverse Effects

Some of the key adverse effects of clomiphene are mentioned in Figure 12.

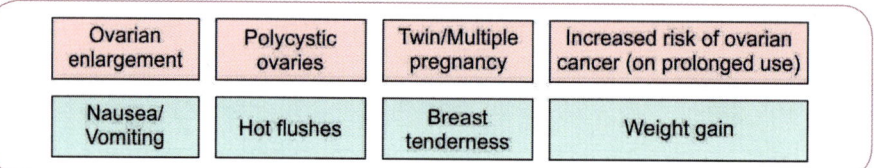

Figure 12: Adverse effects of clomiphene

Clinical Uses

○ **Female infertility**
  ▫ Clomiphene is mainly used to treat female infertility due to anovulation. It is of no use in primary ovarian or pituitary failure.
  ▫ Used as a cyclic therapy—50 mg once daily for 5 days starting from 5th day of the cycle. Treatment is repeated monthly.
  ▫ Long-term cyclic therapy (i.e. beyond a total of about 6 cycles) is not recommended.
○ **Male infertility**
  ▫ It can also be used to treat male infertility.
  ▫ It leads to increased GnRH secretion, resulting in increased testosterone secretion and spermatogenesis.
○ *In vitro* **fertilization**
  ▫ Used as an adjunctive drug along with gonadotropins to cause maturation of several ova and their harvesting.

■ TAMOXIFEN

Tamoxifen has both estrogenic and antiestrogenic actions depending on the tissue type. It was the first SERM to be introduced.

The main pharmacological actions of tamoxifen are mentioned in Figure 13.

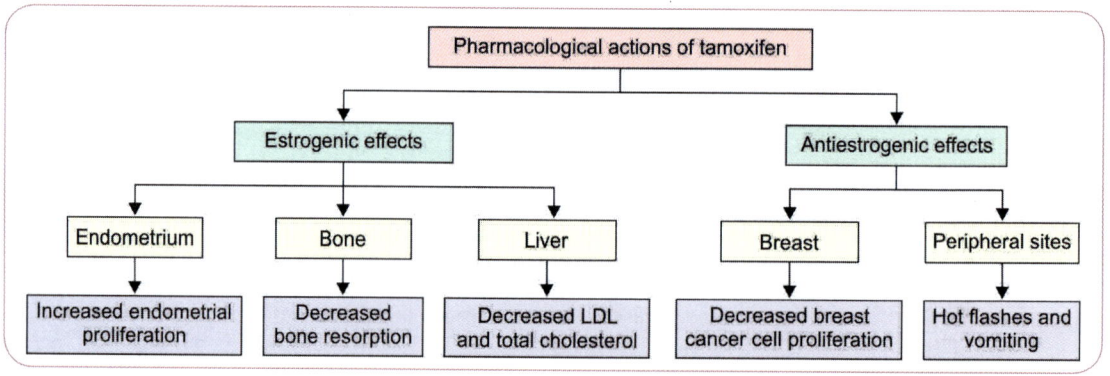

Figure 13: Pharmacological actions of tamoxifen

Pharmacokinetics

Tamoxifen is given orally. It exhibits biphasic elimination half-lives: 7–14 hours and 4–11 days. Due to a long half-life, the steady state plasma levels are achieved in 3–4 weeks.

It is metabolized in the liver to an active metabolite 4-hydroxytamoxifen. Although tamoxifen is a potent drug, the metabolite 4-hydroxytamoxifen is much more potent than tamoxifen as an antiestrogen.

Therefore, drugs that block the conversion of tamoxifen to its more potent metabolite 4-hydroxytamoxifen impacts its therapeutic efficacy in breast cancer.

It undergoes enterohepatic circulation.

Adverse Effects

Tamoxifen has a much lower toxicity than other anticancer drugs. The key adverse effects include:
○ Hot flashes, nausea and vomiting

o   Increased risk of endometrial cancer
o   Increased risk of venous thromboembolism

Clinical Uses

o   Treatment of breast cancer (in both pre- and postmenopausal women)
o   Prevention of breast cancer in high-risk women.

RALOXIFENE

Raloxifene is another drug with both estrogenic and antiestrogenic actions depending on the tissue type. It does not stimulate endometrial proliferation and therefore, the risk of endometrial cancer is not increased.

It has an antiresorptive effect in the bone and decreases the number of vertebral fractures by up to 50%.

The main pharmacological actions of raloxifene are mentioned in Figure 14.

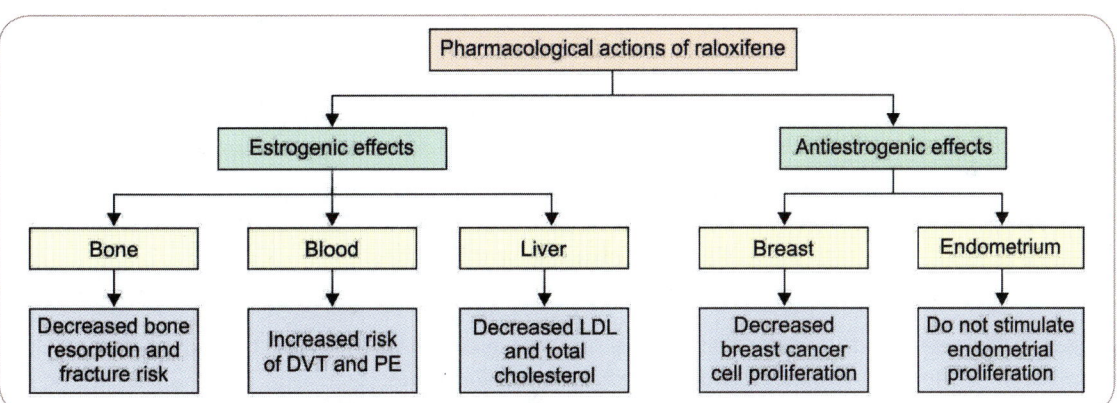

Figure 14: Pharmacological actions of raloxifene

Abbreviations: DVT, deep vein thrombosis; PE, pulmonary embolism.

Raloxifene is given orally. It has a poor bioavailability due to high first-pass metabolism. It has a long half-life of 28 hours and is eliminated in the feces.

The adverse effects are hot flashes, leg cramps, and a 3-fold increased risk of venous thromboembolism. It does not increase the risk of endometrial cancer.

It is used for treatment and prevention of osteoporosis in postmenopausal women.

ORMELOXIFENE

It is a SERM with antiestrogenic actions in breast and uterus. It is used for the treatment of dysfunctional uterine bleeding associated with anovulatory cycles that occurs near menopause.

It has also been used as a nonhormonal oral contraceptive.

The adverse effects are nausea, weight gain and headache.

PROGESTINS

PROGESTERONE

The natural progestin is progesterone.

It is produced by the corpus luteum of ovary in the 2nd half (luteal/secretory phase) of the menstrual cycle. LH stimulates progesterone secretion during the normal cycle.

During pregnancy, progesterone is produced by the placenta.

In addition to its hormonal effects, progesterone serves as a precursor for the synthesis of estrogen, testosterone and adrenal steroids.

A variety of synthetic progestins with high oral activity have been developed. They are either progesterone derivatives (21 carbon) or 19-nortestosterone derivatives (18 carbon) (Figure 15).

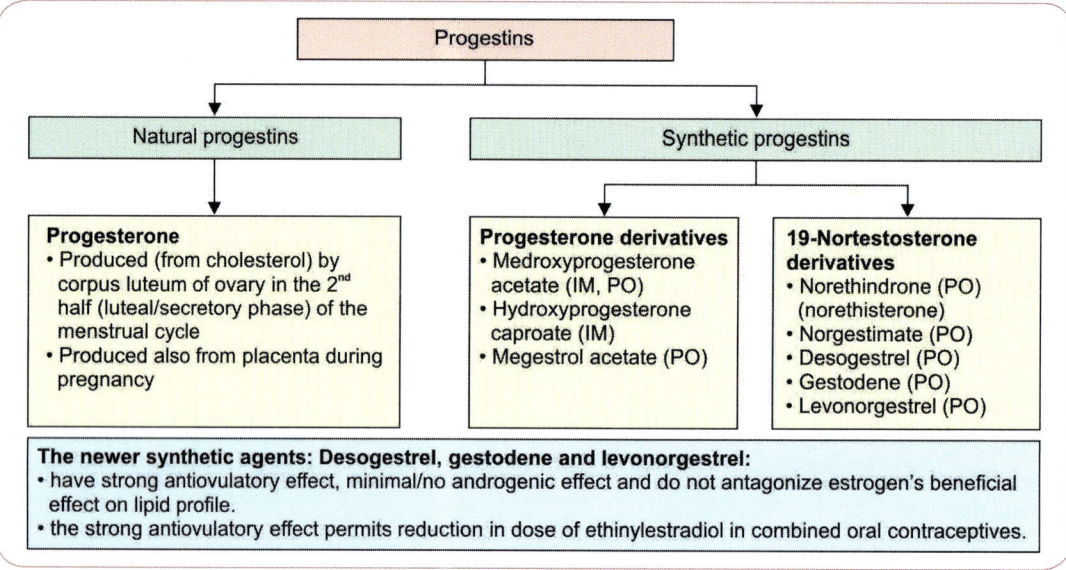

Figure 15: Classification of progestins

Pharmacokinetics

Progesterone is not effective orally due to high first-pass metabolism. However, high dose of micronized progesterone is effective orally. Progesterone has a half-life of 5–7 minutes.

Most of the synthetic progestins are orally effective and their plasma half-life ranges from 10 to 24 hours. Their duration of action ranges from 1 to 3 days.

Pharmacological Actions

The pharmacological actions of progestins are mentioned in Table 4.

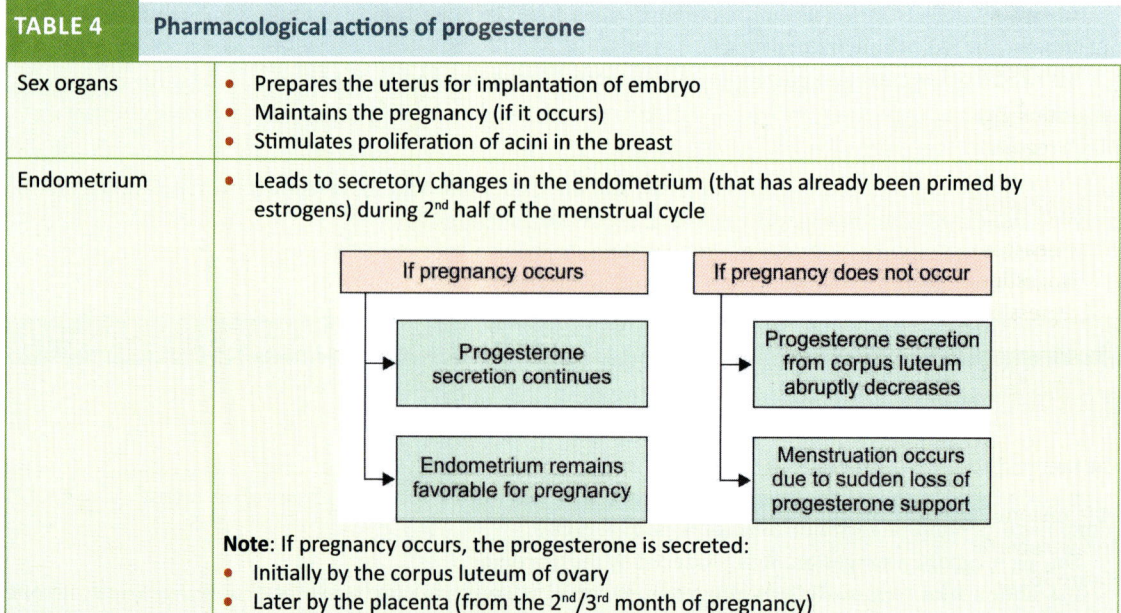

TABLE 4	Pharmacological actions of progesterone
Sex organs	• Prepares the uterus for implantation of embryo • Maintains the pregnancy (if it occurs) • Stimulates proliferation of acini in the breast
Endometrium	• Leads to secretory changes in the endometrium (that has already been primed by estrogens) during 2nd half of the menstrual cycle

Note: If pregnancy occurs, the progesterone is secreted:
- Initially by the corpus luteum of ovary
- Later by the placenta (from the 2nd/3rd month of pregnancy)

Contd...

Cervix	• Makes cervical secretions thick, viscous and acidic; hence, decreases sperm penetration
Fallopian tubes and myometrium	• Reduces rhythmic contractions of tubes and myometrium
Metabolic	• Increases LDL levels • Decreases HDL levels • Decreases glucose tolerance on long-term use • Mild salt-water retention and edema • Increases body temperature slightly (0.5°C or 1°F)

Adverse Effects

The key adverse effects of progestins include headache, depression, edema, weight gain, breast engorgement, depression, irregular bleeding, decrease libido, acne and hirsutism. Long-term use may increase the risk of breast cancer.

Clinical Uses

Progestins are most commonly used as contraceptive therapy (given either alone or with an estrogen) and post-menopausal hormone replacement therapy (given along with an estrogen).

These and the other uses of progestins are discussed below:

Contraception

Progestins are used in contraception as combined pill (i.e. estrogen + progestin), minipill, postcoital pill, injectables, implants etc. These are discussed later in the chapter.

Hormone Replacement Therapy

In patients with an intact uterus, progestins are given in combination with estrogens for HRT. This is because progestin decreases the risk of endometrial cancer associated with unopposed estrogen therapy.

Note: In hysterectomized patients (where uterus has been removed), estrogen alone is given for HRT and progestins are not given. This is because there is no risk of endometrial cancer. In such a scenario, progestins should be avoided as they may counter the beneficial effects of estrogens on lipid parameters.

Dysfunctional Uterine Bleeding

Progestins given in large doses quickly arrests bleeding. The cyclical treatment may be continued subsequently which regularizes menstrual flow.

Endometriosis

This disease is characterized by dysmenorrhea, menorrhagia and infertility.

Progestins given on a continuous basis induces an anovulatory, hypoestrogenic condition resulting in atrophy and regression of lesions.

ANTIPROGESTINS

MIFEPRISTONE

Mifepristone is a strong competitive antagonist to progesterone and has luteolytic action. It also has antiglucocorticoid and antiandrogenic actions. The pharmacological actions of mifepristone are mentioned in Figure 16.

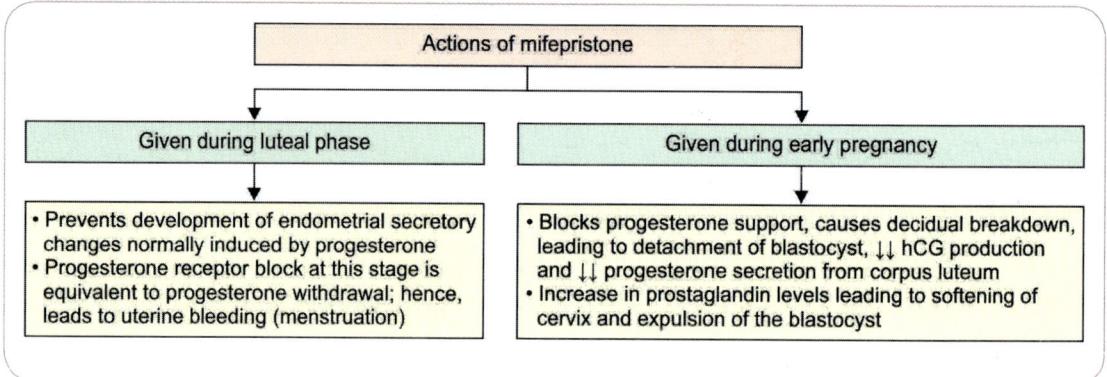

Figure 16: Pharmacological actions of mifepristone

Mifepristone is effective orally and has a long plasma half-life of 20-40 hours. It undergoes metabolism in the liver and enterohepatic circulation.

Clinical Uses

Termination of Pregnancy

Mifepristone is used for the termination of early pregnancy (of up to 7 weeks). It is used in combination with prostaglandins such as misoprostol.

A single 600 mg oral dose of mifepristone, followed 48 hours later by a single 400 mg oral dose of misoprostol is commonly used (Figure 17). In place of oral misoprostol, 1 mg vaginal pessary of gemeprost may also be used. The success rate is >90%.

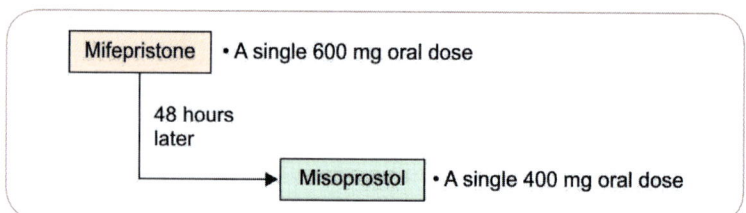

Figure 17: Regimen for termination of pregnancy

Postcoital (Emergency) Contraception

A single 600 mg dose of mifepristone given within 72 hours of unprotected intercourse, is a highly effective method of emergency contraception. It interferes with implantation by causing decidual sloughing.

Induction of Labor

It blocks the uterine relaxant effect of progesterone and may induce labor. It is used in cases of intrauterine fetal death.

Cervical Ripening

It may be used for cervical ripening prior to surgical abortion or induction of labor.

HORMONAL CONTRACEPTIVES

Hormonal contraception is currently the most popular method for contraception.

The hormonal preparations lead to a reversible suppression of fertility. The fertility with these agents can be suppressed as and when required, and for as long as desired. Both oral and parenteral preparations are available.

CLASSIFICATION

Two types of preparations are used as oral contraceptives:
1. Combination of estrogen and progestins (monophasic, biphasic or triphasic)
2. Progestin-only without estrogen component

The injectable contraceptives and implants mostly contain progestin-only component.

The various types of hormonal contraceptive preparations are mentioned in Figure 18.

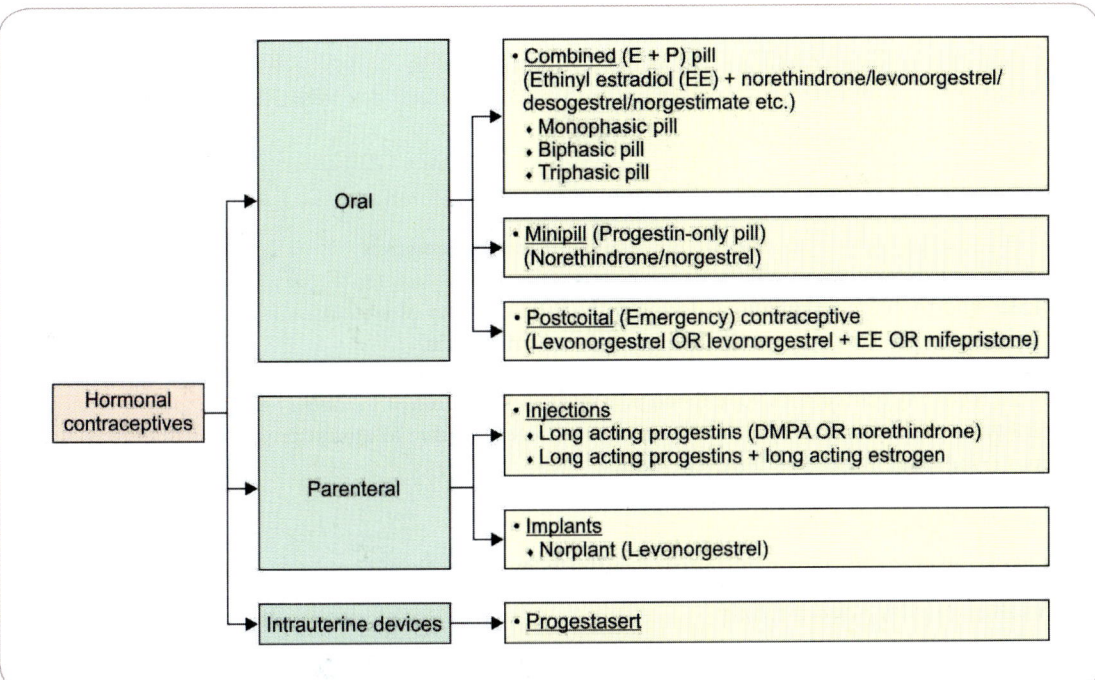

Figure 18: Types of hormonal contraceptives

Combined Pill (Combined Estrogen and Progestin Pill)

The combined oral contraceptives contain both an estrogen and a progestin.

They are the most effective (efficacy 98–99.9%) and the most commonly used drugs for contraception (Figure 19).

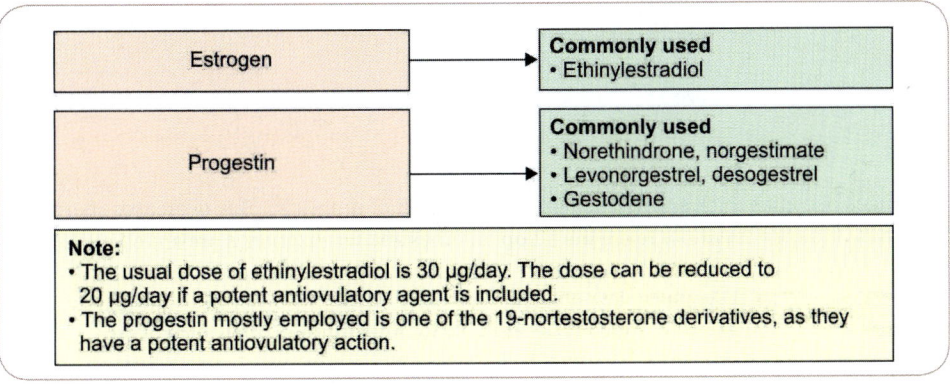

Figure 19: Commonly used drugs for contraception

The combined oral contraceptives are marketed in the form of monophasic, biphasic or triphasic pills (Figure 20).

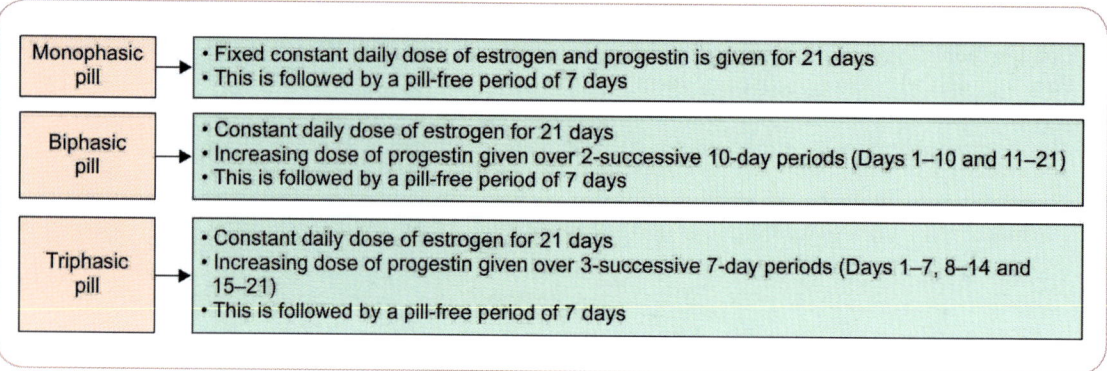

Monophasic pill	• Fixed constant daily dose of estrogen and progestin is given for 21 days • This is followed by a pill-free period of 7 days
Biphasic pill	• Constant daily dose of estrogen for 21 days • Increasing dose of progestin given over 2-successive 10-day periods (Days 1–10 and 11–21) • This is followed by a pill-free period of 7 days
Triphasic pill	• Constant daily dose of estrogen for 21 days • Increasing dose of progestin given over 3-successive 7-day periods (Days 1–7, 8–14 and 15–21) • This is followed by a pill-free period of 7 days

Figure 20: Combined oral contraceptives

The biphasic and triphasic preparations decrease the total quantity of steroids administered and mimics the estrogen/progestin ratio that occur during the normal menstrual cycle.
- The amount of estrogen in these combined pills usually ranges from 20 μg/day to 30 μg/day.
- The amount of progestin in these combined pills usually ranges from 0.15 mg/day to 1.0 mg/day.

In all the 3 types of preparations, predictable menstrual bleeding (due to abrupt progestin withdrawal) usually occurs during the 7-day pill-free period every month.

Mechanism of Action

The combined pill produces contraceptive action by the following mechanisms:

Hypothalamic-pituitary-ovarian Axis

The combined pill acts by inhibiting ovulation from the ovaries. This is the most important mechanism. The ovulation is inhibited by the following mechanism:

Estrogen and progestin act synergistically to reinforce the normal hypothalamopituitary negative feedback mechanism. This results in a decrease of FSH and LH release from the pituitary. LH surge does not happen in the mid-cycle and hence, follicles fail to develop, and ovulation does not occur (Figure 21).

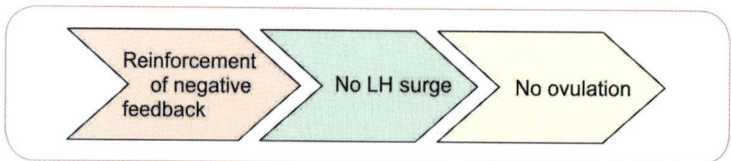

Figure 21: Ovulation inhibiting effect of combined pill

Cervix

The cervical mucus becomes thick and viscous under the action of progestin. This decreases sperm penetration through the cervix. The sperms cannot reach the fallopian tubes and fertilization is prevented.

Endometrium

The endometrium is rendered in a state which is not suitable for implantation of the blastocyst.

Uterus and Fallopian Tubes

The contractions of uterus and cervix are increased which may inhibit fertilization.

Minipill (Progestin-only pill)

- Minipill contains progestin-only in a very low dose.
- The common progestin used is norethindrone.
- The efficacy of minipill is 96%. Hence, these are less effective than combined pills.
- These are taken continuously for 28 days without any gap or pill-free period.
- The mechanism of action is:
    - Altering the cervical mucus to make it thick and viscous
    - Endometrial changes to prevent implantation
    - Inhibition of ovulation (in 60–80% of cycles)
- Minipills are indicated in women who are smokers, intolerant to estrogen or in whom estrogen is contraindicated.

Postcoital Pill (Emergency Contraception)

- The drugs commonly employed are high doses of either levonorgestrel, levonorgestrel + ethinylestradiol, or mifepristone.
- The drugs are used following unprotected/accidental intercourse such as rape or condom rupture.
- The drugs are to be taken as soon as possible, but preferably within 72 hours of an unprotected intercourse.
- The common drug regimens for emergency contraception are mentioned in Figure 22.

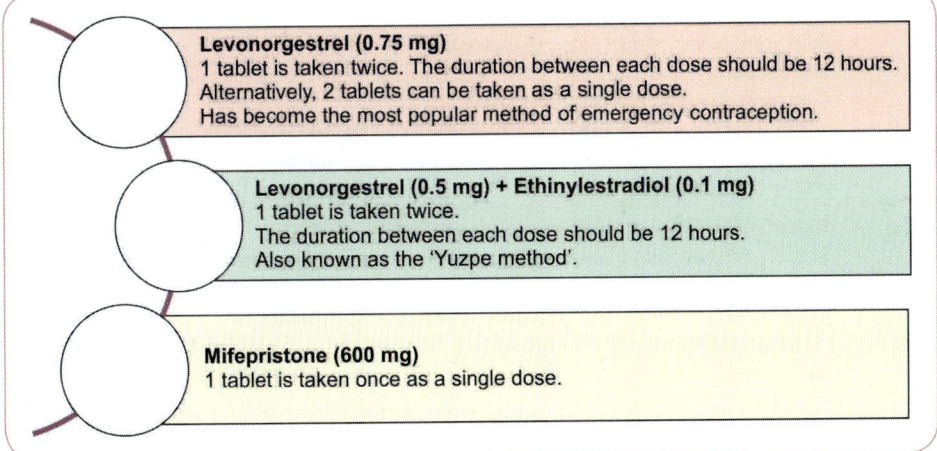

Figure 22: Emergency contraception

Injectable Contraceptives

The injectable contraceptives were developed so that the daily ingestion of pills can be avoided, and patient compliance can be improved. They are administered as intramuscular (IM) injections.

These are used in patients who are not compliant to daily drug intake, who are intolerant to estrogens, or who have contraindications to estrogen containing products.

The following points are noteworthy regarding the injectable preparations (Table 5):

TABLE 5	Injectable contraceptives
Agents used	• Depot medroxyprogesterone acetate (DMPA) ▪ 150 mg IM once every 3 months ▪ Common brand name—Depo-provera • Norethindrone enanthate (NET-EN) ▪ 200 mg IM once every 2 months ▪ Common brand name—Noristerat
Advantages	• Need for daily ingestion of pills is avoided; patient compliance is improved • Do not contain estrogen component—risk of endometrial carcinoma is decreased
Limitations	• Commonly causes menstrual irregularities, headache, weight gain, mood changes and decreased bone mineral density • After discontinuation of the drug, the return of fertility may take 6–12 months or longer • Due to the risk of osteoporosis and fractures on long-term use, the drug should not be used for >2 years, unless the patient is unable to tolerate other options

Implants

These are drug delivery methods in which the drugs are implanted under the skin. This ensures slow, long-term release of the hormone.

There are 2 implants commonly used as contraceptives. These are mentioned in Table 6.

TABLE 6	Implants
Norplant	• Subcutaneous implant containing levonorgestrel • Six (6)-specially designed capsules, each containing 36 mg levonorgestrel (total 216 mg) • Contraceptive effect lasts up to 5 years • Fertility is immediately restored after removal of the implant • Progestin adverse effects may occur (e.g. headache, weight gain, mood changes, acne) • Highly efficacious agent
Implanon	• Subcutaneous implant containing etonogestrel • Single, rod-shaped implant containing 68 mg synthetic progestin etonogestrel • Contraceptive effect lasts up to 3 years • Fertility is immediately restored after removal of the implant • Progestin adverse effects may occur (e.g. headache, weight gain, mood changes, acne)

Device

- It is a small, often T-shaped device that is inserted and placed inside the uterine cavity. There is a slow, long-term release of the hormone.
- It releases the hormone levonorgestrel.
- Contraceptive effect lasts up to 5 years.
- Fertility is immediately restored after removal of the implant.
- Progestin adverse effects may occur (e.g. headache, weight gain, mood changes, acne).
- It should not be used in women having pelvic inflammatory disease and with a history of ectopic pregnancy.
- The hormonal device is thought to be more effective than other common forms of reversible contraception, such as birth control pills, because no particular action is required after insertion.

ADVERSE EFFECTS

Most of the adverse effects are dose dependent and are observed with high-dose preparations. Hence, to decrease the incidence of adverse effects, low-dose preparations have been developed.

The current understanding is that the low-dose preparations have minimal adverse effects.

There is an increased occurrence of adverse effects in women who have risk factors such as age >35 years, smoking, hypertension and diabetes.

The key adverse effects that may occur with the use of hormonal contraceptives are mentioned in Figure 23.

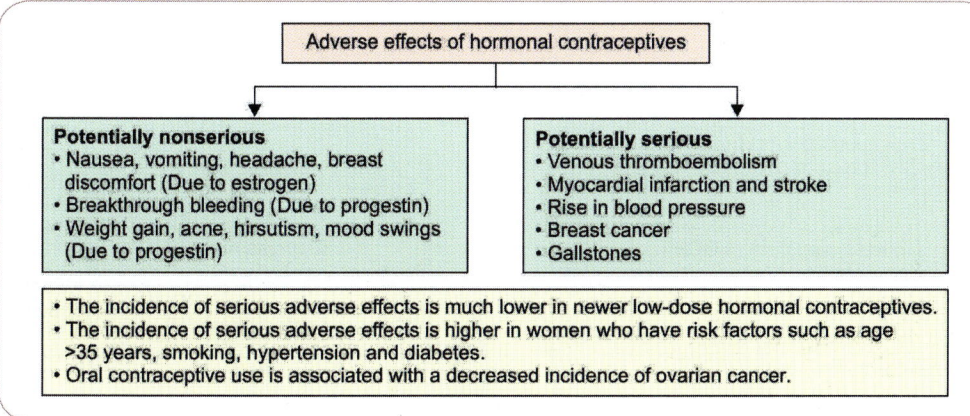

Figure 23: Adverse effects of hormonal contraceptives

CONTRAINDICATIONS

The current low-dose contraceptives are generally considered safe in most healthy women; however, these may lead to several thromboembolic, cardiovascular and malignant adverse effects if risk factors (such as age >35 years, smoking, hypertension and diabetes) are present.

The following clinical conditions are therefore considered as contraindications for combined oral contraceptives and progestin-only contraceptives (Figure 24).

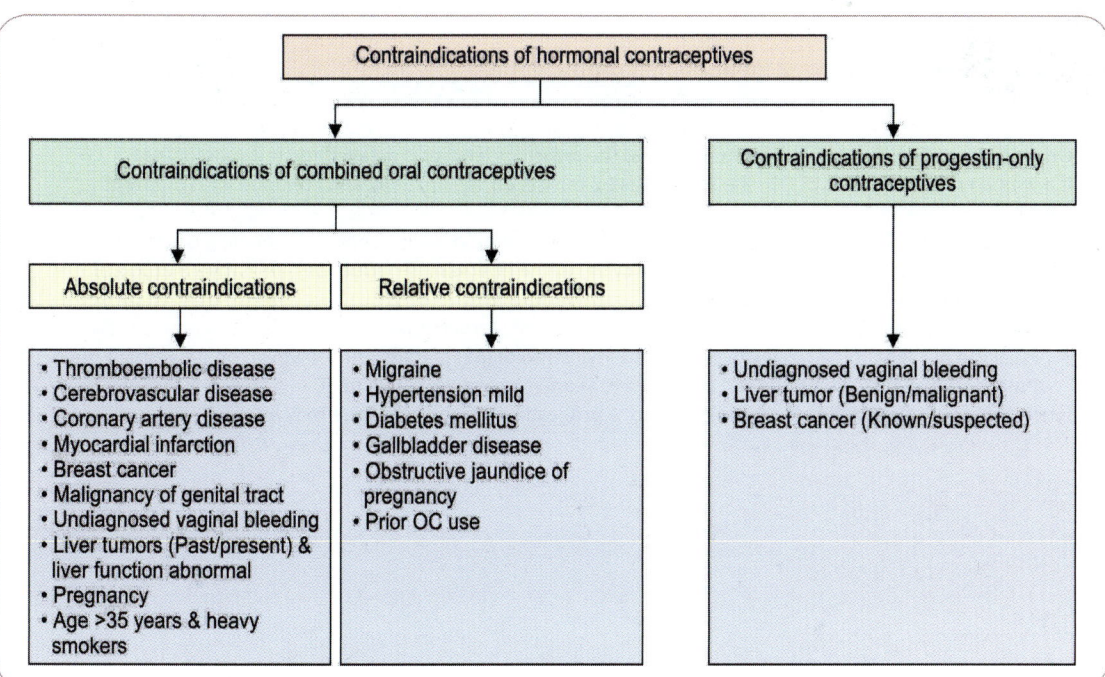

Figure 24: Contraindications of hormonal contraceptives

DRUG INTERACTIONS

Important drug interactions that may lead to oral contraceptive failure are mentioned in Figure 25.

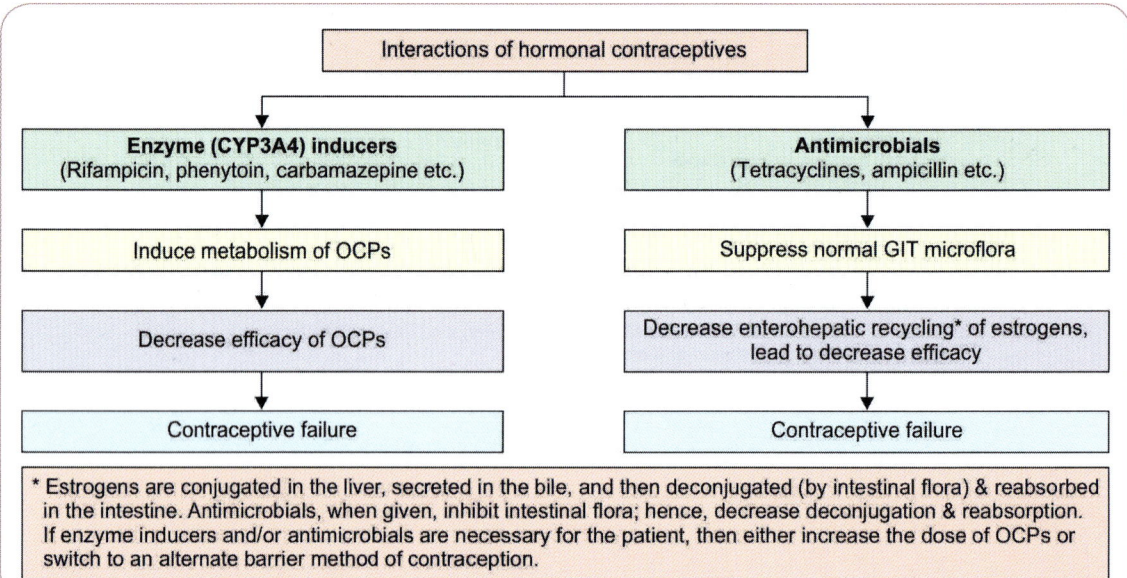

Figure 25: Drug interactions of hormonal contraceptives

POINTS TO CONSIDER REGARDING HORMONAL CONTRACEPTIVES (TABLE 7)

TABLE 7	Points to consider for hormonal contraceptives

- On discontinuation of oral contraceptives, the fertility usually completely returns within 1–2 months.
- On discontinuation of injectable contraceptives, the return of fertility is delayed for several months.
- If a woman misses 1 tablet of OC, she should take 2 tablets on the next day and continue with the routine course.
- If a woman misses 2 tablets of OC, then the current course should be discontinued. The new course should be started on the 1st day of the next menstrual cycle. In the intervening period, an alternative method of contraception should be used.
- The treatment should be started with the minimum dose of steroids that provides effective contraception.
  - Usually, a pill containing progestin + 30 µg ethinylestradiol (EE) is sufficient. However, obese women may require 50 µg while lighter women and age >40 years may require 20 µg of EE.
- In women where estrogens are contraindicated, a progestin-only contraceptive may be used.

ASSESS YOURSELF (Examination Questions of Various Universities)

1. Enumerate hormonal contraceptives. Explain the mechanism of action, adverse effects, drug interactions and contraindications of hormonal contraceptives.
2. Enumerate selective oestrogen receptor modulators (SERMs). Write briefly the mechanism of action in correlation with their therapeutic uses.
3. What are the indications and adverse effects of progesterones.
4. Discuss the rationale of using:
   a. Clomiphene in infertility
   b. Tamoxifen in breast cancer
   c. Mifepristone in termination of early pregnancy
   d. Mifepristone and misoprostol in medical termination of pregnancy

5. Write short notes on:
   a. Emergency contraception
   b. Combined pill
   c. Minipill
   d. Injectable contraceptives
   e. Tamoxifen
   f. Adverse effects of oral contraceptives
6. Explain why:
   a. Progesterone is not added in hormone replacement therapy, in women who have undergone hysterectomy
   b. Rifampicin, when given reduces the efficacy of oral contraceptives
7. Name one SERM used in the treatment of osteoporosis.

MULTIPLE CHOICE QUESTIONS

1. Which of the following drug is a SERM useful for treatment of osteoporosis? *(AIIMS Nov 2010)*
   a. Raloxifene   b. Bisphosphonate
   c. Strontium   d. Estradiol
2. Which of the following drug is used in the treatment of estrogen dependent breast carcinoma? *(AIIMS Nov 2010)*
   a. Tamoxifen   b. Methotrexate
   c. Paclitaxel   d. Adriamycin
3. Which of the following progesterone is used in emergency contraception? *(AIIMS May, Nov 2009)*
   a. Levonorgestrel
   b. Micronized progesterone
   c. Norgesterone
   d. Depot medroxyprogesterone acetate
4. Hormone replacement therapy is helpful in all of the following conditions except:
   a. Vaginal atrophy   *(AIIMS May 2007)*
   b. Flushing
   c. Coronary heart disease
   d. Osteoporosis
5. Mifepristone (RU-486) is the most commonly used drug for medical abortion and emergency contraception. Pharmacologically the drug is a:

   a. Antiprogesterone   *(Recent Question 2016)*
   b. Progestin analogue
   c. PGE1 analogue
   d. PGE2 analogue
6. Tamoxifen is: *(Recent Question 2016)*
   a. SSRI   b. SERM
   c. SNRI   d. DNRI
7. DMPA is given once in *(Recent Question 2016)*
   a. 3 months   b. 6 months
   c. 9 months   d. 45 days
8. Mechanism of action of oral contraceptive pill can be all except: *(Recent Question 2016)*
   a. Hostile to sperm penetration
   b. Anovulatory cycle
   c. Failure of blastocyst implantation
   d. Blockade of fimbrial ostia
9. All are true about estrogen except:
                         (Recent Question 2016)
   a. Causes cholestasis
   b. Used in treatment of gynecomastia
   c. Used in HRT
   d. Increased risk of breast cancer
10. SERM are all except: *(WBPG 2012)*
    a. Reserpine   b. Clomiphene
    c. Tamoxifen   d. Toremifene

Ans.

| 1. | (a) | 2. | (a) | 3. | (a) | 4. | (c) | 5. | (a) | 6. | (b) |
| 7. | (a) | 8. | (d) | 9. | (b) | 10. | (a) | | | | |

38 Androgens and Antiandrogens

ANDROGENS

Testosterone is the primary androgen secreted in men. It is produced by the Leydig cells of the testes.

The testes has 2 components:
- Leydig cells (Interstitial cells)—testosterone synthesis occurs
- Sertoli cells—spermatogenesis occurs

Regulation of Secretion

The testosterone secretion is regulated by the following:
- GnRH secreted from the hypothalamus
- Luteinizing hormone (LH) and follicle-stimulating hormone (FSH) secreted from the pituitary

The FSH is responsible for spermatogenesis and LH is responsible for the secretion of testosterone. In addition, high testosterone concentration locally also is required for continuous sperm production from Sertoli cells (Figure 1).

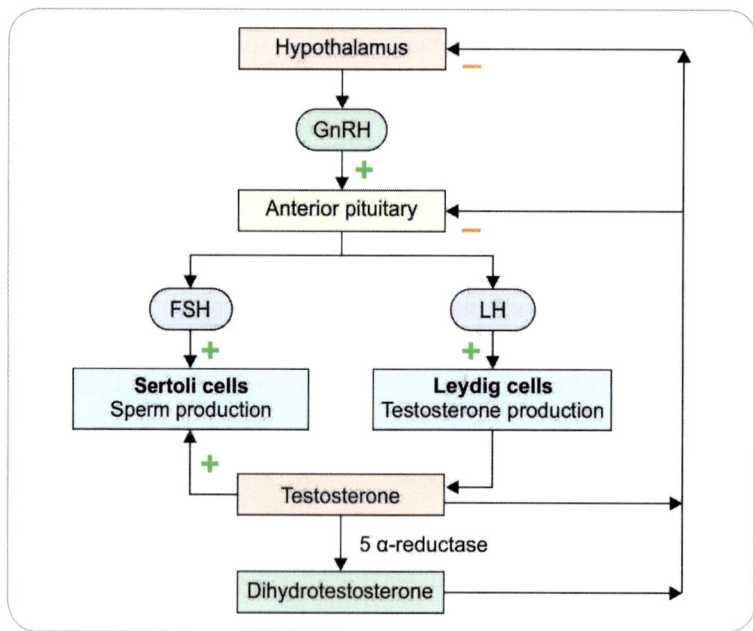

Figure 1: Regulation of testosterone secretion

Classification of Androgens

Natural

Testosterone is daily produced by the testes, some part of which is converted (in the extraglandular tissues) to the more potent androgen dihydrotestosterone by the enzyme 5 α-reductase.

Adrenal cortex produces small amounts of dehydroepiandrosterone (DHEA) and androstenedione. These are known as 'weak androgens' because they have a much lower potency, as compared to testosterone.

Synthetic

Testosterone is not active orally because of high first-pass metabolism in the liver. The duration of IM testosterone is also extremely short. To counter these limitations, synthetic androgens were developed. The synthetic androgens include:

- *Testosterone esters*—testosterone enanthate (IM), testosterone cypionate (IM), testosterone propionate (IM), testosterone undecanoate (oral, IM)
- *17 α-alkylated derivatives*—methyltestosterone (oral), fluoxymesterone (oral)

The classification of androgens is mentioned in Figure 2.

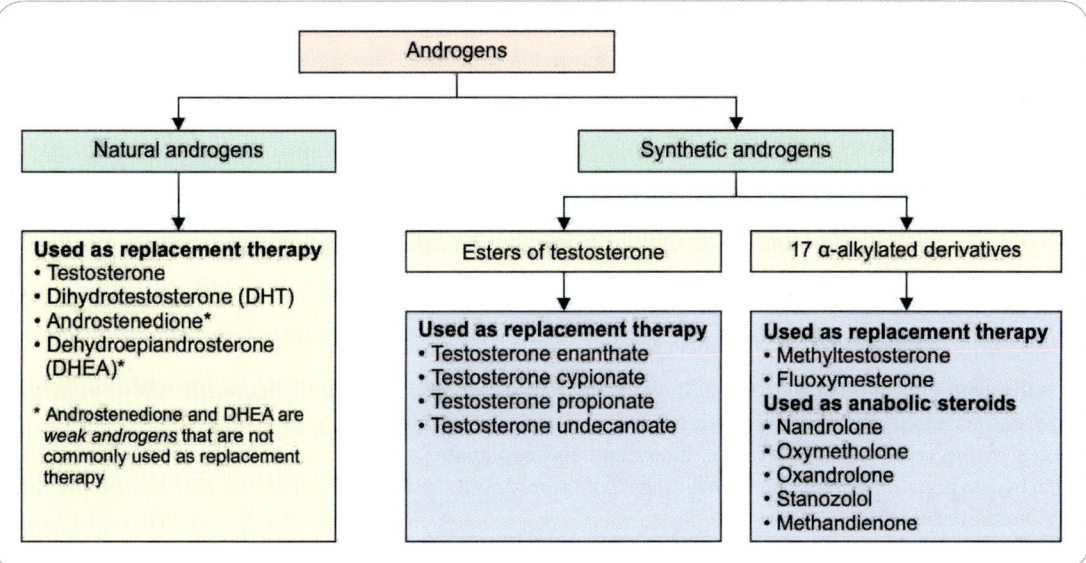

Figure 2: Classification of androgens

Physiological Actions

Testosterone has androgenic as well as anabolic actions. The main androgenic actions are growth/maturation of sex organs and secondary sex characteristics. The main anabolic actions are increase in skeletal muscle mass and strength (Figure 3).

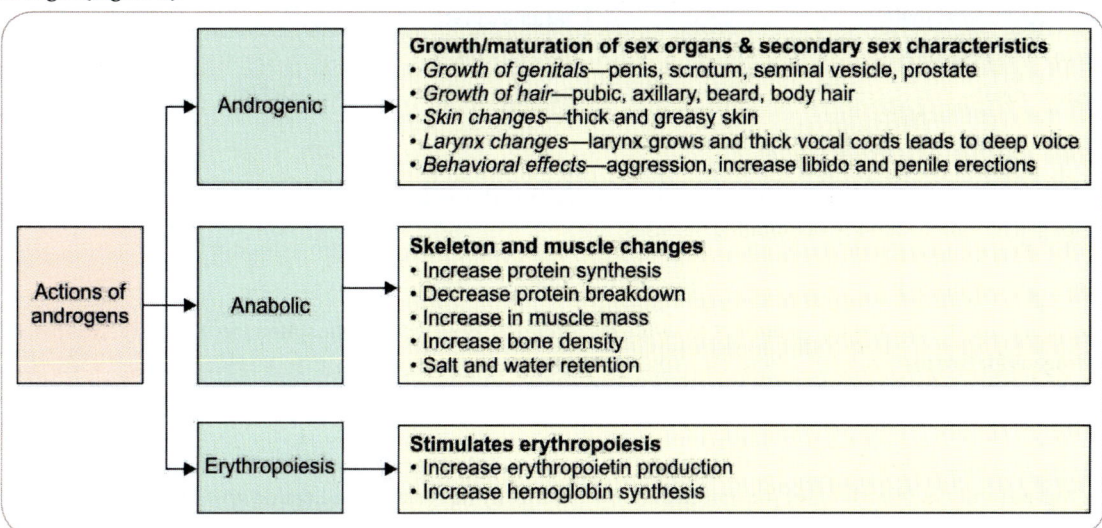

Figure 3: Actions of androgens

Pharmacokinetics

Testosterone is inactive orally because of high first-pass metabolism in the liver. Hence, esters of testosterone have been developed which are mostly given by IM route.

Adverse Effects

The key adverse effects of testosterone are mentioned below:
- In women, virilization occurs resulting in increased body hair, menstrual irregularities and deepening of voice
- In children, precocious puberty and shortening of stature (due to premature epiphyseal closure)
- *Cholestatic jaundice*—occurs with 17 α-alkylated derivatives and not with testosterone esters. It occurs in a dose dependent manner and is reversible on therapy discontinuation.
- *Gynecomastia*—may occur due to peripheral conversion of testosterone to estrogens
- *Edema*—uncommon but may occur in patients with heart and kidney disease

Precautions and Contraindications

- Pregnancy—masculinization of the female fetus may occur
- Cancer of prostate and male breast
- Cardiac and renal disease—edema occurs which may aggravate the underlying condition

Clinical Uses

Replacement Therapy in Male Hypogonadism

This is the main indication of androgens. These drugs are useful both in primary hypogonadism (due to testicular failure) and secondary hypogonadism (due to hypothalamic/pituitary failure).

Long-acting testosterone esters (i.e. enanthate and cypionate) and transdermal testosterone preparations (which bypass hepatic first-pass metabolism) are commonly used. Testosterone propionate is not used because of short duration of action.

The androgen preparations commonly used for replacement therapy are mentioned in Table 1.

TABLE 1	Androgen preparations used for replacement therapy
Preparation	**Route**
Methyltestosterone	Oral
Fluoxymesterone	Oral
Testosterone enanthate	Intramuscular
Testosterone cypionate	Intramuscular
Testosterone	Transdermal

Debilitating Diseases and Aging

Androgens have been used along with exercise and dietary measures, to reverse protein loss after surgery, trauma, prolonged immobilization or debilitating diseases.

Senile Osteoporosis

Androgens may be used in the treatment of senile osteoporosis; however, bisphosphonates have largely replaced androgens for this use.

Hereditary Angioneurotic Edema (HAN)

This is a hereditary disorder characterized by deficiency of complement C1 esterase inhibitor. The 17 α-alkylated androgens (and not testosterone) prevent the attacks of HAN by increasing the hepatic synthesis of complement C1 esterase inhibitor.

ANABOLIC STEROIDS

These are synthetic androgens which have higher anabolic effect and lower androgenic effect. They promote protein synthesis, increase muscle mass and increase appetite leading to weight gain. They induce a sense of general well-being in the person.

The anabolic effects are similar to that of testosterone and are mediated by the same androgen receptors.

The commonly used anabolic steroids are nandrolone (IM), stanozolol (oral), oxandrolone (oral), oxymetholone (oral) etc.

The anabolic: androgenic activity of testosterone is 1:1 while that of anabolic steroids is between 1:3 and 1:10 (Table 2).

TABLE 2	Androgens with relative Androgenic: Anabolic activity
Androgens	**Androgenic: Anabolic activity**
Testosterone	1:1
Methyltestosterone	1:1
Testosterone enanthate	1:1
Testosterone cypionate	1:1
Testosterone propionate	1:1
Fluoxymesterone	1:2
Oxymetholone	1:3
Nandrolone	1:2.5–1:4
Stanozolol	1:4–1:5
Oxandrolone	1:3–1:10

Clinical Uses

o Catabolic conditions
  □ Anabolic steroids are used in recovery from chronic illness, surgery, trauma, burns and debilitating illnesses. They increase nitrogen balance in the short-term and induce weight gain and a sense of well-being.
o Chronic wasting associated with HIV infection and cancer
o Postmenopausal and senile osteoporosis—Bisphosphonates are preferred
o Catabolic state secondary to long-term corticosteroid use

Adverse Effects

The adverse effects of anabolic steroids are similar to that of androgens. Anabolic steroids are commonly misused by athletes for improving their performance.

Anabolic Steroid Misuse in Sports

Anabolic steroids are commonly misused by athletes and sport persons for increasing their physique (muscle mass and strength) and improving their physical performance.

The anabolic steroid user usually consumes a dose much higher than the therapeutic dose. This leads to a number of adverse effects including the following:
o Testicular atrophy, impotence, gynecomastia in males
o Hirsutism, alopecia, acne, deepening of voice, menstrual irregularities in females
o Epiphyseal closure and premature cessation of growth in adolescents
o Increased aggression, psychotic symptoms
o Cholestatic jaundice, hepatic failure
o Coronary artery disease, ventricular arrhythmias

The anabolic effects of these steroids are transient, and the person is subject to a high risk of serious adverse effects. Their use is referred to as doping and therefore, is banned by most major sporting bodies.

These substances have been included in the list of "Dope test" performed on athletes before competitive sports.

DANAZOL

The following are noteworthy regarding danazol:
- Orally active ethisterone derivative
- Weak androgenic, progestational and glucocorticoid activities
- Inhibits the mid-cycle FSH and LH surge; inhibition of ovarian and testicular function
- Used in endometriosis, fibrocystic breast disease and menorrhagia
- Adverse effects include amenorrhea, hot flushes, muscle cramps and androgenic effects

ANTIANDROGENS

Various types of androgen antagonists have been developed. They are used for prostate disorders, male pattern baldness and other diseases. They act through different mechanisms such as inhibition of testosterone synthesis, inhibition of testosterone conversion to a more active form dihydrotestosterone, or inhibition of androgen receptors (Figure 4).

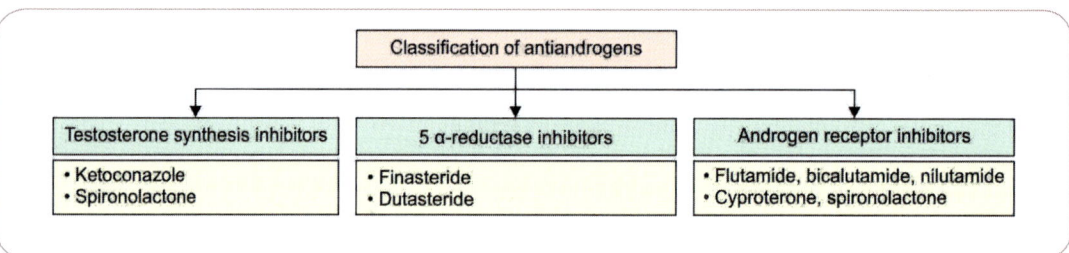

Figure 4: Classification of antiandrogens

The sites of action of antiandrogen drugs is depicted in Figure 5.

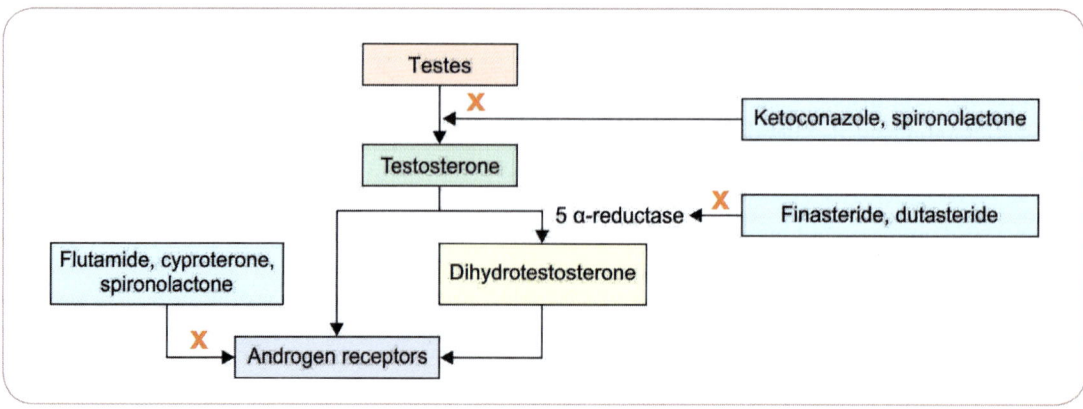

Figure 5: Sites of action and mechanism of antiandrogen drugs

Testosterone Synthesis Inhibitors

Ketoconazole is an antifungal drug that in high doses, inhibits the synthesis of testosterone and adrenal steroids. The toxicity at higher doses limits its use as an antiandrogen.

Spironolactone is an aldosterone antagonist and a K^+-sparing diuretic. It inhibits testosterone synthesis (inhibits 17α-hydroxylase) and is also a competitive blocker of androgen receptors. The main adverse effects include hyperkalemia and gynecomastia.

5 α-Reductase Inhibitors

These are competitive inhibitors of the enzyme 5 α-reductase which converts testosterone to its more active form dihydrotestosterone (DHT). DHT is mainly responsible for androgenic action in many tissues such as prostate, skin and hair follicles (Figure 6).

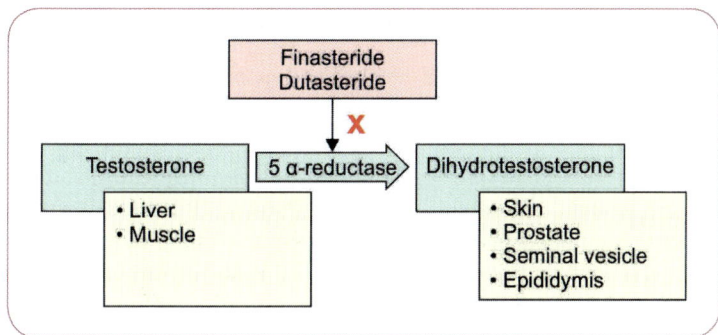

Figure 6: Mechanism of action of 5 α-reductase inhibitors

Finasteride is used in benign prostatic hyperplasia (BPH). It decreases plasma and prostatic dihydrotestosterone levels. Given orally, it decreases prostatic size and increases peak urinary flow rate. The drug has to be given continuously for sustained benefit. Stopping the drug leads to regrowth of the prostate gland.

Finasteride is less effective in relieving symptoms as compared to surgery or α_1-blockers. It is more effective when used in combination with α_1-blockers.

Finasteride is also effective in male pattern baldness.

The adverse effects include decrease libido, impotence, decrease volume of ejaculate, rash and lip swelling.

Dutasteride has a slower onset and a longer duration of action, as compared to finasteride. It is used in BPH.

Androgen Receptor Inhibitors

Cyproterone acetate competitively blocks the androgen receptors on target tissues. It has marked progestational activity which inhibits LH and FSH release, resulting in more effective antiandrogenic effect. It is used to treat hirsutism in females and excessive sexual drive in males.

Flutamide competitively blocks the androgen receptors on target tissues.

It also blocks the androgen receptors in pituitary, blocks the feedback inhibition resulting in an increase in LH and testosterone secretion. Therefore, it is used along with a GnRH agonist to decrease LH and testosterone secretion.

It is used to treat metastatic prostate cancer in males and hirsutism in females. The adverse effects include gynecomastia, breast tenderness, hepatotoxicity and gastrointestinal effects.

Bicalutamide is a more potent and longer acting congener of flutamide.

It is used in metastatic prostate cancer. It is better tolerated than flutamide with lesser hepatotoxic and gastrointestinal effects than flutamide.

DRUGS USED IN ERECTILE DYSFUNCTION

Erectile dysfunction (ED) means an inability of the man to attain and maintain penis erection with sufficient rigidity to permit sexual intercourse. It usually occurs in men >65 years of age. It can be due to vascular, neurological, hormonal, psychogenic or pharmacologic factors.

The drugs used in the management of ED are discussed below:

ANDROGENS

Transdermal testosterone or parenteral testosterone esters are effective only when androgen deficiency is the cause of ED.

PHOSPHODIESTERASE-5 (PDE-5) INHIBITORS

The PDE-5 inhibitors commonly used are sildenafil, tadalafil and vardenafil.

Mechanism of Action

During sexual stimulation, nitric oxide (NO) is released from the parasympathetic nonadrenergic noncholinergic (NANC) nerves. NO activates guanylyl cyclase which forms cGMP from GTP. Increased cGMP levels lead to smooth muscle relaxation in corpora cavernosa of penis. This results in vascular filling and penile erection.

PDE-5 on the other hand is responsible for the hydrolysis of cGMP to GMP resulting in bringing back the penis to the flaccid state.

PDE-5 inhibitors inhibit PDE-5 leading to sustained increase in cGMP levels resulting in sustained erection (Figure 7).

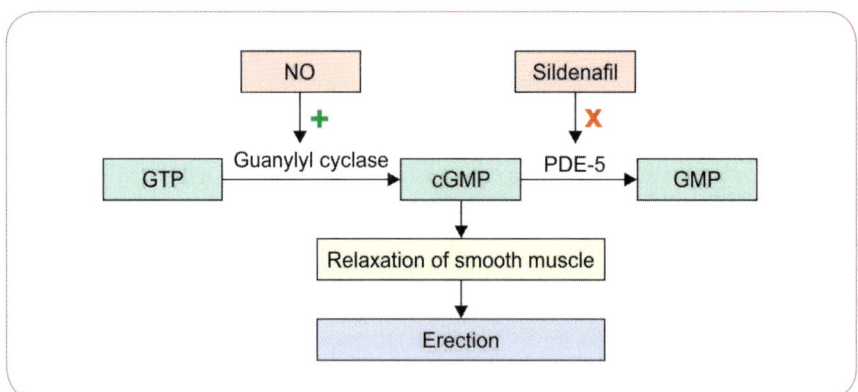

Figure 7: Mechanism of action of PDE-5 inhibitors

SILDENAFIL

Sildenafil is an orally active drug. It selectively inhibits PDE-5 resulting in increased cGMP levels, vascular relaxation in corpora cavernosa and increased penile erection. It does not cause penile erection in the absence of sexual activity.

The oral bioavailability is 40%, peak levels are attained in 1–2 hours and the half-life is around 4 hours. It is metabolized by CYP3A4 and an active metabolite is produced.

Adverse Effects

The adverse effects include the following:
- Vasodilatation effects—headache, flushing, dizziness, nasal congestion, hypotension etc.
- Disturbance in color vision mainly blue green discrimination

This occurs because sildenafil also weakly inhibits PDE-6 which is present in retina and is important in color vision. In a few cases, nonarteritic anterior ischemic optic neuropathy (NAION) may occur.

Drug Interactions

- **Sildenafil with organic nitrates:** Sildenafil markedly potentiates the vasodilator action of nitrates. Concurrent use of both may result in severe hypotension and a few myocardial infarctions have been reported. There should be a gap of at least >6 hours between nitrate and sildenafil use.
- **Sildenafil with CYP3A4 inhibitors:** CYP3A4 inhibitors such as ketoconazole, erythromycin, cimetidine, verapamil etc. may increase the plasma levels of sildenafil and potentiate its action.

Precautions and Contraindications

Sildenafil is contraindicated in patients with coronary artery disease, retinitis pigmentosa and those consuming nitrates.

It is to be cautiously used in patients with peptic ulcer, liver and kidney disease, patients consuming CYP3A4 inhibitors and patients with multiple myeloma, sickle cell anemia and leukemia (may predispose to priapism).

Clinical Uses

- Erectile dysfunction
- Pulmonary arterial hypertension

TADALAFIL AND VARDENAFIL

Tadalafil is a more potent and longer acting congener of sildenafil. It less frequently causes visual disturbances. Vardenafil has similar pharmacokinetics as sildenafil. The other pharmacological features of both are similar to sildenafil.

PGE$_1$ ANALOGUE (ALPROSTADIL)

Alprostadil is the most commonly used drug in patients who do not respond to PDE-5 inhibitors. It is injected directly into the corpora cavernosa of the penis or placed in the urethra as a suppository. It produces erection that lasts for 1–2 hours. Penile fibrosis and priapism are rare.

PAPAVERINE/PHENTOLAMINE

Papaverine injections have been used with or without phentolamine to produce penile erections. They are injected directly into the corpora cavernosa of the penis. Priapism occurs in 3–15% of patients and if not promptly treated, it may lead to permanent damage in the form of penile fibrosis. It is rarely used now. It is a reserve drug for patients not responding to sildenafil and alprostadil.

ASSESS YOURSELF (Examination Questions of Various Universities)

1. Mention four anabolic steroids and discuss their therapeutic uses.
2. Discuss the rationale of using:
   a. Flutamide in prostatic cancer
   b. Finasteride in benign prostatic hypertrophy
3. Write short notes on:
   a. Anabolic steroids
   b. 5-α reductase inhibitors

c. Phosphodiesterase-5 inhibitors
d. Drugs used in erectile dysfunction
e. Uses and misuses of anabolic steroids
4. Explain why:
   a. Anabolic steroids should not be used indiscriminately.
   b. Sildenafil should not be used concurrently with organic nitrates

MULTIPLE CHOICE QUESTIONS

1. Flutamide is used in CA
   (Recent Question 2016)
   a. Cervix   b. Prostate
   c. Kidneys   d. Liver
2. Danazol has which of the following action:
   (Recent Question 2016)
   a. Weak androgenic   b. Progestational
   c. Anabolic   d. All the above
3. Finasteride acts by blocking:
   (Recent Question 2016)
   a. α-receptors
   b. 5 α-reductase enzyme
   c. Androgen receptors
   d. β-receptors

4. The 5α-reductase inhibitor that has been found to be effective both in benign prostatic hypertrophy and male pattern baldness is:
   (Recent Question 2016)
   a. Flutamide   b. Finasteride
   c. Prazosin   d. Minoxidil
5. Most potent androgen is:
   (Recent Question 2016)
   a. Dihydrotestosterone
   b. Testosterone
   c. Dehydroepiandrosterone
   d. Epiandrosterone
6. Which of the following is antiandrogenic drug?
   (Recent Question 2016)
   a. Bicalutamide   b. Oxymetholone
   c. Raloxifene   d. Stanozolol

Ans.

| 1. (b) | 2. (d) | 3. (b) | 4. (b) | 5. (a) | 6. (a) |

Thyroid Hormone and Antithyroid Drugs

The thyroid gland is an endocrine gland located at front of the neck, below the Adam's apple. The thyroid gland secretes thyroid hormones, which enables normal growth and maturation, by maintaining an optimum metabolic rate.

THYROID HORMONES

The thyroid gland secretes 3 hormones: thyroxine (T_4), triiodothyronine (T_3) and calcitonin (Table 1).

TABLE 1	Thyroid hormones	
Thyroxine (T_4)	**Triiodothyronine (T_3)**	**Calcitonin**
• Produced by follicular cells of thyroid • Considered as thyroid hormone	• Produced by follicular cells of thyroid • Considered as thyroid hormone	• Produced by interfollicular C cells of thyroid • Not considered as thyroid hormone • Regulates Ca^{2+} and PO_4^{2-} metabolism

REGULATION OF THYROID HORMONES

The thyroid function (secretion of T_3 and T_4) is regulated by thyroid stimulating hormone or thyrotropin (TSH) which is secreted by the anterior pituitary gland. The secretion of TSH in turn, is regulated by thyrotropin releasing hormone (TRH) secreted by the hypothalamus.

T_3 and T_4 inhibits the secretion of TSH (at pituitary) and TRH (at hypothalamus) by a negative feedback mechanism as depicted in Figure 1.

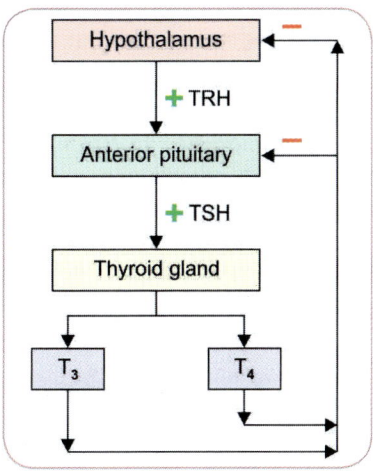

Figure 1: Regulation of thyroid secretion

The deficiency of thyroid hormones leads to cretinism in children and myxedema in adults. Cretinism is characterized by mental retardation because thyroid hormone is essential for normal brain development in children. An increased secretion of thyroid hormones leads to thyrotoxicosis (Figure 2).

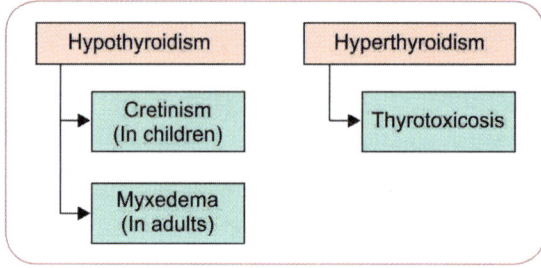

Figure 2: Thyroid disorders

SYNTHESIS OF THYROID HORMONES

The synthesis and release of thyroid hormones (from the thyroid gland) occurs by the following steps:

Iodide Trapping

It is the process of transport of iodide ions (I^-) into thyroid follicular cells. It is an active transport process and takes place by a membrane protein 'Na/I symporter' (NIS).

The iodide uptake is stimulated by TSH and inhibited by thiocyanates and perchlorates.

Oxidation and Iodination

The iodide ion is oxidized to iodine by the enzyme peroxidase. The peroxidase enzyme is inhibited by thioamide drugs (propylthiouracil [PTU] and carbimazole/methimazole).

The iodine combines with tyrosine (in thyroglobulin) to form MIT (monoiodotyrosine) and DIT (diiodotyrosine) without any enzymatic intervention.

Coupling

Coupling is a process where MIT and DIT combine to form T_3 and T_4 as follows:
- $MIT + DIT = T_3$
- $DIT + DIT = T_4$

The coupling reaction is catalyzed by the same peroxidase enzyme that is involved in the step of oxidation.

The peroxidase enzyme is inhibited by thioamide drugs (propylthiouracil and carbimazole/methimazole).

Hormone Release

Thyroglobulin is broken down (proteolysis) to release T_3, T_4, MIT and DIT. The T_3 and T_4 are released in the circulation while MIT and DIT are reutilized after deiodination.

This process is stimulated and controlled by TSH. The hormone release is inhibited by high level of iodides.

Peripheral Conversion (T_4 to T_3)

Most of the hormone released in the circulation is T_4; however, T_4 is less potent than T_3. The peripheral conversion from T_4 to T_3 mostly occurs in the liver and kidney.

This peripheral conversion is inhibited by the following drugs:
- Propylthiouracil (and not carbimazole/methimazole)
- Propranolol, amiodarone and glucocorticoids

The synthesis and release of thyroid hormones as well as the drugs affecting them is depicted in Figure 3.

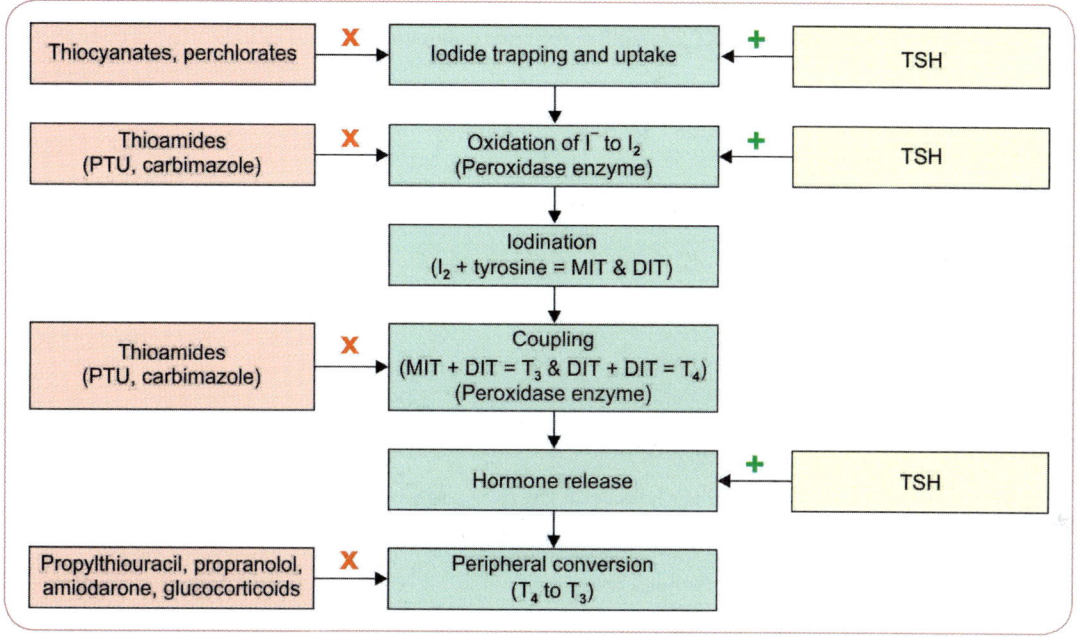

Figure 3: Synthesis and release of thyroid hormones

MECHANISM OF ACTION

The mechanism of action of thyroid hormones is comparable to that of steroid hormones. However, the following points are noteworthy regarding thyroid hormones:
- T_4 needs to be converted to T_3 inside the cell, before T_3 can bind to the nuclear receptors.
- In contrast to the steroid receptors (which are present in the cytoplasm), the thyroid receptors are located in the **nucleus** of the cell.

The mechanism of action of thyroid hormones is mentioned in Figure 4.

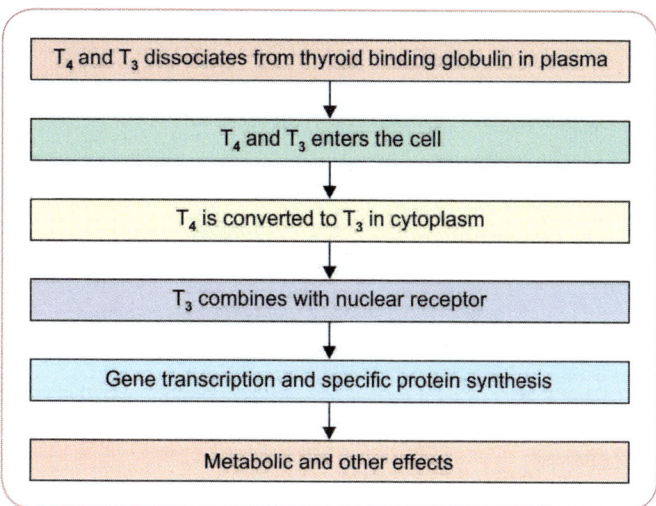

Figure 4: Thyroid hormones: Mechanism of action

PHARMACOLOGICAL ACTIONS OF THYROID HORMONES

The actions of thyroid hormones T_3 and T_4 are similar and can be illustrated in the features of hyperthyroidism and hypothyroidism (Table 2).

TABLE 2	Features of hyperthyroidism and hypothyroidism	
Function	**Hyperthyroidism**	**Hypothyroidism**
Metabolism	• Increased basal metabolic rate (BMR)	• Decreased basal metabolic rate
• Carbohydrate metabolism	• Increased glucose levels: diabetes like state	• Hypoglycemia in severe cases
• Protein metabolism	• Negative nitrogen balance; tissue wasting • Increased protein breakdown	• Positive nitrogen balance; weight gain
• Fat metabolism	• Decreased cholesterol and LDL levels	• Increased cholesterol and triglycerides
Cardiovascular system	• Increased heart rate, cardiac output and stroke volume • High-output heart failure • Arrhythmia, angina	• Decreased heart rate, cardiac output and stroke volume • Low-output heart failure • Pericardial effusion
CNS	• Anxiety, nervousness, excitability	• Lethargy, sluggishness • Mental retardation in cretinism
Skeletal muscle	• Weakness, muscle fatigue, tremor, increased tone	• Stiffness, muscle fatigue
GIT	• Increased appetite • Diarrhea	• Decreased appetite • Constipation
Eyes and face	• Retraction of upper lid with stare, exophthalmos, diplopia	• Drooping of eyelids, puffy face, large tongue
Skin and hair	• Warm, moist skin • Heat intolerance • Fine, thin hair	• Pale, puffy skin • Cold intolerance • Dry, brittle hair

T_3 AND T_4: IMPORTANT DIFFERENCES

The important differences between T_3 and T_4 are mentioned in Table 3.

TABLE 3	Differences between T_3 and T_4
T_3 (Triiodothyronine)	**T_4 (Thyroxine)**
• More potent	• Less potent
• Faster onset of action	• Slower onset of action
• Short half-life (1–2 days)	• Long half-life (6–7 days)
• Less amount present in circulation	• More amount present in circulation

Hence, the following can be inferred:
○ T_3 is the active hormone
○ T_4 is the major circulating hormone, as it is the main hormone released from thyroid

CLINICAL USES

Replacement therapy in various hypothyroid states, is the most important clinical use of thyroid hormones. The specific instances are further discussed:

Cretinism

Thyroid deficiency during fetal life results in congenital cretinism which is characterized by irreversible mental retardation and dwarfism.

Treatment of the newborn with levothyroxine therefore, should be started as soon as possible, to prevent mental retardation in the child and to ensure normal growth.

The response to thyroid hormones is dramatic in that the mental retardation is prevented and the growth normalizes.

Adult Hypothyroidism (Myxedema)

Adult hypothyroidism is treated by replacement therapy with levothyroxine (T_4). Levothyroxine is preferred over T_3 because:
- T_4 is better tolerated
- T_4 has a longer half-life
- T_4 requires once-daily dosing

Adult Hypothyroidism with Coronary Artery Disease

In patients with coronary artery disease, low levels of thyroid hormones have a protective effect on the heart (against increasing demands). Correcting hypothyroidism quickly can precipitate an attack of ischemia and myocardial infarction. Hence, the treatment is started with low doses of levothyroxine (12.5–25 µg/day), and then it is gradually increased.

Adult Hypothyroidism without Coronary Artery Disease

These patients can be treated with full replacement doses of levothyroxine (50–100 µg/day).

Myxedema Coma

The following are noteworthy regarding myxedema coma:
- Medical emergency
- End-state of long standing untreated myxedema
- May be precipitated by stress, infections or medications
- **Clinical features:**
  - Weakness, stupor, hypothermia, hypoventilation, hypoglycemia, hyponatremia, shock and death
- **Treatment:**
  - Immediate treatment is required as there is a high mortality rate (up to 60%)
  - All drugs should be given IV—there is poor absorption from other routes
  - Rapid thyroid replacement is critical
  - **Levothyroxine (T_4) is the drug of choice:** Loading dose (200–500 µg) followed by daily maintenance dose (100 µg)
  - Hydrocortisone to treat associated adrenal insufficiency
  - Ventilatory support
  - Correction of electrolyte imbalance
  - Rewarming with blankets.

Benign Thyroid Nodule

Some benign functioning nodules regress/decrease when TSH levels are suppressed by administering T_4.

Papillary Carcinoma of Thyroid

There may be a temporary tumor size reduction when TSH levels are suppressed by administering T_4.

ANTITHYROID DRUGS

These drugs lower the level of thyroid hormones and are used in the treatment of hyperthyroidism/thyrotoxicosis. These drugs either inhibit thyroid hormone synthesis, or release, or both.

CLASSIFICATION OF ANTITHYROID DRUGS

The classification of antithyroid drugs is mentioned in Figure 5.

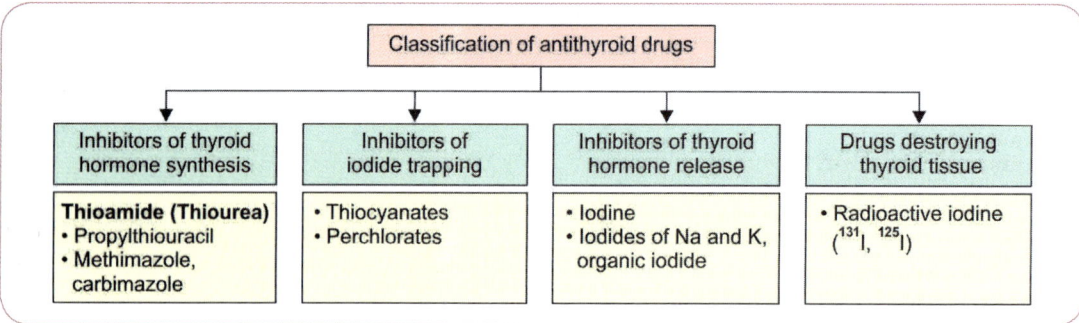

Figure 5: Classification of antithyroid drugs

Thioamides/Thioureas (Inhibitors of Thyroid Hormone Synthesis)

The 3 thioamides used as antithyroid drugs are propylthiouracil, methimazole and carbimazole.

Mechanism of Action

The thioamides inhibits the peroxidase enzyme. This results in the following actions:
- Prevents the oxidation of iodide ion to iodine. Hence, iodination of tyrosine (to form MIT and DIT) is prevented.
- Inhibits the coupling of iodotyrosine residues (MIT and DIT) to form T_3 and T_4.

In addition, propylthiouracil (but not carbimazole/methimazole) inhibits the peripheral conversion of T_4 to T_3.

Pharmacokinetics

The thioamides are well absorbed orally. They are widely distributed in the body and are concentrated in the thyroid. They cross placental barrier and are secreted in breast milk. They are metabolized in liver and the metabolites are excreted in urine. Carbimazole gets converted to methimazole after absorption.

Propylthiouracil has a shorter half-life and dosing is required every 4–8 hours; whereas carbimazole can be administered as a single daily dose.

Propylthiouracil is the preferred drug during pregnancy because it is more strongly bound to plasma proteins and therefore, less readily crosses the placenta. Surgery and ^{131}I are contraindicated during pregnancy.

The comparison between propylthiouracil and carbimazole is depicted in Table 4.

TABLE 4	Comparison between propylthiouracil and carbimazole
Propylthiouracil	**Carbimazole**
• Less potent	• More potent
• Highly plasma protein bound	• Less plasma protein bound
• Short half-life (1–2 hours)	• Long half-life (6–10 hours)
• Short duration of action (4–8 hours)	• Long duration of action (12–24 hours)
• Multiple daily doses required	• Single daily dose required
• Inhibits peripheral conversion of T_4 to T_3	• Do not inhibit peripheral conversion of T_4 to T_3
• No active metabolite	• Active metabolite is methimazole
• Low passage across placenta	• Low passage across placenta

Adverse Effects

The most common adverse effect is mild maculopapular pruritic skin rash. The other adverse effects include gastrointestinal intolerance, joint pain, headache, paresthesia and hepatitis. Hypothyroidism and goiter may occur due to overtreatment with these drugs, but is reversible.

The following adverse effects need special mention:

- ○ **Propylthiouracil-associated hepatitis:** Due to a black box warning (by the FDA) of severe hepatitis, propylthiouracil is considered as a reserve drug for use in:
    - ❑ 1st trimester of pregnancy
    - ❑ Thyroid storm
    - ❑ Patients with adverse events to carbimazole

    Propylthiouracil should not be used in children unless other options are not available.
- ○ **Agranulocytosis:** It is the most dangerous complication. It usually occurs during the first few weeks or months of therapy. It develops rapidly, so regular blood counts are of little use. These drugs should be immediately stopped on the development of sore throat and fever, which are the first signs of agranulocytosis. It is rapidly reversible on drug discontinuation.

    Cross-sensitivity of developing the reaction is 50% between propylthiouracil and carbimazole; hence, switching these drugs after the development of this reaction is not recommended.

Clinical Uses

Long-term Treatment of Thyrotoxicosis

Carbimazole/methimazole are the preferred drugs as they have a long half-life, are longer acting and have lesser adverse effects.

Preoperative Preparation in Thyrotoxicosis

Surgery is not safe in thyrotoxic patients. Hence, all patients must be rendered euthyroid prior to surgery.

Carbimazole is used for achieving euthyroidism prior to thyroid surgery. Iodide is given for 7–10 days before surgery to decrease the vascularity of the thyroid gland. All the antithyroid drugs should be discontinued after surgery.

Along with ^{131}I Therapy

They are used along with radioactive iodine to hasten recovery while waiting for the effects of radiation therapy.

Thyroid Storm (Thyrotoxic Crisis)

Propylthiouracil is used along with propranolol, iodides, corticosteroids and supportive measures. Propylthiouracil is the preferred drug in thyrotoxicosis because it inhibits the peripheral conversion of T_4 to T_3.

Anion Inhibitors (Inhibitors of Iodide Trapping)

These drugs block iodide trapping and hence, block its uptake into the thyroid gland. The examples include thiocyanate, perchlorate, pertechnetate and nitrate.

They are highly toxic agents and have unpredictable actions; hence, they are no longer used clinically.

Iodine and Iodides (Inhibitors of Thyroid Hormone Release)

They are the oldest drugs used in hyperthyroidism. They are the fastest acting thyroid inhibitors. Nowadays, they are rarely used as solo therapy.

Iodides inhibit almost all steps in thyroid hormone synthesis. They decrease the iodination and synthesis of iodotyrosines (MIT, DIT) and iodothyronines (T_3, T_4). However, the most prominent action is the inhibition of hormone release. Iodides decrease the size and vascularity of the hyperplastic thyroid gland.

Escape Phenomenon

With daily administration, the peak inhibitory effects of iodides are observed in 10–15 days. Subsequently, in 4–8 weeks (in individuals with normal thyroid function), the thyroid gland escapes from this inhibitory effect and iodide organification resumes. The hyperthyroidism may then return with a much greater effect.

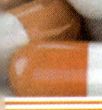

The following effects may be seen with iodide administration: Wolff-Chaikoff effect and Jod-Basedow effect (Table 5).

TABLE 5	Wolff-Chaikoff and Jod-Basedow effect
Iodides/Iodine administration	
Wolff-Chaikoff effect	Jod-Basedow effect
• Iodine induced hypothyroidism • Occurs in normal or hyperthyroid state • Excess iodine acutely inhibits iodination of tyrosine residues • Is a transient 2-day phenomenon	• Iodine induced hyperthyroidism • Occurs in iodine deficient hypothyroid state • Thyroid hormone synthesis increases excessively due to high iodine exposure

Preparations

○ Lugol's iodine (5% iodine in 10% KI solution)
○ Ipodate sodium and Iopanoic acid

Clinical Uses

Preoperative Preparation

The iodides are given for 10 days prior to surgery because it decreases the size of gland, makes it less firm and less vascular, so that it is easier to operate upon with less bleeding and complications.

Thyroid Storm

Iodides are given to treat severe thyrotoxicosis when a quick decrease in circulating levels of T_3 and T_4 are required.

Carbimazole is additionally given to make the patient euthyroid and *propranolol* may be additionally given for rapid control of symptoms.

Prophylaxis of Endemic Goiter

Iodides are given in the form of 'iodized salt'.

Antiseptic

Tincture of iodine is used.

Adverse Effects

The adverse effects may be divided into acute and chronic toxicity (Table 6).

TABLE 6	Adverse effects of iodides
Acute toxicity	Hypersensitivity, angioedema, laryngeal edema, cutaneous hemorrhages, fever, lymphadenopathy, arthralgia, eosinophilia etc.
Chronic toxicity (Iodism)	Salivation, sneezing, eye irritation, swelling of the lids, burning in the mouth, headache, productive cough, gastric irritation, skin lesions etc. These symptoms disappear after stopping iodides. Hypothyroidism and goiter may occur on long-term use of high doses. Use during pregnancy may cause fetal goiter.

Radioactive Iodine

The radioactive isotope used therapeutically is [131]I. The isotope used for diagnostic scan is [123]I.

[131]I is rapidly concentrated by the thyroid and emits γ and β rays from within the follicles. The β rays cause necrosis of the follicular cells leading to fibrosis. This results in correction of the hyperthyroid state.

Clinical Uses

It is used in hyperthyroidism due to Grave's disease or toxic multinodular goiter.

It is administered orally as capsule or solution. The average total dose is 4–15 millicurie. The response is slow which starts after 2 weeks and then increases gradually.

^{131}I is the treatment of choice in older patients, in those having heart diseases (e.g. heart failure, angina) and in whom surgery is contraindicated.

Advantages

- Treatment is simple and convenient. Hospitalization is not required.
- No surgical risk of injury to recurrent laryngeal nerve and parathyroid glands.
- Hyperthyroidism is permanently cured.

Disadvantages

- **Hypothyroidism:** There is a high chance of delayed hypothyroidism
- **Slow acting:** Long time-period for the response to occur
- Not suitable in:
  - **Pregnancy**—fetal thyroid destruction occur; may lead to cretinism
  - **Children and young patients:** They are very likely to become hypothyroid later; may require lifelong thyroid treatment.

Beta Adrenergic Blockers

Propranolol (and other nonselective β blockers) are an important form of therapy for thyrotoxicosis. The most widely used β blocker is propranolol.

They rapidly decrease the symptoms that occur due to sympathetic overstimulation (e.g. tremor, palpitation, tachycardia, sweating, nervousness). They do not affect thyroid function. Propranolol in addition also inhibits the peripheral conversion of T_4 to T_3.

They are used in the following situations:

- To provide symptomatic relief until the effect of carbimazole or ^{131}I appear
- Preoperative preparation before thyroidectomy
- Thyroid storm (thyrotoxic crisis)

Thyroid Storm (Thyrotoxic Crisis)

It is a medical emergency characterized by sudden acute increase of all the symptoms of thyrotoxicosis. Immediate vigorous treatment is required. The salient features and the treatment of thyrotoxic crisis is mentioned in Table 7.

TABLE 7	Thyroid storm (Thyrotoxicosis)
Features	**Treatment**
• Acute, life threatening, hypermetabolic emergency • Occurs due to excessive release of thyroid hormones • Fever, tachycardia, hypertension, GIT abnormalities, mental confusion (apart from hyperthyroid features) • Precipitated by sepsis, drugs, diabetic ketoacidosis, trauma, surgery etc. • Almost invariably fatal if left untreated; rapid diagnosis and aggressive treatment are critical	• Nonselective β blockers: Propranolol, esmolol • Diltiazem (If β blockers are contraindicated) • Propylthiouracil blocks hormone synthesis • Oral iodides (Inhibits hormone release; ipodate decreases peripheral $T_4 \to T_3$) • Hydrocortisone IV (Corrects any adrenal insufficiency, if present and also decreases peripheral $T_4 \to T_3$) • Supportive care (Cooling, hydration antibiotics etc.)

Drugs Acting on the Endocrine Physiology

SECTION H

1. Classify antithyroid drugs. Explain the mechanism of action, pharmacokinetics, adverse effects and therapeutic uses of any one drug inhibiting thyroid synthesis.
2. What is the rationale of using propranolol in thyrotoxicosis.
3. List important differences between propylthiouracil and carbimazole.
4. Write short notes on:
   a. Thyroid storm
   b. Myxedema coma
   c. Propylthiouracil
   d. Lugol's iodine
   e. Radioactive iodine
   f. Iodine and iodide preparations
5. Explain why Lugol's iodine is given for a few days prior to surgery in thyrotoxicosis.

MULTIPLE CHOICE QUESTIONS

1. All of the following are rare but serious/fatal side effects of thioanamide group of antithyroid drugs except: *(AIIMS Nov 2016)*
   a. Agranulocytosis
   b. Aplastic anemia
   c. Liver toxicity
   d. Lung fibrosis

2. Conversion of T_4 to T_3 is inhibited by all except: *(AIIMS Nov 2011)*
   a. Propranolol
   b. Propylthiouracil
   c. Amiodarone
   d. Methimazole

3. The first line antithyroid drug is methimazole, and the antithyroid drug which is safest in pregnancy is propylthiouracil. Which among the following is the fastest acting antithyroid drug? *(Recent Question 2016)*
   a. Sodium iodide
   b. Propylthiouracil
   c. Methimazole
   d. Carbimazole

4. Which drug prevent peripheral conversion of T_4 to T_3 *(Recent Question 2016)*
   a. Propylthiouracil
   b. Propranolol
   c. Iodides
   d. Diltiazem

5. Which of the following drug does not act on thyroid? *(Recent Question 2016)*
   a. Propranolol
   b. Propylthiouracil
   c. Sodium iodide
   d. Thiocyanate

6. Lugol's Iodine contains: *(Recent Question 2016)*
   a. 5% iodine and 10% Kl
   b. 10% iodine and 20% Kl
   c. 10% iodine and 15% Kl
   d. 5% iodine and 15% Kl

7. True about propylthiouracil: *(Recent Question 2016)*
   a. Inhibit peripheral conversion of T_4 to T_3
   b. Crosses placenta and secreted in breast milk
   c. Active metabolite formed inside the body
   d. 5 times more potent than carbimazole

8. Thyroid storm-management all except: *(Recent Question 2016)*
   a. Propylthiouracil
   b. Lugol's iodine
   c. Steroids
   d. Thyroid surgery

9. A patient on treatment with carbimazole develops sore throat. Immediate investigation to be done is: *(Recent Question 2016)*
   a. Renal function tests
   b. Thyroid function test
   c. Complete blood count
   d. Liver function tests

10. Propylthiouracil is used in all except: *(Recent Question 2016)*
    a. Thyroid storm
    b. Life threatening thyrotoxicosis
    c. First trimester pregnancy
    d. Agranulocytosis caused by methimazole

Ans.

| 1. (d) | 2. (d) | 3. (a) | 4. (a) | 5. (a) | 6. (a) |
| 7. (a) | 8. (d) | 9. (c) | 10. (d) | | |

40 Insulin, Oral Antidiabetic Drugs and Glucagon

Diabetes mellitus (DM) is a metabolic disorder characterized by hyperglycemia. The symptoms in diabetes can include:

- Polyuria—increased urine production
- Polydipsia—increased thirst
- Polyphagia—excessive eating

The underlying cause is a deficiency of insulin which can be relative or absolute. The deficiency of insulin affects the metabolism of carbohydrates, proteins and fats.

TYPE 1 DIABETES

Type 1 diabetes was also earlier known as insulin-dependent diabetes mellitus (IDDM) or juvenile-onset diabetes mellitus. Onset of type 1 diabetes is usually in childhood and adolescence.

In type 1 diabetes, there is an autoimmune mediated destruction of pancreatic beta cells. This leads to a reduced production of insulin and insulin deficiency in the body.

The cause of autoimmune mediated destruction of beta cells is not completely understood and is believed to be due to multiple factors including environmental, genetic susceptibility, viruses etc.

Therapy with insulin is mandatory in patients with type 1 diabetes.

TYPE 2 DIABETES

Type 2 DM was earlier known as noninsulin dependent diabetes mellitus (NIDDM). Type 2 diabetes is associated with a resistance to insulin. Onset of type 2 DM is usually in adulthood.

Type 2 DM is usually associated with obesity and weight gain. Type 2 diabetes is more common than type 1 diabetes.

INSULIN

Insulin is synthesized in the β cells of pancreatic islets. Banting and Best discovered insulin in 1921.

The synthesis of insulin occurs in the β cells of pancreatic islets as preproinsulin (single chain peptide with 110 amino acids) which is converted to proinsulin (by removal of 24 amino acids). Removal of C peptide from proinsulin leads to the formation of insulin.

Insulin is a two-chain polypeptide that has 51 amino acids. The A chain has 21 amino acids and the B chain has 30 amino acids. The two peptide chains are connected by two disulfide bonds.

INSULIN SECRETION

Insulin is secreted at a basal rate of approximately 1 U/hour by the pancreas. Larger quantities are released from the pancreas after every meal. The following factors regulate the secretion of insulin from the β cells (Table 1):

- Chemical
  - Release of insulin is triggered by the entry of glucose in the β cells of pancreas. The entry of glucose is through the glucose transporter (GLUT-2).
  - Amino acids, fatty acids and ketones can also trigger the release of insulin
  - Glucose is the main regulator of insulin release and it can also stimulate synthesis of insulin from the pancreas

❑ Oral glucose is more effective in causing insulin release as compared to IV glucose. This is possibly due to glucose-induced generation of incretins (chemical signals) from the GIT. Incretins cause anticipatory release of insulin from the pancreatic β cells.

TABLE 1	Regulation of insulin secretion	
Chemical	**Neural**	**Hormonal**
• Release triggered by glucose	• α_2 adrenergic stimulation → Decrease insulin release	• Glucagon → Release of insulin and somatostatin
• Other triggers are amino acids, fatty acids and ketones	• β_2 adrenergic stimulation → Increase insulin release	• Somatostatin → Inhibits release of insulin and glucagon
• Glucose is the main factor and uses GLUT 2 transporter	• Cholinergic stimulation (By ACh or vagal) → Increase insulin release	• Insulin → Inhibits secretion of glucagon

o Neural
  ❑ Primary site of central regulation of insulin is in the hypothalamus
  ❑ α_2 adrenergic stimulation → Decrease insulin release
  ❑ β_2 adrenergic stimulation → Increase insulin release
  ❑ Cholinergic stimulation (By ACh or vagal) → Increase insulin release
o Hormonal
  ❑ Glucagon → Causes release of insulin and somatostatin
  ❑ Somatostatin → Inhibits release of insulin and glucagon
  ❑ Insulin → Inhibits secretion of glucagon
  ❑ Other hormones such as growth hormone, corticosteroids, thyroxine modify the release of insulin

▌METABOLIC ACTIONS

Insulin enhances the storage of glucose and fat in the body and hence, the main metabolic effects are anabolic. These effects impact the metabolism of glucose, proteins and fats and take place predominantly in the liver, muscle and adipose tissue. Insulin promotes the entry of glucose in cells of the body.

The key metabolic effects of insulin are mentioned in Figure 1.

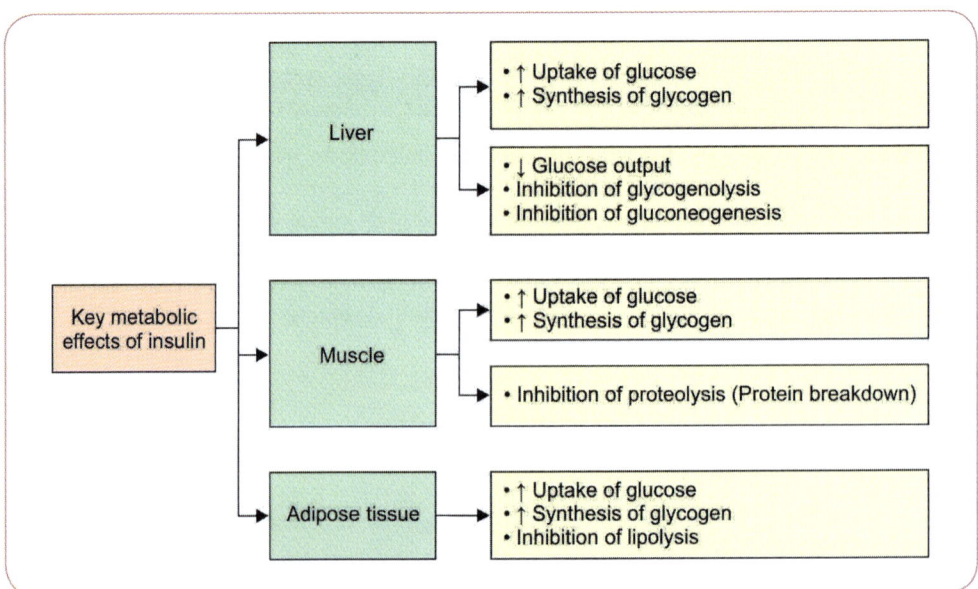

Figure 1: Key metabolic effects of insulin

PHARMACOKINETICS

Insulin is a peptide and gets degraded in the GIT. Hence, it is not administered orally. Parenterally administered insulin is metabolized mainly in the liver.

MECHANISM OF ACTION

Insulin acts by binding to tyrosine kinase receptors present on the cellular membranes. These receptors consist of 2 α subunits which are extracellular and 2 β subunits that are transmembrane proteins.

PREPARATIONS OF INSULINS

Conventional Preparations of Insulin

These are obtained from beef or pork.
- Pork insulin
  - Differs from human insulin by one amino acid
- Beef insulin
  - Differs from human insulin by three amino acids

Both beef and pork derived insulins are antigenic as they contain ~1% of other proteins. Beef derived insulins are more antigenic than the pork derived insulins.

Highly Purified or Monocomponent Insulins

These insulins were made by applying purification techniques such as ion-exchange chromatography to conventional pork insulins. These highly purified or monocomponent insulins have the following advantages:
- Less antigenic than conventional insulin preparations
- Lower incidence of insulin resistance
- Lower incidence of lipodystrophy at the site of injection
- More stable

Human Insulins

Human insulins are produced by recombinant DNA technology using *E. coli* and yeast. They have the same amino acid sequence as insulin (produced by the human body). They are least antigenic and have a very low incidence of insulin resistance or lipodystrophy.

Example include regular human insulin.

Insulin Analogues

These are made by recombinant DNA technology. The sequence of amino acids is slightly different as compared to human insulins. The pharmacokinetic profile of insulin analogues is modified, but the pharmacodynamic effects are similar to insulin. Insulin analogues offer more stability and consistency. Examples include insulin glargine, insulin aspart etc.

Preparations of Insulin and Insulin Analogues based upon Onset and Duration of Action

Insulin preparations can be categorized by their time to onset and duration of action (Table 2). It should be noted that the pharmacokinetic parameters for insulin vary across patients and can be impacted by multiple variables including—injection site and the technique, amount of blood flow to the injection site, amount of subcutaneous fat etc.

TABLE 2	Insulin preparations	
	Types of Insulin	**Comments**
Rapid acting	• Inulin lispro • Insulin aspart • Insulin glulisine	• Can be mixed with regular insulin and neutral protamine hagedorn (NPH) insulin
Short acting	• Regular (soluble) insulin	• Can be used via SC, IV route • Can be mixed with all preparations except insulin glargine • Duration of action is 6–8 hours
Intermediate acting	• Insulin zinc suspension (Lente) • Neutral protamine hagedorn (NPH) or isophane insulin	• Can be mixed with regular insulin
Long acting	• Protamine zinc insulin (PZI) • Insulin glargine • Insulin detemir • Insulin degludec	• Protamine zinc insulin can be mixed with regular insulin • Insulin glargine cannot be mixed with any other insulin because it has an acidic pH (pH 4.0)

SPECIAL INSULIN DELIVERY SYSTEMS

Insulin Pen

○ Are prefilled insulin delivery devices
○ Can be used as an alternative to syringes
○ Advantage include ease during traveling

Insulin Pump

○ Used for continuous delivery of insulin via the subcutaneous route
○ Insulin pump can be set-up to deliver insulin at a basal rate and also can provide a premeal bolus dose
○ Disadvantages include increased cost of external device, risk of skin infections, risk of pump malfunction that may impede/stop delivery of insulin and lead to complications
○ Requires frequent monitoring of blood glucose and maintaining vigilance regarding pump function

ADVERSE EFFECTS OF INSULIN THERAPY

The adverse effects of insulin therapy include the following (Table 3):
○ Hypoglycemia
○ Allergic reactions
○ Insulin resistance
○ Lipodystrophy
○ Edema

TABLE 3	Adverse effects of insulin therapy
1. Hypoglycemia	
Most common and a potentially dangerous complication. Irreversible neurological damage can occur in prolonged hypoglycemia.	
Hypoglycemia can occur in any patient with diabetes and can be due to administration of a large dose of insulin, missing or delaying a meal, or performing vigorous physical exercise.	

Contd...

Clinical manifestations include	• Symptoms due to counter regulatory sympathetic stimulation ▪ Sweating, palpitations, tachycardia, anxiety, tremors • Symptoms due to neuroglucopenia (↓ glucose in brain) ▪ Confusion, headache, fatigue, dizziness, behavioral changes ▪ Severe cases can result in seizures, unconsciousness, coma Hypoglycemia unawareness → patients with long standing diabetes mellitus may not become aware of the hypoglycemic episodes
Treatment includes	• Glucose—oral or IV • Glucagon or adrenaline—if patient cannot take oral glucose and IV glucose is not available
2. Allergic reactions	• Not commonly observed and are due to contaminants • Can manifest as rashes, anaphylaxis
3. Insulin resistance	Increased requirement of insulin (Conventionally >200 U/day) in a patient of diabetes mellitus. • **Acute insulin resistance** ▪ Seen in conditions such as infection, surgery, trauma, stress, corticosteroid therapy, ketoacidosis ▪ Management includes treatment of the underlying condition and administration of high doses of insulin ▪ Insulin requirement becomes normal once the underlying condition is treated • **Chronic insulin resistance** ▪ Usually observed in patients who are on prolonged therapy with beef or pork insulin ▪ Develops due to the presence of antibodies that can bind to insulin ▪ More common in patients of type 2 DM ▪ May respond to switching to more purified insulins
4. Lipodystrophy	• Injection site lipodystrophy can develop upon prolonged use • Use of purified insulin preparations can prevent the development of lipodystrophy
5. Edema	• May be observed at the initiation of insulin therapy and is due to retention of salt and water

DRUG INTERACTIONS

Some of the drug interactions with insulin are mentioned below:
- β blockers inhibit symptoms due to counter regulatory sympathetic stimulation and can prolong hypoglycemia. It can lead to masking of the warning signs of hypoglycemia such as palpitations, tremors etc.
- Drugs such as corticosteroids, thiazides, oral contraceptives increase blood glucose levels and can decrease the efficacy of insulin.

CLINICAL USES

The clinical uses of insulin include the following:
- Type 1 diabetes mellitus
- Type 2 diabetes mellitus (in conditions where the blood sugar level is not controlled by diet, exercise, oral anti-diabetic drugs etc.)
- Diabetic ketoacidosis
- Hyperosmolar (nonketotic hyperglycemic) coma
- Stressful conditions such as surgery, trauma and infections in diabetic patients
- Diabetes in pregnancy

MANAGEMENT OF DIABETIC KETOACIDOSIS (DIABETIC COMA)

Diabetic ketoacidosis is a medical emergency and requires prompt management.

It is more common in patients with type 1 diabetes mellitus and rare in patients with type 2 diabetes mellitus.

Conditions such as infections, trauma, stress etc. are often the precipitating factors. Clinical manifestations include dehydration, nausea, vomiting, hypotension, hyperventilation, impaired consciousness and coma. The key measures in the management of diabetic ketoacidosis are mentioned in Table 4.

TABLE 4	Diabetic ketoacidosis
1.	Regular insulin • Intravenous bolus followed by infusion
2.	Fluid replacement • Intravenous fluids—initially normal saline is infused, followed by 5% glucose in ½ N saline
3.	Potassium • Hypokalemia can occur during insulin therapy and acidosis correction. ECG monitoring and serum potassium measurements should be performed.
4.	Sodium bicarbonate (if required)
5.	Phosphate (if required)
6.	Antibiotics (to treat any infections, if present)
7.	Supportive management of airway, breathing, circulation, fluid and electrolyte balance

MANAGEMENT OF HYPEROSMOLAR (NONKETOTIC HYPERGLYCEMIC) COMA

Hyperosmolar hyperglycemic coma is a medical emergency and requires prompt management.

It is seen in patients with type 2 diabetes mellitus. The patient presents with hyperglycemia, dehydration and hyperosmolality. There is no ketosis. The principles of management are similar to that of diabetic ketoacidosis; however, the patient requires faster fluid replacement and alkali therapy is usually not needed.

ORAL ANTIDIABETIC DRUGS

The oral antidiabetic drugs can be classified as follows (Table 5):

TABLE 5	Classification of oral antidiabetic drugs	

1.	Sulfonylureas	• First generation
		  ▪ Tolbutamide, chlorpropamide
		• Second generation
		  ▪ Glyburide (Glibenclamide), glipizide, gliclazide, glimepiride

2.	Biguanides	• Metformin
3.	Meglitinide analogue	• Repaglinide
4.	d-phenylalanine derivative	• Nateglinide
5.	Thiazolidinediones	• Pioglitazone, rosiglitazone
6.	Alpha-glucosidase inhibitors	• Acarbose, miglitol, voglibose
7	Other drugs/Newer drugs	• Glucagon-like peptide-1 (GLP-1) receptor agonists → Exenatide, liraglutide • Dipeptidyl peptidase-4 (DPP-4) inhibitors → Saxagliptin, sitagliptin, alogliptin, linagliptin • Amylin analogue → Pramlintide • Sodium-glucose co-transporter 2 (SGLT-2) inhibitors → Canagliflozin, dapagliflozin

SULFONYLUREAS

The mechanism of action of first and second-generation sulfonylureas is similar. The second-generation sulfonylureas (e.g. glibenclamide, glipizide) are more potent than the first-generation sulfonylureas (e.g. tolbutamide, chlorpropamide).

Mechanism of Action

Sulfonylureas cause hypoglycemia by the following action:
o   Stimulate insulin secretion by acting on sulfonylurea receptors on the pancreatic β cells. Hence, they are known as insulin secretagogues.

Sulfonylureas are not effective in patients with type 1 diabetes mellitus because they require the presence of functioning pancreatic β cells. At least 30% of the functioning pancreatic β cells are required for their therapeutic effect.

Pharmacokinetics

o   Sulfonylureas are well absorbed following oral administration. Metabolism occurs in the liver and metabolites are excreted in the urine.
o   They are highly bound to plasma proteins (90–99%).

Adverse Effects

The key adverse effects of sulfonylureas are mentioned below:
o   Hypoglycemia
    □   Can be potentially life-threatening
    □   Higher incidence in elderly and in patients with underlying liver and renal disease
    □   Chlorpropamide has a high propensity to cause hypoglycemia due to long duration of action
o   Weight gain
o   Hypersensitivity
    □   Rashes, allergic reactions, leukopenia
o   Other adverse effects
    □   Nausea, vomiting, headache, diarrhea
    □   Chlorpropamide → intolerance to alcohol (disulfiram like action), dilutional hyponatremia, cholestatic jaundice
o   Pregnancy → sulfonylureas are not considered safe during pregnancy

Drug Interactions

Some of the key interactions of sulfonylureas are mentioned below:
o   Phenytoin, phenobarbitone, rifampicin can reduce the effect of sulfonylureas by enhancing their metabolism
o   Corticosteroids, thiazides and oral contraceptives can increase blood sugar levels and decrease the effects of sulfonylureas
o   Sulfonamides and salicylates can enhance the effect of sulfonylureas by displacing them from plasma protein binding sites. This can lead to hypoglycemia.
o   Cimetidine, sulfonamides and warfarin can inhibit the metabolism of sulfonylureas and increase their level. This can lead to hypoglycemia.
o   Propranolol can have the following effects in patients:
    □   Inhibit glycogenolysis (blockade of hepatic β_2 receptors)
    □   Mask the compensatory symptoms due to hypoglycemia (e.g. palpitations, tachycardia, tremors)

Clinical Uses

Sulfonylureas are used in patients of type 2 diabetes mellitus.

BIGUANIDES—METFORMIN

Mechanism of Action

The mechanism of action of metformin includes:
○ Reduction of hepatic gluconeogenesis → main action
○ Enhances the utilization of glucose in fat and skeletal muscle
○ Decreases the intestinal absorption of glucose

Metformin does not evoke the release of insulin. Hence, it rarely causes hypoglycemia.

Pharmacokinetics

Metformin is well absorbed orally. It does not bind to plasma proteins. It is not metabolized and is excreted unchanged in the urine.

Adverse Effects

○ Gastrointestinal effects (Nausea, diarrhea, abdominal pain, metallic taste) are most common—occurs in approx. 20% of patients
○ Lactic acidosis
  ❑ Rare but serious complication
○ Vitamin B_{12} deficiency can occur on long-term use of metformin as it can interfere with B_{12} absorption
○ Contraindicated in patients with renal, hepatic, respiratory and cardiovascular disease, hypotensive states and chronic alcoholics.

Clinical Uses

Metformin is used in patients of type 2 diabetes mellitus.

MEGLITINIDE ANALOGUE (REPAGLINIDE)/D-PHENYLALANINE DERIVATIVE (NATEGLINIDE)

The mechanism of action of these drugs is similar to sulfonylureas. They cause the release of insulin from the pancreas. They are known as insulin secretagogues.

The onset of action is rapid, and the duration of action is shorter. They can therefore be used multiple times in a day to control postprandial hyperglycemia, as compared with the once or twice daily dosing of sulfonylureas.

Adverse effects of repaglinide include weight gain and hypoglycemia; while those of nateglinide include nausea, dizziness and flu-like symptoms. These drugs should be avoided in patients with hepatic disease.

They are clinically used in patients of type 2 diabetes mellitus and are used to control postprandial hyperglycemia.

THIAZOLIDINEDIONES—PIOGLITAZONE, ROSIGLITAZONE

These drugs are insulin sensitizers—increase the sensitivity of peripheral tissues (adipose tissue, skeletal muscle, liver) to insulin.

They are agonists for the nuclear receptor peroxisome-proliferation-activating receptor-γ (PPAR-γ).

Binding of the drugs to nuclear receptor PPAR-γ leads to the transcription of various insulin responsive genes. They enhance lipogenesis, increase the entry of glucose into adipose tissue and muscle and decrease hepatic gluconeogenesis.

The adverse effects include the following:

- Weight gain and edema are common adverse effects
- Increase in plasma volume, nausea, vomiting
- Heart failure may be precipitated or aggravated
- Liver toxicity—periodic monitoring of hepatic function is recommended
- Contraindicated in patients of heart failure or hepatic disease
- Increased risk of bone fracture
- Increase risk of bladder cancer

They are clinically used in patients of type 2 diabetes mellitus.

ALPHA-GLUCOSIDASE INHIBITORS—ACARBOSE, MIGLITOL, VOGLIBOSE

Alpha-glucosidase is an intestinal enzyme that is involved in the digestion of starch and disaccharides.

Acarbose, miglitol and voglibose inhibit alpha-glucosidase enzyme. This delays the digestion and absorption of carbohydrates leading to a reduction in postprandial glucose levels.

These drugs are mild antihyperglycemic agents and are used as adjuvant therapy in obese patients of type 2 diabetes mellitus.

Adverse effects include flatulence and diarrhea.

GLUCAGON-LIKE PEPTIDE-1 RECEPTOR AGONISTS—EXENATIDE, LIRAGLUTIDE

These drugs are analogues of glucagon like peptide-1 (GLP-1) and exert their effect by binding to GLP-1 receptors. GLP-1 is an incretin and is released from the GIT after meals. It has the following effects:

- Improve glucose dependent insulin secretion
- Decrease glucagon secretion
- Decrease gastric emptying time
- Suppression of appetite

The GLP-1 is not used therapeutically as it has a short half-life and is inactivated by dipeptidyl peptidase-4 (DPP-4) enzyme. However, the GLP-1 receptor agonists (which are resistant to DPP-4) can be used therapeutically.

The GLP-1 receptor agonists are indicated for management of type 2 diabetes mellitus. They are often used as adjunct medications. They are injected subcutaneously. Adverse effects include nausea, vomiting and pancreatitis.

DIPEPTIDYL PEPTIDASE-4 INHIBITORS—SAXAGLIPTIN, SITAGLIPTIN, ALOGLIPTIN, LINAGLIPTIN

These drugs inhibit the dipeptidyl peptidase-4 (DPP-4) enzyme and prevent the inactivation glucagon like peptide (GLP-1). This leads to an increased release of insulin and decreased release of glucagon.

It is clinically used in patients of type 2 diabetes mellitus. Adverse effects include headache, rhinitis, pancreatitis and allergic reactions.

SYNTHETIC AMYLIN ANALOGUE—PRAMLINTIDE

Pramlintide is an amylin analogue. It has the following effects:

- Reduction of glucagon secretion
- Reduced gastric emptying
- Suppression of appetite

It is clinically used in both type 1 and type 2 diabetes mellitus. It is injected subcutaneously. Adverse effects include nausea, headache and hypoglycemia.

SODIUM-GLUCOSE COTRANSPORTER 2 INHIBITORS—CANAGLIFLOZIN, DAPAGLIFLOZIN

These drugs inhibit sodium-glucose cotransporter 2 (SGLT2) and have the following effects:
- Inhibition of renal glucose reabsorption
- Glycosuria
- Reduced plasma glucose levels

They are clinically used in type 2 diabetes mellitus. Adverse effects include genitourinary infections, osmotic diuresis and increased thirst.

GLUCAGON

Glucagon has 29 amino acids and is secreted by the α cells of the pancreas.

It causes hyperglycemia by the following effects:
- Increased gluconeogenesis
- Increased glycogenolysis
- Reduced utilization of glucose in adipose tissue and muscle

The clinical uses of glucagon include the following:
- Hypoglycemia—glucagon is used in emergency for severe hypoglycemia when the patient cannot take oral glucose and IV glucose is not available (Glucagon has a secondary role).
- Cardiogenic shock—in patients with β blocker overdose. Glucagon has a cardiac stimulant effect.
- Radiology of the intestine—Due to its ability to relax the intestines, glucagon is used in radiology to facilitate radiography of the intestine.

ASSESS YOURSELF (Examination Questions of Various Universities)

1. Classify and enumerate insulin preparations. Discuss the adverse effects and clinical uses of insulin.
2. Classify oral antidiabetic drugs. Discuss the mechanism of action and adverse effects of metformin.
3. Enumerate the drugs used for treatment of diabetes mellitus. Discuss the mechanism of action, adverse effects and clinical uses of sulfonylureas.
4. Discuss the management of diabetic ketoacidosis.

5. Write short notes on:
   a. Repaglinide
   b. Biguanides
   c. Glibenclamide
   d. Thiazolidinediones
   e. Insulin sensitizers
   f. Adverse effects of insulin
6. Discuss in brief the pharmacological basis for the use of:
   a. Pioglitazone in diabetes mellitus
   b. Potassium supplementation in diabetic ketoacidosis

MULTIPLE CHOICE QUESTIONS

1. Drug used in both type 1 and 2 DM
   (Recent Question 2016)
   a. Bromocriptine   b. Colesevelam
   c. Pramlintide   d. Exenatide
2. Pramlintide is   *(Recent Question 2016)*
   a. Synthetic amylin analogue
   b. Inhibitor of DPP 4
   c. GLP 1 analogue
   d. PPAR gamma
3. Rosiglitazone mechanism of action is:
   (Recent Question 2016)
   a. Acts as PPAR gamma agonist
   b. Inhibitor of alpha glucosidase
   c. Acts as amylin analogue
   d. Acts as dipeptidyl peptidase inhibitor
4. Incretin like function is seen in:
   (Recent Question 2016)
   a. Exenatide
   b. Miglitol
   c. Pioglitazone
   d. Repaglinide

5. Drug used in postprandial sugar control is:
   (Recent Question 2016)
   a. Alpha glucosidase inhibitors
   b. Biguanides
   c. Sulfonylurea
   d. Repaglinide
6. Which of the following antidiabetic drugs can cause vitamin B_{12} deficiency?
   (Recent Question 2016)
   a. Glipizide   b. Acarbose
   c. Metformin   d. Pioglitazone
7. Tolbutamide acts by increasing:
   (Recent Question 2016)
   a. Insulin receptors   b. Glucose entry
   c. Glucose absorption   d. Insulin secretion
8. Common side effect of thiazolidinediones is:
   (Recent Question 2016)
   a. Dysgeusia
   b. Hypoglycemia
   c. Water retention with weight gain
   d. Anemia

Ans.

1. (c)	2. (a)	3. (a)	4. (a)	5. (d)	6. (c)
7. (d)	8. (c)				

41

Drugs Affecting Calcium Balance

▌CALCIUM

Calcium is an essential constituent of the body. It is required for various biological functions. Most of the calcium (99%) is stored in the bones.

The plasma calcium levels are mainly regulated by the following hormones:
- Parathormone (PTH)
- Calcitonin
- Calcitriol (Vitamin D)

These hormones regulate plasma calcium levels by controlling its intestinal absorption, bone exchanges and excretion from the kidneys. Other hormones such as corticosteroids, androgens, thyroxine etc. also play a role in calcium metabolism.

The normal plasma level of calcium ranges from 9 mg/dL to 11 mg/dL.

Functions

Calcium regulates (and is required for) the following physiological functions:
- Excitability of nerves and muscles
- Contraction of all types of muscles (cardiac, skeletal and smooth)
- Formation of bones and teeth
- Release of neurotransmitters
- Maintenance of cell membrane integrity and regulation of cell membrane permeability
- Functions as an intracellular messenger
- Blood coagulation

Preparations

Calcium salts are available as parenteral or oral preparations (Table 1).

TABLE 1	Preparations of calcium
Parenteral	• Calcium gluconate (IV) → Nonirritating and is the preferred salt • Calcium chloride (IV) → Highly irritant, can lead to tissue necrosis
Oral	• Calcium carbonate → Tasteless and nonirritant, used as antacid • Calcium dibasic phosphate → Used as an antacid • Calcium lactate

Adverse Effects

Calcium is generally well tolerated. Adverse effects include constipation, bloating etc.

Clinical Uses

- Dietary supplements to correct deficiency in:
  - Pregnancy, lactation, menopausal women
  - Growing children
- Tetany → Intravenous calcium gluconate is used for immediate management

- Antacid → Calcium carbonate is used as an antacid
- Osteoporosis → Has an adjuvant role in the prevention and treatment of osteoporosis
- Empirical role → Dermatoses, paresthesia (calcium gluconate has been used as intravenous therapy)

PARATHYROID HORMONE

Parathyroid hormone (Parathormone) is a polypeptide with 84 amino acids that is secreted by the chief cells of parathyroid gland.

Plasma calcium level is the main regulator of PTH secretion. A reduction in plasma Ca^{2+} level leads to increased secretion of PTH and vice versa.

↓ Plasma Ca^{2+} → ↑ Release of PTH	↑ Plasma Ca^{2+} → ↓ Release of PTH

Functions

The PTH exerts its effects on multiple organs including bone, kidneys and the intestine (Figure 1).

The PTH receptor is a G-protein coupled receptor that leads to an increase in intracellular cAMP and calcium levels.

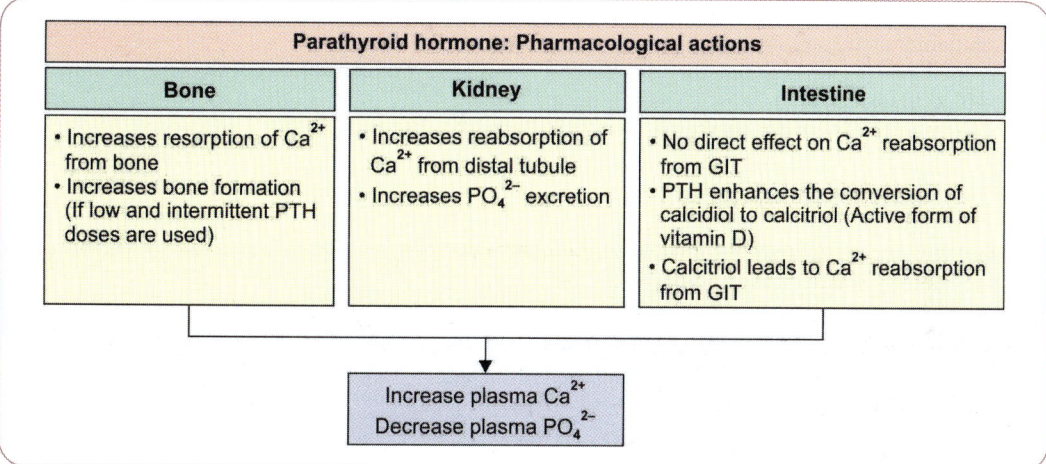

Figure 1: Functions of parathyroid hormone

Hyperparathyroidism

It is a medical condition associated with an increased level of PTH in the body.

One of the common causes of hyperparathyroidism is parathyroid tumor. The clinical manifestations of hyperparathyroidism include—hypercalcemia, bone fragility leading to fractures, renal stones, fatigue, constipation.

Treatment involves management of the underlying condition including surgery.

Pharmacological management includes the use of calcimimetics such as cinacalcet.

Cinacalcet

It is a calcimimetic drug that directly reduces the levels of PTH by the following actions:

- It enhances the sensitivity of the calcium sensing receptor (in the parathyroid gland) to calcium.
- By enhancing the sensitivity of calcium sensing receptor to calcium, cinacalcet lowers the calcium concentration at which PTH release is suppressed.
- This results in a decrease in the levels of PTH leading to a reduction in plasma calcium levels.

The indications of cinacalcet include the following:
○ Secondary hyperparathyroidism in patients with renal disease
○ Parathyroid carcinoma (to reduce hypercalcemia)

Hypoparathyroidism

It is a medical condition associated with decreased level of PTH in the body.

Causes

The causes of hypoparathyroidism include:
○ Postsurgical e.g. following surgery for thyroid, other neck surgeries
○ Autoimmune
○ Hereditary
○ Postradiation therapy

Clinical Features

○ Tetany, paresthesia, seizures, arrhythmias, psychiatric disorders
○ Growth retardation, decreased mental development

Treatment

○ Calcium and vitamin D to correct hypocalcemia
○ Recombinant human parathormone (subcutaneous use)
  ❑ It is indicated as an adjunct to calcium and vitamin D (to control hypocalcemia in patients with hypoparathyroidism)
  ❑ It has a potential risk of osteosarcoma

BISPHOSPHONATES

Bisphosphonates are pyrophosphate analogues. They inhibit bone resorption mediated by osteoclast. They increase bone density and decrease fracture risk.

The bisphosphonates are classified into 3 generations based on the order of their increasing potency (1st generation have lowest potency [and are rarely used now] while 3rd generation have highest potency).

The classification of bisphosphonates is mentioned in Table 2.

TABLE 2	Classification of bisphosphonates	
First generation	**Second generation**	**Third generation**
• Etidronate • Tiludronate	• Pamidronate • Alendronate • Ibandronate	• Risedronate • Zoledronate

Mechanism of Action

Bisphosphonates decrease osteoclast-mediated bone resorption by the mechanisms mentioned in Table 3.

TABLE 3	Bisphosphonates: Mechanism of action
Increase in osteoclastic apoptosis	**Inhibition of cholesterol synthetic pathway**
Bisphosphonates (BPN) have high Ca^{2+} affinity in the bone ↓ BPN are released along with Ca^{2+} ions from the bone surface ↓ BPN are taken up by osteoclasts ↓ Increase in osteoclast apoptosis	Inhibit mevalonate pathway in cholesterol synthesis ↓ Suppression of normal osteoclast function **Note:** This is an additional important mechanism in 2nd and 3rd generation BPNs.

Pharmacokinetics

All bisphosphonates are poorly absorbed after oral administration (bioavailability ~5%). Food further decreases the bioavailability. Hence, these drugs should be taken in an empty stomach in the morning (30 minutes before food) with plenty of water.

Some part of administered bisphosphonate gets adsorbed to bone and remains there for a long period of time (months to years). The free drug is excreted unchanged by the kidneys.

Pamidronate and zoledronate are given only intravenously; ibandronate can be given both orally and intravenously, while the others are given only orally.

Adverse Effects

Oral bisphosphonates commonly cause gastrointestinal toxicity including nausea, vomiting, heartburn, esophageal erosions etc. To prevent esophageal erosions, the following measures are taken:

- Administer with plenty of water
- Remain upright and not to lie down for at least 30 minutes after swallowing the drug

Other adverse effects may include thrombophlebitis of the injected vein, fever, flu-like reaction etc.

A specific adverse effect is osteonecrosis of the jaw that occurs after long-term therapy with higher intravenous (IV) doses.

Clinical Uses

The bisphosphonates are used in the following situations:

Postmenopausal Osteoporosis

The 2nd and 3rd generation bisphosphonates are used in prevention as well as treatment of postmenopausal osteoporosis. They conserve bone mineral density and decrease the incidence of hip and vertebral fractures.

Steroid-induced Osteoporosis

The 2nd and 3rd generation bisphosphonates are used.

Paget's Disease

The bisphosphonates inhibit osteolysis and decrease bone pain and other symptoms. They may induce long-lasting remissions. They are frequently used in combination with calcitonin. The treatment should not exceed a duration of 6 months per course. The treatment may again be repeated after a gap of 6 months, if required.

Hypercalcemia of Malignancy

The drugs mostly preferred in hypercalcemia of malignancy are intravenous bisphosphonates (pamidronate and zoledronate). They act by blocking osteoclast activity and subsequently decreasing bone resorption.

Initially supportive treatment should be given (IV fluids along with furosemide and intramuscular calcitonin) because severe hypercalcemia is an emergency and bisphosphonates takes some time to act.

Osteoytic Bone Lesions

Intravenous bisphosphonates (pamidronate and zoledronate) are the preferred drugs in this condition.

VITAMIN D

Vitamin D is a prohormone. It is converted in the body to several active metabolites that function as hormones.

Vitamin D is either obtained from the diet (mainly from fish liver oils, yeast and dairy products) or it is synthesized in the skin by exposure to direct sunlight (ultraviolet B radiation).

Vitamin D exists in 2 main forms:

- D_2 (Ergocalciferol): Dietary source

○ D$_3$ (Cholecalciferol): Synthesized in the skin under UVB exposure

The vitamin D synthetic pathway is mentioned in Figure 2.

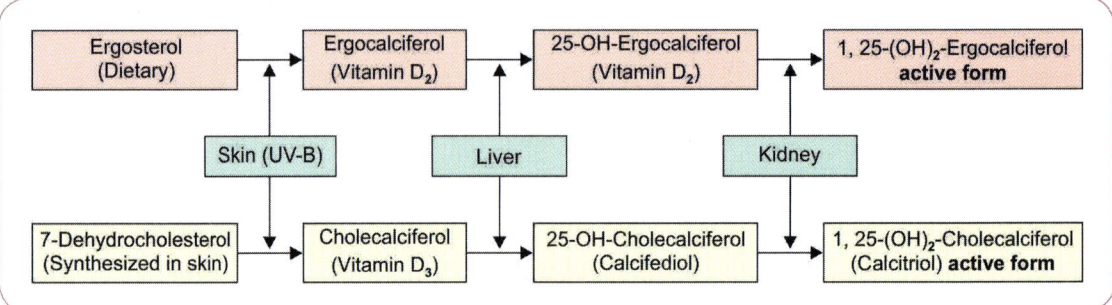

Figure 2: Vitamin D synthetic pathway

Vitamin D along with parathyroid hormone plays a key role in the regulation of plasma calcium levels and bone formation.

Pharmacological Actions

The main sites of action of vitamin D are intestine, bone and kidney. The net effect of vitamin D is an increase in plasma calcium and phosphate levels (Figure 3).

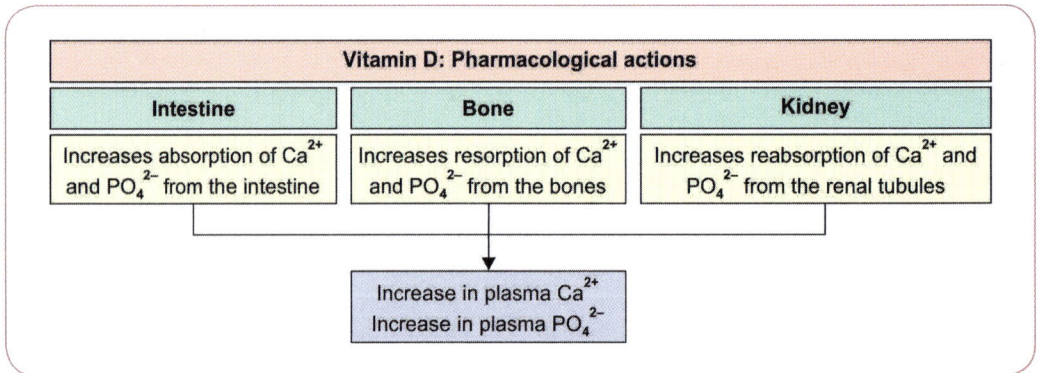

Figure 3: Pharmacological actions of vitamin D

Vitamin D Deficiency and Hypervitaminosis D

Vitamin D deficiency results in rickets in children and osteomalacia in adults.

The disease mechanism involves deficient intestinal absorption of calcium and phosphate leading to decreased plasma calcium and phosphate levels. Parathyroid hormone becomes elevated as a compensatory measure.

The elevated PTH maintains normal plasma calcium levels at the expense of bone i.e. PTH pulls out calcium from the bone to maintain plasma calcium levels.

Hypervitaminosis D occurs mainly due to long-term ingestion of large doses of vitamin D. The manifestations occur due to increased plasma calcium levels and deposition of calcium in the tissues. The symptoms include hypercalcemia, fatigue, diarrhea, polyuria, renal stones etc. The treatment includes withdrawing the vitamin, low calcium diet, administration of fluids and corticosteroids.

Vitamin D Preparations

The various vitamin D preparations are mentioned in Table 4.

TABLE 4	Vitamin D preparations
Calciferol/Ergocalciferol (Vitamin D_2)	• Available as oral capsules • Used for treatment of nutritional rickets and osteomalacia
Cholecalciferol (Vitamin D_3)	• Available as granules for oral therapy • Used for treatment of nutritional rickets and osteomalacia
Calcitriol (Active vitamin D_3)	• Available as oral capsules and injections for parenteral use • Used in renal bone disease, vitamin D dependent rickets, vitamin D resistant rickets, hypoparathyroidism etc.
Alfacalcidol	• Prodrug, converted in the liver to the active form i.e. vitamin D_3 (Calcitriol) • Same indications/uses as those of calcitriol
Calcipotriol	• An analogue of calcitriol, used in psoriasis topically

Clinical Uses

Vitamin D and its analogues are used in the following conditions:

Prophylaxis and Treatment of Nutritional Deficiency of Vitamin D

The preparation of choice is cholecalciferol/calciferol.

Vitamin D Dependent Rickets

These are X-linked genetic disorders. There is a deficiency of renal hydroxylase enzyme, which converts 25-OH-cholecalciferol to the active form calcitriol. These are treated with calcitriol or alfacalcidol in normal doses.

Vitamin D Resistant Rickets

These are X-linked hereditary disorders in which there is a disorder of calcium and phosphate metabolism wherein the vitamin D metabolism is normal. These are treated with phosphate and large doses of calcitriol or alfacalcidol.

Renal Rickets

This occurs in chronic renal failure wherein the conversion of 25-OH-cholecalciferol to the active form calcitriol, does not take place. These are treated with calcitriol or alfacalcidol in normal doses.

Postmenopausal or Senile Osteoporosis

Administration of calcitriol (Vitamin D_3) + calcium improves calcium balance in elderly males and postmenopausal females. This reduces the risk of fractures.

Hypoparathyroidism

In this condition, there is decreased calcium levels and increased phosphate levels in the plasma. Calcitriol or alfacalcidol are used in the treatment.

Psoriasis

Calcipotriol, an analogue of calcitriol, is used topically in psoriasis.

CALCITONIN

It is a hypocalcemic hormone produced by parafollicular 'C' cells of the thyroid. The actions of calcitonin are usually opposite to that of parathyroid hormone. Hence, it decreases plasma calcium and phosphate levels by direct action on bone and the kidneys (Figure 4).

The secretion of calcitonin is stimulated by an increase in plasma calcium and is inhibited by a decrease in plasma calcium.

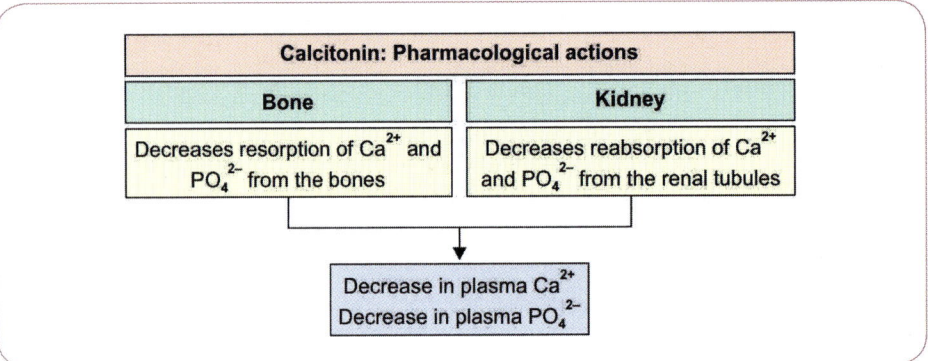

Figure 4: Pharmacological actions of calcitonin

Adverse Effects

The adverse effects of calcitonin include nausea, bad taste, flushing and tingling of fingers.

Clinical Uses

Hypercalcemic Conditions

Calcitonin is used in conditions such as hyperparathyroidism, hypervitaminosis D, hypercalcemia of malignancy and osteolytic bone metastasis. It is a weak hypocalcemic drug; hence, it is used as an adjuvant to bisphosphonates for the first few days because it takes 1–2 days for the actions of bisphosphonates to manifest.

Paget's Disease

Bisphosphonates are the preferred drugs. Calcitonin is used as an adjuvant or a second-line reserve drug.

Postmenopausal Osteoporosis

Calcitonin is given along with calcium and vitamin D. A nasal spray formulation has become available.

TERIPARATIDE

The salient features of teriparatide are mentioned below:
- It is a recombinant form of human parathyroid hormone.
- It is used for the treatment of postmenopausal osteoporosis.
- It is administered subcutaneously daily.
- It is the first drug that stimulates bone formation; other drugs inhibit bone resorption.
- It promotes bone formation by stimulating osteoblasts.

DENOSUMAB

The salient features of denosumab are mentioned below:
- It is a monoclonal antibody.
- It inhibits receptor activator of nuclear factor for KB ligand (RANKL).
- It inhibits the formation and function of osteoclast.
- It is used for the treatment of postmenopausal osteoporosis.
- It is administered subcutaneously every 6 months.
- The adverse effects include joint and muscle pains, increase risk of infections, osteonecrosis of the jaw, hypocalcemia and atypical fracture.

TREATMENT OF OSTEOPOROSIS

The classification of drugs used in the treatment of osteoporosis is mentioned in Table 5.

TABLE 5	Drugs used in osteoporosis
Bisphosphonates	
• First generation	• Etidronate, tiludronate
• Second generation	• Pamidronate, alendronate, ibandronate
• Third generation	• Risedronate, zoledronate
Selective estrogen receptor modulator (SERM)	
Raloxifene	
Calcitonin	
Teriparatide	
Denosumab	

Drugs Acting on the Endocrine Physiology

SECTION H

ASSESS YOURSELF (Examination Questions of Various Universities)

1. Enumerate bisphosphonates. Discuss the mechanism of action, adverse effects and clinical uses of bisphosphonates.
2. Discuss the pharmacological basis for the use of alendronate in osteoporosis.
3. Explain why the patients need to be adequately instructed before starting therapy with alendronate.

4. Write short notes on:
   a. Pharmacotherapy of osteoporosis
   b. Therapeutic uses of vitamin D
   c. Calcitonin
   d. Parathormone

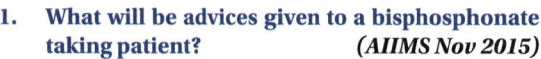

MULTIPLE CHOICE QUESTIONS

1. What will be advices given to a bisphosphonate taking patient? (*AIIMS Nov 2015*)
   a. Take tab before food with full glass of water
   b. Take tab after food with full glass of water
   c. Stop if gastroesophageal discomfort persists
   d. Stop if consistent bone pain persists

2. Bisphosphonates are used in all except:
   (*AIIMS Nov 2007*)
   a. Malignancy
   b. Vitamin D excess
   c. Postmenopausal osteoporosis
   d. Hypercalcemia

3. Denosumab, a monoclonal antibody against RANK ligand is used for the treatment of:
   (*AIIMS Nov 2006*)
   a. Rheumatoid arthritis
   b. Osteoporosis
   c. Osteoarthritis
   d. Systemic lupus erythematosus

4. Teriparatide acts by:
   (*Recent Question Dec 2016*)
   a. Increasing osteoblastic activity
   b. Decreasing osteoclastic activity
   c. Decreasing osteoclastic and increasing osteoblastic activity
   d. Increasing calcium

5. Bisphosphonates act by:
   (*Recent Question 2016*)
   a. Increasing osteoid formation
   b. Increasing mineralization of osteoid

   c. Decreasing osteoclast mediated resorption of bone
   d. Decreasing PTH secretion

6. Which of the following drug causes osteonecrosis by giving IV route? (*Recent Question 2016*)
   a. Zoledronate   b. Dalteparin
   c. Calcitriol   d. Zidovudine

7. Parathyroid hormone (*Recent Question 2016*)
   a. Decreases bone resorption
   b. Increases bone resorption
   c. Enhances phosphate reabsorption from kidney
   d. Decreases calcium reabsorption from kidney

8. Intranasal calcitonin is given in:
   (*Recent Question 2016*)
   a. Paget's disease
   b. MEN syndrome
   c. Hypercalcemia
   d. Postmenopausal osteoporosis

9. All of the following decrease bone resorption in osteoporosis except: (*Recent Question 2016*)
   a. Alendronate   b. Etidronate
   c. Strontium   d. Teriparatide

10. Bisphosphonate is: (*Recent Question 2016*)
    a. Risedronate   b. Raloxifen
    c. Tamoxifen   d. Teriparatide

Ans.

1. (a)	2. (b)	3. (b)	4. (a)	5. (c)	6. (a)
7. (b)	8. (d)	9. (d)	10. (a)		

42

Drugs Acting on the Uterus

UTERINE STIMULANTS (OXYTOCICS, ECBOLICS)

Uterine stimulants or oxytocics stimulate the contraction of the uterus.

Classification of uterine stimulants is depicted in Table 1.

TABLE 1	Classification of uterine stimulants	
Oxytocin	**Ergot derivatives**	**Prostaglandins**
• It is posterior pituitary hormone	• Ergometrine • Methylergometrine	• PGE_2, $PGF_{2\alpha}$, 15-methyl $PGF_{2\alpha}$ • Misoprostol

OXYTOCIN

It is a hormone that is synthesized in the supraoptic and paraventricular nuclei of hypothalamus and secreted by the posterior pituitary gland. The synthesis and release of oxytocin is shown in Figure 1.

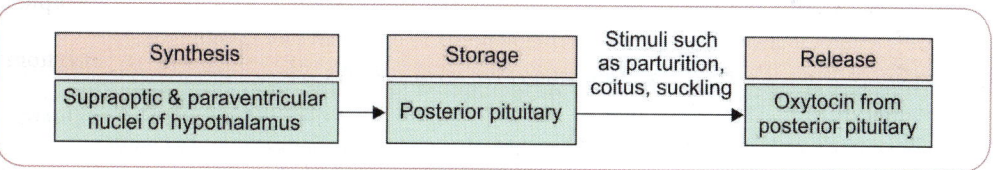

Figure 1: Synthesis and storage of oxytocin

Pharmacological Actions

The pharmacological actions of oxytocin are mentioned in Figure 2.

Oxytocin exerts its actions by binding to the G protein coupled receptors on the uterus. This results in generation of IP_3 and release of calcium. It also causes an increased release of prostaglandins and leukotrienes.

Pharmacokinetics

Oxytocin is inactive orally as it is a peptide. It is available for parenteral use (IM or IV). It has a plasma half-life of ~6 minutes.

1 U of oxytocin = 2 µg of oxytocin. Synthetic preparation of oxytocin is used commercially.

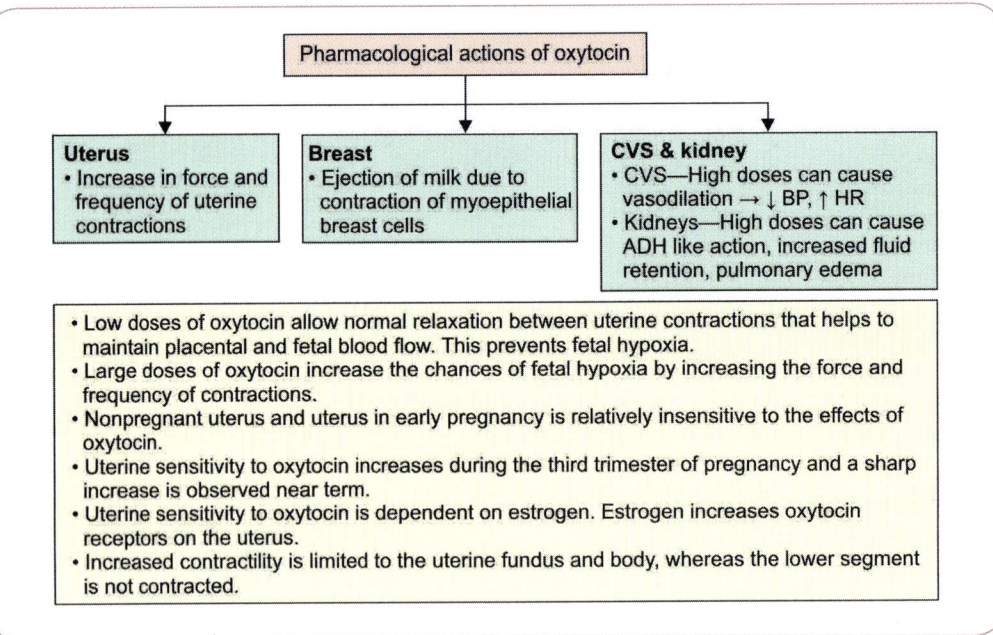

Figure 2: Pharmacological actions of oxytocin

Clinical Uses

Induction of Labor/Augmentation of Dysfunctional Labor (Uterine Inertia)

- Slow intravenous (IV) infusion of oxytocin is given for induction of labor. Monitoring of the infusion rate, uterine contractions, fetal heart rate, maternal blood pressure and heart rate should be done.
- Augmentation of labor is done if the contractions are weak and the progression of labor is unsatisfactory (uterine inertia).
- Oxytocin is the preferred drug (as compared to ergometrine or prostaglandins) for the induction of labor and augmentation of dysfunctional labor (uterine inertia) because of the following reasons:
  - Oxytocin has a short half-life (~6 minutes). This allows a better control over the intensity of the action and quick termination of action can be done in case of uterine hyperstimulation or fetal distress.
  - Fetal descent during labor is not compromised since the lower segment of uterus is not contracted.
  - Low concentrations of oxytocin allow normal relaxation between uterine contractions that helps to maintain placental and fetal blood flow. This prevents fetal hypoxia.
  - Consistent augmentation of the uterine contractions.

Oxytocin infusion should be administered by experienced and qualified professionals. It is important to exclude conditions such as cephalopelvic disproportion, placenta previa, fetal distress, transverse lie etc. prior to oxytocin infusion.

Postpartum Hemorrhage (PPH)

- Oxytocin is useful in PPH because it contracts the uterine muscles leading to compression of the blood vessels passing through the myometrium, resulting in stoppage of the bleeding.
- It is administered parenterally (IM or IV).

Breast Engorgement

- Intranasal spray of oxytocin may be used for this purpose.

Adverse Effects

- ○ Uterine hyperstimulation
  - ❑ Administration at too high doses can result in an increase in the force and frequency of uterine contractions. This can lead to uterine rupture, fetal distress, hypoxia and fetal death.
- ○ Water intoxication
  - ❑ Administration of high doses of oxytocin along with an increased fluid administration (over an extended duration of time), can lead to water intoxication.
  - ❑ May manifest clinically as headache, nausea, vomiting, drowsiness, electrolyte imbalance, seizure, loss of consciousness. It can be potentially fatal.

CARBETOCIN

Carbetocin is a long acting oxytocin analogue. It is used for the prevention of postpartum hemorrhage (uterine atony) following delivery by cesarean section. It is not used for the induction of labor.

ERGOT DERIVATIVES—(ERGOMETRINE AND METHYLERGOMETRINE)

Ergometrine (ergonovine) and methylergometrine (methylergonovine) are used in obstetric practice (Table 2).

TABLE 2	Ergometrine and methylergometrine	
Ergometrine	**Methylergometrine**
Natural ergot derivative	Semisynthetic derivative
Less potent action on uterus	More potent (~1.5 times) action on uterus
Less preferred in obstetric practice	More preferred in obstetric practice

Pharmacological Actions

The pharmacological actions of ergometrine are mentioned in Figure 3.

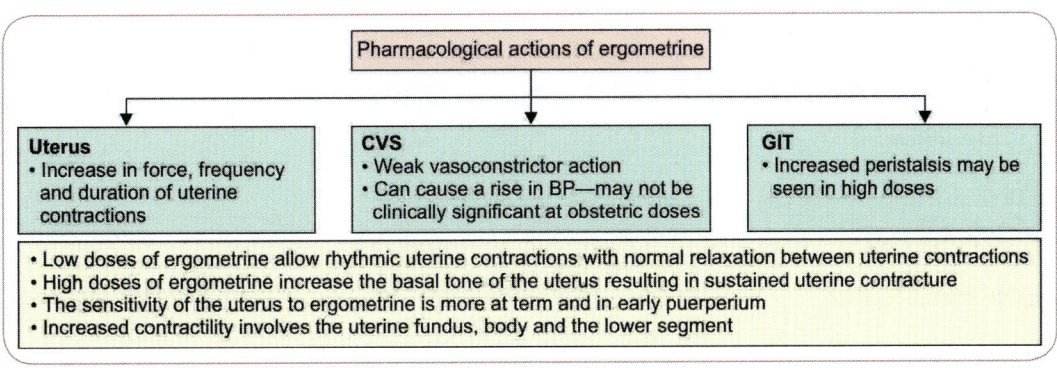

Figure 3: Pharmacological action of ergometrine

Pharmacokinetics

Both ergometrine and methylergometrine can be administered orally and parenterally (IM, IV). Onset of action is rapid. Plasma half-life is 1–2 hours.

Clinical Uses

Prevention and Control of Postpartum Hemorrhage

○ Ergometrine and methylergometrine are administered following the delivery of anterior shoulder of the infant.
○ Rationale of using these drugs for postpartum hemorrhage (PPH) is that they produce a sustained tonic contraction of the uterine muscles that compresses the uterine blood vessels and stops the bleeding (Figure 4).

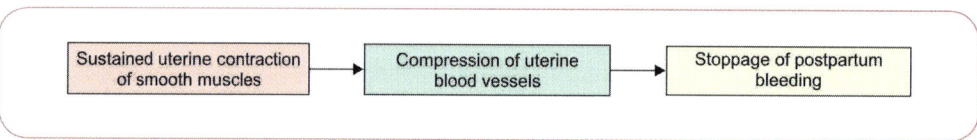

Figure 4: Rationale of ergometrine and methylergometrine in PPH

Prevention of Uterine Atony after Cesarean Section/Instrumental Delivery

Ensure Normal Involution of Uterus

○ Indicated in women where a risk of delayed involution is anticipated (multiparous pregnancy). However, it is not indicated for routine use in all cases because the normal uterine involution is not hastened.

Adverse Effects

The adverse effects of ergot derivatives are mentioned below:
○ Nausea and vomiting—occurs due to direct effect on CNS emetic centers
○ Prolonged vasospasm—coronary vasospasm, peripheral vascular disease, hypertension
○ Muscle weakness, muscle pain, tingling and numbness of fingers
○ Inhibition of prolactin release due to dopaminergic action can lead to reduced milk secretion

Contraindications

The ergot derivatives are contraindicated in the following clinical situations:
○ Pregnancy and before the third stage of labor (Prior to the delivery of the anterior shoulder).
  ❑ This is because of the risk of developing prolonged and powerful uterine contractions that can result in uterine rupture, fetal distress, hypoxia and fetal death. In multiple births, ergometrine and methylergometrine should not be administered before the delivery of the last child.
○ Other contraindications include:
  ❑ Severe hypertension, preeclampsia, eclampsia
  ❑ Uterine inertia (primary or secondary)
  ❑ Cardiac diseases
  ❑ Hepatic or renal diseases
  ❑ Occlusive vascular diseases
  ❑ Sepsis

PROSTAGLANDINS

○ PGE_2 (Dinoprostone) and PGE_1 (Misoprostol) are used in the induction of labor because they promote cervical dilation and ripening.
○ Both these drugs can also be used for termination of pregnancy.
○ The main adverse effect is uterine hyperstimulation.

UTERINE RELAXANTS (TOCOLYTICS)

Uterine relaxants or tocolytics are drugs that reduce the motility of the uterus. They inhibit the contractions of the uterus and are used to suppress labor.

These drugs are clinically used in the following situations:
- To delay or postpone labor
- Threatened abortion
- Dysmenorrhea

Some of the tocolytics used are mentioned in Table 3.

TABLE 3	Tocolytics
Classification	**Examples**
β_2 agonists	• Ritodrine, terbutaline, salbutamol
Oxytocin receptor antagonist	• Atosiban
Calcium channel blockers	• Nifedipine
Other drugs	• NSAIDs (Indomethacin) • Progesterone • Magnesium sulfate • Nitroglycerin • Halothane

β_2 ADRENERGIC AGONISTS

Drugs such as ritodrine, terbutaline, salbutamol can cause uterine relaxation.

They can also cause adverse effects such as tachycardia, arrhythmias, hyperglycemia and hypokalemia. Hence, they should be avoided in women with diabetes or cardiac disease.

OXYTOCIN RECEPTOR ANTAGONIST

Atosiban is a synthetic analogue of oxytocin that inhibits uterine contractions by competitively blocking uterine oxytocin receptors.

It is administered intravenously via infusion. Adverse effects include nausea, headache, dizziness and injection site reactions.

CALCIUM CHANNEL BLOCKERS

Nifedipine blocks the transmembrane calcium transport and decreases the levels of intracellular calcium. This prevents uterine contractions.

Nifedipine can be administered orally. Adverse effects include hypotension and tachycardia. They should be used with caution in women with underlying cardiac disease due to the risk of cardiac complications.

OTHER DRUGS

Magnesium sulfate is used for the prevention and treatment of convulsions in preeclampsia and eclampsia. It has also been used to delay preterm labor since it suppresses uterine contractions. It is administered intravenously via infusion. Adverse effects include arrhythmias, respiratory depression, muscle weakness and CNS depression.

Prostaglandin synthesis inhibitors can inhibit preterm labor. Adverse effects include suppression of platelet function and closure of ductus arteriosus (*in utero*).

ASSESS YOURSELF (Examination Questions of Various Universities)

1. Enumerate tocolytic drugs. Discuss briefly pharmacological actions, adverse effects and clinical uses of oxytocin.
2. Discuss the pharmacological actions of oxytocin on uterus.
3. Explain why oxytocin is preferred over methylergometrine for the induction of labour.
4. Explain the rationale of using methylergometrine for postpartum haemorrhage.
5. Write short notes on:
   a. Oxytocin
   b. Tocolytics
   c. Methylergometrine

MULTIPLE CHOICE QUESTIONS

1. What is the action of oxytocin in small doses, when used as intravenous infusion in a full term uterus? *(MHCET 2006)*
   a. Relaxes uterus
   b. Induces uterine contractions
   c. Causes cervical dilatation
   d. All

2. True about atosiban: *(MHCET 2006)*
   a. Is an oxytocin receptor antagonist
   b. Is an progesterone receptor antagonist
   c. Is least effective in inhibiting preterm uterine contractions
   d. Is an antitocolytic drug

Ans.

1. (b)   2.   (a)

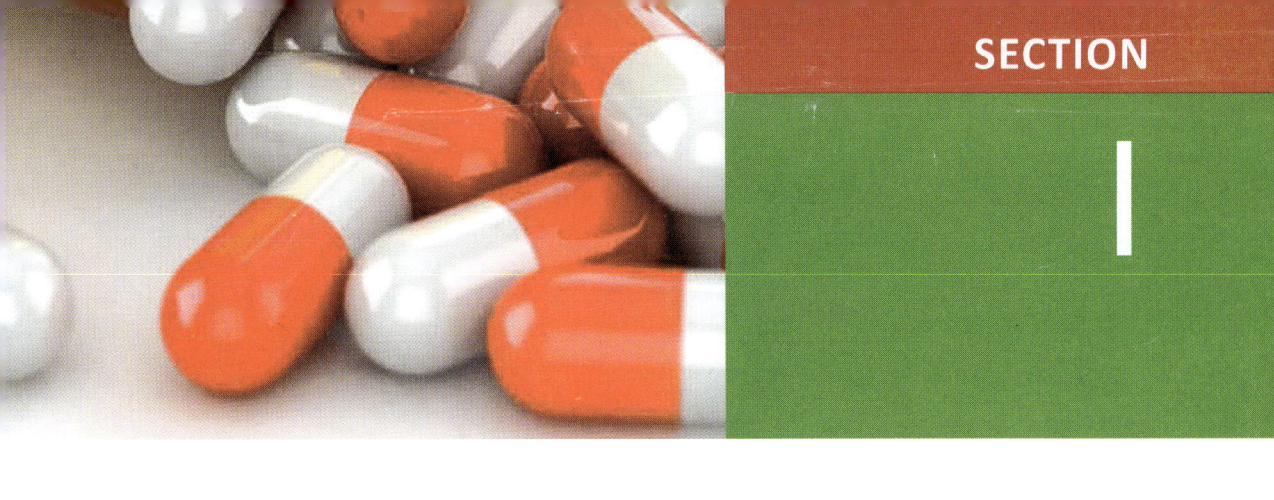

I

Drugs Acting on the Renal System

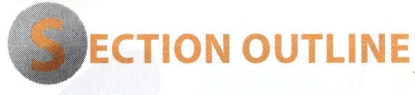

SECTION OUTLINE

○ Diuretics and Antidiuretic Drugs

RENAL ANATOMY AND PHYSIOLOGY

The kidneys play an important role in the elimination of waste products, maintenance of fluid and electrolyte balance and hormone synthesis (Figure 1).

Functions of kidney	Structure of kidney	Functional unit of kidney
Elimination of waste products (uric acid, urea, creatinine)	Cortex (outer part)	Nephron is the functional unit
Maintenance of acid base, electrolyte and fluid balance	Medulla (inner part)	1.3 million nephrons per kidney
Hormone synthesis (angiotensin, erythropoietin, prostacyclin, hydroxylation of Vitamin D)	Pelvis which empties into the ureter	Site of action of many diuretic drugs

Figure 1: Renal anatomy and physiology

RENAL NEPHRON

The nephron is the functional unit of the kidney. The key functions of the nephron and the site of action of various diuretic drugs is mentioned in Figure 2 and Table 1.

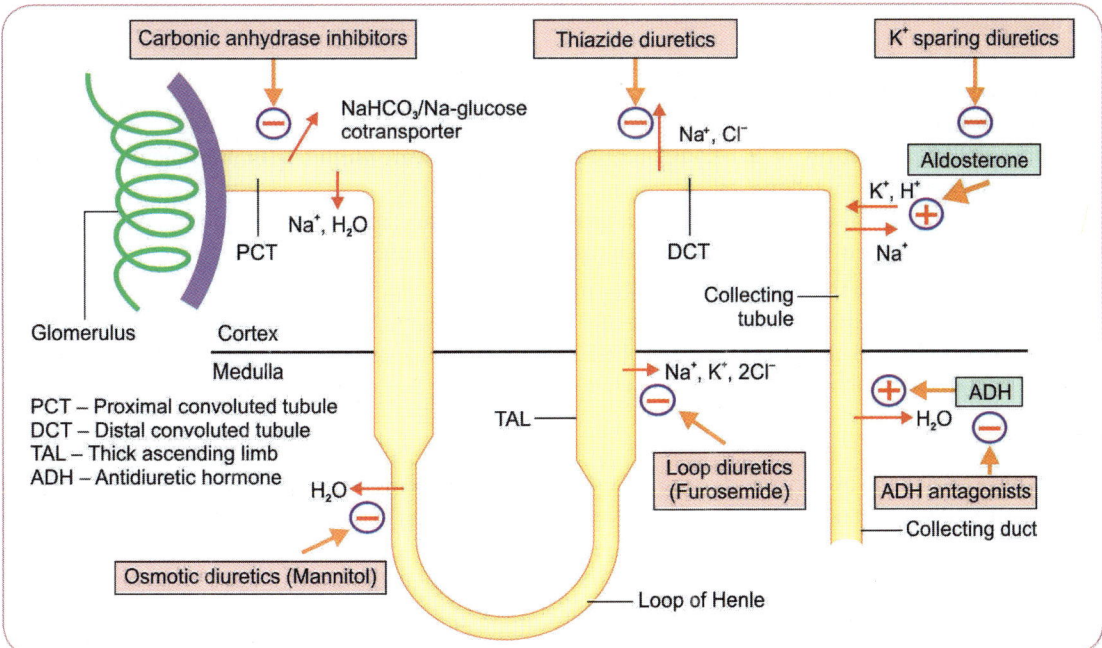

Figure 2: The nephron and sites of action of diuretics

TABLE 1	The nephron and sites of action of diuretics	
Region of nephron	Key function(s)	Drugs with main site of action
Glomerulus and Bowman's capsule	Hydrostatic pressure in glomerular capillaries filters water and electrolytes into Bowman's capsule and into the proximal convoluted tubule (PCT)	• No diuretic with a major action
Proximal convoluted tubule	• Reabsorption of sodium, potassium, calcium, magnesium, $NaHCO_3$, glucose, amino acids • About 65–70% sodium is reabsorbed • Isosmotic reabsorption of sodium $\rightarrow$ every molecule of sodium that is reabsorbed is also accompanied by a molecule of water	• Carbonic anhydrase inhibitors (e.g. acetazolamide)
Thick ascending limb of Henle	• Active reabsorption of Na^+, K^+, Cl^- • Secondary reabsorption of Mg^{2+}, Ca^{2+}	• Loop diuretics (e.g. furosemide)
Distal convoluted tubule	• Active reabsorption of Na^+, Cl^- • Reabsorption of Ca^{2+}	• Thiazide diuretics (e.g. chlorothiazide)
Cortical collecting tubule	• Reabsorption of Na^+, coupled with secretion of K^+, H^+	• K^+ sparing diuretics (e.g. spironolactone)
Medullary collecting duct	• ADH controlled reabsorption of H_2O	• ADH antagonists (e.g. tolvaptan)

DIURETICS

LOOP DIURETICS (HIGH CEILING DIURETICS)

o Furosemide
o Bumetanide
o Torsemide
o Ethacrynic acid

These drugs inhibit the activity of Na^+-K^+-$2Cl^-$ cotransporter in the thick ascending limb of the loop of Henle. Hence, they are known as 'loop diuretics'.

Loop diuretics are also called 'high-ceiling diuretics' because they are highly efficacious, i.e. the maximal sodium excreting capacity of loop diuretics is much higher than that of other classes.

The high efficacy of loop diuretics is due to the following factors:

o Around 25% of the filtered Na^+ is reabsorbed by the thick ascending limb of the loop of Henle.
o The nephron distal to the thick ascending limb (i.e. distal tubule and collecting duct) do not have the reabsorptive capacity to rescue (absorb) the solutes rejected by thick ascending limb.

Mechanism of Action

Loop diuretics inhibit the Na^+-K^+-$2Cl^-$ cotransporter in the thick ascending limb of the loop of Henle. This leads to a decrease in reabsorption of Na^+, K^+ and Cl^- ions. They are secreted in the proximal tubule, reach the thick ascending limb, and act from the luminal side of the membrane.

Increased amounts of Na⁺ therefore, reach the distal tubule. In the distal tubule, more Na⁺ is exchanged for K⁺ leading to K⁺ loss and hypokalemia.

Inhibition of the Na⁺-K⁺-2Cl⁻ cotransporter leads to abolition of the transepithelial potential difference resulting in inhibition of Ca^{2+} and Mg^{2+} absorption. Hence, Ca^{2+} and Mg^{2+} excretion is increased.

They also have weak carbonic anhydrase inhibiting activity leading to an increased HCO_3^- and PO_4^{3-} excretion (Figure 3).

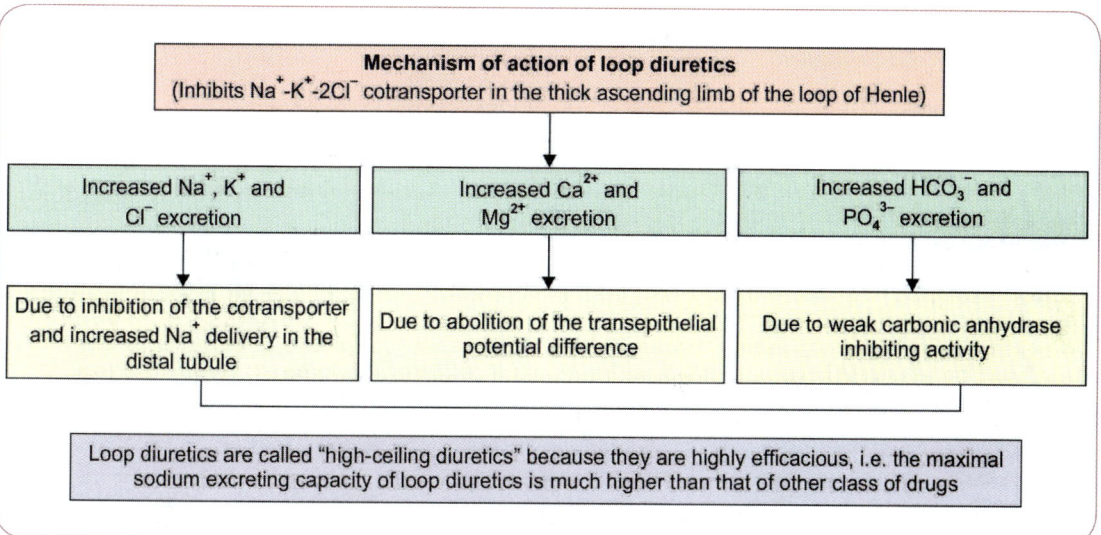

Figure 3: Mechanism of action of loop diuretics

Hemodynamic Effects

Loop diuretics have the following actions:
- Increase renal blood flow. There is redistribution of blood to the midcortical zone. Glomerular filtration rate usually does not change due to compensatory mechanisms.
- Prompt increase in systemic venous capacitance leading to a decrease in left ventricular filling pressure. This is the reason it provides instant relief in pulmonary edema, even before the start of its diuretic action.

Both the actions are mediated by an increase in prostaglandin (PG) synthesis.

Pharmacokinetics

Loop diuretics are well-absorbed orally. They are all available as oral formulations; furosemide and bumetanide are also available as IV and IM formulations.

Furosemide has a quick onset of action (2–5 minutes by IV route; 10–20 minutes by IM route and 20–40 minutes by oral route). The duration of action is 2–3 hours.

These drugs are highly bound to plasma proteins; hence, they are filtered at glomerulus only to a very limited extent. However, their action is from the luminal side of the tubule. Therefore, to reach the lumen of the tubule, they are actively secreted in the proximal tubule by organic acid transport system.

Adverse Effects

The key adverse effects of loop diuretics are mentioned in Figure 4.

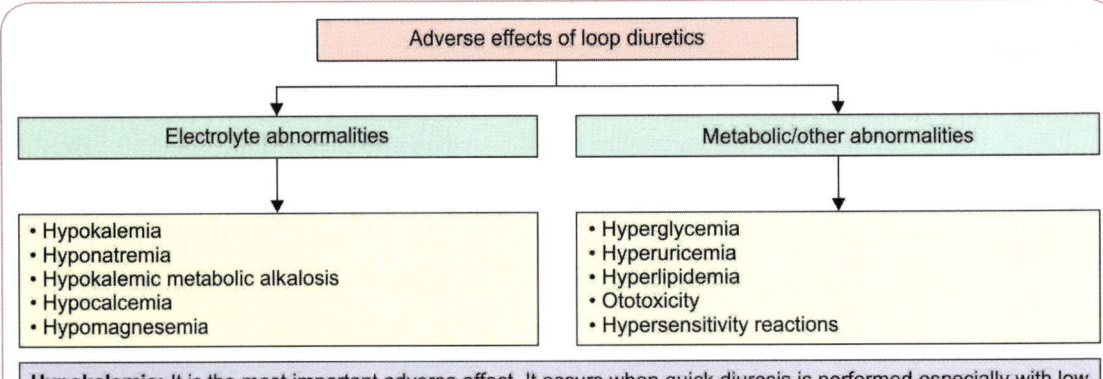

Figure 4: Adverse effects of loop diuretics

Drug Interactions

The key drug interactions with loop and thiazide diuretics are mentioned in Table 2.

TABLE 2	Drug interactions of loop and thiazide diuretics
Furosemide and aminoglycosides	• Both the drugs are ototoxic. Results in additive ototoxicity.
Furosemide/thiazides and digoxin	• These diuretics cause hypokalemia. Hypokalemia increase digoxin binding to Na+-K+-ATPase. This results in digoxin toxicity.
Furosemide and NSAIDs	• NSAIDs inhibit PG synthesis and therefore inhibit PG-mediated hemodynamic changes of loop diuretics. • Chronic use of NSAIDs decrease the antihypertensive effects of loop diuretics and thiazides.
Furosemide/thiazides and lithium	• These diuretics cause enhanced reabsorption of lithium in proximal tubule, resulting in increased serum lithium levels.
Furosemide/thiazides and probenecid	• Probenecid competitively inhibits tubular secretion of furosemide and thiazide—diminishes their action by reducing the luminal concentration.

Clinical Uses

- **Acute pulmonary edema:** Loop diuretics are the preferred drugs in the treatment of pulmonary edema, where they are given intravenously, and they act by the mechanism mentioned in Figure 5.

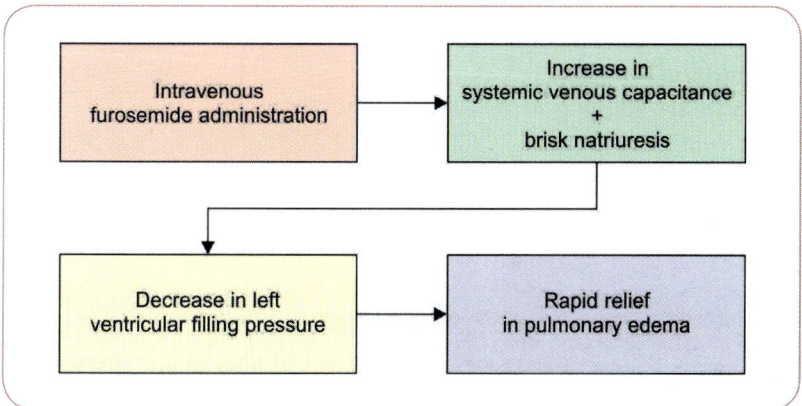

Figure 5: Loop diuretics in acute pulmonary edema

- **Acute/chronic edema due to congestive heart failure, liver cirrhosis and renal disease:** Diuretics are used for most other types of edema. Loop diuretics are preferred because of rapid onset of action especially when given intravenously. Thiazides may be given during the maintenance phase but are often ineffective.

    The edema of nephrotic syndrome is often refractory to other diuretics, and loop diuretics are the only drugs effective for reducing the massive edema of nephrotic syndrome. The edema of chronic kidney disease requires higher doses of loop diuretics.
- **Hypertension:** Loop diuretics are used in hypertension only when the following conditions are present: renal insufficiency, congestive heart failure or in hypertensive emergencies.

    Loop diuretics are not preferred in uncomplicated hypertension because of a higher potency and a shorter duration of action. Thiazides are preferred in such situations.
- **Cerebral edema:** The preferred drug for cerebral edema is IV mannitol; however, furosemide may be combined for better efficacy.
- **Hypercalcemia:** Loop diuretics promote Ca^{2+} excretion. Hence, they may be used along with isotonic saline for the treatment for hypercalcemia.

THAZIDES AND THIAZIDE LIKE DIURETICS (MEDIUM EFFICACY DIURETICS)

- Benzothiadiazine (thiazides)-Hydrochlorothiazide, benzthiazide
- Thiazide like diuretics (lacks thiazide structure, but have the same mechanism of action)-Chlorthalidone, metolazone, indapamide, xipamide

These are sulfonamide derivatives that act on the early distal tubule by inhibiting the Na^+-Cl^- symport.

Mechanism of Action

Thiazide and thiazide like diuretics inhibit the Na^+-Cl^- symport in the early part of distal convoluted tubule. This leads to diuresis of concentrated (hyperosmolar) urine with increased excretion of Na^+ and Cl^- (**Figure 6**).

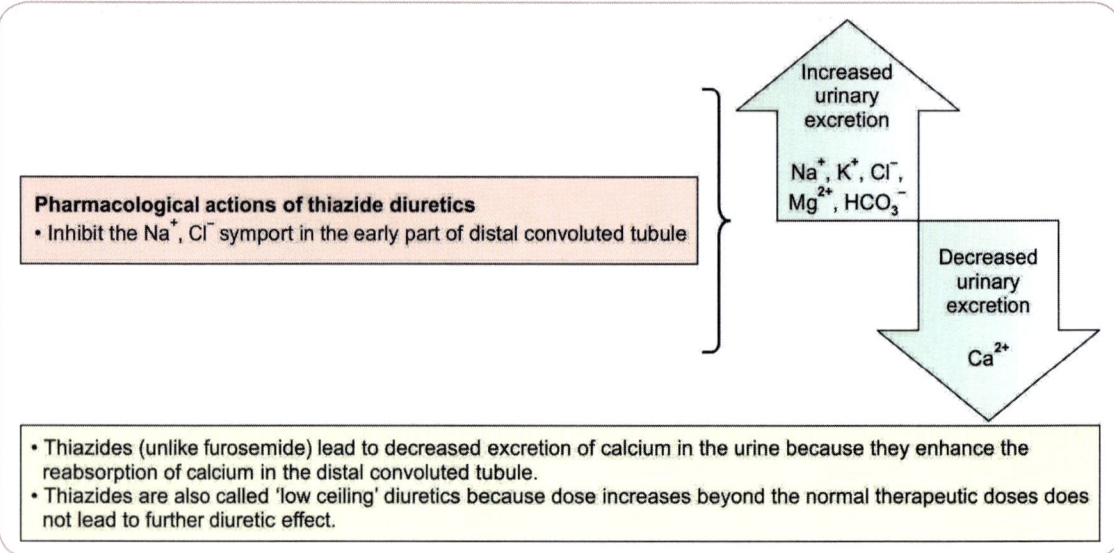

Figure 6: Pharmacological actions of thiazides

Pharmacokinetics

Thiazides are orally effective and have a prolonged duration of action.

Adverse Effects

The adverse effects of thiazides and thiazide like diuretics are mentioned in Figure 7.

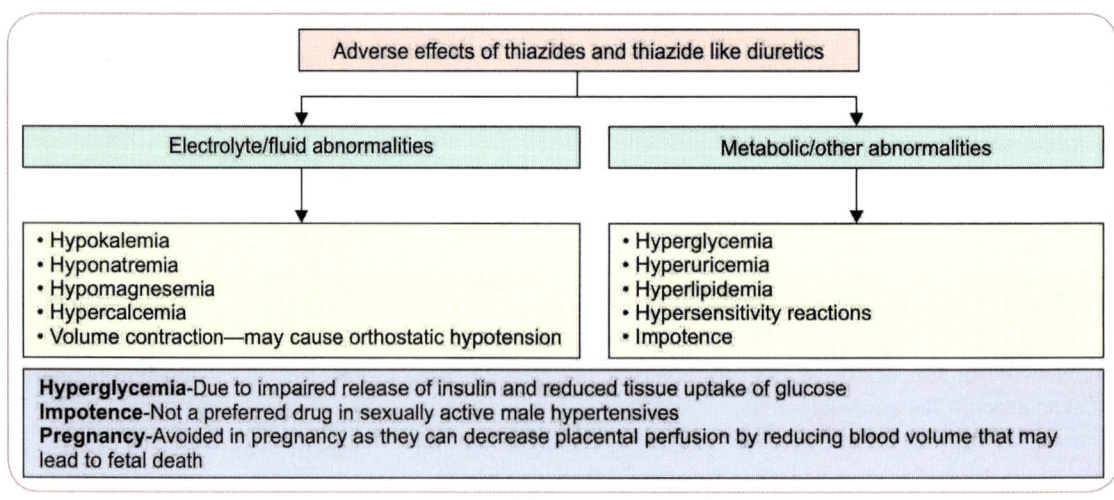

Figure 7: Adverse effects of thiazides and thiazide like diuretics

Clinical Uses

○ **Hypertension:** Thiazides have the following advantages:
  ❑ Inexpensive and well tolerated by elderly patients
  ❑ Prolonged duration of action; hence, multiple doses are minimized
  ❑ Reduced excretion of calcium; hence, can decrease the incidence of fracture in elderly patients
  ❑ Synergistic effect when used in combination with other antihypertensive drugs

- **Heart failure:**
  - Diuretics act by reducing the circulating volume (by promoting salt and water excretion)
  - Loop diuretics (furosemide) are preferred as compared to thiazides
- **Diabetes insipidus:**
  - Thiazides leads to diuresis of concentrated (hyperosmolar) urine
- **Hypercalciuria:**
  - Thiazides leads to decreased calcium excretion in the urine, because they enhance the reabsorption of calcium in the distal convoluted tubule
  - Useful in patients with calcium oxalate stones

THIAZIDE LIKE DIURETICS—CHLORTHALIDONE, METOLAZONE, INDAPAMIDE

- Chlorthalidone-has a long duration; hence, can be used as once a day therapy for hypertension
- Metolazone-more potent than thiazides
- Indapamide-long duration of action

POTASSIUM SPARING DIURETICS

- Aldosterone antagonists—spironolactone, eplerenone
- Inhibitors of renal epithelial Na^+ channels (Directly acting)—triamterene, amiloride

Aldosterone Antagonists—Spironolactone, Eplerenone

These drugs reduce Na^+ absorption in the collecting tubules.

Spironolactone: It is a synthetic steroid and acts as a competitive antagonist to aldosterone.

Eplerenone: It is a spironolactone analogue with a higher selectivity for the mineralocorticoid receptor and is much less active on the androgen and progestogen receptors. Hence, it has a favorable endocrine adverse event profile as compared to spironolactone.

Mechanism of Action

The mechanism of action of aldosterone antagonists is mentioned in Figure 8.

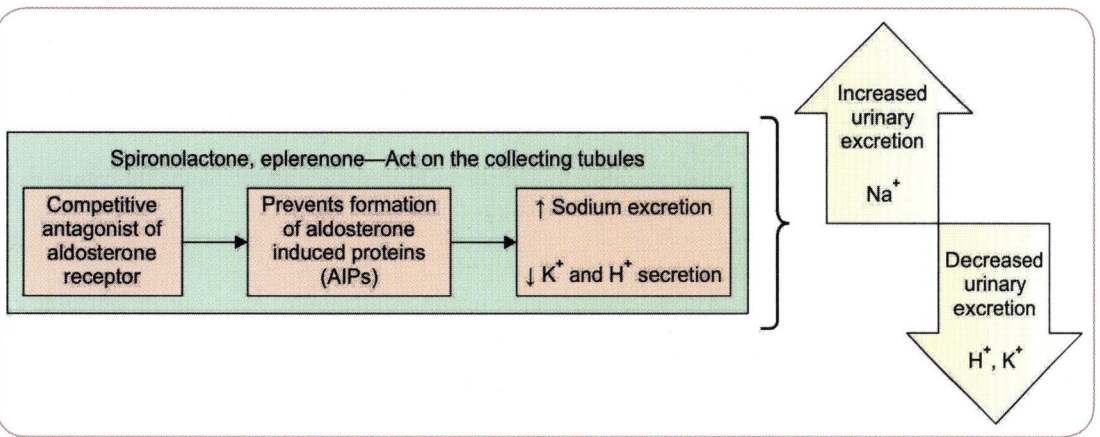

Figure 8: Pharmacological actions of aldosterone antagonists

Pharmacokinetics

Spironolactone is well absorbed after oral administration. It is metabolized completely in the liver to active metabolites. The most important active metabolite is canrenone. Spironolactone has a half-life of 1–2 hours while canrenone has a half-life of 18 hours.

Adverse Effects

The adverse effects of spironolactone include:

- **Hyperkalemia:** Increased risk in patients with renal disease or patients who are on ACE inhibitors, angiotensin receptor blockers ARBs, NSAIDs or β-blockers.
- Antiandrogenic effect leading to gynecomastia, decreased libido and menstrual abnormalities.
- GIT abnormalities such as nausea and vomiting.

Clinical Uses

- Secondary hyperaldosteronism
  - It is seen in conditions such as hepatic cirrhosis and nephrotic syndrome
  - Spironolactone is considered a preferred diuretic in patients of hepatic cirrhosis
- Heart failure
  - Aldosterone antagonists are used to counteract the hypokalemia caused by loop diuretics
  - These drugs decrease morbidity and mortality in patients of severe heart failure on therapy with other drugs. They also prevent ventricular remodeling.
- Hypertension
  - Prevent excessive depletion of potassium and hence, are usually given along with thiazide diuretics
  - Augment the antihypertensive effect of diuretics
  - Antagonize the potassium excreting and sodium retaining action of aldosterone

INHIBITORS OF RENAL EPITHELIAL Na⁺ CHANNELS—TRIAMTERENE, AMILORIDE

Mechanism of Action

These drugs block Na⁺ transport channels in the collecting tubules resulting in increased Na⁺ excretion and increased K⁺ retention.

Adverse Effects

- Hyperkalemia is the most important adverse effect. These drugs should not be used with potassium supplements, ACE inhibitors, ARBs or NSAIDs.
- Other adverse effects include nausea, vomiting and muscle cramps.

Clinical Uses

- They are not very effective diuretics and are used along with thiazide or loop diuretics to prevent excessive depletion of potassium
- They augment the antihypertensive effect of diuretics
- Amiloride is also used in lithium-induced nephrogenic diabetes insipidus because it blocks the transport of lithium through the Na⁺ transport channels in the collecting tubules

CARBONIC ANHYDRASE INHIBITORS

Acetazolamide

Acetazolamide is the prototype of carbonic anhydrase (CA) inhibitors.

CA inhibitors nowadays have limited utility as diuretics because of lower efficacy, as well as the availability of higher efficacious loop and thiazide diuretics.

Mechanism of Action

Carbonic Anhydrase Enzyme

Carbonic anhydrase is an enzyme that catalyzes the following reversible reaction:

$$CO_2 + H_2O \leftrightarrow H_2CO_3$$

Carbonic anhydrase is mainly present in the epithelial cells of proximal tubule (PT). In the proximal tubule, carbonic anhydrase catalyzes the reactions mentioned in the Figure 9.

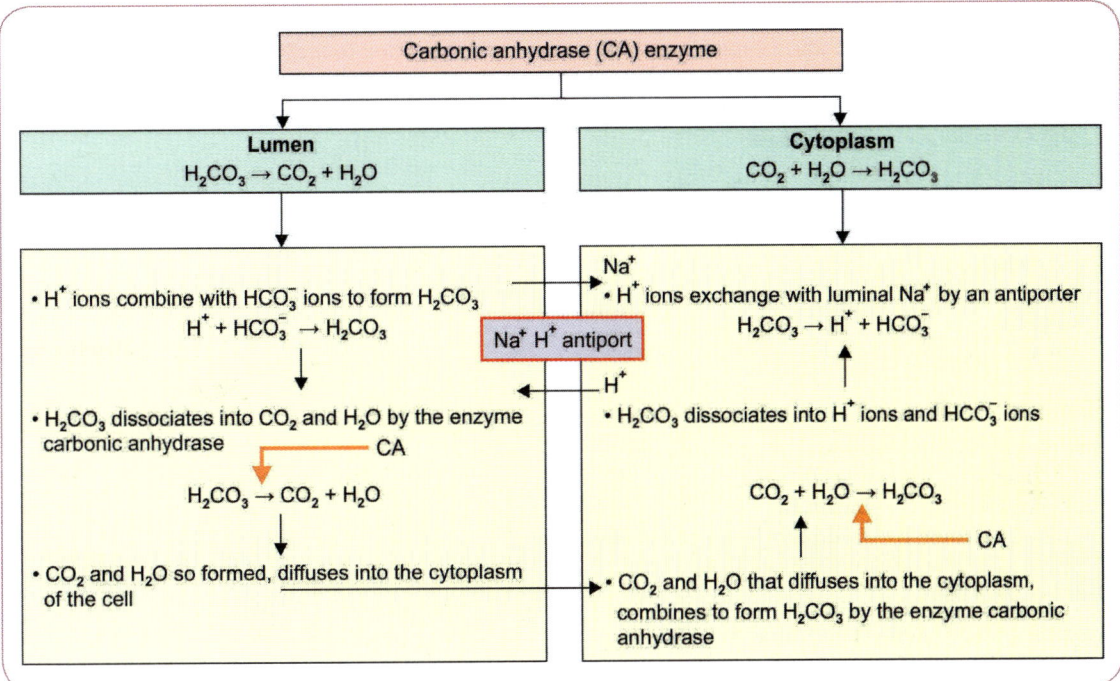

Figure 9: Carbonic anhydrase enzyme

Acetazolamide has the following actions:
- Inhibits the formation of H_2CO_3 in the cytoplasm
- Prevents the formation of H^+ and HCO_3^- ions (from H_2CO_3) in the cytoplasm
- Na^+-H^+ exchange at the luminal membrane is prevented
- H^+ ions are not available to move out from the cytoplasm into the lumen
- Na^+ ions are not able to move in from the lumen into the cytoplasm
- HCO_3^- ions cannot be neutralized to H_2CO_3 in the lumen because H^+ ions are not available

The above actions result in the following:
- Loss of Na^+ and HCO_3^- ions in the urine
- In the DCT, Na^+ ions are exchanged for K^+ ions

The above changes finally lead to the following:
- Loss of Na^+, K^+ and HCO_3^- ions in the urine resulting in diuresis and alkaline urine

Adverse Effects

The adverse effects include metabolic acidosis (mild), hypokalemia, drowsiness, paraesthesia and hypersensitivity reactions (fever, rashes, nephritis).

It is contraindicated in patients with liver disease because it may precipitate hepatic coma by decreasing urinary elimination of NH_3.

Clinical Uses

- **Glaucoma:** CA inhibitors decrease the production of aqueous humor and reduce intraocular pressure. They are useful in patients with chronic open angle glaucoma.

- Topical CA inhibitors such as dorzolamide and brinzolamide have the advantage of not causing renal or systemic effects.
- **Mountain sickness:** Acetazolamide is used for symptomatic relief as well as for prophylaxis of acute mountain sickness. The benefit is derived probably due to a decrease in CSF formation and a decrease in the pH of CSF.
- **Alkalinization of urine:** Acetazolamide is used for urine alkalinization to facilitate the excretion of certain acidic drugs, cystine and uric acid calculi.
- **Epilepsy:** It is used as an adjuvant in absence seizures in cases where the primary drugs are not effective.
- **Hypokalemic periodic paralysis**

OSMOTIC DIURETICS

- Mannitol
- Isosorbide
- Glycerol
- Urea

Mannitol

It has the following properties:
- Pharmacologically inert substance
- Freely filtered at the glomerulus
- Undergoes limited reabsorption by the renal tubule

Pharmacokinetics

Mannitol must be administered intravenously.

Mechanism of Action

The main site of action is the loop of Henle with action also in the proximal tubules.
- Mannitol is confined to the extracellular compartment and has an osmotic effect that causes fluid to shift from the intracellular to the extracellular compartment.
- It is freely filterable at the glomerulus and very little is reabsorbed back from the kidney tubule. It remains confined to the kidney tubules and exerts an osmotic effect which prevents fluid reabsorption from the glomerular filtrate and causes diuresis. It also increases electrolyte excretion, especially sodium, potassium and chloride.
- Mannitol increases renal blood flow that reduces the tonicity in the renal medulla that also inhibits reabsorption of water.

Adverse Effects

The key adverse effects of mannitol include:
- **CNS toxicity:** It can manifest as confusion, lethargy and coma. These may be due to high serum mannitol concentrations, serum hyperosmolarity, electrolyte and acid/base balance abnormality including hyponatremia
- Acute oligoanuric renal failure
- Risk of hypervolemia

Contraindications

The contraindications of mannitol include:
- Severe dehydration
- Acute tubular necrosis, anuria
- Severe heart failure
- Severe pulmonary congestion or pulmonary edema → can expand the ECF volume leading to volume overload
- Active intracranial bleeding

Clinical Uses

○ To reduce intracranial or intraocular pressure in conditions such as head injury, stroke or acute congestive glaucoma:
  ❑ Reduction of intracranial pressure-by exerting osmotic pressure, mannitol leads to movement of fluid from the brain tissue; hence, causes a reduction in the brain volume and intracranial pressure
  ❑ Reduction of intraocular pressure-leads to movement of fluid from the aqueous humor; hence, causes a reduction in the intraocular pressure
○ To induce diuresis in the prevention and/or treatment of the oliguric phase of acute renal failure before irreversible renal failure becomes established:
  ❑ This may be in conditions of shock, severe trauma, cardiac surgery and hemolytic reactions

ANTIDIURETIC DRUGS

Vasopressin (Antidiuretic hormone, ADH) and its analogues have two key functions:
○ Vasoconstriction of the blood vessels leading to a rise in blood pressure
○ Water reabsorption from the renal collecting tubules

The salient features of vasopressin and its analogues are mentioned in Figure 10.

Salient Features

Vasopressin (Antidiuretic hormone, ADH)		
What is vasopressin (ADH)	**Actions of ADH**	**Adverse effects of vasopressin and vasopressin analogues**
Nonapeptide hormone	Mediated via V_1 and V_2 receptors	**V_1 receptor mediated**
Synthesized in the hypothalamus and released by the posterior pituitary	**V_1 receptors** • Blood vessels—vasoconstriction • Hepatocytes—glycogenolysis • Platelets—aggregation • GIT—increased peristalsis	• Pallor, abdominal pain, diarrhea myocardial infarction • Precipitation of angina due to coronary artery vasoconstriction—to be used with extreme caution in patients with hypertension and coronary artery disease
Triggers for the release of ADH are: • Increase in plasma osmolarity • Contraction of ECF volume	**V_2 receptors** • Collecting tubules of kidneys—Increases water reabsorption (Antidiuretic effect) • Vascular endothelium—release of factor VIII and vWF	**V_2 receptor mediated** • Fluid retention, hyponatremia
• Antidiuretic action is mediated through the V_2 receptors, located in the collecting tubules of the kidneys		

Vasopressin and vasopressin analogues				
Vasopressin	**Desmopressin**	**Terlipressin**	**Felypressin**	**Lypressin**
• Short duration of action • Nonselective V_1 and V_2 action • Administered via parenteral and intranasal route	• Longer duration of action ($t_{1/2}$-2 hours) • V_2 selective action • Administered via parenteral, oral and intranasal routes	• Prodrug of vasopressin • More potent than vasopressin • Selective V_1 action • Preferred for management of variceal bleeding	• Short duration of action • Mainly V_1 action and used with local anesthetic drugs to prolong their action	• Less potent than vasopressin, but has a prolonged duration of action

Figure 10: Vasopressin (Antidiuretic hormone, ADH) and its analogues

Clinical Uses

The clinical uses of vasopressin and its analogues are mentioned in Figure 11.

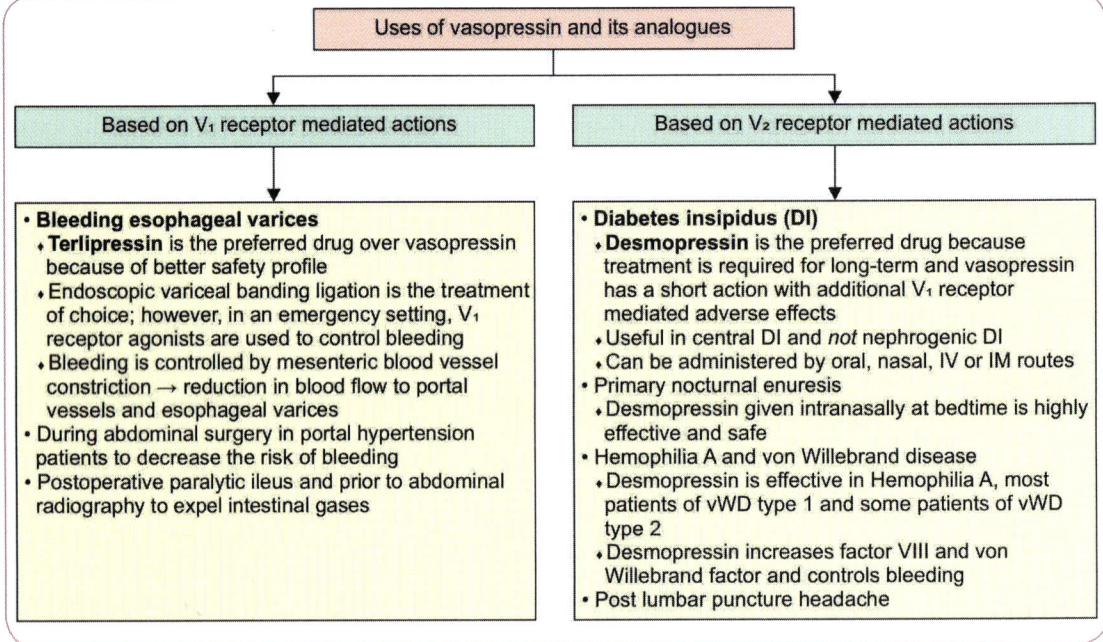

Figure 11: Uses of vasopressin and its analogues

SYNDROME OF INAPPROPRIATE ANTIDIURETIC HORMONE SECRETION (SIADH)

SIADH is characterized by inappropriate release of antidiuretic hormone resulting in the following:
- Impaired water excretion
- Hyponatremia
- Hypoosmolality

Causes

- **CNS conditions:** Brain abscess, head injury, encephalitis, meningitis
- **Neoplasia:** Lung cancer, pancreatic cancer
- **Pulmonary disease:** Pneumonia, asthma
- **Drugs:** Chlorpropamide, carbamazepine, vincristine

Treatment

- Restriction of fluid intake
- Treatment of the underlying cause
- Drug therapy
  - Demeclocycline—inhibits the action of ADH in the collecting tubule
  - Vasopressin (ADH) antagonists—conivaptan, tolvaptan

ASSESS YOURSELF (Examination Questions of Various Universities)

1. Classify diuretics. Discuss the mechanism of action, adverse effects, and clinical uses of loop diuretics.
2. What is the pharmacological basis for use of furosemide in pulmonary oedema.
3. Discuss the mechanism of action and clinical uses of carbonic anhydrase inhibitors.
4. Discuss briefly on:
   a. High-ceiling diuretics
   b. Potassium-sparing diuretics

   c. Adverse effects and clinical uses of thiazides
   d. Mechanism of action, contraindications and clinical uses of mannitol
   e. Mechanism of action and therapeutic uses of spironolactone
5. Explain why:
   a. Spironolactone is combined with furosemide
   b. Thiazides are used in patients with renal stones

MULTIPLE CHOICE QUESTIONS

1. The site of action of the loop diuretic furosemide is   *(AIIMS May 2014)*
   a. Thick ascending limb of loop of Henle
   b. Descending limb of loop of Henle
   c. Proximal tubule
   d. Distal tubule

2. Thiazides can cause: *(AIIMS Nov 2009)*
   a. Hyperkalemic paralysis b. Hypouricemia
   c. Hypolipidemia   d. Impotence

3. Hypercalcemia is caused by all except:
                               (AIIMS Nov 2007)
   a. Loop diuretics   b. Lithium
   c. Vitamin D intoxication d. Thiazides

4. Thiazide diuretics causes all except:
                               (AIIMS Nov 2007)
   a. Hyperglycemia
   b. Increased calcium excretion
   c. Useful in congestive heart failure
   d. Decreased uric acid excretion

5. Regarding furosemide true statement is:
                               (AIIMS Nov 2007)
   a. Acute pulmonary edema is an indication
   b. Acts on PCT
   c. Mild diuresis
   d. Given only by parental route

6. Mannitol is not useful for:
   a. Glaucoma   *(Recent Question 2016)*
   b. Raised ICT

   c. Impending renal failure
   d. Pulmonary edema

7. Following are the side effects of thiazides except: *(Recent Question 2016)*
   a. Hypokalemia   b. Hypocalcemia
   c. Hepatic coma   d. Impotence

8. Mechanism of action thiazide is:
                               (Recent Question 2016)
   a. Na^+Cl^- symport inhibitor
   b. Na^+K^+ symport inhibitor
   c. Carbonic anhydrase inhibitor
   d. Osmotic diuresis

9. Complication of long-term thiazide administration: *(Recent Question 2016)*
   a. Metabolic alkalosis
   b. Metabolic acidosis
   c. Hypermagnesemia
   d. Hypocalcemia

10. Vasopressin cannot correct:
                               (Recent Question 2016)
    a. Nephrogenic DI
    b. Neurogenic DI
    c. Gl bleeding
    d. Nocturnal enuresis

11. Lithium induced diabetes insipidus respond to:
                               (Recent Question 2016)
    a. Diclofenac   b. Vasopressin
    c. Amiloride   d. Indapamide

Ans.

1.	(a)	2.	(d)	3.	(a)	4.	(b)	5.	(a)	6.	(d)
7.	(b)	8.	(a)	9.	(a)	10.	(a)	11.	(c)		

12. Most common complication of loop diuretics:
(Recent Question 2016)
a. Hypocalcemia   b. Hypokalemia
c. Hyperkalemia   d. Hypercalcemia

13. Drug causing metabolic acidosis:
(Recent Question 2016)
a. Acetazolamide   b. Thiazide
c. Torsemide   d. Spironolactone

14. All the following adverse effects can be caused by loop diuretics except:
(Recent Question 2016)
a. Hypercalcemia   b. Hyperglycemia
c. Hypomagnesemia   d. Hyperuricemia

15. Drug causing gynecomastia is:
(Recent Question 2016)
a. Spironolactone   b. Rifampicin
c. Penicillin   d. Bumetanide

16. Amiloride can cause hyperkalemia due to its action on: *(Recent Question 2016)*
a. Electrogenic K^+ channels
b. Electrogenic Na^+ channels
c. Non electrogenic Na^+ -Cl^- symporter
d. H^+ – K^+ – ATPase

17. Selective V2 receptor agonist useful for the treatment of central diabetes insipidus is:
(Recent Question 2016)
a. Arginine vasopressin   b. Desmopressin
c. Lypressin   d. Terlipressin

18. Desmopressin can be used for all of the following conditions except:
(Recent Question 2016)
a. Neurogenic diabetes insipidus
b. Nephrogenic diabetes insipidus
c. Bed wetting in children
d. Bleeding due to hemophilia

19. Furosemide should not be administered with NSAIDs because latter: *(Recent Question 2016)*
a. Prevent platelet aggregation
b. Inhibit prostacyclin synthesis
c. Decrease sodium reabsorption
d. Increase the secretion of furosemide in urine

20. All of the following diuretics inhibit Na^+ -K^+-$2Cl^-$ symporter, except: *(Recent Question 2016)*
a. Furosemide   b. Thiazide
c. Ethacrynic acid   d. Mersalyl

21. Drug causing deafness is:
(Recent Question 2016)
a. Thiazide   b. Spironolactone
c. Ethacrynic acid   d. Triamterene

22. Which of the following is aldosterone antagonist? *(Recent Question 2016)*
a. Eplerenone
b. Deoxycorticosterone
c. Fenoldopam
d. Furosemide

23. Canrenone is a metabolite of:
(Recent Question 2016)
a. Ampicillin   b. Spironolactone
c. Furosemide   d. Acetazolamide

24. Acetazolamide can be used in all except:
a. Epilepsy   *(Recent Question 2016)*
b. Acute mountain sickness
c. Cirrhosis
d. Glaucoma

25. Furosemide causes all except:
a. Hyperglycemia   *(Recent Question 2016)*
b. Hypomagnesemia
c. Hypokalemia
d. Acidosis

26. Loop diuretics act by: *(PGI Dec 2008)*
a. Inhibition of Na^+-Cl^- Symport
b. Inhibition of Na^+-K^+-2 Cl^- cotransport
c. Inhibition of Na^+-K^+ ATPase
d. Inhibition of H^+-K^+ ATPase
e. Inhibition of renal epithelial Na^+ channel

27. Drug causing osmotic diuresis is:
(NIMHANS 2013)
a. Mannitol   b. Isosorbide
c. Glycerol   d. All of the above

28. Potassium sparing diuretic is: *(TN PG 2008)*
a. Furosemide   b. Indapamide
c. Spironolactone   d. Benzthiazide

29. Which of the following is an aldosterone antagonist? *(MH CET 2010 2007)*
a. Eplerenone   b. Amiloride
c. Triamterene   d. All of the above

30. Spirolactone is contraindicated with enalapril because it causes: *(WB PG 2007)*
a. Hyperkalemia   b. Hypercalcemia
c. Hypernatremia   d. Hypokalemia

Ans.											
12.	(b)	13.	(a)	14.	(a)	15.	(a)	16.	(b)	17.	(b)
18.	(b)	19.	(b)	20.	(b)	21.	(c)	22.	(a)	23.	(b)
24.	(c)	25.	(d)	26.	(b)	27.	(d)	28.	(c)	29.	(a)
30.	(a)										

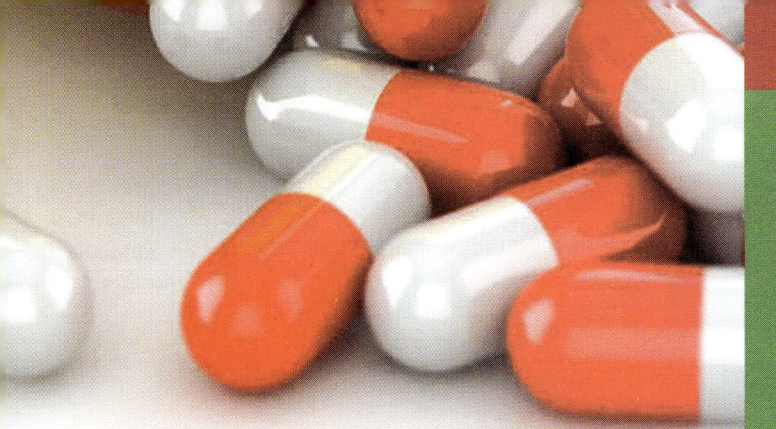

Drugs Acting on Blood and Blood Formation

SECTION OUTLINE

○ Hematinics and Erythropoietin
○ Drugs Affecting Coagulation, Bleeding and Thrombosis

Hematinics and Erythropoietin

Hematinics are nutrients that are needed for the formation of blood cells. The key hematinics include iron, vitamin B_{12} and folic acid and are used in the treatment of anemia.

Some of the causes of anemia are mentioned in Table 1.

TABLE 1	Causes of anemia
Causes	**Examples**
Blood loss	GI bleeding, worm infestation
Deficiency of nutrients	Iron, vitamin B_{12} or folate deficiency
Bone marrow depression	Radiation, malignancies, anticancer medications
Increased destruction of RBCs	Hemolytic anemia: Can be due to autoimmune disorders, infections, drugs etc.

IRON

Iron is an essential substance in the body. It is a vital constituent of hemoglobin (Hb), myoglobin and various enzymes such as cytochrome and catalases that are involved in oxygen transfer. The total body iron in an adult is 2.5–5 g (Table 2).

TABLE 2	Iron distribution and sources		
Total body iron	2.5–5 g (adult)		
Distribution of iron	Hemoglobin	66%	
	Ferritin and hemosiderin (storage)	25%	
	Parenchymal iron	6%	
	Myoglobin	3%	
Sources of iron	Liver, egg yolk, dry fruits, meat, chicken, fish and spinach		
Daily requirement of iron	Adult male: 0.5–1 mg Adult female (menstruating): 1–2 mg Pregnancy: 3–5 mg		

IRON ABSORPTION AND TRANSPORT

Iron content of an average daily diet is 10–20 mg. Iron in the diet can be of two types: heme iron and inorganic iron. Although the absorption of heme iron is better, it is generally not a major part of the diet. Most of the iron absorption occurs in the upper part of intestine (duodenum and upper jejunum). Iron is transported in a complex with transferrin and stored in bone marrow, liver or spleen (Figure 1).

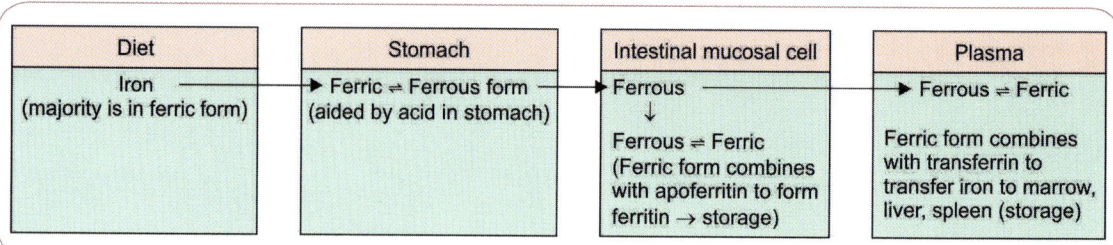

Figure 1: Iron absorption and transport

The factors that facilitate iron absorption include an acidic environment (stomach) and the presence of reducing substances such as ascorbic acid. Iron deficiency states also enhance the absorption of iron. Meat facilitates absorption of iron by increasing acid secretion. Meat is also a source of iron.

The factors that reduce iron absorption are alkalis such as antacids as they prevent the reduction of iron to the ferrous form. Phosphates, phytates and tetracyclines reduce the absorption of iron by forming insoluble iron complexes in the stomach.

IRON PREPARATIONS

Iron preparations can be oral or parenteral. Oral iron preparations are preferred in the treatment of iron deficiency anemia (Figure 2).

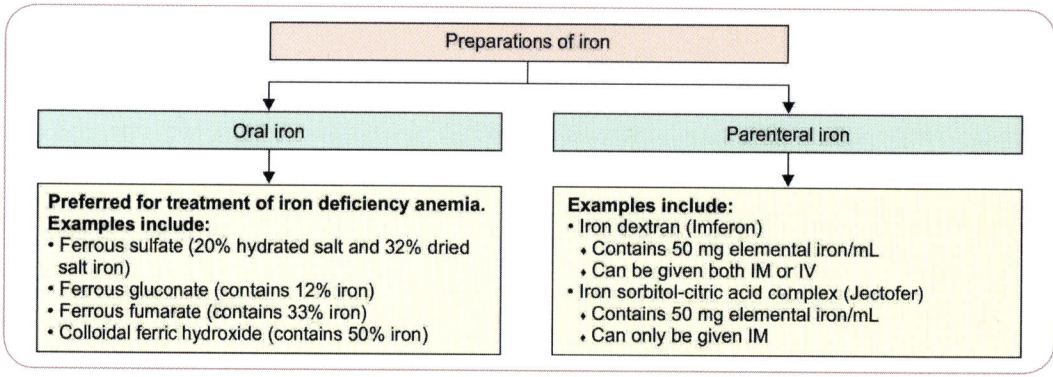

Figure 2: Preparations of iron

Oral Iron Therapy

Oral iron therapy is preferred for the treatment of iron deficiency anemia. It is important to know the elemental iron content of the preparations.

Adverse effects of oral iron preparations include epigastric pain, nausea, vomiting, staining of teeth (with liquid preparations), metallic taste, constipation (possibly due to astringent action of iron) and diarrhea (possibly due to irritant action or iron).

Parenteral Iron Therapy

The indications of parenteral iron therapy include the following:
○ Inability to tolerate oral iron due to adverse effects such as GI upset
○ Inability to absorb oral iron in conditions such as malabsorption, inflammatory bowel disease etc.
○ Severe iron deficiency with chronic bleeding
○ Administered along with erythropoietin therapy. The absorption of oral iron may not be fast enough to meet the iron demand due to rapid erythropoiesis induced by erythropoietin

○ Noncompliance with oral iron therapy

The dose calculation of parenteral iron is as follows:

$$\text{Iron requirement (mg)} = 4.4 \times \text{body weight (kg)} \times \text{Hb deficit (g/dL)}$$

The calculation also includes iron that is required for the replenishment of iron stores.

Adverse effects of parenteral iron preparations include the following:

○ **Local site reactions:** Include staining of the skin, pain at the site of intramuscular (IM) injection, sterile abscess. The IM injections are given deep IM using a Z track technique in the gluteal region. This is done to avoid staining of the skin.

○ **Systemic reactions:** Include pyrexia, headache, vomiting. Parenteral administration of iron preparations can cause hypersensitivity reactions including serious and potentially fatal anaphylactic/anaphylactoid reactions. Hence, administration of parenteral iron should be done in an environment where full resuscitation facilities are available along with the trained personnel for evaluation and management of anaphylactic reactions. Injection of the test dose is done to identify sensitive patients.

CLINICAL USES OF IRON

The clinical uses of iron include the following:

1. Treatment of iron deficiency anemia (microcytic hypochromic anemia)
   - ❑ This anemia is usually observed due to dietary deficiency, pregnancy, chronic blood loss or due to inadequate absorption from the GIT.
   - ❑ An increase in the Hb level by 0.5–1 g/dL is considered a satisfactory response to iron therapy.
   - ❑ Therapy should be continued till Hb levels become normal (usual time taken is 1–3 months of therapy) followed by 2–3 months of therapy to replenish the iron stores.
   - ❑ Oral iron therapy is preferred for the treatment of iron deficiency anemia. Parenteral iron therapy is used for specific indications as mentioned earlier.
2. Prophylaxis of iron deficiency anemia
   - ❑ Usually indicated during pregnancy and infancy. Folic acid is administered from the first trimester to prevent neural tube defects.
   - ❑ Prophylactic iron therapy may also be required in patients of chronic illness, menorrhagia etc.
3. Megaloblastic anemia
   - ❑ Treatment with vitamin B_{12}/folic acid in patients of megaloblastic anemia results in brisk hemopoiesis. This may lead to iron deficiency if the stores of iron are inadequate. Hence, therapy with iron may be required if the iron status is deficient.

ACUTE IRON POISONING

The occurrence of acute iron poisoning is mainly in young children. Clinical features include vomiting, hematemesis, diarrhea, abdominal pain, cyanosis, acidosis, seizures, coma and death. Prompt management is required and involves specific therapy and general management (Figure 3).

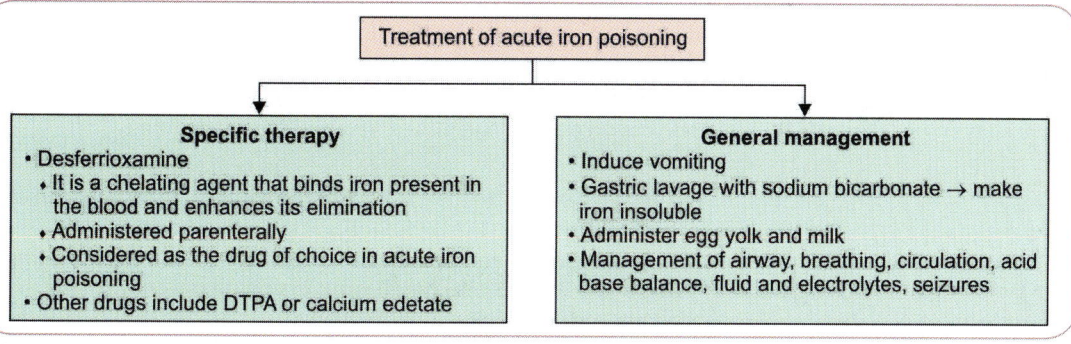

Figure 3: Treatment of acute iron poisoning

MATURATION FACTORS—VITAMIN B$_{12}$ AND FOLIC ACID

Vitamin B$_{12}$ and folic acid are required for DNA synthesis in the body. Deficiency of vitamin B$_{12}$ or folic acid leads to megaloblastic anemia.

■ VITAMIN B$_{12}$

Vitamin B$_{12}$ is a cobalt containing compound that belongs to a family of cobalamins.

Sources

The dietary sources include liver, egg yolk, meat, cheese and kidneys. Legumes are the only vegetable source of vitamin B$_{12}$. This is due to microorganisms contained in the roots of legumes.

Metabolic Functions

Vitamin B$_{12}$ is closely related to the metabolism of folic acid and deficiency can result in megaloblastic anemia. Deoxyadenosylcobalamin (DAB$_{12}$) and methylcobalamin (methyl-B$_{12}$) are active coenzymatic forms of vitamin B$_{12}$ that are generated in the body. The key metabolic functions of vitamin B$_{12}$ are mentioned in Table 3.

TABLE 3	Metabolic functions of vitamin B$_{12}$
1.	**Conversion of homocysteine to methionine** • Methionine is required as a methyl (CH$_3$) group donor in the synthesis of proteins and in various metabolic reactions • Methylcobalamin transfers a CH$_3$ group to homocysteine, thus generating cobalamin and methionine • Cobalamin is converted back to methylcobalamin by taking a CH$_3$ group from Methyl THFA (CH$_3$-tetrahydrofolate), thus generating tetrahydrofolate (THFA). Vitamin B$_{12}$ deficiency results in trapping of folate (folate trap) in the form of methyl THFA and hence, a deficiency of biologically active THFA arises. This affects the synthesis of purines and pyrimidines as folate dependent one carbon transfer reactions cannot be carried out.
2.	**Conversion of malonic acid to succinic acid** → Useful in carbohydrate and lipid metabolism
3.	**Conversion of methionine to S-adenosylmethionine** → Involved in the synthesis of phospholipids and myelin
4.	**Required for cell growth and multiplication**

Pharmacokinetics

Physiological amounts of dietary vitamin B$_{12}$ forms a complex with intrinsic factor (IF) in the stomach. IF is a glycoprotein secreted by the parietal cells of the stomach. The complex of IF + vitamin B$_{12}$ is absorbed from the terminal ileum. Following absorption, vitamin B$_{12}$ is transported in the blood to the various tissues in the body by glycoproteins called transcobalamin-II. Any excess amount of vitamin B$_{12}$ is stored in the liver.

Vitamin B$_{12}$ is primarily excreted in the bile and undergoes significant enterohepatic circulation. Depletion of normal body stores of vitamin B$_{12}$ takes 3–5 years in cases of complete absence of dietary vitamin B$_{12}$.

Causes and Clinical Manifestations of Vitamin B$_{12}$ Deficiency

The causes of vitamin B$_{12}$ deficiency are mentioned below:
○ Pernicious anemia → autoimmune disorder in which there is destruction of gastric parietal cells which results in lack of intrinsic factor generation in the body. This prevents the absorption of B$_{12}$ in the body.
○ Gastric mucosal damage → chronic gastritis, gastric carcinoma, gastrectomy
○ Bowel resection, malabsorption

- ○ Blind loop syndrome, fish tape worm infestation
- ○ Pregnancy and lactation → due to increased demand
- ○ Deficient intake (uncommon as the daily requirement of vitamin B$_{12}$ is very low).

The clinical manifestations of vitamin B$_{12}$ deficiency are mentioned in Table 4.

TABLE 4	Clinical manifestations of vitamin B$_{12}$ deficiency
1.	**Megaloblastic anemia**
2.	**Neurological manifestations** • Subacute combined degeneration of the spinal cord • Paresthesia, peripheral neuritis and neuropathy • Diminished memory, alterations in mood, hallucinations
3.	**Others** • Glossitis, atrophy of tongue, gastrointestinal problems

Vitamin B$_{12}$ Preparations

- ○ Cyanocobalamin
  - ❑ Available for oral, IM or SC administration
  - ❑ Should not be administered IV due to the risk of anaphylaxis
- ○ Hydroxocobalamin
  - ❑ Available for IM administration
- ○ Methylcobalamin (oral administration)

Adverse Effects

Vitamin B$_{12}$ is generally well tolerated; allergic reactions including anaphylaxis can occur.

Clinical Uses

Some of the clinical uses of vitamin B$_{12}$ are mentioned in Table 5.

TABLE 5	Clinical uses of vitamin B$_{12}$
1.	**Treatment of vitamin B$_{12}$ deficiency** (e.g. pernicious anemia and in other conditions with defective absorption of vitamin B$_{12}$) • Parenteral therapy (IM or SC) is used because orally administered vitamin B$_{12}$ would not be effective due to defective absorptive mechanisms. • Significant response to therapy is often observed with patients reporting well-being and improvement in appetite. Neurological improvement may take a longer time. • Folic acid and iron are often added along with vitamin B$_{12}$ because rapid erythropoiesis may unmask the deficiency of folic acid and iron. • Oral vitamin B$_{12}$ is not absorbed in patients of pernicious anemia due to deficiency of intrinsic factor. • In patients of pernicious anemia with vitamin B$_{12}$ deficiency, folic acid alone should not be given because worsening or precipitation of the neurological defects may occur, even though an improvement may be observed in the hematological parameters. This is because the existing small amounts of vitamin B$_{12}$ in the body are diverted to hematopoiesis.
2.	**Tobacco amblyopia**
3.	**Prophylaxis of vitamin B$_{12}$ deficiency** → only if specific predisposing factors are present (e.g. gastrectomy patients)

▌ FOLIC ACID

It is also known as pteroylglutamic acid (PGA). It consists of pteridine, para-aminobenzoic acid and glutamic acid.

Sources

The sources of folic acid include green leafy vegetables, egg, meat, milk and liver.

Metabolic Functions

Folic acid is inactive and gets converted to tetrahydrofolic acid (THFA) which is the active form (Figure 4).

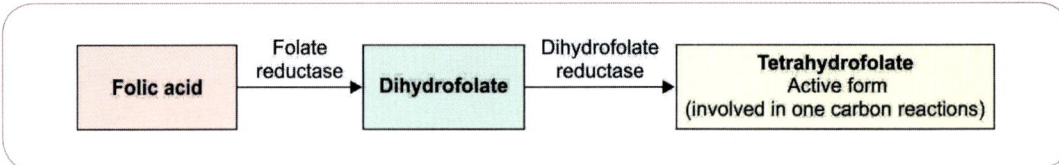

Figure 4: Folic acid

Some of the metabolic functions of folic acid are mentioned below:
- Conversion of homocysteine → methionine
- Thymidylate generation
- Synthesis of purines
- Involved in histidine metabolism

Folic acid plays an important role in the synthesis of DNA, purines, pyrimidines, choline, amino acids etc.

Pharmacokinetics

Folic acid is present in the diet as polyglutamates which is converted to monoglutamates mainly in the upper intestine. It gets reduced to THFA primarily in the jejunum. It is absorbed from proximal small intestine and is transported in the blood as methyl THFA.

The main site of storage is in the liver.

Causes and Clinical Manifestations of Folic Acid Deficiency

Some of the causes of folic acid deficiency are mentioned below:
1. Nutritional deficiency
2. Chronic alcoholism
   - Cause of deficiency includes reduced intake and interference with the release of folic acid from the liver
3. Increased requirement
   - Pregnancy, lactation, periods of rapid growth
   - Hemolytic anemia
4. Malabsorption
   - Celiac disease, tropical sprue
5. Drugs
   - Oral contraceptives
   - Anticonvulsants—phenytoin, phenobarbitone
   - Methotrexate, trimethoprim

The clinical manifestations of folic acid deficiency are mentioned in Table 6.

TABLE 6	Clinical manifestations of folic acid deficiency
1.	**Megaloblastic anemia** • Anemia due to deficiency of folic acid and vitamin B_{12} is generally indistinguishable
2.	**Neural tube defects** • Neural tube defects such as spina bifida occurs in the neonate, due to deficiency of folic acid in the mother
3.	**Others** • Glossitis, enteritis, diarrhea • General debility, weight loss, sterility

Folic Acid Preparations

○ Folic acid
○ Folinic acid (calcium leucovorin)

Adverse Effects

Folic acid is generally well tolerated; hypersensitivity reactions can occur.

Clinical Uses

Some of the clinical uses of folic acid are mentioned in Table 7.

TABLE 7	Clinical uses of folic acid
Megaloblastic anemias (due to)	• Nutritional deficiency • Increased requirement in pregnancy, lactation, periods of rapid growth, hemolytic anemia • Malabsorption syndromes—celiac disease, tropical sprue • Prolonged therapy with anticonvulsants—phenytoin, phenobarbitone • Pernicious anemia 　▪ Folic acid is usually added to vitamin B_{12} therapy because rapid erythropoiesis may unmask the deficiency of folic acid. 　▪ Folic acid should not be given alone in patients with vitamin B_{12} deficiency because worsening or precipitation of the neurological defects may occur even though an improvement may be observed in the hematological parameters. This is because the existing small amounts of vitamin B_{12} in the body are diverted to hematopoiesis.
Prophylaxis of folate deficiency	• Supplementation during pregnancy is done to decrease the risk of neural tube defects.
Methotrexate toxicity	• Methotrexate inhibits dihydrofolate reductase and hence, tetrahydrofolate is not formed. • Folinic acid (leucovorin, citrovorum factor) is an active form of folic acid which does not need to be reduced by dihydrofolate reductase. Hence, it can reduce the toxicity of methotrexate.
Cytotoxic therapy with 5-fluorouracil	• Coadministration of folinic acid and 5-fluorouracil can lead to an increased efficacy of 5-fluorouracil.

ERYTHROPOIETIN

It is a glycoprotein hormone that is a produced by the peritubular cells of the kidney.

Erythropoietin (EPO) is produced primarily by the kidneys in response to hypoxia and stimulates erythropoiesis by acting on the bone marrow.

Adverse Effects

The adverse effects of EPO include the following:
○ Increase in blood pressure, hematocrit, peripheral vascular resistance
○ Arterial and venous thrombosis, embolism
○ Cerebrovascular accidents
○ Nausea, vomiting, headache
○ Flu-like symptoms

Clinical Uses

The clinical uses of EPO include the following:
○ Anemia associated with chronic renal failure (CRF)
○ Anemia in patients receiving cancer chemotherapy
○ Zidovudine-induced anemia in patients with AIDS

SECTION J ■ Drugs Acting on Blood and Blood Formation

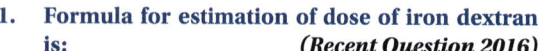

ASSESS YOURSELF (Examination Questions of Various Universities)

1. Enumerate various oral and parenteral Iron preparations. Mention indications for parenteral iron therapy and discuss in brief about treatment of iron poisoning.
2. What are the adverse effects of oral iron
3. Parenteral iron therapy
4. Explain why folic acid is given along with Vitamin B12 to treat megaloblastic anemia
5. Explain why folic acid should not be used alone in pernicious anaemia

MULTIPLE CHOICE QUESTIONS

1. Formula for estimation of dose of iron dextran is: *(Recent Question 2016)*
   a. $4.3 \times (100 - Hb\%) \times$ body wt
   b. $1.3 \times (100 - Hb\%) \times$ body wt
   c. $2.3 \times (100 - Hb\%) \times$ body wt
   d. $3.3 \times (100 - Hb\%) \times$ body wt

2. Erythropoietin is mainly produced in: *(Recent Question 2016)*
   a. Liver
   b. Kidney
   c. Intestine
   d. Bone

3. Methotrexate should be given with which of the following to decrease its side effects? *(Recent Question 2016)*
   a. Folic acid
   b. Cyanocoblamin
   c. Thiamine
   d. Folinic acid

4. Folic acid: *(TNPG 2006)*
   a. Consists of pteridine, paraaminobenzoic acid and glutamine
   b. Maximum absorption occurs at jejunum
   c. Involves in one carbon transfer
   d. All of the above

Ans.

1. (a)   2. (b)   3. (d)   4. (d)

45 Drugs Affecting Coagulation, Bleeding and Thrombosis

Hemostasis is stopping of blood loss or blood flow from a damaged blood vessel. It involves complex interactions between the damaged vessel wall, platelets and coagulation factors.

The coagulation cascade consists of extrinsic pathway, intrinsic pathway and the common pathway that lead to the formation of an insoluble fibrin clot (Figure 1).

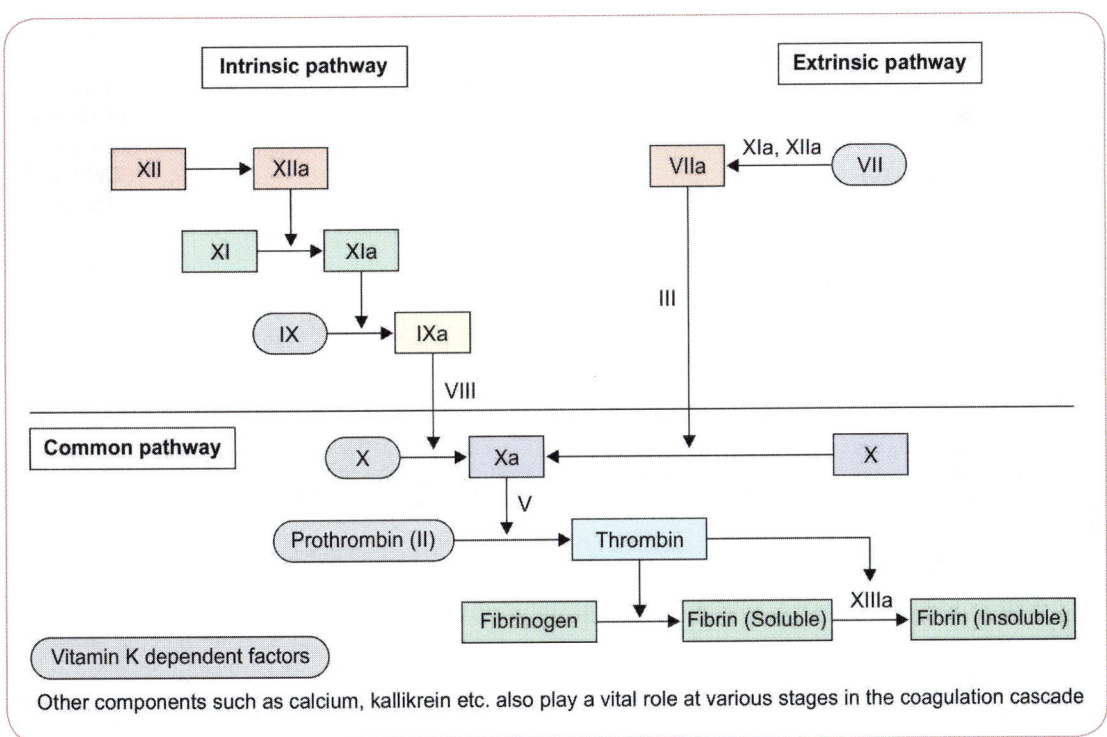

Figure 1: Coagulation cascade

COAGULANTS

Coagulants are substances that cause the blood to clot. Coagulants are useful in the management of hemorrhagic conditions.

Generally, the factors needed for coagulation are provided by the transfusion of whole blood or plasma and are considered as preferred therapy for the management of hemorrhagic conditions. The drugs used in the management of hemostasis are mentioned in Table 1.

TABLE 1	Drugs used for hemostasis
Vitamin K	• Vitamin K$_1$—Phytonadione (plant origin, fat soluble) • Vitamin K$_3$— Menadione (synthetic, fat soluble); menadione sodium bisulfite (synthetic, water soluble)
Other drugs	• Fibrinogen, antihemophilic factor, desmopressin, ethamsylate, rutin

VITAMIN K

It is a fat-soluble vitamin that is required for the synthesis of coagulation factors (prothrombin [II], VII, IX and X) in the liver. It is required for gamma carboxylation of glutamic acid residues of the coagulation factors.

Sources

The sources of vitamin K include green leafy vegetables (spinach, cabbage), liver and cheese.

Pharmacokinetics

Fat soluble forms of vitamin K require bile salts for absorption. They are absorbed via lymph from the intestine. Water soluble forms are absorbed directly from the intestine. It is temporarily stored and metabolized in the liver and excretion is via bile and urine.

Causes of Vitamin K Deficiency and Clinical Manifestations

Vitamin K deficiency states are observed in the following conditions:
○ Hepatic disease
○ Malabsorption
○ Prolonged therapy with antimicrobials leading to alteration of intestinal flora
○ Obstructive jaundice
Clinical manifestations include bleeding tendencies such as hematuria, ecchymosis, GIT bleeding etc.

Clinical Uses

Vitamin K is used in the prophylaxis and treatment of bleeding resulting from deficiency of clotting factors in the following conditions:
1. Overdose of oral anticoagulants → vitamin K$_1$— phytonadione is the preferred preparation because it is rapidly acting
2. Prolonged therapy with antimicrobials
3. Obstructive jaundice or malabsorption
4. Hepatic disease (e.g. hepatitis, cirrhosis)
5. Neonates—all neonates have decreased capacity to synthetize clotting factors and also have a deficiency of vitamin K that results in low levels of clotting factors. The deficiency is exaggerated in premature babies. Menadione is not to be used for this indication.
6. Dietary deficiency

Adverse Effects

The adverse reactions of vitamin K include the following:
○ Allergic reactions, flushing, dyspnea, hypotension and fatalities can occur.
○ Menadione and its water-soluble salts may induce hemolysis in patients, particularly in neonates and in patients with glucose-6-phosphate dehydrogenase (G6PD) deficiency.

❑ Menadione and its water-soluble salts can precipitate kernicterus in the newborn by increasing bilirubin levels due to hemolysis and inhibition of glucuronide conjugation of bilirubin.

○ Menadione and its water-soluble salts are not commonly used for any indication due to decreased efficacy and increased toxicity.

ANTIHEMOPHILIC FACTOR

It contains clotting factor VIII with von Willebrand's factor and is obtained from human plasma. It is given by intravenous (IV) infusion and is used in hemophiliacs.

ETHAMSYLATE

It increases capillary wall stability and reduces capillary bleeding probably by exerting antihyaluronidase activity. It does not have antifibrinolytic activity. It is available for oral and parenteral administration. It is used to prevent and treat capillary bleeding in postpartum hemorrhage, post abortion, menorrhagia, post-tooth extraction, hematuria, epistaxis etc. The adverse effects may include rashes, headache and hypotension.

DESMOPRESSIN

It is an analogue of vasopressin. It is used to control bleeding in hemophilia A and von Willebrand's disease.

LOCAL HEMOSTATICS (STYPTICS)

These are substances used to control bleeding from the blood capillaries and minute blood vessels at local sites, e.g. tooth socket, abrasions etc.

Some of the styptics are mentioned in Table 2.

TABLE 2	Local hemostatics (Styptics)
Styptics	**Features**
Thrombin	• It is obtained from bovine plasma. • Can be applied as a dry powder topically to control bleeding in hemophiliacs.
Fibrin	• It is obtained from human plasma and can be used to control bleeding during surgical procedure.
Gelatin foam	• It is available as an absorbable material (sponge or foam). • It controls bleeding by providing a meshwork which activates clotting.
Adrenaline	• It is a vasoconstrictor (α_1 action). • It is applied at the bleeding site by soaking a sterile cotton pack in adrenaline. • It is avoided in hypertension, ischemic heart disease, arrhythmia etc.
Astringents	• Astringents precipitate proteins at the local site and control bleeding. • Examples include tannic acid, metallic salts etc.
Hemocoagulase	• It is obtained from the venom of *Bothrops atrox* (viper). • It is a powerful hemostatic and converts fibrinogen to fibrin.

ANTICOAGULANTS

Anticoagulants are drugs that are used to prevent or decrease the coagulability of blood. A classification of anticoagulants is mentioned in Figure 2.

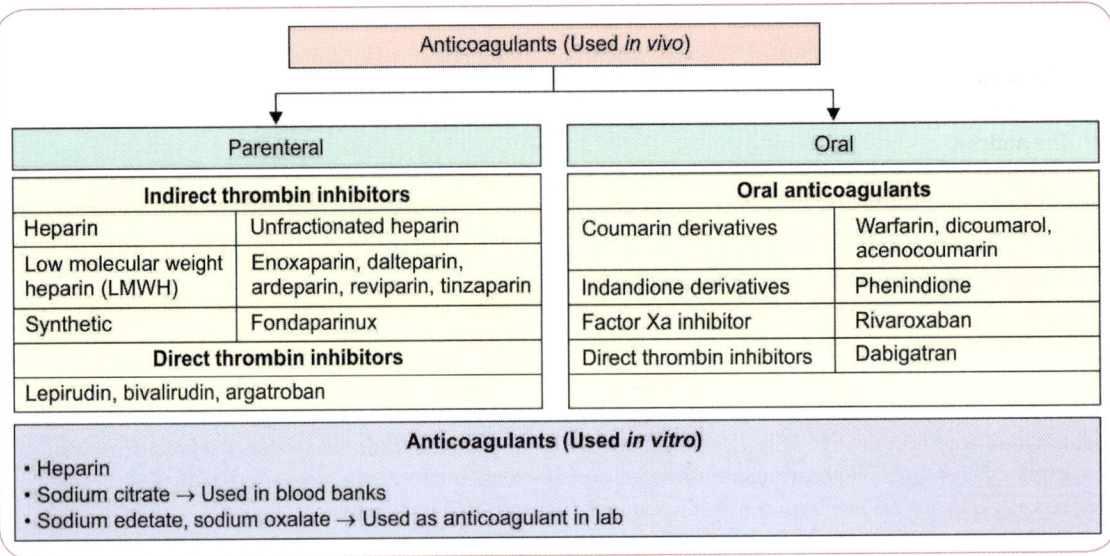

Figure 2: Classification of anticoagulants

PARENTERAL ANTICOAGULANTS (INDIRECT THROMBIN INHIBITORS)

HEPARIN

Heparin was discovered by McLean who was a medical student. It was later named as 'heparin' by Howell and Holt because it was obtained from liver.

Heparin is a naturally occurring mixture of sulfated mucopolysaccharides with a high molecular weight (MW) between 10000 and 20000.

Heparin is a strong electronegative substance and is the strongest organic acid in the body. It naturally occurs in the mast cells particularly in lung, liver etc.

Heparin is commercially obtained from pig intestinal mucosa or ox lung.

Mechanism of Action

Heparin (also referred as unfractionated heparin, UFH) is an injectable and a very rapidly acting anticoagulant.

It acts indirectly by binding to and increasing the activity of antithrombin III. The heparin-antithrombin III complex then rapidly inactivates the clotting factors Xa, IIa, IXa, XIa, XIIa, and XIIIa.

The anticoagulant effect of heparin is mainly caused due to inactivation of factors Xa and IIa. In contrast, low molecular weight heparins predominantly inactivate factor Xa, while fondaparinux only inactivates factor Xa.

Other Actions

Heparin causes release of lipoprotein lipase from the vessel wall leading to triglyceride hydrolysis of VLDL and chylomicrons. At higher doses, heparin inhibits platelet aggregation and prolongs bleeding time.

Pharmacokinetics

Heparin is not absorbed orally because of its high ionization (negative charge) and large molecular size. Hence, it must be given parenterally (intravenously [IV] or subcutaneously [SC]).

The anticoagulant effect occurs immediately after IV injection, but 1–2 hours after SC injection. It does not cross blood-brain barrier or placental barrier and is the preferred anticoagulant during pregnancy.

It is metabolized in the liver by heparinase and the metabolites are excreted by the kidney.

Mode of Administration

Heparin is given by intravenous infusion, or by subcutaneous injection. The intramuscular route is not used as it may lead to hematoma.

The anticoagulation therapy is routinely monitored by measuring the activated partial thromboplastin time (aPTT). The aim is to maintain the aPTT at 1.5 to 2.5 times of the normal control.

Adverse Effects

Some of the key adverse effects are mentioned in Figure 3.

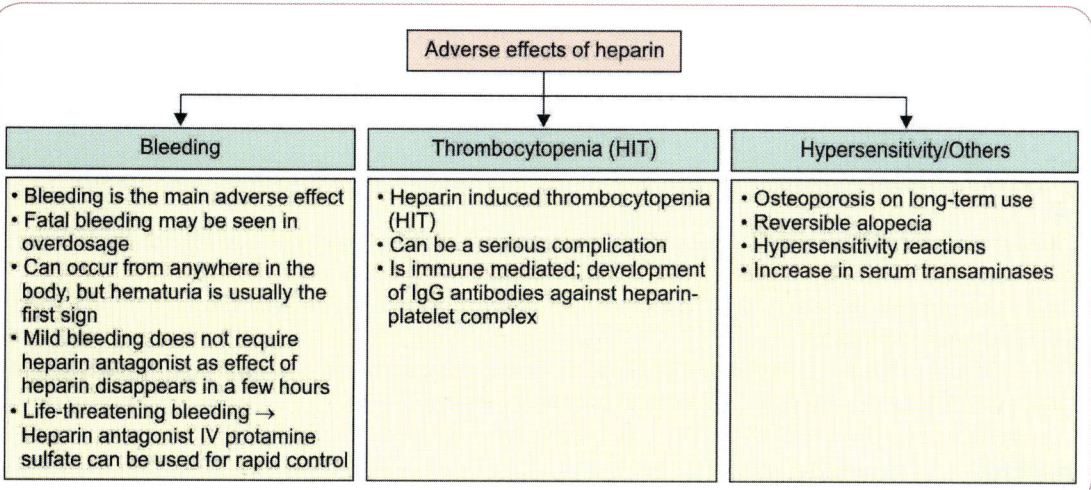

Figure 3: Adverse effects of heparin

Heparin-induced Thrombocytopenia (HIT)

The following are noteworthy points regarding HIT:
○ Serious complication of heparin therapy
○ It can lead to thromboembolic complications (venous thromboembolism is more common, but arterial thrombosis can also occur)
○ It is caused by development of IgG antibodies that bind to heparin-platelet factor 4 complexes and promoting a prothrombotic state
○ It is more frequent with unfractionated heparin (UFH) than with low molecular weight heparin (LMWH)
○ Withdrawal of all heparin compounds (i.e. both UFH and LMWH) is required. Warfarin should be avoided as it may aggravate venous limb gangrene or skin necrosis. A direct thrombin inhibitor can be administered.

Contraindications

The contraindications of heparin therapy includes the following:

Bleeding disorders, hemophiliacs, HIT, severe hypertension, gastrointestinal ulcers, alcoholics, cirrhosis, kidney failure, tuberculosis, bacterial endocarditis, malignancies etc.

LOW MOLECULAR WEIGHT HEPARINS (LMWH)

Heparins have been fractionated to low molecular weight forms (MW 3000–7000) by several techniques.

Examples of LMWH include enoxaparin, dalteparin, tinzaparin, reviparin etc. The LMWHs are given by subcutaneous injection.

The anticoagulation mechanism of LMWH is different from UFH, in that LMWH mainly inactivate factor Xa with lesser effect on factor IIa.

Patients on LMWHs usually do not require aPTT monitoring. However, patients with renal insufficiency and pregnant or obese patients may require monitoring by measurement of factor Xa activity.

The advantages of LMWH over UFH are mentioned in Figure 4.

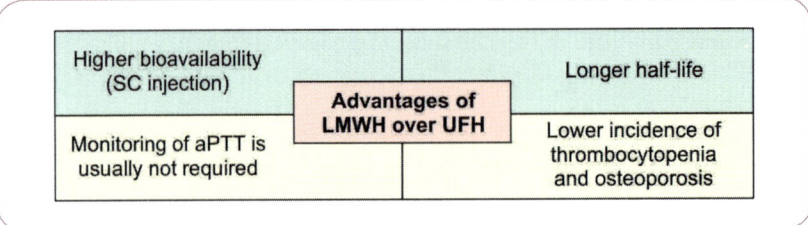

Figure 4: Advantages of LMWH over UFH

The clinical uses and adverse effects of LMWH are the same as that of other anticoagulants.

FONDAPARINUX

It is a synthetic anticoagulant. It selectively binds to antithrombin III and inactivates only factor Xa. It does not require routine monitoring by laboratory tests. It is administered by subcutaneous route.

It is excreted in the urine and has a half-life of approximately 17 hours. Fondaparinux is contraindicated in patients with kidney failure.

The incidence of HIT is less as compared to heparin. There is no specific antidote for fondaparinux.

It is used for deep vein thrombosis (DVT) and pulmonary embolism (PE).

The key differences between UFH, LMWH and fondaparinux are mentioned in Table 3.

TABLE 3	Differences between UFH, LMWH and Fondaparinux		
Parameters	Heparin	LMWH	Fondaparinux
Origin	Biological	Biological	Synthetic
Coagulation factor(s) targeted	Xa & IIa	Xa (main effect) & IIa (lesser effect)	Xa
Bioavailability (%)	30	90	100
Plasma half-life (hours)	1	4	17
Renal excretion	No	Yes	Yes
Effect of antidote	Complete	Partial	No effect
Thrombocytopenia (antiplatelet action)	<5%	<1%	<1%

HEPARIN ANTAGONIST—PROTAMINE SULFATE

It is a strongly basic low molecular weight compound obtained from salmon sperm. It is given intravenously at a slow rate.

It tightly binds to heparin and rapidly neutralizes its effects. The dose guidance is that 1 mg of protamine is required for every 100 units of heparin remaining in the patient.

It is not routinely required because the half-life of heparin being very short, heparin discontinuation itself may solve the problem in many cases. However, it is required in certain situations where termination of heparin's action is urgently required such as after cardiac or vascular surgery.

Excess protamine administration should be avoided because after neutralizing heparin, the excess protamine has anticoagulant effect of its own. It is a basic drug and can cause release of histamine. Protamine can lead to hypersensitivity reactions.

Minimal amount required for heparin neutralization should be given to the patient.

It completely neutralizes heparin, partly neutralizes LMWH and does not neutralize fondaparinux.

PARENTERAL ANTICOAGULANTS (DIRECT THROMBIN INHIBITORS)

LEPIRUDIN AND BIVALIRUDIN

Lepirudin is a recombinant hirudin (hirudin is a direct thrombin inhibitor present in the salivary glands of leech). It directly inhibits thrombin. It is administered intravenously, has a short half-life (around 1.3 hours) and is excreted by the kidneys. It is used as an anticoagulant for the treatment of thrombotic events in patients with heparin induced thrombocytopenia (HIT). Monitoring of aPTT is required during therapy. No specific antidote is available.

Bivalirudin is a synthetic peptide that directly inhibits thrombin by a similar mechanism as lepirudin. It is administered intravenously and has a short half-life of around 25 minutes in patients with normal kidney function. It is used during coronary angioplasty or cardiopulmonary bypass surgery as an alternative to heparin.

ARGATROBAN

It is a synthetic compound that directly inhibits thrombin. It is administered intravenously, has a short half-life (around 40–50 minutes), is metabolized in the liver and excreted in the bile. It is used (as an alternative to lepirudin) for the prophylaxis and treatment in patients with HIT. It is also used in patients at risk of developing HIT. Monitoring of aPTT is required during therapy. Dose reduction is required in patients with liver dysfunction.

ORAL ANTICOAGULANTS

COUMARIN DERIVATIVES—WARFARIN (VITAMIN K ANTAGONISTS)

Coumarin derivatives (warfarin and its congeners) are commonly used as oral anticoagulants. They are antagonists of vitamin K.

They act only *in vivo* (i.e. inside the body) and not *in vitro*. This is because they inhibit the synthesis of vitamin K dependent clotting factors in the liver.

A comparison of the pharmacological properties of heparin (parenteral anticoagulant) and warfarin (oral anticoagulant) is mentioned in Table 4.

TABLE 4	Comparison of heparin and warfarin	
Features	**Heparin**	**Warfarin**
Source	Natural	Synthetic
Activity	*In vivo* and *in vitro*	*In vivo* only
Route	Parenteral (IV/SC)	Oral
Onset of action	Immediate	Delayed
Duration of action	Short (3–6 hours)	Long (3–6 days)
Mechanism	Inactivates clotting factors Xa, IIa, IXa, XIa, XIIa, and XIIIa	Inhibits synthesis of clotting factors II, VII, IX and X
Monitoring	By aPTT	By INR
Safer in pregnancy	Yes	No
Drug interaction	Lesser and not clinically significant	More and clinically significant
Clinical use	Initiation therapy for anticoagulation	Maintenance therapy for anticoagulation
Antagonist	Protamine sulfate	Vitamin K

Mechanism of Action

Clotting factors II, VII, IX and X are synthesized in the liver in the inactive (descarboxy) form. Vitamin K (as a cofactor) is required for the activation of these inactive clotting factors by the following mechanism:

The inactive descarboxy form of clotting factors II, VII, IX and X become activated when they are carboxylated by the enzyme γ-glutamyl transferase. In the same carboxylation reaction, vitamin K hydroquinone (reduced vitamin K) is converted to vitamin K epoxide (oxidized vitamin K).

Reduced vitamin K needs to be continuously regenerated from oxidized vitamin K for the carboxylation reaction to occur and continued generation of activated clotting factors.

The generation of reduced vitamin K from oxidized vitamin K is catalyzed by the enzyme vitamin K epoxide reductase.

Warfarin has a similar structure to that of vitamin K. Hence, warfarin competitively inhibits the enzyme vitamin K epoxide reductase. This leads to inhibition of reduced vitamin K (vitamin K hydroquinone) regeneration. This finally results in prevention of the activation step (decarboxylation) of clotting factors II, VII, IX and X (Figure 5).

The activated clotting factors cannot be generated leading to anticoagulant action.

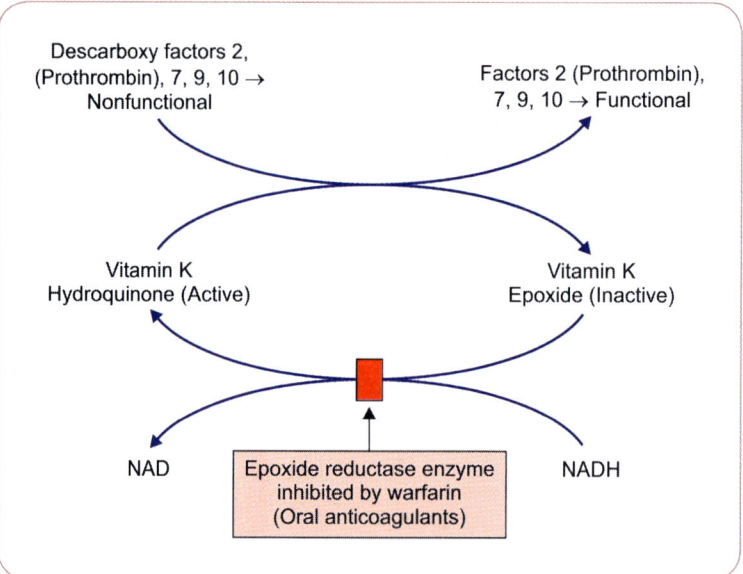

Figure 5: Mechanism of action of oral anticoagulants

The approximate half-lives of individual clotting factors are as follows: VII (6 hours), IX (24 hours), X (36 hours) and II (50 hours). Although the synthesis of clotting factors decreases within 2–4 hours, the anticoagulant effect appears only after 1–3 days. This is because the clotting factors already present in the plasma decline gradually. Therefore, there is a delay between initiation of warfarin therapy and anticoagulant effect.

Hence, warfarin is active *in vivo* and not *in vitro* because it inhibits the epoxide reductase enzyme and interferes with the synthesis of vitamin K dependent coagulation factors in the liver.

Pharmacokinetics

Warfarin is nearly completely absorbed after oral administration and is 99% bound to plasma proteins. It can also be administered intravenously. The intramuscular injection is not recommended due to the risk of hematoma formation.

It crosses the placental barrier. It is metabolized in the liver mainly by CYP2C9 and the inactive metabolites are excreted in urine and stool. The plasma half-life is long and varies between 25 and 60 hours (mean of around 40 hours) and the duration of action is 2–5 days.

Adverse Effects

The adverse effects of warfarin include the following:

Bleeding

Bleeding is a very significant and common adverse effect of warfarin therapy.

Bleeding can occur at any site in the body, e.g. gastrointestinal, urinary tract, pulmonary, intracranial, hepatic, cutaneous etc.

The following measures are taken for the treatment of bleeding:
- Warfarin withdrawal
- Vitamin K_1 (as an antidote)

  The effect of vitamin K_1 is delayed for at least 6–24 hours because it takes such time for the new clotting factors to be synthesized in the liver, and released in circulation. Oral and intravenous vitamin K_1 are given for mild and severe bleeding respectively.
- Fresh blood transfusion/fresh frozen plasma

  These are administered in severe bleeding when a rapid reversal of warfarin effect is required. They supply active clotting factors immediately and replenish the lost blood.

It is therefore crucial to regularly monitor INR and adjust the dose of warfarin. The INR is measured by the following:

$$INR = \left(\frac{PT_{pt}}{PT_{ref}} \right)^{ISI}$$

Abbreviations: INR, International normalized ratio; PT_{pt}, Prothrombin time of patient; PT_{ref}, Prothrombin time of reference; ISI, International sensitivity index.

Skin Necrosis

Warfarin-induced skin necrosis is a rare complication where the skin lesions usually occur 3-10 days after therapy initiation. The lesions generally occur on the extremities. There is extensive thrombosis of the microvessels, which sometimes become necrotic and may require debridement and amputation.

Teratogenicity

Warfarin is teratogenic and should not be given during pregnancy. It may cause fetal hemorrhage, birth defects and intrauterine death.
- If given during the 1st trimester, it may cause fetal warfarin syndrome—hypoplasia of nose, eye sockets and stippled epiphyseal calcification
- If given during the 2nd or 3rd trimester, it may cause CNS abnormalities

Warfarin and its congeners are contraindicated during pregnancy. Heparin and LMWH are the preferred drugs during pregnancy.

Other Adverse Effects

Other adverse effects include alopecia, diarrhea, dermatitis, urticaria, anorexia, and abdominal cramps.

Warfarin can precipitate venous limb gangrene and skin lesions if given to patients with HIT. Hence, warfarin is not to be given in HIT until thrombocytopenia has resolved.

Contraindications

The contraindications of warfarin are similar to those mentioned earlier for heparin. Additionally, warfarin and its congeners are contraindicated in pregnancy.

Drug Interactions

Many drugs interact with warfarin at the pharmacokinetic or pharmacodynamic level. They either increase warfarin effect resulting in bleeding or decrease warfarin effect leading to therapeutic failure.

Some of the key drug interactions are mentioned in Figure 6.

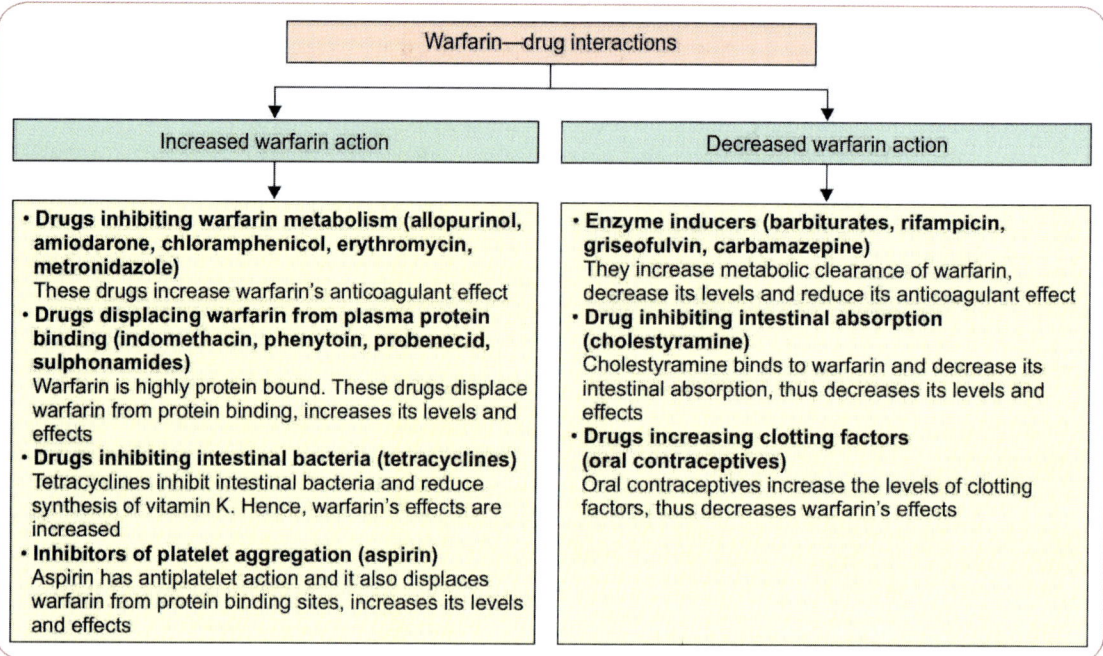

Figure 6: Drug interactions of warfarin

Clinical Uses of Anticoagulants (Parenteral and Oral)

The primary aim of anticoagulant therapy is to:
- Prevent formation of an intravascular thrombus
- Prevent extension of an already formed thrombus
- Prevent embolic complications

The anticoagulants do not dissolve an already formed thrombus.

The anticoagulant therapy with heparin (LMWH or UFH) and warfarin are started together. Heparin is discontinued after 4–7 days while warfarin is continued as a maintenance therapy.

Heparin is given for the initial 4–7 days to provide cover for warfarin to achieve its full therapeutic effect (*Note*: Warfarin has a delayed onset of action as it inhibits synthesis of new clotting factors in the liver, but has no effect on the circulating clotting factors).

Deep Vein Thrombosis (DVT) and Pulmonary Embolism (PE)

Venous thrombi are primarily fibrin thrombi; hence, anticoagulants are very effective in the treatment and prophylaxis of DVT and PE.

The anticoagulants are used in the treatment and prophylaxis of DVT and PE in high-risk situations such as:
- Patients undergoing major surgery/postoperative patients
- Bedridden, elderly, leg fracture, poststroke, postpartum etc.

Myocardial Infarction (MI)

Arterial thrombi are primarily platelet thrombi and therefore, anticoagulants are of limited value. However, they may be used in providing benefit by preventing thrombi generation at infarction site and venous thrombi in deep veins.

Heparin followed by warfarin is used after coronary artery recanalization by fibrinolytic therapy. Heparin is also used during coronary angioplasty.

Unstable Angina

Heparin used on a short-term basis reduces the occurrence of MI in patients with unstable angina.

Atrial Fibrillation (AF)

Heparin and warfarin are used in stroke prevention in patients with AF. Anticoagulants are given for 3–4 weeks prior to and after attempting cardioversion of AF to sinus rhythm.

Other Uses

These include disseminated intravascular coagulation (in some situations), vascular surgery and prosthetic heart valves.

DIRECT THROMBIN INHIBITORS—DABIGATRAN AND RIVAROXABAN

Dabigatran is a novel direct thrombin inhibitor. Rivaroxaban is a novel factor Xa inhibitor.

Routine lab monitoring is not required for both the drugs. Both are used for the prevention of venous thromboembolism after hip replacement surgery.

FIBRINOLYTIC DRUGS AND ANTIFIBRINOLYTIC DRUGS

FIBRINOLYTIC DRUGS

These drugs are used to lyse (dissolve) the thrombi in the occluded blood vessels.

The clinically relevant fibrinolytic drugs are streptokinase, urokinase, alteplase, reteplase and tenecteplase.

These drugs activate the conversion of plasminogen to plasmin. Plasmin hydrolyzes fibrin to form fibrin degradation products and therefore dissolve clots (Figure 7).

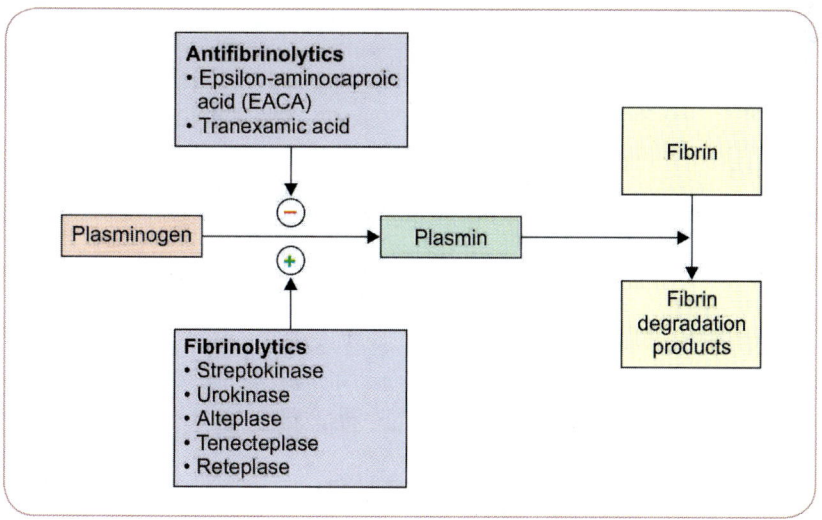

Figure 7: Fibrinolytics and antifibrinolytics

Generally, clot dissolution or fibrinolysis occurs with greater efficacy if therapy is initiated early after clot formation. The key pharmacological properties of streptokinase, urokinase and alteplase are mentioned in Figure 8.

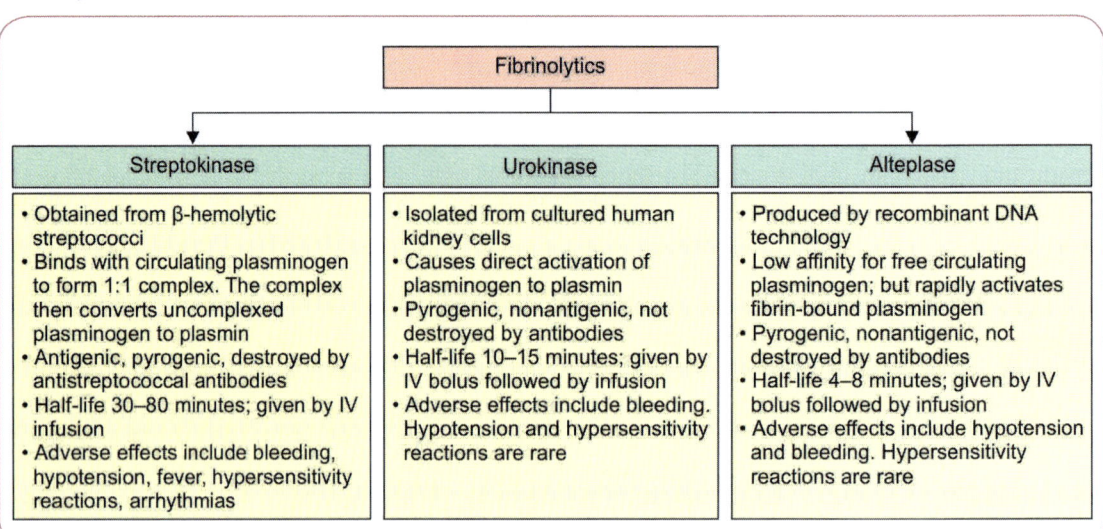

Figure 8: Fibrinolytics—pharmacological properties

Reteplase and tenecteplase are longer acting drugs as compared to alteplase. Both are produced by recombinant DNA technology.

Clinical Uses

Acute Myocardial Infarction

Acute myocardial infarction (MI) is the main indication of fibrinolytics. They act by dissolving the clot and restoring the patency of coronary artery. The time lag in starting the therapy is crucial in acute MI. This is because the clot becomes resistant to lysis as time passes by.

The earlier the treatment is administered, the greater is the benefit. Alteplase, reteplase and streptokinase should be given as early as possible (ideally within the 1st hour—the golden hour).

Deep Vein Thrombosis

Fibrinolytics benefit by preventing the occurrence of pulmonary embolism, reducing pain and swelling, improving perfusion of the limbs.

Pulmonary Embolism

Fibrinolytics are indicated in massive life-threatening pulmonary embolism for clot lysis.

Some of the contraindications to fibrinolytic therapy include active bleeding or bleeding diathesis, recent trauma, surgeries, uncontrolled or severe hypertension, recent ischemic stroke, history of intracranial hemorrhage etc.

ANTIFIBRINOLYTIC DRUGS

These drugs are used to block the conversion of plasminogen to plasmin. Therefore, they block the fibrinolytic activity.

Epsilon Aminocaproic Acid (EACA)

It is a lysine analog. It competes for the lysine binding sites of plasminogen and plasmin, thereby blocking the interaction of plasmin with fibrin.

It is a potent inhibitor of fibrinolysis and it reverses the conditions associated with excessive fibrinolysis. The main complication is that the thrombi that form during its treatment are then not lysed.

It is given orally or intravenously. It is used mainly to control bleeding in overdose of fibrinolytics, surgery (prostatectomy, tooth extraction in hemophiliacs), postpartum hemorrhage, abruptio placentae etc. It rarely causes muscle necrosis and myopathy.

Tranexamic Acid

The mechanism of action and indications are the same as that of EACA. It is however 7 times more potent than EACA. It is given orally or intravenously and the adverse effects include nausea, headache and diarrhea.

ANTIPLATELET DRUGS

Antiplatelet drugs inhibit the aggregation of platelets.

CLASSIFICATION OF ANTIPLATELET DRUGS

The antiplatelet drugs can be classified based on the mechanism of action (Table 5).

TABLE 5	Antiplatelet drugs
Thromboxane A$_2$ synthesis inhibitor	Low dose aspirin
Phosphodiesterase inhibitor	Dipyridamole
GPIIb/IIIa receptor antagonist	Abciximab, tirofiban, eptifibatide
Purinergic receptor antagonists	Ticlopidine, clopidogrel, prasugrel, ticagrelor, cangrelor

Platelets have a very important role in the hemostatic mechanism. The damage of vascular endothelium leads to the activation of platelets, that causes release of mediators resulting in platelet aggregation.

THROMBOXANE A$_2$ SYNTHESIS INHIBITOR

Low Dose Aspirin

Low dose aspirin irreversibly inactivates (acetylates) the cyclooxygenase 1 (COX-1) enzyme and therefore reduces the production of thromboxane A$_2$ by the platelets. Low dose aspirin has a clinically useful antiplatelet action due to the following factors:

○ Irreversible inactivation of the COX enzyme in the platelets
○ Lack of nucleus in the platelets → platelets cannot synthetize new COX enzymes
○ Antiplatelet action of aspirin lasts for the life time of platelets (~7–10 days)

Aspirin in higher doses reduces the synthesis of both thromboxane A$_2$ and prostacyclin (prostaglandin I$_2$) leading to potentially reduced antiplatelet efficacy.

The antiplatelet efficacy of aspirin is observed at doses ranging from 50 mg to 320 mg daily.

Adverse effects include increased bleeding tendencies, hemorrhage, gastric irritation and hypersensitivity reactions.

▌ PHOSPHODIESTERASE INHIBITOR

Dipyridamole

Dipyridamole is a phosphodiesterase inhibitor that leads to an increase in cAMP level in the platelets resulting in reduced platelet aggregation. Dipyridamole also has a vasodilatory effect.

It is used in combination with warfarin to reduce the incidence of thromboembolism in patients with prosthetic cardiac valves.

▌ PURINERGIC RECEPTOR ANTAGONISTS

Ticlopidine, Clopidogrel, Prasugrel, Cangrelor, Ticagrelor

These drugs block the purinergic ($P2Y_{12}$) receptors on the platelets. This leads to an inhibition of ADP-mediated platelet aggregation.

Ticlopidine, clopidogrel and prasugrel cause an irreversible blockade of the platelet receptor ($P2Y_{12}$). Cangrelor and ticagrelor cause a reversible blockade of the platelet receptor ($P2Y_{12}$).

The onset of action of prasugrel is faster compared to ticlopidine and clopidogrel.

Adverse effects of ticlopidine include nausea, diarrhea, bleeding, severe neutropenia and thrombocytopenia. Clopidogrel is better tolerated than ticlopidine and may have a lower incidence of neutropenia and thrombocytopenia.

▌ GPIIb/IIIa RECEPTOR ANTAGONIST

Abciximab, Eptifibatide, Tirofiban

These drugs block GPIIb/IIIa receptors located on the surface of platelets. These receptors are mainly for fibrinogen, fibronectin and von Willebrand's factor and serve as the final common pathway for platelet aggregation.

Abciximab is a fragment of a chimeric monoclonal antibody. It is indicated in adults as an adjunct to heparin and acetylsalicylic acid for:
- Percutaneous coronary intervention
- Unstable angina

Eptifibatide is obtained from the venom of rattle snake.

▌ CLINICAL USES OF ANTIPLATELET DRUGS

The antiplatelet drugs increase the risk of bleeding including intracranial hemorrhage.

The clinical uses of antiplatelet drugs include the following:
1. Acute coronary syndrome including:
   - Acute myocardial infarction—ST elevation myocardial infarction (STEMI) and non-ST elevation myocardial infarction (NSTEMI)
   - Unstable angina
2. Coronary artery disease
3. Transient ischemic attack
4. Prosthetic cardiac valves, coronary angioplasty, placement of stents
5. Peripheral vascular disease

Combination therapy with multiple antiplatelet drugs may be considered in appropriate situations.

ASSESS YOURSELF (Examination Questions of Various Universities)

1. Enumerate anticoagulant drugs. Write the mechanism of action, uses and adverse effects of heparin.
2. Low molecular weight heparins
3. What are fibrinolytic agents? Give examples, mechanisms and their uses
4. Rationale for use of aspirin in low doses as an antiplatelet agent
5. Therapeutic use and adverse effects of warfarin
6. Why warfarin is not effective in vitro as anticoagulant
7. Therapeutic status of fondaparinux in deep vein thrombosis
8. Differences between heparin and warfarin

MULTIPLE CHOICE QUESTIONS

1. All of the following are GpIIb/IIIa receptor inhibitor except: *(AIIMS May 2016)*
   a. Abciximab
   b. Prasugrel
   c. Eptifibatide
   d. Tirofiban
2. Antidote for overdose of fibrinolytic therapy: *(AIIMS Nov 2015)*
   a. Heparin
   b. Epsilon aminocaproic acid
   c. Protamine
   d. Warfarin
3. Which of the following does not act on ADP? *(Recent Question Dec 2016)*
   a. Prasugrel
   b. Ticlopidine
   c. Clopidogrel
   d. Aspirin
4. Teratogenic effect of Warfarin is: *(Recent Question Dec 2016)*
   a. Absent nasal bone
   b. Midfacial hypoplasia
   c. Neural tube defects
   d. Cardiac anomalies
5. Anticoagulant with both *in vitro* and *in vivo* activity is: *(Recent Question Dec 2016)*
   a. Heparin
   b. Warfarin
   c. Apixaban
   d. Dabigatran
6. Which is not an antiplatelet drug: *(Recent Question Dec 2016)*
   a. Aspirin
   b. Streptokinase
   c. Clopidogrel
   d. Ticlopidine
7. Fibrinolytic that is antigenic: *(Recent Question 2016)*
   a. Streptokinase
   b. Urokinase
   c. Alteplase
   d. Tenecteplase
8. Agent used for treatment of heparin induced thrombocytopenia: *(Recent Question 2016)*
   a. Lepirudin
   b. Abciximab
   c. Warfarin
   d. Alteplase
9. Drug not acting on P2y12 receptor is: *(Recent Question 2016)*
   a. Ticlopidine
   b. Clopidrogrel
   c. Dipyridamole
   d. Prasugrel
10. Streptokinase causes increase in: *(Recent Question 2016)*
    a. Plasmin
    b. Thrombin
    c. Kallikrein
    d. Angiotensin II
11. Not Vitamin K dependent clotting factor is: *(Recent Question 2016)*
    a. II
    b. VII
    c. VIII
    d. IX
12. True about HIT syndrome are all except: *(Recent Question 2016)*
    a. LMW heparin should not be used for treatment
    b. It causes both arterial and venous thrombosis
    c. More common with fractionated heparin
    d. Occurs commonly in about a week of heparin therapy
13. Vitamin K dependent clotting factors are: *(Recent Question 2016)*
    a. Factor IX and X
    b. Factor IV
    c. Factor XII
    d. Factor I
14. Drug used in heparin overdose is: *(Recent Question 2016)*
    a. Protamine sulfate
    b. Phylloquinone
    c. Ticlopidine
    d. Clopidogrel

Ans.

1. (b)	2. (b)	3. (d)	4. (b)	5. (a)	6. (b)
7. (a)	8. (a)	9. (c)	10. (a)	11. (c)	12. (c)
13. (a)	14. (a)				

15. Vitamin K is a cofactor in:

(Recent Question 2016)
- a. Carboxylation
- b. Hydroxylation
- c. Deamination
- d. Hydrolysis

16. A patient of thrombosis of veins has been receiving coumarin therapy for three years. Recently she developed bleeding tendency. How will you reverse the effect of coumarin therapy?

(Recent Question 2016)
- a. Protamine injection
- b. Vitamin K injection
- c. Infusion of fibrinogen
- d. Whole blood transfusion

17. Urgent reversal of warfarin induced bleeding can be done by the administration of:

(Recent Question 2016)
- a. Cryoprecipitate
- b. Platelet concentrates
- c. Fresh frozen plasma
- d. Packed red blood cells

18. Heparin acts via activation of:

(Recent Question 2016)
- a. Antithrombin III
- b. Factor VIII
- c. Factor II and X
- d. Factor V

19. Abciximab is: *(Recent Question 2016)*
- a. Antibody against IIb/IIIa receptors
- b. Antibody against Ib/IX receptors
- c. Topoisomerase inhibitor
- d. Adenosine inhibitor

20. All are seen with heparin therapy except:

(Recent Question 2016)
- a. Skin necrosis
- b. Thrombosis and thrombocytopenia
- c. Osteoporosis
- d. Alopecia

21. A useful thrombolytic agent that leads to plasmin activation is: *(Recent Question 2016)*
- a. Vitamin K
- b. Heparin
- c. Streptokinase
- d. Aspirin

22. Heparin injection releases which of the following: *(JIPMER 2014)*
- a. Lipoprotein lipase
- b. Nitric oxide
- c. cGMP
- d. Hormone sensitive lipase

23. Heparin treatment is monitored by:

(JIPMER 2008)
- a. aPTT
- b. PT
- c. CT
- d. BT

24. INR monitoring is done for: *(WBPG 2014)*
- a. Heparin
- b. Warfarin
- c. Lepirudin
- d. Enoxaparin

25. Protamine sulfate is not effective against:

(WBPG 2012)
- a. Fondaparinux
- b. Enoxaparin
- c. Dalteparin
- d. Low molecular heparin

26. Heparin acts via which of the following adjuvants? *(AIIMS May 2018)*
- a. Antithrombin III
- b. Protein C
- c. Protein S
- d. Thrombomodulin

Ans.

15. (a)	**16.** (b)	**17.** (c)	**18.** (a)	**19.** (a)	**20.** (a)
21. (c)	**22.** (a)	**23.** (a)	**24.** (b)	**25.** (a)	**26.** (a)

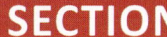

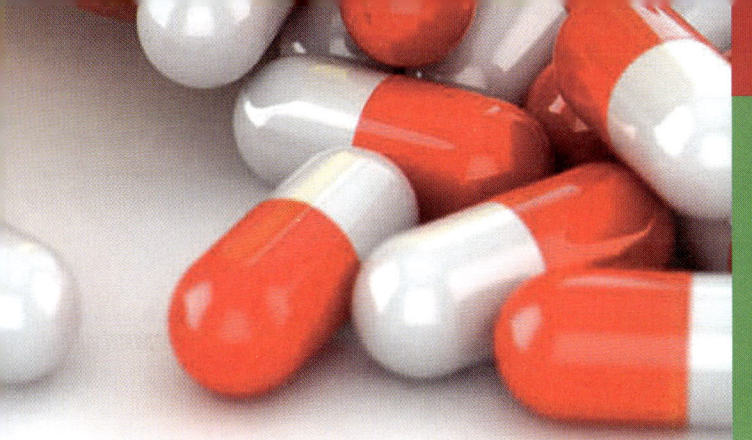

Drugs Acting on the Gastrointestinal System

46

Drugs Used for Acid Peptic Disease

Acid peptic disease occurs in the gastrointestinal tract. Usually, a balance is maintained between the aggressive factors (such as gastric acid secretion) and the mucosal defenses of the gastroduodenal system. Erosion and subsequently peptic ulcer develops due to disruption of this balance (Table 1).

TABLE 1	Aggressive and protective factors for peptic ulcer
Aggressive factors	**Protective (defensive) factors**
• Gastric acid, pepsin, bile, *H. pylori*, NSAIDs	• Gastric mucus, bicarbonate, mucosal blood flow, prostaglandins

Some of the predisposing factors for the development of peptic ulcer include *H. pylori* infection, NSAIDs, lifestyle factors (stress, smoking), burns (Curling's ulcer), systemic illness, sepsis and genetic factors.

CLASSIFICATION OF DRUGS

The classification of drugs used for the management of peptic ulcers is mentioned in Table 2.

TABLE 2	Drugs used for management of peptic ulcers
Drugs causing reduction of gastric acid secretion • Proton pump inhibitors → Omeprazole, pantoprazole, lansoprazole, rabeprazole • H_2 receptor antagonists (H_2 blockers) → Cimetidine, ranitidine, roxatidine, famotidine • Prostaglandin analogue → Misoprostol • Anticholinergics → Piperazine, telenzepine	
Drugs causing neutralization of gastric acids (antacids) • Systemic antacids → Sodium bicarbonate, sodium citrate • Nonsystemic antacids → Magnesium hydroxide, magnesium trisilicate, aluminum hydroxide gel, calcium carbonate	
Ulcer protectives • Sucralfate • Colloidal bismuth subcitrate (CBS)	
Anti *H. pylori* drugs • Amoxicillin, metronidazole, clarithromycin, tetracycline—part of triple therapy or quadruple therapy regimens	

PROTON PUMP INHIBITORS

Omeprazole

It is a proton pump inhibitor (PPI) and can be considered as a prototype drug.

Mechanism of Action

Omeprazole causes an irreversible inactivation of the gastric proton pump (H^+/K^+-ATPase enzyme) which is the final step in the secretion of gastric acid. This leads to inhibition of acid secretion from the gastric parietal cells.

Omeprazole diffuses from the blood into the gastric parietal cell. It gets concentrated in the cell canaliculi. In the acidic pH (pH < 5), it gets converted into a sulfenic acid and a sulfenamide configuration. The sulfenamide form binds covalently with the H^+/K^+-ATPase enzyme and inhibits it irreversibly.

As they inhibit the final step in gastric acid secretion, PPIs are effective in inhibiting acid secretion at rest or following various types of stimulation such as food.

Pharmacokinetics

- Omeprazole has a high plasma protein binding. It is metabolized in the liver and excreted in the urine.
- Omeprazole should be taken orally, empty stomach, approximately 30 minutes prior to a meal because:
  - Secretion of acid is stimulated by food. Secretion of acid is required for the activation of omeprazole (PPIs).
  - Bioavailability of omeprazole is decreased by food.
- Omeprazole has a short half-life, but has a prolonged duration of action due to irreversible inhibition of the H^+/K^+-ATPase. Hence, suppression of gastric acid is observed up to 24 hours.
- Omeprazole suppresses 80–90% of the 24-hour acid secretion. Gastric acid secretion gradually starts over 3–5 days following drug cessation.

Adverse Effects..

The adverse effects of omeprazole include the following:
- Nausea, headache, diarrhea, constipation, abdominal pain
- Following can occur during long-term therapy:
  - Atrophic gastritis
  - Osteoporosis, bone fractures
  - Reduced absorption of vitamin B_{12}
  - Increased risk of specific infections (e.g. *Clostridium difficile*, hospital acquired pneumonia)
  - Compensatory hypergastrinemia, increased risk of gastric tumors
  - Erectile dysfunction, gynecomastia

Drug Interactions

Some of the interactions of omeprazole are mentioned below:
- Metabolism of drugs such as diazepam, phenytoin and warfarin is inhibited by omeprazole. Hence, their plasma levels may be increased.
- Metabolism of omeprazole is inhibited by clarithromycin; hence, plasma levels of omeprazole may be increased.

Clinical Uses

Some of the clinical uses of PPIs are mentioned in Table 3.

TABLE 3	Clinical uses of proton pump inhibitors
Peptic ulcer • PPIs are the preferred drugs for peptic ulcer, due to rapid onset of action and faster ulcer healing • Can lead to healing of duodenal ulcers (2–4 weeks) and gastric ulcer (4–8 weeks) • Preferred drugs for NSAID-induced gastric and duodenal ulcers	
Stress ulcer	
Bleeding peptic ulcer • Clot formation and healing is enhanced due to suppression of gastric acid secretion; intravenous therapy with PPIs (pantoprazole, rabeprazole) is preferred	
Zollinger-Ellison syndrome • Due to gastrin secreting tumor leading to hypersecretion of gastric acid • Surgical management may be required	
Gastroesophageal reflux disease (GERD)	
Aspiration pneumonia prophylaxis • Used for preoperative prophylaxis of aspiration pneumonitis in patients who are administered anesthesia	

Lansoprazole

○ More potent than omeprazole

Pantoprazole

○ Can be administered intravenously
○ More acid stable

■ H$_2$ RECEPTOR ANTAGONISTS (H$_2$ BLOCKERS)

These drugs are competitive antagonists of H$_2$ receptors located on the parietal cells. They suppress all phases of gastric acid secretion. They suppress acid secretion by stimuli such as histamine, food, acetylcholine, gastrin and alcohol.

H$_2$ receptor antagonists suppress 60–70% of the 24-hour acid secretion—have a lower potency than PPIs.

H$_2$ receptor antagonists also have an antiulcerogenic effect. Cimetidine was the first clinically used H$_2$ receptor antagonist and is considered as the prototype drug. However, cimetidine is now not commonly used due to its adverse effect profile.

Cimetidine

Pharmacokinetics

Cimetidine is well absorbed orally and undergoes first-pass hepatic metabolism. Presence of food in the stomach does not interfere with absorption of cimetidine.

Adverse Effects

The adverse effects of cimetidine include the following:
○ Headache, dizziness, dry mouth
○ CNS → Confusion, convulsions, coma can occur in elderly patients or in those with renal disease
○ Bolus intravenous (IV) administration can cause cardiac arrhythmias, including arrest—hence, administration should be via slow infusion
○ Cimetidine (but not other H$_2$ blockers) has antiandrogenic effect by displacing dihydrotestosterone from its receptor. It can lead to increased prolactin levels, gynecomastia, impotence, loss of libido and decrease in sperm count.
○ Hepatic dysfunction including increased aminotransferases

Drug Interactions

Some of the interactions of cimetidine are mentioned below:
○ Absorption of H$_2$ receptor antagonists is reduced by antacids. Hence, a 2-hour gap in administration should be maintained.
○ Cimetidine decreases hepatic blood flow and inhibits various cytochrome P450 enzymes in the liver. Increased levels of drugs such as phenytoin, theophylline, metronidazole, sulfonylureas, warfarin, lidocaine etc. can occur due to inhibition of their metabolism by cimetidine.

Ranitidine

The key differences between ranitidine and cimetidine are mentioned in Table 4.

TABLE 4	Ranitidine and cimetidine	
	Ranitidine (H$_2$ receptor blocker)	Cimetidine (H$_2$ receptor blocker)
Potency	More potent (5 times)	Less potent
Duration of action	Longer	Shorter
24-hour acid suppression	Greater	Lesser
Antiandrogenic effect, ↑ prolactin levels	No	Yes
Effects such as gynecomastia, impotence, decrease in sperm count	No	Yes
Incidence of CNS effects such as confusion, convulsions etc.	Less (due to poor penetration into brain)	More
Effect on hepatic metabolism of drugs	Less—most of the drug interactions are not clinically significant	More
Adverse effect profile	Better	Worse

Famotidine

- More potent than ranitidine
- No antiandrogenic effect

Roxatidine

- Profile is similar to ranitidine
- More potent than ranitidine
- No antiandrogenic effect

Clinical Uses

Some of the clinical uses of H$_2$ receptor blockers are mentioned in Table 5.

TABLE 5	Clinical uses of H$_2$ receptor blockers
Peptic ulcer • Used in patients of gastric and duodenal ulcers • PPIs are preferred drugs for peptic ulcer as they have a rapid onset of action and promote faster ulcer healing	
Stress ulcers and gastritis • Can occur in conditions such as severe trauma, burns, critically ill patients, hepatic coma etc.	
Zollinger-Ellison syndrome • Due to gastrin secreting tumor leading to hypersecretion of gastric acid • Surgical management may be required	
Gastroesophageal reflux disease	
Aspiration pneumonia prophylaxis • Used for preoperative prophylaxis of aspiration pneumonitis in patients who are administered anesthesia	

■ PROSTAGLANDIN ANALOGUE

Misoprostol

- It is an analogue of naturally occurring prostaglandin E$_1$.

- It has the following effects:
  - Inhibits gastric acid secretion
  - Increases bicarbonate and mucus secretion
  - Increases mucosal blood flow
  - Cytoprotective effect
- Adverse effects include diarrhea, abdominal pain and uterine bleeding. It is contraindicated in pregnancy because it stimulates uterine contractions and is associated with abortion, fetal death and congenital defects.
- The clinical uses include prophylaxis and treatment of NSAID-induced ulcers.
- It is not frequently used because of the need for four-times daily dosing and its adverse effect profile.

ANTICHOLINERGICS

These drugs are selective M_1 blockers and they decrease the volume of gastric acid secretion. They are not frequently used due to the availability of drugs with better efficacy and tolerability.

ANTACIDS

Antacids are weak bases and they neutralize gastric acid. They increase the gastric pH. They do not reduce the secretion of gastric acid.

Antacids can lead to acid rebound by causing a rise in the gastric pH (pH > 4). This causes release of gastrin leading to increased secretion of gastric acid. Gastric motility is also increased.

Systemic Antacids

Sodium Bicarbonate

- It is water soluble and neutralizes gastric acid.
- Disadvantages include:
  - Systemic absorption can lead to alkalosis
  - Release of CO_2 in the stomach can lead to distension of the abdomen, ulcer perforation
  - Acid rebound
  - Increase sodium load can precipitate heart failure
- Clinical uses include symptomatic relief of heart burn, urine alkalization and treatment of acidosis.

Nonsystemic Antacids

Nonsystemic antacids are insoluble compounds. They produce the corresponding chloride salt in the stomach. Chloride reacts with bicarbonate in the intestine; hence, systemic alkalosis does not occur because bicarbonate is not available for absorption.

Magnesium Trisilicate

- Has low solubility
- Magnesium salts cause diarrhea

Aluminum Hydroxide Gel

- Aluminum salts cause constipation; they relax smooth muscle and have mucosal astringent effect.
- Potency (acid neutralizing capacity) of aluminum hydroxide gel slowly decreases upon storage as it gradually polymerizes into less reactive forms.
- Regular use of aluminum hydroxide can lead to hypophosphatemia by binding to phosphate in the intestine and inhibiting its absorption. This can lead to osteomalacia. Aluminum hydroxide can also be clinically used in patients of hyperphosphatemia.
- Aluminum toxicity can occur in patients of renal failure that may lead to encephalopathy and osteoporosis.

Antacid Combinations

The reasons for antacid combinations along with their potential benefits are mentioned in Table 6.

TABLE 6	Combination of antacids
Reason for combination of antacids	**Potential benefits**
• Magnesium hydroxide (fast acting) and aluminum hydroxide (slow acting)	Fast and sustained effect
• Magnesium salts cause diarrhea and increase gastric emptying • Aluminum salts cause constipation and decrease gastric emptying	Minimal effect on the bowel movements
• Reduction in the dose of individual components	Decrease incidence of systemic adverse effects

Drug Interactions

Some of the interactions with antacids are mentioned below:
○ Decreased absorption of drugs such as tetracyclines, fluoroquinolones, ketoconazole, H_2 blockers, phenytoin and diazepam. This is because antacids increase the pH of the stomach and form complexes with various drugs. Hence, a gap of 2 hours should be maintained between administration.

Clinical Uses

The clinical uses of antacids include:
○ Nonulcer dyspepsia, heartburn
○ Gastroesophageal reflux.

ULCER PROTECTIVES

Sucralfate

It is an aluminum salt of sulfated sucrose.

Sucralfate polymerizes in the acidic pH (pH < 4) of the stomach and forms a gel like substance. This gel like substance adheres to the base of the ulcer and acts as a physical barrier that protects the ulcer from substances such as acid and pepsin. Deposition of the dietary proteins on this layer also adds to the protection.

Sucralfate decreases gastric emptying and does not have any acid neutralizing effect.

Sucralfate should not be administered along with drugs such as PPIs, H_2 blockers and antacids because sucralfate needs acidic pH to work. Sucralfate interferes with the absorption of drugs such as phenytoin, digoxin, tetracyclines, ketoconazole and fluoroquinolones.

Clinical uses include peptic ulcers, gastritis and prevention of stress ulcers. It has a limited role in peptic ulcers as it requires multiple daily dosing as well as the availability of better efficacy drugs such as PPIs.

Adverse effects include constipation, nausea and risk of hypophosphatemia.

Colloidal Bismuth Subcitrate (CBS)

The mechanism of action is unclear, but the following are postulated:
○ Stimulation of PGE_2 production → Increase secretion of bicarbonate and mucus
○ Formation of a glycoprotein-bismuth complex that acts as a barrier to acid by coating the ulcer
○ Antimicrobial activity against *H. pylori* → Detaches the bacteria from the mucosa and kills it
Colloidal bismuth subcitrate is part of the therapy regimens against *H. pylori* in peptic ulcer patients.

Adverse effects include diarrhea and blackening of tongue and stools. Osteodystrophy and encephalopathy may occur on prolonged use.

ANTI *H. pylori* DRUGS

H. pylori is a gram-negative bacterium. It is a gastric pathogen that can survive in acidic environment of the stomach. It has been associated with gastritis, peptic ulcer disease and gastric carcinoma.

H. pylori has high urease activity and produces ammonia.

A combination of antibiotics and a proton pump inhibitor are used for the treatment. Some of the anti *H. pylori* regimens are mentioned in Figure 1. Amoxicillin should not be administered to patients who are allergic to penicillins.

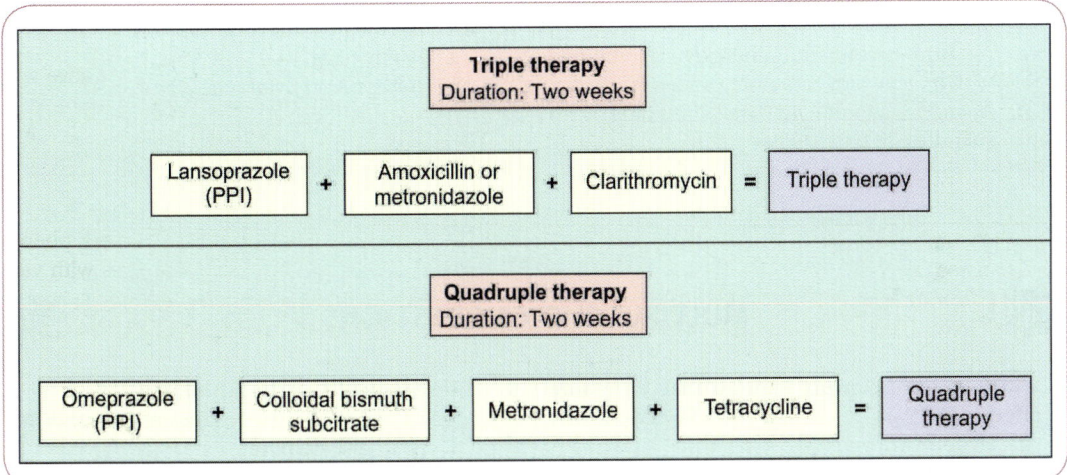

Figure 1: Anti *H. pylori* regimens

Post the completion of the antibiotic based regimens, PPIs should be continued for 4–6 weeks to promote healing of the ulcer.

PHARMACOTHERAPY FOR GASTROESOPHAGEAL REFLUX DISEASE

The drugs that can be used in patients of gastroesophageal reflux disease (GERD) are mentioned in Table 7.

TABLE 7	Pharmacotherapy for GERD
Proton pump inhibitors (e.g. omeprazole) • PPIs are highly effective in GERD • Increase gastric pH, provide symptomatic benefit and promote healing of esophageal lesions	
H₂ receptor antagonists (H₂ blockers) (e.g. ranitidine) • Increase gastric pH and can promote healing of esophageal lesions • Less effective than PPIs	
Antacids • Only used for temporary symptomatic benefit	
Prokinetic medications (e.g. metoclopramide, cisapride) • Are useful as they increase lower esophageal sphincter (LES) tone, gastric emptying and esophageal clearance • No effect on gastric pH and do not promote healing of esophageal lesions	
Sodium alginate • Forms a froth on the gastric contents. It acts as a barrier to contact with gastric acid.	

SECTION K ■ Drugs Acting on the Gastrointestinal System

ASSESS YOURSELF (Examination Questions of Various Universities)

1. Classify drugs used in the treatment of peptic ulcer. Discuss the mechanism of action, adverse effects and clinical uses of proton pump inhibitors.
2. Discuss the mechanism of action, pharmacokinetics, adverse effects and clinical uses of ranitidine.
3. Explain why:
   a. Aluminium containing antacids are combined with magnesium containing antacids
   b. Antacids should not be combined with sucralfate in peptic ulcer

c. Ranitidine is preferred over cimetidine in peptic ulcer
4. List the demerits of misoprostol as an antiulcer drug.
5. Write short notes on:
   a. Sucralfate
   b. *Anti-Helicobacter pylori drugs*
6. Discuss the pharmacotherapy of:
   a. Peptic ulcer
   b. *Helicobacter pylori infection*

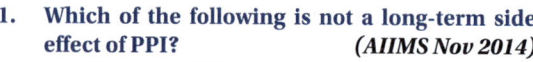

MULTIPLE CHOICE QUESTIONS

1. Which of the following is not a long-term side effect of PPI? *(AIIMS Nov 2014)*
   a. Hypothyroidism
   b. Pelvic fracture
   c. Increased risk of pneumonia
   d. Increased risk of *C. difficile* infection
2. Drug not used in *H. pylori* is:
   (AIIMS May 2008, Nov 2006)
   a. Metronidazole
   b. Omeprazole
   c. Mosapride
   d. Amoxicillin
3. Which of the following agents is beneficial in NSAID induced gastric ulcer?
   (Recent Question 2016)
   a. PGE_1 agonist
   b. PGE_2 agonist
   c. PGD_2 agonist
   d. PGF_{2a} agonist
4. Proton pump inhibitors are most effective when they are given: *(Recent Question 2016)*
   a. After meals
   b. Shortly before meals
   c. Along with H_2 blockers
   d. During prolonged fasting periods

5. Esomeprazole acts by inhibiting:
   (Recent Question 2016)
   a. $H^+ K^+$ ATPase pump
   b. $H^+ Na^+$ ATPase pump
   c. H^+ pump
   d. Any of the above
6. Antacid drug that typically causes diarrhea is:
   (Recent Question 2016)
   a. Sodium bicarbonate
   b. Magnesium hydroxide
   c. Calcium bicarbonate
   d. Aluminium hydroxide
7. All are H_2 blockers except:
   (Recent Question 2016)
   a. Omeprazole   b. Cimetidine
   c. Famotidine   d. Ranitidine
8. Antacids should not be given along with:
   (Recent Question 2016)
   a. Sucralfate
   b. H_2 blockers
   c. Proton pump inhibitors
   d. Prostaglandins
9. Which of the following is PPI?
   (Recent Question 2016)
   a. Ranitidine   b. Lansoprazole
   c. Misoprostol   d. Amoxicillin

Ans.

| 1. (a) | 2. (c) | 3. (a) | 4. (b) | 5. (a) | 6. (b) |
| 7. (a) | 8. (a) | 9. (b) | | | |

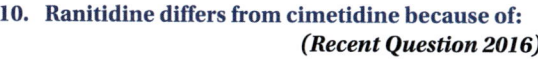

10. **Ranitidine differs from cimetidine because of:**
    (Recent Question 2016)
    a. Ranitidine does not have antiandrogenic side effect
    b. Shorter half-life
    c. More side effects
    d. Less potent

11. **A patient of peptic ulcer disease was prescribed ranitidine and sucralfate in the morning hours. Why is this combination incorrect?**
    (Recent Question 2016)
    a. Ranitidine combines with sucralfate and prevents its action

    b. Combination of these two drugs produce serious side effects like agranulocytosis.
    c. Ranitidine increases gastric pH so that sucralfate is unable to act
    d. Sucralfate inhibits the absorption of ranitidine

12. **Gynecomastia and infertility is caused by?**
    (Recent Question 2016)
    a. Flutamide
    b. Cimetidine
    c. Ranitidine
    d. Methotrexate

Ans.

10. (a)	11. (c)	12. (b)

47

Drugs Used for Constipation

Laxatives are drugs that are used in the prevention or treatment of constipation. Laxatives facilitate the evacuation of stools (Table 1).

TABLE 1	Laxatives and purgatives	
	Laxative (Aperient)	Purgative (Cathartic)
Effect on bowel evacuation	Mild effect leading to evacuation of formed, soft stools	Stronger effect leading to evacuation of unformed, watery stools
Many drugs function as laxatives at low doses and as purgatives at high doses		

CLASSIFICATION OF DRUGS

The classification of drugs used for the management of constipation is mentioned in Table 2.

TABLE 2	Classification of drugs used in constipation
Bulk forming agents	• Dietary fiber: Bran, methylcellulose, psyllium, ispaghula
Stool softener	• Docusates, liquid paraffin
Stimulant purgatives	• Phenolphthalein, bisacodyl, sodium picosulfate • Senna, castor oil
Osmotic purgatives	• Magnesium sulfate, magnesium hydroxide • Sodium sulfate, sodium phosphate • Lactulose • 5-HT$_4$ agonist → Tegaserod
Others	• Lubiprostone

BULK FORMING AGENTS

Bulk forming agents such as bran increase the water content and bulk of stool by absorbing water in the intestine. This leads to softening of stool, stimulation of peristalsis and evacuation of bowels.

Bran contains 40% fiber. Pectin (type of dietary fiber) can decrease LDL cholesterol levels by binding to bile acids and facilitating their excretion in stool.

Methylcellulose is a semisynthetic derivative of cellulose. Psyllium and ispaghula contain natural mucilage that absorbs water.

Bran is unpalatable and large amounts need to be consumed. Bulk forming agents should be taken with lots of water. Intestinal obstruction can occur if they are swallowed dry.

Bran does not soften stool that is already present in the intestine—hence, it is not useful in patients who are already constipated. Gastrointestinal (GIT) discomfort such as bloating, flatulence and abdominal distension can occur. Patients with intestinal stenosis, adhesions or those at risk of intestinal obstruction should not be administered these agents.

Clinical uses include functional constipation, irritable bowel syndrome and prevention of straining during defecation.

STOOL SOFTENER

Some of the salient features of docusates and liquid paraffin are mentioned in Table 3.

TABLE 3	Docusates and liquid paraffin
Docusates	• Are anionic surfactants • Cause accumulation of fluids by decreasing surface tension of stool → Lead to stool softening • Can lead to disruption of the mucosal barrier of the intestine and therefore, increase the absorption of drugs such as liquid paraffin → Coadministration should not be done • Adverse effects include GIT discomfort such as abdominal pain; hepatotoxicity (can occur on prolonged use)
Liquid paraffin	• Pharmacologically inert substance • Lubricates and softens stools • Disadvantages include: ▪ Has an oily consistency; unpleasant to swallow ▪ Prolonged use can lead to deficiency of fat soluble vitamins as they are excreted in stools ▪ May lead to foreign body granuloma in intestine, lymph nodes, liver and spleen ▪ May lead to lipid pneumonia if small amounts enter the lungs while swallowing ▪ Oil leakage past the anal sphincter can occur, leading to soiling of clothes

STIMULANT PURGATIVES

The general mechanism of action of stimulant purgatives is as follows:
- Increased amount of water and electrolytes in the intestinal lumen by:
  - Inhibition of Na^+-K^+ ATPase in the intestinal mucosa → Decreased intestinal absorption of Na^+ and water
  - Increased synthesis of prostaglandins and increased activity of cAMP → Increased intestinal secretion
- Action on the myenteric plexus to enhance intestinal motility

Large doses can lead to water and electrolyte imbalance; colonic atony can occur on prolonged use. They should not be used during pregnancy as they can cause stimulation of the uterus. They should also not be given to patients with intestinal obstruction.

Some of the salient features of stimulant purgatives are mentioned in Table 4.

TABLE 4	Stimulant purgatives
Phenolphthalein	• It is an indicator and is not used due to adverse effects • Can lead to tumors in mice
Bisacodyl	• Colon is the main site of action • Has an irritant effect on the colonic mucosa • Available for oral use and also as a suppository • Adverse effects include allergic reactions, Stevens-Johnson syndrome • Clinical uses include bowel evacuation prior to surgery or colonoscopy
Sodium picosulfate	• Has an irritant effect on the colonic mucosa and also stimulates the myenteric plexus • Clinical uses include bowel evacuation prior to surgery or colonoscopy
Senna	• Anthraquinone derivative • Has an irritant effect on the colonic mucosa and also stimulates the myenteric plexus • Adverse effects include skin rashes; prolonged use can lead to colonic atony and melanosis (colonic pigmentation)
Castor oil	• Obtained from seeds of *Ricinus communis* • Not frequently used due to unpleasant taste, abdominal cramps and risk of dehydration after constipation. Damage to the intestinal mucosa can occur upon prolonged use.

OSMOTIC PURGATIVES

The general mechanism of action of osmotic purgatives (also known as saline purgatives) is as follows:
○ Increase in the volume of colonic content by osmotic action, to retain water in the intestinal lumen
○ This leads to distension of the intestinal lumen and indirectly causes peristalsis leading to bowel evacuation

Some of the salient features of magnesium and sodium osmotic purgatives are mentioned in Table 5.

TABLE 5	Magnesium and sodium osmotic purgatives	
Magnesium salts	**Sodium salts**	
E.g. Magnesium sulfate (Epsom salt), magnesium hydroxide (Milk of magnesia)	E.g. Sodium sulfate (Glauber's salt), sodium phosphate	
Apart from osmotic action, magnesium salts also release cholecystokinin that may help in purgation	Avoided in patients of heart failure, and other conditions where sodium retention is to be avoided	
Contraindicated in patients with renal dysfunction		

- Osmotic purgatives are not used in treatment of constipation as they can cause after constipation.
- Prolonged use can lead to fluid and electrolyte imbalance.
- Osmotic purgatives can be used for bowel preparation prior to surgery and colonoscopy, some patients with poisoning (drug/food).

Lactulose

○ It is a synthetic disaccharide of fructose and galactose.
○ Lactulose is an osmotic purgative and leads to retention of water resulting in peristalsis and bowel evacuation
○ Adverse effects include abdominal discomfort and flatulence
○ It is clinically used for:
❏ Treatment of constipation
❏ Reduction of ammonia levels in patients of hepatic encephalopathy (Figure 1)

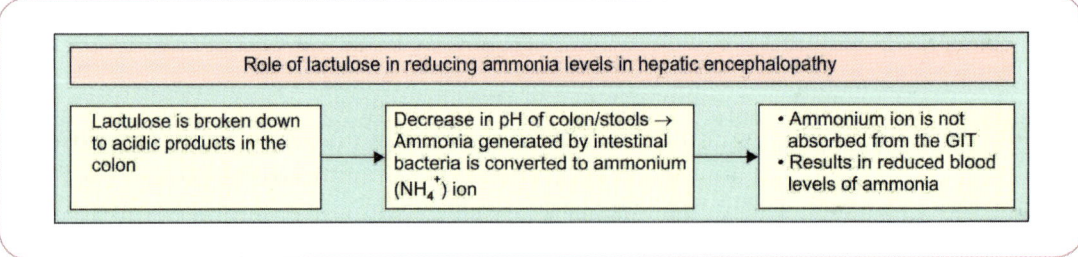

Figure 1: Lactulose in patients of hepatic encephalopathy

Tegaserod

○ It is a 5-HT$_4$ agonist
○ It increases the release of acetylcholine and calcitonin gene related peptide (CGRP) leading to peristalsis and increase in colonic secretion
○ The adverse effects include diarrhea, headache and flatus
○ Clinical uses include irritable bowel syndrome and chronic constipation.

OTHER PURGATIVES

Lubiprostone

- Stimulates the chloride channels in the small intestine → Increases the secretion of chloride rich fluid in the intestine → Increases intestinal motility and reduces intestinal transit
- Clinical uses include chronic constipation and irritable bowel syndrome
- Should not be used during pregnancy, and in women of childbearing potential not using contraception.

CLINICAL USES OF LAXATIVES

Some of the clinical uses of laxatives are mentioned in Table 6.

TABLE 6	Clinical uses of laxatives

Functional constipation	• Spastic constipation (Irritable bowel)
	  ▪ Preferred laxative → Dietary fiber, bulk forming agents
	  ▪ Stimulant purgatives are contraindicated
	• Atonic constipation
	  ▪ Bulk forming agents are preferred
	Nonpharmacologic measures should be tried

Patients confined to bed (e.g. postsurgical, stroke)	• Prevention of constipation
	  ▪ Bulk forming agents (preferred)
	  ▪ Lactulose, docusates
	• Treatment of constipation
	  ▪ Soap water or glycerine enema
	  ▪ Senna, bisacodyl

Bowel preparation prior to surgery or colonoscopy	• Saline purgatives • Senna, bisacodyl
Prevent straining during defecation (e.g. eye surgeries, CVS disease, hernia)	• Bulk forming agents • Lactulose, docusates
Post-therapy with anthelmintic drugs (e.g. for tapeworm)	• Saline purgatives • Senna
Patients with poisoning (food/drug)	• Saline purgatives

CONTRAINDICATIONS OF LAXATIVES

Laxatives are contraindicated in the following situations:
- Organic constipation (secondary) resulting from intestinal obstruction, strictures, carcinomas, endocrine conditions (e.g. hypothyroidism, hypercalcemia), drugs (e.g. sedatives, opiates)
- Patients with undiagnosed vomiting or pain in the abdomen

It is important to identify and treat the underlying cause of constipation or bowel abnormalities.

ASSESS YOURSELF (Examination Questions of Various Universities)

1. **Classify purgatives. Discuss the mechanism of action and pharmacological features of osmotic purgatives.**
2. **Write short notes on:**
   a. Liquid paraffin
   b. Lactulose
   c. Bulk forming laxatives

3. **Explain the rationale of using lactulose in patients with hepatic encephalopathy.**

MULTIPLE CHOICE QUESTIONS

1. **Stimulant purgatives are contraindicated in:**
   (Recent Question 2016)
   a. Bed ridden patients
   b. Before abdominal radiography
   c. Subacute intestinal obstruction
   d. All of these

2. **Bisacodyl is:** *(Recent Question 2016)*
   a. Bulk forming
   b. Stool softener
   c. Stimulant purgative
   d. Osmotic purgative

3. **Drug useful in hepatic encephalopathy is:**
   (Recent Question 2016)
   a. Magnesium sulfate   b. Lactulose
   c. Bisacodyl   d. Bisphosphonates

4. **Laxative acting by opening of chloride channels**
   (Recent Question 2016)
   a. Docusate   b. Anthraquinone
   c. Lubiprostone   d. Bisacodyl

5. **Aloe, senna, and cascara are:**
   (Recent Question 2016)
   a. Laxatives   b. Emetics
   c. Antidiarrheals   d. Antiemetics

Ans.

1. (c)   2. (c)   3. (b)   4. (c)   5. (a)

48 Emetics and Antiemetics

EMESIS

Emesis is also known as vomiting and consists of the following:
- Nausea → unpleasant feeling of wanting to vomit or feeling of imminent vomiting
- Retching → spasmodic respiratory activity that often follows nausea
- Vomiting → forceful expulsion of gastric and upper gastrointestinal contents via mouth

Vomiting can be triggered by several stimuli such as:
- Pain, anxiety, smell, increased intracranial pressure
- Drugs, radiation, chemotherapy, toxins
- Motion, vestibular or ear disorders
- Gastrointestinal factors such as irritation, stasis, obstruction, infection, trauma

These stimuli can affect various structures involved in vomiting (Figure 1).

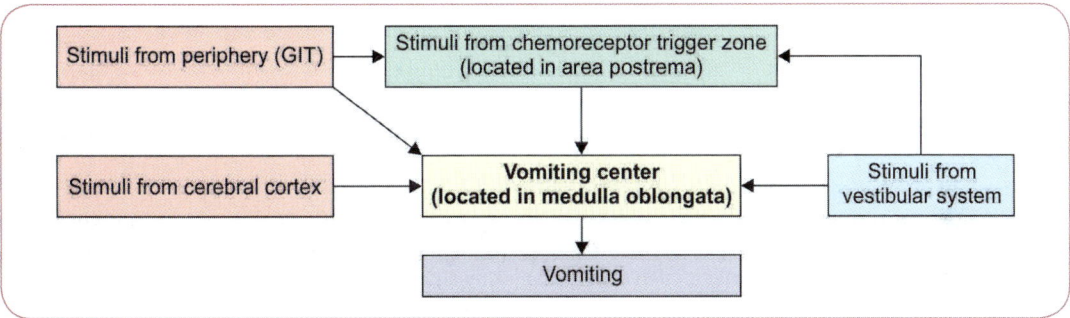

Figure 1: Structures involved in vomiting

EMETICS

The drugs that induce vomiting are called emetics (Table 1). They can be used in specific poisonings, if clinically indicated.

TABLE 1	Emetics
Apomorphine	• Semisynthetic derivative of morphine • Dopamine agonist → acts on the chemoreceptor trigger zone (CTZ)
Ipecacuanha	• Used as syrup ipecac and contains emetine • Stimulates CTZ and cause gastric irritation
Salt solution or powered mustard	• Cause gastric irritation

Contraindications of emetics
- Patients who are unconscious → risk of aspiration
- Patients with corrosive poisoning → further trauma can occur, including perforation
- Patients with kerosene poisoning → risk of aspiration
- Patients with central nervous system (CNS) stimulant poisoning → risk of convulsions

ANTIEMETIC DRUGS

Drugs that prevent or inhibit vomiting are called antiemetics. The classification of antiemetics is mentioned in Table 2.

TABLE 2	Antiemetics
Classification	**Examples**
• Anticholinergics	Scopolamine (hyoscine), dicyclomine
• Antihistaminics (H_1 blockers)	Diphenhydramine, promethazine, cyclizine, doxylamine, dimenhydrinate, meclizine, cinnarizine
• 5-HT_3 (Serotonin) receptor antagonists	Ondansetron, granisetron, palonosetron
• Prokinetic drugs	Metoclopramide, domperidone, mosapride
• Neuroleptics	Prochlorperazine, chlorpromazine, haloperidol
• Neurokinin (NK_1) receptor antagonists	Aprepitant, fosaprepitant
• Adjuvant drugs	Glucocorticoids (dexamethasone, betamethasone) Benzodiazepines (diazepam, lorazepam, alprazolam) Cannabinoids (dronabinol, nabilone)

ANTICHOLINERGICS

Scopolamine (Hyoscine)

- Antiemetic effect of scopolamine is possibly due to:
  - Anticholinergic effect that interferes with the neural transmission from the vestibular system to the vomiting center
- It is used for prevention and treatment of motion sickness
- It is not effective in vomiting from other causes
- Scopolamine is available for oral, parenteral and transdermal patch administration
- It also results in anticholinergic effects such as sedation, drowsiness, urinary retention, dry mouth and blurring of vision

ANTIHISTAMINICS (H_1 BLOCKERS)

- Antiemetic effect is possibly due to:
  - Antihistaminic, anticholinergic and sedative actions
- Clinically used in motion sickness, morning sickness and postoperative vomiting
- It can lead to drowsiness and dry mouth

5-HT_3 (SEROTONIN) RECEPTOR ANTAGONISTS

Ondansetron, Granisetron, Palonosetron

These drugs exert their antiemetic effect by blocking the 5-HT_3 receptors (Figure 2).

Pharmacokinetics

5-HT_3 receptor antagonists can be administered orally or parenterally (intravenous [IV]). They are well-absorbed orally and are metabolized in the liver. Elimination occurs via urine and feces.

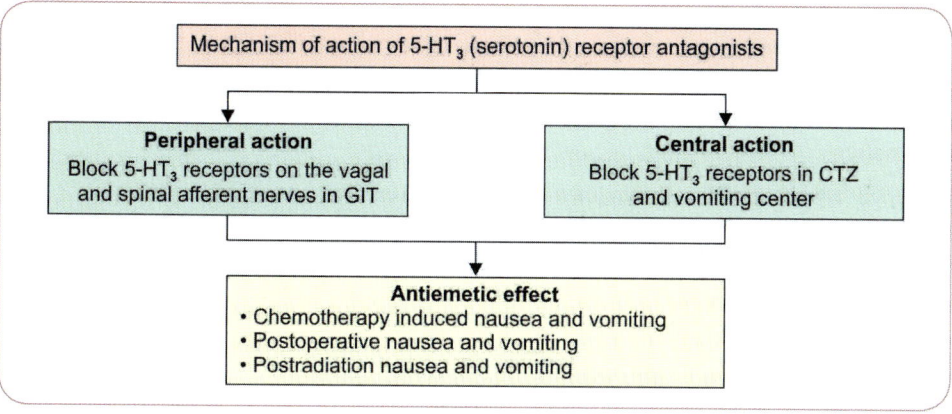

Figure 2: Mechanism of action of 5-HT$_3$ receptor antagonists

Adverse Effects

The adverse effects include hypersensitivity reactions, headache and constipation. QTc prolongation may occur in some patients.

Clinical Uses

The clinical uses of 5-HT$_3$ receptor antagonists include the prevention and treatment of:
- Chemotherapy induced nausea and vomiting
  - Efficacy can be increased by administering along with drugs such as dexamethasone, aprepitant and diazepam
- Postoperative nausea and vomiting
- Postradiation nausea and vomiting

PROKINETIC AGENTS

Prokinetic agents increase gastrointestinal motility and enhance gastric emptying. Metoclopramide and domperidone are clinically used as antiemetic drugs.

Metoclopramide

Metoclopramide is a prokinetic agent and is used as an antiemetic drug.

Mechanism of Action

Metoclopramide has complex mechanism of action (Table 3). It has prokinetic and antiemetic effects.

TABLE 3	Mechanism of action of metoclopramide
D$_2$ receptor blockade	**Gastrointestinal tract (GIT)** • Increased release of acetylcholine → ↑ Gastric emptying, ↑ Lower esophageal sphincter (LES) tone **Central action (CTZ)** • Antiemetic effect
5-HT$_4$ agonist effect	**Gastrointestinal tract** • Increased release of acetylcholine → ↑ Gastric emptying, ↑ Lower esophageal sphincter (LES) tone
5-HT$_3$ receptor antagonism	• Blockade of 5-HT$_3$ receptors in the GIT and CTZ • Central effect (CTZ) is observed at high doses

The actions of metoclopramide can be summarized as:
- ○ Gastrointestinal (Upper GI tract) → Prokinetic effect, ↑ Gastric peristalsis, ↑ LES tone, relaxation of pylorus, ↑ peristalsis of small intestine
- ○ Central nervous system → antiemetic effect

Pharmacokinetics

Metoclopramide is absorbed orally, metabolized in the liver and excreted mainly via urine.
It crosses the blood brain barrier.

Adverse Effects

Some of the key adverse effects and drug interactions of metoclopramide are mentioned in Table 4.

TABLE 4	Adverse effects and drug interactions of metoclopramide
Neurological	• Extrapyramidal symptoms (e.g. tremors, rigidity, acute dystonia) • Drug-induced parkinsonism • Dizziness, drowsiness, sedation
Endocrine	• Hyperprolactinemia, galactorrhea, gynecomastia, menstrual abnormalities • Usually observed during prolonged therapy
Others	• Diarrhea, hypersensitivity reactions
Drug interactions	• Metoclopramide and levodopa → metoclopramide can antagonize the antiparkinsonian effect of levodopa. This is because metoclopramide can cross the blood brain barrier and cause blockade of D_2 receptors. • Metoclopramide has a prokinetic effect and hence, it can enhance the absorption of drugs such as diazepam

Clinical Uses

The clinical uses of metoclopramide include the following:
- ○ **Antiemetic**
  - ❑ Postoperative nausea and vomiting
  - ❑ Nausea and vomiting associated with diseases (e.g. migraine), drugs, radiation
  - ❑ Chemotherapy-induced nausea and vomiting
  - ❑ It is less effective in motion sickness
- ○ **Gastroesophageal reflux disease (GERD)**
  - ❑ Symptomatic benefit in mild cases
  - ❑ Less effective than other drugs such as H_2 blockers and proton pump inhibitors
- ○ **Prokinetic agent (enhance gastric emptying)**
  - ❑ In patients undergoing duodenal intubation
  - ❑ Symptomatic benefit in gastroparesis
  - ❑ Emergency surgery requiring general anesthesia in patients who may have recently consumed food

Domperidone

- ○ Domperidone is a D_2 receptor blocker
- ○ Does not readily cross the blood brain barrier; lower incidence of extrapyramidal effects
- ○ Adverse effects include dry mouth, headache, diarrhea, prolactin release, galactorrhea, menstrual abnormalities, QTc prolongation, extrapyramidal disorder
- ○ Clinically used for relief of nausea and vomiting

Some of the key differences between metoclopramide and domperidone are mentioned in Table 5.

TABLE 5	Metoclopramide and domperidone
Metoclopramide	**Domperidone**
Higher antiemetic efficacy	Lower antiemetic efficacy
Crosses the blood brain barrier	Does not readily cross the blood brain barrier
Higher incidence of extrapyramidal disorders	Lower incidence of extrapyramidal disorders
Metoclopramide can antagonize the therapeutic anti-parkinsonism effect of levodopa or bromocriptine. Hence, it is not used in the treatment of levodopa- or bromocriptine-induced vomiting.	Domperidone can oppose the emetic effects of levodopa or bromocriptine, but does not significantly affect the therapeutic antiparkinsonism effects of these drugs. Hence, it is preferred for the treatment of levodopa or bromocriptine induced vomiting.

Mosapride

- It is a prokinetic agent but is not used as an antiemetic drug
- It has 5-HT$_4$ agonist (primary effect) and 5-HT$_3$ antagonist effects
- Clinical uses include gastroesophageal reflux disease

NEUROLEPTICS (D$_2$ BLOCKERS)

- The neuroleptic drugs include prochlorperazine, chlorpromazine, haloperidol
- Antiemetic effect is possibly due to:
  - D$_2$ receptor blockade in the CTZ
  - Antihistaminic and anticholinergic actions
- Clinically used in nausea and vomiting associated with diseases, drugs, radiation and chemotherapy induced nausea and vomiting
- Adverse effects include sedation, muscle dystonia and extrapyramidal symptoms
- Prochlorperazine is frequently used and has specific antiemetic and antivertigo effect

NEUROKININ (NK$_1$) RECEPTOR ANTAGONISTS

- The NK$_1$ receptor antagonists include aprepitant and fosaprepitant
- Antiemetic effect is possibly due to:
  - Antagonism of neurokinin (NK$_1$) receptors in the brain
- Clinically used in the prevention of nausea and vomiting associated with moderately and highly emetogenic chemotherapy
- Can be used along with drugs such as dexamethasone and ondansetron to increase antiemetic efficacy
- Adverse effects include fatigue, dizziness and flatulence
- Fosaprepitant is a prodrug of aprepitant

ADJUVANT DRUGS

Glucocorticoids (Dexamethasone, Betamethasone)

- These are used along with drugs such as ondansetron or metoclopramide to increase the antiemetic effect.

Benzodiazepines (Diazepam, Lorazepam, Alprazolam)

- Antiemetic effect is possibly due to antianxiety, sedative and amnesic properties.

Cannabinoids (Dronabinol, Nabilone)

- Dronabinol → (Δ^9-tetrahydrocannabinol [THC]) is a psychoactive substance and is the major component in marijuana. It is uncommonly used as an antiemetic in chemotherapy-induced nausea and vomiting. Adverse effects include hallucinations, euphoria, sedation, dry mouth and drug dependence.

ASSESS YOURSELF (Examination Questions of Various Universities)

1. Enumerate different classes of antiemetic drugs. Discuss the mechanism of action, adverse effects and clinical uses of metoclopramide.
2. Mention two drugs of different groups used in vomiting with their mechanism of action.
3. List important differences between metoclopramide and domperidone.
4. Write short notes on:
   a. Prokinetic drugs
   b. Metoclopramide
   c. Ondansetron

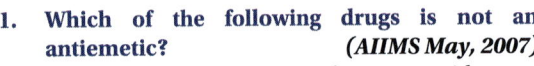

MULTIPLE CHOICE QUESTIONS

1. Which of the following drugs is not an antiemetic? *(AIIMS May, 2007)*
   a. Ondansetron
   b. Domperidone
   c. Metoclopramide
   d. Cinnarizine

2. All are antiemetic except: *(Recent Question 2016)*
   a. Ondansetron
   b. Metoclopramide
   c. Chlorpromazine
   d. Bismuth

3. Ondansetron acts by inhibiting which of the following receptors: *(Recent Question 2016)*
   a. 5-HT_1
   b. 5-HT
   c. 5-HT_3
   d. 5-HT_4

4. Mosapride is a: *(Recent Question 2016)*
   a. 5HT_4 agonist
   b. 5HT_3 agonists
   c. 5HT_3 antagonists
   d. 5HT_4 antagonists

5. Hyperprolactinemia is a side effect of: *(Recent Question 2016)*
   a. Bromocriptine
   b. Levodopa
   c. Amantadine
   d. Metoclopramide

6. Which of the following is a true match among antiemetics? *(NIMHANS 2011)*
   a. Domperidone-5-HT_2 antagonist
   b. Ondansetron selective-5HT_3 antagonist
   c. Metoclopramide-5HT_1 antagonist
   d. Meclizine-5HT_4 antagonist

7. NK1 receptor antagonist: *(TNPG 2011)*
   a. Aprepitant
   b. Apoferritin
   c. Apraclonidine
   d. Aripiprazole

8. Metoclopramide is useful for all except: *(TNPG 1998)*
   a. GERD
   b. Vomiting
   c. Galactorrhea
   d. Emergency GA

Ans.

1. (d)	2. (d)	3. (c)	4. (a)	5. (d)	6. (b)
7. (a)	8. (c)				

Drugs Used for Diarrhea

Diarrhea is an unusual increase in the number, volume or liquidity of stools.
Some of the causes of diarrhea are mentioned in Table 1.

TABLE 1	Causes of diarrhea
Causes	**Examples**
Infections • Viral infections • Bacterial infections • Parasitic infections	• Rotavirus • *Salmonella, Shigella, E. coli, V. cholerae, C. difficile* • *Giardia lamblia, Entamoeba histolytica*
Medications	• Antibiotics • Laxatives
Inflammatory bowel disease	• Ulcerative colitis • Crohn's disease
Malabsorption syndrome	• Celiac sprue
Tumors	• Carcinoid syndrome • Carcinoma colon
Others	• Hyperthyroidism

The management of diarrhea in a patient consists of the management of symptoms (diarrhea) and the management of underlying cause(s). It is useful to differentiate between acute and chronic diarrhea.
The key principles in the management of diarrhea are as follows:
○ Rehydration therapy
  ❑ Oral rehydration therapy
  ❑ Intravenous rehydration therapy
○ Nutritional and supportive management
○ Drugs
  ❑ Absorbants
  ❑ Antisecretory and antimotility agents
  ❑ Antimicrobials

The relative importance of each of the above therapies in the management of a diarrhea patient depends upon various factors such as the severity of diarrhea, underlying cause(s) and the general condition of the patient.

REHYDRATION THERAPY

ORAL REHYDRATION THERAPY

A significant cause of morbidity and mortality in patients of diarrhea is dehydration.

Oral rehydration therapy is a safe, effective and an inexpensive method to prevent or treat dehydration in patients of diarrhea.

Oral rehydration therapy does not stop diarrhea, but can prevent or treat dehydration, and maintain fluid and electrolyte balance. In many cases, diarrhea often ceases spontaneously. Oral rehydration therapy is considered the preferred therapy in patients of diarrhea.

WHO—Oral Rehydration Salts (ORS)

The WHO—ORS is used to prevent or treat dehydration in patients of diarrhea. The composition of new WHO-ORS is mentioned in Table 2.

TABLE 2	New WHO oral rehydration salts			
Sodium chloride	2.6 g/L	Sodium	75 mmol/L
Potassium chloride	1.5 g/L	Glucose, anhydrous	75 mmol/L
Glucose, anhydrous	13.5 g/L	Chloride	65 mmol/L
Trisodium citrate	2.9 g/L	Potassium	20 mmol/L
		Citrate	10 mmol/L
Total osmolality		245 mOsm/L	

- **Glucose** → Facilitates the absorption of sodium and water from the small intestine
- **Sodium and potassium** → For replacement of the loss of these ions during diarrhea/vomiting
- **Citrate** → For correction of acidosis due to diarrhea and dehydration

Administering zinc to children with acute diarrhea for 10–14 days may lead to a decrease in the duration and severity of diarrheal episodes. It may also prevent future episodes of diarrhea for 2–3 months.

Oral rehydration therapy may also be used to maintain hydration in situations such as burns, trauma or heatstroke.

INTRAVENOUS REHYDRATION THERAPY

Patients with severe dehydration require therapy with intravenous fluids to correct and maintain fluid and electrolyte balance.

DRUGS—ABSORBANTS, ANTISECRETORY AND ANTIMOTILITY AGENTS

Some of the key features of these drugs are mentioned in Table 3.

TABLE 3	Absorbants, antisecretory and antimotility agents
Absorbants	
	• Bulk forming agents • Alter the consistency of stools • For example, ispaghula, psyllium • Used in irritable bowel syndrome, diarrhea associated with ileostomy, colostomy
Antisecretory agents	
Octreotide	• Synthetic analogue of somatostatin • Clinically used for symptomatic relief (diarrhea) in patients of carcinoid tumors and VIPoma (vasoactive intestinal peptide secreting tumors), refractory diarrhea in patients of AIDS

Contd...

Racecadotril	<ul><li>It is a prodrug that is hydrolyzed to its active metabolite thiorphan</li><li>Thiorphan is an inhibitor of enkephalinase, an enzyme present in the small intestine</li><li>Inhibition of enkephalinase leads to an increase in the level of enkephalins, which are agonists of δ opioid receptors. This results in a decrease in intestinal hypersecretion.</li><li>It does not alter the duration of intestinal transit</li><li>Clinical use includes complementary symptomatic management of acute secretory diarrhea. It can be used in children.</li></ul>
Other drugs	<ul><li>Sulfasalazine, mesalazine</li></ul>
Antimotility agents (Opioids)—also have antisecretory action	
Mechanism of action <ul><li>These drugs are opioids and act on the opioid receptors in the GIT</li><li>Primary actions are —↑ tone of small intestine, ↓ propulsive peristalsis, ↑ intestinal transit time and ↓ intestinal secretions</li><li>Tolerance to the constipating effect of opioids is not observed</li></ul>	
Codeine	<ul><li>Leads to constipation</li><li>Potential for abuse</li></ul>
Loperamide	<ul><li>Opioid analogue</li><li>Significant action on µ receptors in the GIT</li><li>Mechanism → ↑ tone of small intestine, ↓ propulsive peristalsis, ↑ intestinal transit time, ↓ intestinal secretions and ↑ tone of anal sphincter</li><li>Poor penetration in the CNS and hence, has no abuse potential</li><li>Longer duration of action, as compared to codeine and diphenoxylate</li><li>Adverse effects → Nausea, flatulence, abdominal pain, rashes, paralytic ileus, toxic megacolon—contraindicated in children less than 4 years of age</li><li>Clinical uses include symptomatic treatment of acute diarrhea and chronic diarrhea in adults</li></ul>
Diphenoxylate	<ul><li>Related to pethidine and is a synthetic opioid</li><li>It has antidiarrheal action</li><li>Diphenoxylate has abuse potential and hence, atropine is added in subtherapeutic doses to discourage abuse</li><li>Adverse effects include malaise, somnolence, hallucinations, allergic reactions, paralytic ileus and toxic megacolon. Atropinic adverse effects can include cardiac abnormalities and respiratory depression.</li><li>Used as an adjunctive drug in acute diarrhea. Also used in colostomy or ileostomy patients to control stool formation.</li></ul>
Antimotility drugs are contraindicated in acute infectious diarrhea because they can delay the excretion of pathogen from the intestine and increase the severity of the disease. This can lead to further invasion of the intestinal mucosa by the pathogen, and may result in worsening of the disease. Antimotility drugs can increase the intraluminal pressure and hence, are contraindicated in patients of acute ulcerative colitis.	

DRUGS—ANTIMICROBIALS

Antimicrobials are only required in specific situations and due consideration should be given to local treatment protocol/guidelines along with the condition of the patient and the type of diarrhea. Some of the pathogens with examples of antibiotics that may be used in the treatment are mentioned in Table 4.

TABLE 4	Antimicrobials
V. cholerae	• Tetracycline, doxycycline • Cotrimoxazole, ciprofloxacin
Shigella	• Ciprofloxacin, norfloxacin
C. jejuni	• Norfloxacin, erythromycin
C. difficile	• Metronidazole, vancomycin
E. histolytica, G. lamblia	• Metronidazole
E. coli	• Ciprofloxacin

DRUG THERAPY FOR INFLAMMATORY BOWEL DISEASE

Inflammatory bowel disease (IBD) is a chronic inflammatory condition of the gastrointestinal tract, characterized by remissions and relapses. IBD includes Crohn's disease and ulcerative colitis (UC).

The clinical features include diarrhea, abdominal pain, GI bleeding, anemia and various extraintestinal symptoms.

The management of IBD is mentioned in Table 5.

TABLE 5	Therapy for inflammatory bowel disease
Supportive care	• Stress management • Dietary management
Aminosalicylates	• Sulfasalazine, mesalamine, olsalazine, balsalazide
Glucocorticoids	• Prednisolone, hydrocortisone, methylprednisolone, budesonide
Immunosuppressant drugs	• Azathioprine, methotrexate, 6-mercaptopurine
Biologic agents	• Infliximab, adalimumab
Antibiotics	• Metronidazole, ciprofloxacin

AMINOSALICYLATES

Sulfasalazine

Sulfasalazine consists of 5-ASA (5-aminosalicylic acid) and sulfapyridine that is linked by an azo bond. 5-ASA has anti-inflammatory action that is beneficial in patients of inflammatory bowel disease. Apart from IBD, sulfasalazine is also used in the management of rheumatoid arthritis (Figure 1).

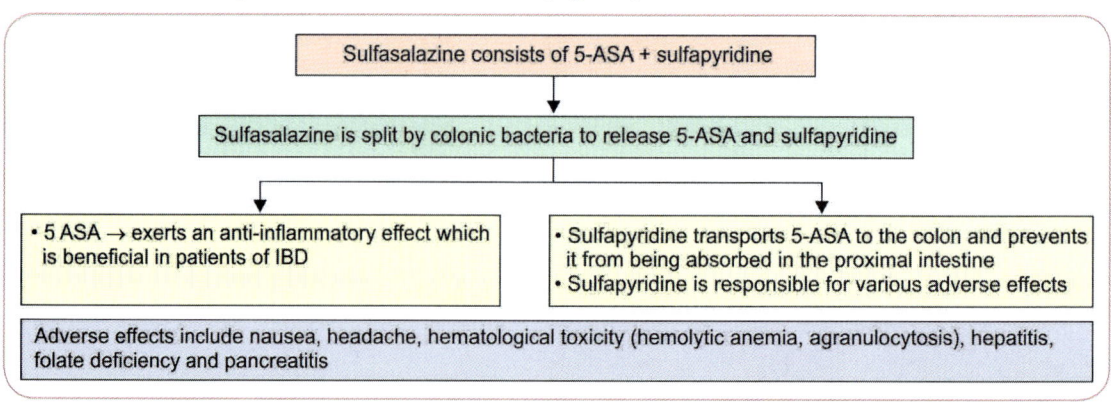

Figure 1: Sulfasalazine in inflammatory bowel disease

Mesalamine (Mesalazine)

○ It is 5-aminosalicylic acid.
○ It is administered as specific formulations (e.g. delayed release) to prevent its absorption in the upper intestine
○ Upon release in the terminal ileum and colon, mesalamine (5-ASA) exerts an anti-inflammatory effect which is beneficial in patients of inflammatory bowel disease.
○ Adverse effects include headache, nausea, abdominal pain and diarrhea. Mesalamine has been observed to be associated with nephrotoxicity (interstitial nephritis).
○ It is also available as suppositories.

Olsalazine

○ It is split into 2 molecules of 5-ASA by the colonic bacteria.

Balsalazide

○ It consists of 5-ASA linked to an inert carrier molecule. 5-ASA is released in the colon to exert the therapeutic effect.

GLUCOCORTICOIDS

Glucocorticoids are used for short-term use such as acute flare-ups in many patients of IBD.

Hydrocortisone (IV, enema), prednisolone (oral) or budesonide (oral) can be used.

The adverse effects include adrenocortical suppression, osteoporosis, gastric ulcers, infections etc.

IMMUNOSUPPRESSANT DRUGS

These drugs cause generalized immunosuppression. They can be used in patients with moderate to severe IBD.

The adverse effects include gastrointestinal toxicity, myelosuppression and hepatotoxicity.

BIOLOGIC AGENTS

These drugs have anti-TNF-α activity and cause suppression of immune function. They are used in patients with moderate to severe IBD.

The adverse effects include hypersensitivity, neurological reactions, potential for reactivation of infections such as tuberculosis and fungal infections, and risk of malignancies.

ANTIBIOTICS

Antimicrobials such as metronidazole and ciprofloxacin can be used in patients of Crohn's disease.

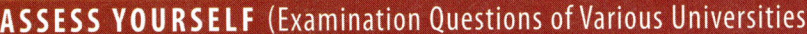

ASSESS YOURSELF (Examination Questions of Various Universities)

1. Discuss the pharmacotherapy of inflammatory bowel disease.
2. Write short notes on:
   a. Oral rehydration therapy
   b. Sulfasalazine

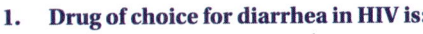

MULTIPLE CHOICE QUESTIONS

1. **Drug of choice for diarrhea in HIV is:**
   (Recent Question 2016)
   a. Loperamide
   b. Somatostatin
   c. Octreotide
   d. Codeine

2. **A 45 years old male patient a known case of Crohn's disease presents with recent flare-ups suggestive of fistulas. He was admitted and treated with immune-suppressive. Unfortunately, he got reactivation of his tuberculosis as a result of the side effects of the treatment. Which of the following immunosuppressive medication is the most likely cause of his TB reactivation?**
   (JIPMER 2016)
   a. Methotrexate
   b. Infliximab
   c. Azathioprine
   d. Mizoribine

3. **A 40-year-old woman with Crohn's disease reports multiple bowel movements with frequent stools. She was previously treated with a mesalamine derivative "Pentasa" and in the latest episode of the disease flare up she did not tolerate the oral steroid therapy with budesonide. What is the next appropriate step in her treatment?**
   (JIPMER 2016)
   a. Hydrocortisone (IV)
   b. Prednisolone (oral)
   c. Azathioprine
   d. Sulfasalazine

4. **Mesalamine is used in:** *(JIPMER 2012)*
   a. Ulcerative colitis
   b. Diabetes
   c. Erectile dysfunction
   d. Tinea corporis

5. **DOC for ulcerative colitis:** *(TNPG 2008)*
   a. Sulfasalazine
   b. Sulfadiazine
   c. Sulfur dioxide
   d. Etanercept

Ans.

| 1. (c) | 2. (b) | 3. (c) | 4. (a) | 5. (a) |

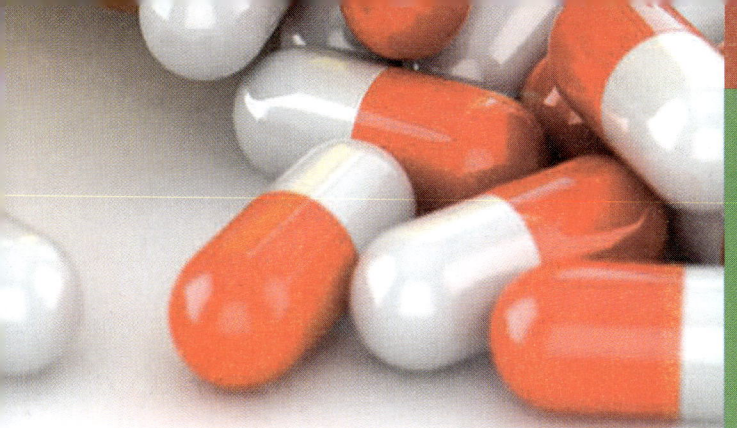

Antimicrobials

SECTION OUTLINE

Antimicrobial Agents: General Considerations

INTRODUCTION

There are many terms used in relation to therapy with antimicrobial agents. Some of them are mentioned below:

Chemotherapy

It is defined as the use of chemical substances/drugs to treat infectious diseases or malignancies, that selectively damages the microorganisms or cancer cells without significantly damaging the host tissues.

Antimicrobial Agents (AMAs)

AMAs are naturally obtained as well as synthetic drugs that acts on and inhibits the microorganisms.
- Natural (obtained from microorganisms)—these are called antibiotics
- Synthetic (synthesized in the laboratory)—these are called antibacterial/antifungal/antiviral agents.

Bacteriostatic Agents

These agents inhibit the growth and multiplication of microorganisms and therefore, limit the spread of infection. The number of microorganisms is not decreased. Examples include sulphonamides and tetracyclines etc.

Bactericidal Agents

These agents kill the microorganisms; therefore, decreases the number of microorganisms. Examples include penicillin and aminoglycosides etc.

> **Note:** At higher concentrations, some bacteriostatic drugs may convert into bactericidal drugs, e.g. sulphonamides, chloramphenicol etc.

Minimum Inhibitory Concentration (MIC)

It is defined as the lowest AMA concentration that prevents visible growth of microorganisms.

Minimum Bactericidal Concentration (MBC)

It is defined as the lowest AMA concentration that kills 99.9% of the microorganisms. A small difference between MIC and MBC suggests that the AMA is bactericidal.

Postantibiotic Effect (PAE)

The PAE is the duration of time required by a microbe to show viable regrowth following the removal of an antibiotic after a brief exposure.

This means that the antibacterial action persists following a brief exposure to antibiotics. It is observed with β lactams, fluoroquinolones and aminoglycosides.

CLASSIFICATION OF ANTIMICROBIAL AGENTS

The antimicrobial drugs can be classified in several ways. Some of them are mentioned in Figures 1, 2 and 3.

Antimicrobials

SECTION L ■

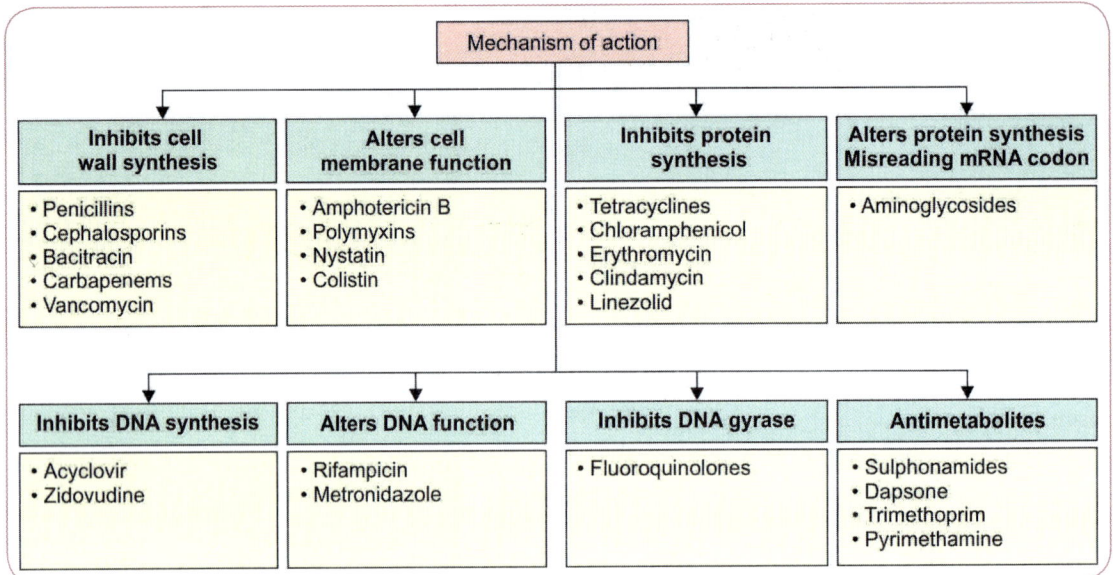

Figure 1: Classification based on mechanism of action

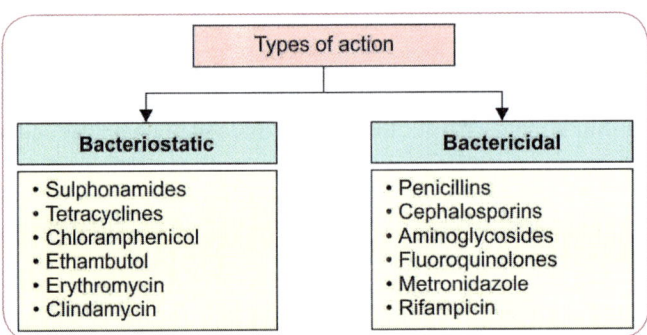

Figure 2: Classification based on types of action

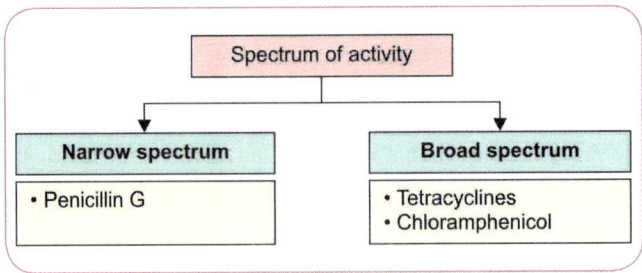

Figure 3: Classification based on spectrum of activity

■ RESISTANCE TO ANTIMICROBIAL AGENTS

Resistance means unresponsiveness of a microorganism to an antimicrobial agent.

A similar term used in humans is 'tolerance', where a higher dose is required (with time) to produce the same pharmacological response.

Resistance can be of 2 types: natural or acquired (Table 1).

TABLE 1	Types of resistance
Natural	• The microbe was always resistant to the AMA • It is usually genetically determined and the microbe lacks the target site or metabolic process affected • Example—Gram-negative bacilli are not affected by penicillin G
Acquired	• The microbe was initially responsive to the AMA • It later becomes resistant due to the use of AMA • Example—Gonococci resistance to sulphonamides and penicillin G

The microbes may develop resistance (to the AMA) by mutation or by gene transfer.

Mutation

It is a change that occurs spontaneously and randomly in the DNA of a microbe.

It is not induced by the AMA *per se*. However, any sensitive microbe colony contains a few mutant microbes, which require a higher AMA concentration for their inhibition.

During the course of AMA therapy, the sensitive microbes die but the mutant microbes (that require a higher drug concentration) survive, and they then get a chance to flourish in the absence of sensitive microbes. This is called selection of the mutants. It will then appear that with time, the sensitive strains have been replaced by mutant strains.

Mutation and resistance can be single step or multistep.

Gene Transfer

The transfer of resistance genes from one microbe to another can occur by the following methods:

Conjugation

It is the transfer of resistance gene from one bacteria to another by direct contact through sex pilus or bridge. Multiple drug resistance usually occurs through conjugation.

It commonly occurs among gram-negative bacilli. The frequent site is the colon where large varieties of gram-negative bacilli come in close contact. Example: *E. coli* resistance to streptomycin, typhoid bacilli resistance to chloramphenicol.

Transduction

It is the transfer of resistance gene from one bacteria to another by a bacteriophage. Bacteriophage is a virus that infects the bacterium. Example: *Staphylococcus aureus* resistance to various AMAs.

Transformation

It is the release of resistance gene into the environment (i.e. the medium), by the resistant bacteria. This is taken up by other sensitive bacteria which then become resistant. Example: *Streptococcus pneumonia* resistance to penicillin G.

Mechanism of Resistance to AMAs

Production of an Enzyme that Inactivates the AMA

The resistant microbe produces an enzyme that inactivates or destroys the AMA. Examples include:
- *Staphylococcus aureus, Neisseria gonorrhoea, Haemophilus influenzae* etc. produce β lactamases that inactivate penicillins and cephalosporins.
- Certain gram-positive and negative bacteria produce enzymes which inactivate chloramphenicol and aminoglycosides.

Inhibiting Drug Accumulation in the Microbe

The drug accumulation inside the microbe is prevented. Examples include:
- **Decreased influx:** Specific channels or 'porins' that initially were used to concentrate the AMA inside the cell, are gradually not formed by the microbe. For example, some gram-negative bacteria block the inflow of hydrophilic AMA such as penicillins.
- **Increased efflux:** Efflux pumps in the cell membrane of many bacteria pump out chemicals and protect them. E.g. resistance of many gram-positive and negative bacteria to tetracyclines, fluoroquinolones, erythromycin etc. occur by this mechanism.

Modification of the Binding Site

The common examples where alteration in the binding protein leads to resistance includes:
- Modification of the penicillin binding protein (PBP) in certain *Streptococcus pneumoniae* that does not bind penicillin.
- Modification of RNA polymerase in certain *Staphylococcus aureus* and *E. coli* that does not bind rifampicin.

Development of an Alternative Metabolic Pathway

As an example, bacteria resistant to sulphonamides start utilizing preformed folic acid instead of synthesizing it from PABA.

Cross Resistance

When a microorganism become resistant to one AMA, it may also simultaneously become resistant to other chemically related AMAs. This phenomenon is known as cross resistance. Cross resistance can be one-way or two-way (Table 2).

TABLE 2	Types of cross resistance
Types of cross resistance	**Example**
One-way	Neomycin → Streptomycin
Two-way	Erythromycin ⇔ Clindamycin

In one-way cross resistance, an organism resistant to neomycin is also resistant to streptomycin; but an organism resistant to streptomycin may still be sensitive to neomycin.

In two-way cross resistance, an organism resistant to erythromycin is resistant to clindamycin and the one resistant to clindamycin is resistant to erythromycin.

Cross resistance is considered as complete when resistance to one member confers resistance to all the other members in the group, e.g. resistance to one sulfonamide results in resistance to all other sulfonamides.

Prevention of Development of Resistance to AMA

The resistance can be prevented by the following measures:
- Preventing indiscriminate, inadequate or prolonged use of an AMA
- Selecting an appropriate AMA
- Employing rapidly acting and narrow-spectrum AMA, wherever possible
- Using proper combination of AMAs, e.g. in tuberculosis, multidrug therapy is employed to prevent the development of resistance.

SUPERINFECTION (SUPRAINFECTION)

It refers to the appearance of a new infection because of the use of antimicrobial therapy. It is caused by a different microbial agent than that of the primary disease.

Most AMAs cause some alteration of normal bacterial flora of the body. This alteration is much more pronounced with broad-spectrum antibiotics—tetracyclines, chloramphenicol, ampicillin, amoxicillin etc.

These AMAs alter the normal microbial flora leading to breakdown of the host defence system. In this situation, pathogenic microorganisms invade the body leading to superinfection.

Mechanism of Superinfection

Superinfection can result by the following mechanisms (Figure 4):

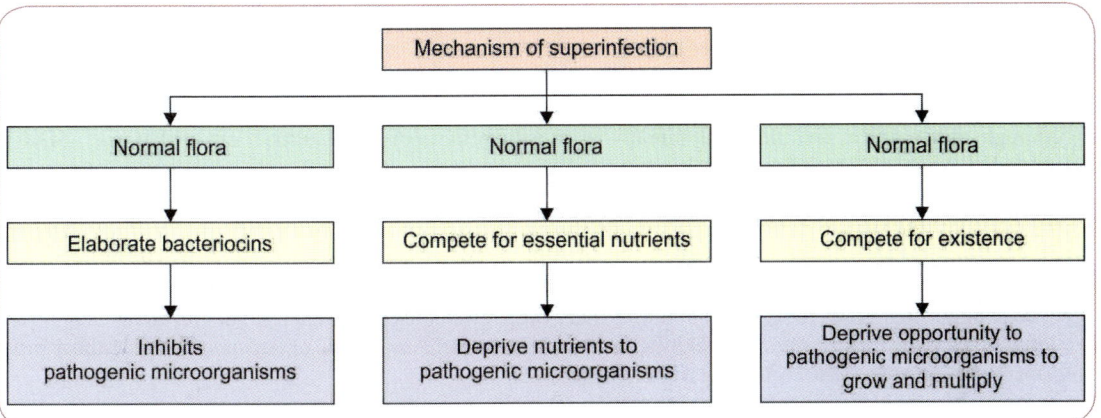

Figure 4: Mechanism of superinfection

Normal flora inhibits the growth of pathogenic microorganisms by the above mechanisms. Hence, in the absence of normal flora, pathogenic microorganisms multiply and grow and result in superinfection.

The sites commonly involved in superinfection are those which usually harbor commensal organisms e.g. intestines, pharynx, respiratory tract, skin, genitourinary tract etc.

The superinfections are much more difficult to treat than the primary infections. The common microorganisms causing superinfections and their treatment are mentioned in Figure 5.

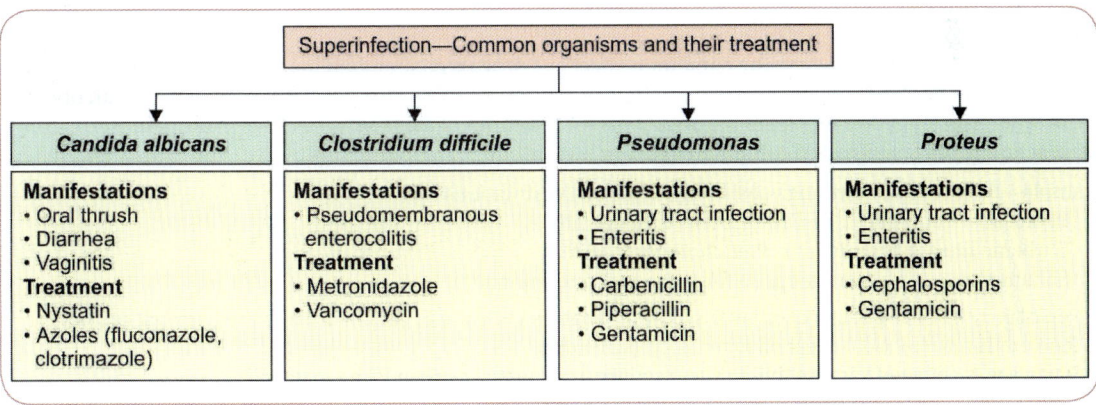

Figure 5: Superinfection—Common organisms and their treatment

Factors Predisposing to Superinfection

Superinfection commonly occurs when the host defense or immune system is compromised. Some of these conditions include:
- Diabetes mellitus
- Prolonged corticosteroid therapy
- Acquired immunodeficiency syndrome (AIDS)
- Malignancies

Actions to Minimize Superinfection

Superinfection can be minimized by:
o Using specific (narrow-spectrum) AMAs
o Avoiding indiscriminate or unnecessary use of AMAs
o Avoiding prolonged use of AMAs.

COMBINED USE OF ANTIMICROBIAL AGENTS

It refers to the simultaneous use of 2 or more AMAs for the treatment of specific infections.

Although single-agent antimicrobial therapy is mostly preferred; combination of 2 or more AMAs is recommended in specific scenarios:

Advantages of Antimicrobial Combinations

To Broaden the Spectrum of Action for Polymicrobial (Mixed) Infections

Infections of abdomen, brain, lung, peritoneum, urinary tract, gynecological, diabetes foot etc. are usually mixed infections. This means that they are caused by a variety of aerobic and anaerobic organisms. Therefore, 2 or more AMAs are required to cover the entire spectrum of organisms.

Example—Metronidazole + ceftriaxone in abdominal sepsis or brain abscess

To Broaden the Spectrum of Action for Initial Treatment of Severe Infections Till Causative Organism is Not Known

For empirical therapy, combination of drugs covering gram-positive and gram-negative organisms is usually employed, because the causative organism is unknown.

Example—Cephalosporin + aminoglycoside + metronidazole for severe abdominal infections

Later, when the causative organism becomes known, the AMA should be chosen as per the organism type and susceptibility.

To Attain Synergism

Synergy refers to a situation where the combined effect of 2 drugs is greater than the sum of their individual effects (i.e. supra-additive effect).

In synergism, one AMA sensitizes the organisms to the actions of the other AMA. This may manifest as stronger lethal action of the combination compared to either AMA alone.

Example—Beta lactam + aminoglycoside in the following situations:
o Penicillin + gentamicin for *Enterococcus* endocarditis*
o Carbenicillin + gentamicin for *Pseudomonas* infection
o Sulfamethoxazole + trimethoprim for *P. jirovecii* pneumonia**

* Penicillin by inhibiting bacterial cell wall synthesis, enables the entry of gentamicin into the bacterial cell, which then exerts a bactericidal effect on *Enterococci* (synergism).
** Synergism is obtained because these drugs produce a sequential block in folate metabolism.

To Prevent Emergence of Resistance

In conditions such as tuberculosis, leprosy, AIDS etc., multiple AMAs are given together to prevent the emergence of resistance.

It is more relevant in chronic infections that require long-term therapy. It is less relevant in acute and brief infections.

To Reduce Adverse Effects

The adverse effects can be reduced only if the combined AMAs are synergistic that permits reduction in dosage.

It is of relevance in cases of AMAs having narrow margin of safety and a high propensity of adverse effects.

Examples:

o Penicillin + streptomycin in SABE
o Amphotericin B + flucytosine in cryptococcal meningitis

Disadvantages of Antimicrobial Combinations

Some of the disadvantages of antimicrobial combinations include:

o Increased toxicity
o Increased frequency of superinfection
o Irrational use of AMA may lead to development of resistance
o Increased cost.

CHEMOPROPHYLAXIS

Chemoprophylaxis is the use of AMAs either to prevent infection in a person who is not yet infected, or to prevent development of symptomatic disease in an already infected person. Chemoprophylaxis may be classified as:

Prophylaxis against Specific Infections

The prophylaxis regimens commonly used against some specific infections are mentioned in Table 3.

TABLE 3	Prophylaxis regimens against specific infections
Disease	**Chemoprophylaxis**
Tuberculosis	• INH (5 mg/kg) alone for 6 months or • INH (5 mg/kg) + rifampicin (10 mg/kg) for 6 months
Meningococcal meningitis	• Rifampicin 600 mg orally, 12 hourly for 4 doses (most effective drug) • Ciprofloxacin 500 mg orally single dose (alternative) • Ceftriaxone 250 mg parenterally single dose (alternative)
Rheumatic fever	• Benzathine penicillin 12 lac IU given every 4 weeks (drug of choice for preventing recurrences)
Endocarditis (drugs given ~1 hour before surgical procedure)	Treatment of choice • Amoxicillin 2 g orally • Ampicillin 2 g IV/IM (if unable to take oral amoxicillin) Penicillin allergy • Clindamycin 600 mg orally • Cephalexin 2 g orally • Azithromycin 500 mg orally Penicillin allergy and unable to take oral medication • Clindamycin 600 mg IV • Cefazolin or ceftriaxone 1 g IV
Malaria	• Chloroquine—300 mg once weekly • Mefloquine—250 mg once weekly
Pneumocystis jirovecii infection	• Cotrimoxazole is used to prevent *P. jirovecii* pneumonia in AIDS patients

Prevention of Infection in High Risk Conditions

Prophylaxis may be used to protect the predisposed patients who are at high-risk for developing the infection. Some examples are mentioned below:

o Prevent endocarditis in patients with damaged heart valves when surgical procedure is undertaken (Figure 6). Clindamycin or amoxicillin may be given a few hours before to a few hours after surgery.

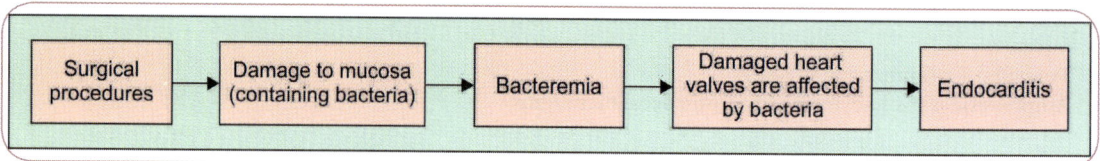

Figure 6: Mechanism of endocarditis in a patient undergoing surgical procedure

○ Prevent urinary tract infections in patients with abnormalities of the urinary tract: nitrofurantoin or cotrimoxazole may be given for prolonged periods.

○ Prevent respiratory tract and other infections in immunocompromised patients (e.g. long-term steroid use, neutropenic, organ transplant patients etc.): beta lactam + aminoglycoside (covering both gram +ve and -ve bacteria) are often used.

SELECTION OF ANTIMICROBIAL AGENTS

Once it is confirmed that the patient would require a systemic AMA, the next step is to select an appropriate AMA from the large number of options available. The AMA selection depends upon the patient's characteristics, the drug's features and the microorganisms involved.

Some of the factors involved in selection of a suitable AMA are mentioned below (Figure 7).

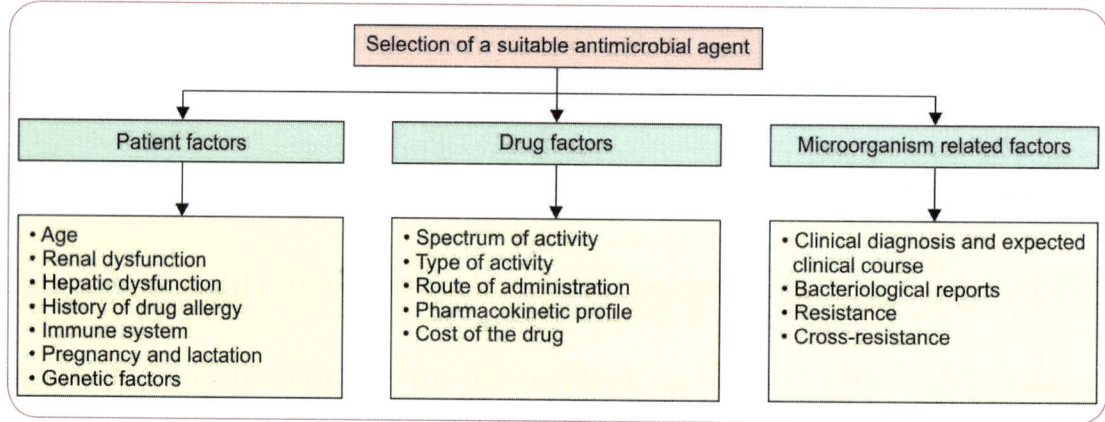

Figure 7: Selection of antimicrobial agents

PATIENT FACTORS

Age

Age affects the kinetics of several AMAs. The common examples are mentioned in Table 4.

TABLE 4	AMA selection - effect of age
Chloramphenicol use in newborn	**Gray baby syndrome** The hepatic metabolism and renal excretion processes in the newborn are poorly developed.
Sulfonamide use in newborn	**Kernicterus** Sulfonamide displaces bilirubin from protein-binding sites resulting in an elevation of plasma bilirubin, which crosses the blood-brain barrier (BBB) to cause kernicterus. This is because the BBB is poorly developed in the newborn, especially if premature.
Aminoglycoside use in the elderly	**Ototoxicity and nephrotoxicity:** Renal function declines with advancing age; hence, clearance of aminoglycoside is decreased in the elderly, resulting in an increased half-life.

Renal Dysfunction

Renal impairment may lead to accumulation of drugs that are eliminated by the kidneys. This leads to toxicity of these drugs.

Therefore, aminoglycosides, cephalosporins, amphotericin B, vancomycin etc. should either be avoided or if used, their dose should be reduced.

Hepatic Dysfunction

Hepatic impairment may lead to accumulation of drugs that are extensively metabolized by the liver.

Therefore, rifampicin, pyrazinamide, erythromycin, tetracyclines etc. should either be avoided or if used, their dose should be reduced.

History of Drug Allergy

Any history of allergy to previous drug exposure should be obtained. In case, a drug has previously caused an allergic reaction, it must be avoided. The AMAs that frequently cause drug allergy are beta lactams, sulphonamides, fluoroquinolones etc.

Immune System

An intact immune system is required for eliminating the infections from the body.

Therefore, in immunocompromised patients (AIDS, neutropenia, leukemia, diabetics etc.), bacteriostatic drugs may not be adequate and bactericidal drugs may be frequently required. Further, higher doses of bactericidal drugs are required for a longer duration to treat infections.

Pregnancy

Most of the AMAs cross the placental barrier. They may therefore adversely affect the developing fetus. The AMAs should by and large, be avoided in pregnancy.

However, penicillins, cephalosporins and erythromycin may be relatively safer as compared to the other AMAs.

Example—Tetracyclines (if used during pregnancy), may cause teeth and bone abnormalities in the newborn, and hepatotoxicity and renal toxicity in the mother.

Genetic Factors

Primaquine, pyrimethamine, sulfonamides, nitrofurantoin, fluoroquinolones etc. may cause hemolysis in patients with G6PD deficiency, and should be avoided.

DRUG FACTORS

Spectrum of Activity

○ **For decisive therapy (when the causative organism is known):** A narrow-spectrum AMA which selectively inhibits the concerned organism is preferred. It is more effective than the broad-spectrum AMA. Also, it is less likely to alter the normal flora of the body.
○ **For empirical therapy (when the causative organism is not known):** A broad-spectrum AMA is preferred so that the causative organism is more likely to be covered under its broad-spectrum. However, as soon as the bacteriological diagnosis is available, it is advisable to shift to the narrow-spectrum AMA that specifically affects the causative organism.

Type of Activity

Bactericidal drugs directly kill bacteria and decrease their number. Bacteriostatic drugs inhibit the growth and multiplication of bacteria (prevents the increase in their number) until the body's immune system eliminates the organism.

In immunocompromised conditions, bactericidal drugs should be used, as the host defenses against the bacteria are impaired.

Route of Administration

Many AMAs are available for oral as well as parenteral administration. However, the AMA is selected based on the site and severity of infection.

For mild infections, an oral AMA is usually preferred; however, for severe infections (e.g. meningitis, sepsis, endocarditis etc.), parenteral AMA is preferred.

Pharmacokinetics

The AMA should penetrate to the site of infection for exerting an antimicrobial effect. This depends on the pharmacokinetic profile of the AMA.

Example—A highly lipid soluble and unionized AMA penetrates the blood-brain barrier (BBB) and is effective in the treatment of brain infections.

Penicillins and aminoglycosides poorly penetrate the BBB (unless the meninges are inflamed and there is a breach in the BBB) while metronidazole, chloramphenicol, ciprofloxacin, ceftriaxone etc. effectively penetrate the BBB.

Cost of the Drug

The cost of therapy should be borne in mind; more expensive AMAs should not be routinely used when less expensive and effective alternatives are available.

MICROORGANISM RELATED FACTORS

Clinical Diagnosis and Expected Clinical Course

In certain situations, the clinical diagnosis can guide the AMA to be selected. This is because the infecting organism and its AMA sensitivity is not variable e.g. syphilis, diphtheria, trachoma etc.

Bacteriological Reports

The bacteriological report is necessary in cases where no guess can be made about the infecting organism or its AMA sensitivity. Examples include meningitis, osteomyelitis, pneumonia, wound infection etc.

In these situations, empirical therapy with broad-spectrum AMAs should be initiated based on the clinical judgement. Later, when the bacteriological report regarding the causative organism becomes available, the AMA should be selected accordingly.

Resistance and Cross-Resistance

The resistance and cross-resistance of the organism (to various AMAs) must be considered while selecting an AMA for treating an infection. Example—while treating staphylococcal infections, if penicillin resistance is present, alternative AMAs should be selected.

COMMON CLASSES OF BACTERIA

The common classes of bacteria are mentioned in Figure 8.

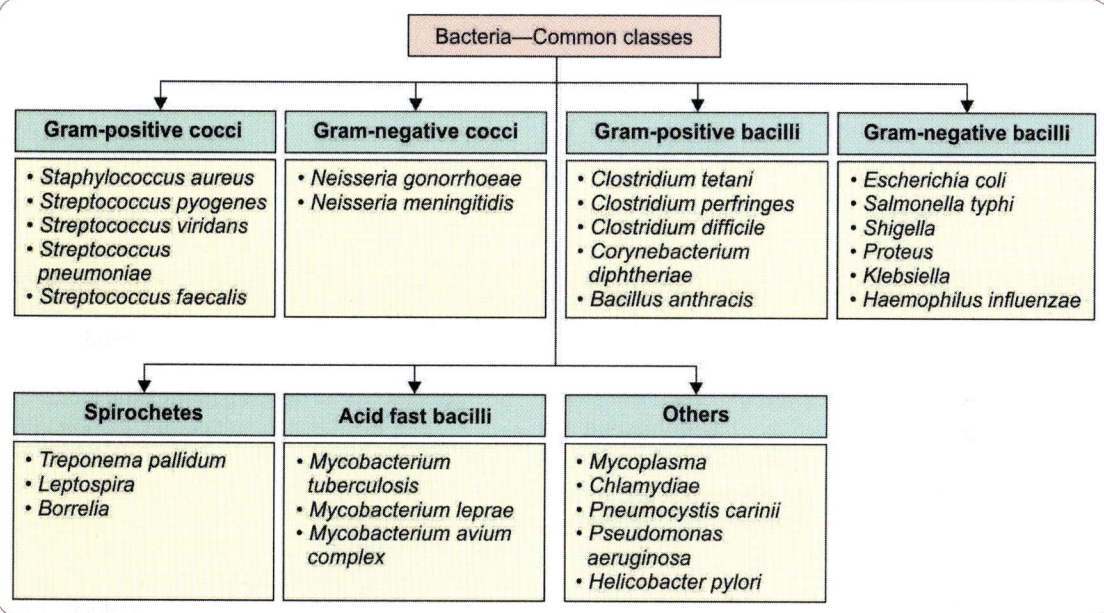

Figure 8: Common classes of bacteria

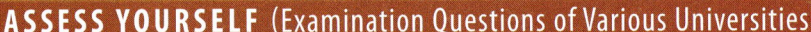

ASSESS YOURSELF (Examination Questions of Various Universities)

1. Drug resistance
2. Superinfections with antimicrobial therapy
3. Chemoprophylaxis
4. Discuss factors important in the choice of antimicrobial regime, giving suitable examples
5. Resistance to antimicrobial agents

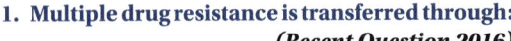

MULTIPLE CHOICE QUESTIONS

1. Multiple drug resistance is transferred through:
   (Recent Question 2016)
   a. Transduction   b. Transformation
   c. Conjugation   d. Mutation

2. Which of the following antibiotics is a cell wall synthesis inhibitor? *(Recent Question 2016)*
   a. Streptomycin
   b. Penicillin G
   c. Erythromycin
   d. Chloramphenicol

3. Gray baby syndrome is caused by:
   (Recent Question 2016)
   a. Chlorpromazine
   b. Chloramphenicol
   c. Phenytoin
   d. Gentamycin

4. A bactericidal drug would be preferred over a bacteriostatic drug in a patient with:
   (Recent Question 2016)
   a. Neutropenia
   b. Cirrhosis
   c. Pneumonia
   d. Heart disease

5. Drug acting by inhibiting cell wall synthesis:
   (Recent Question 2016)
   a. Erythromycin
   b. Cephalosporins
   c. Chloramphenicol
   d. Sulphonamides

Ans.

| 1. | (c) | 2. | (b) | 3. | (b) | 4. | (a) | 5. | (b) |

51 | Sulfonamides and Cotrimoxazole

SULFONAMIDES

Sulfonamides are considered as synthetic derivatives of *para*-amino benzene sulfonamide (sulfanilamide).

Sulfonamide was first clinically used by Domagk in 1930s. He received the noble prize for discovering the therapeutic value of sulfonamide.

Classification

A classification of sulfonamides is mentioned in Figure 1.

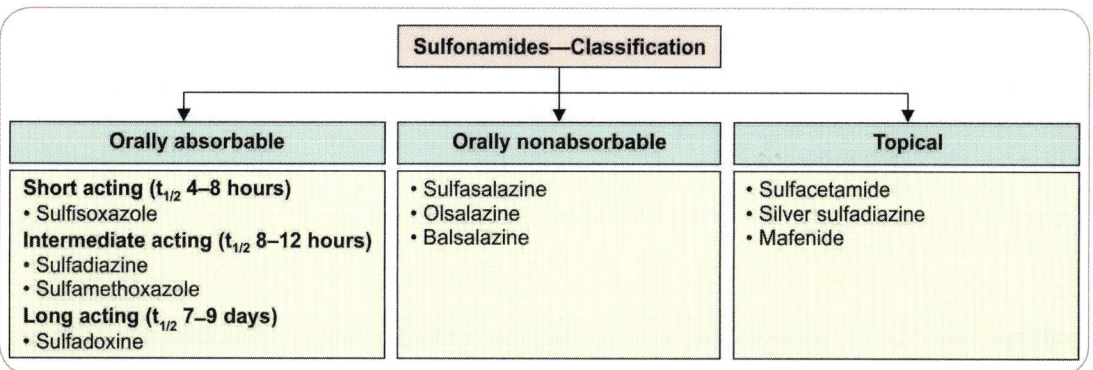

Figure 1: Classification of sulfonamides

Antibacterial Spectrum

Sulfonamides inhibit a wide range of gram-positive and gram-negative bacteria. However, resistance rapidly develops, and many bacteria have now become resistant.

Hence, the utility of sulfonamides has greatly diminished over the years, both because of development of resistance as well as availability of safer and effective alternatives.

The bacteria that may be still sensitive include *Streptococcus pyogenes*, *Haemophilus influenzae*, *Haemophilus ducreyi*, *Nocardia*, *Actinomyces*, *Toxoplasma gondii*, and *Chlamydia trachomatis*.

Mechanism of Action

Bacteria cannot utilize the preformed folic acid from exogenous (outside) sources. They synthesize their own folic acid from *para*-aminobenzoic acid (PABA) for growth and multiplication.

Sulfonamides are structural analogs of PABA; hence, they competitively inhibit the enzyme dihydropteroate synthase, and prevent the formation of folic acid. Sulfonamides are therefore, bacteriostatic drugs (Figure 2).

Host (mammalian) cells cannot synthesize their own folic acid; instead they take up preformed folic acid from the surrounding medium. Hence, sulfonamides selectively inhibit the bacterial cells and not the host cells.

The bacteriostatic effect of sulfonamides can be competitively reversed by PABA. Hence, in the presence of pus and tissue extracts, sulfonamides are not effective (because pus contains PABA, purines and thymidine).

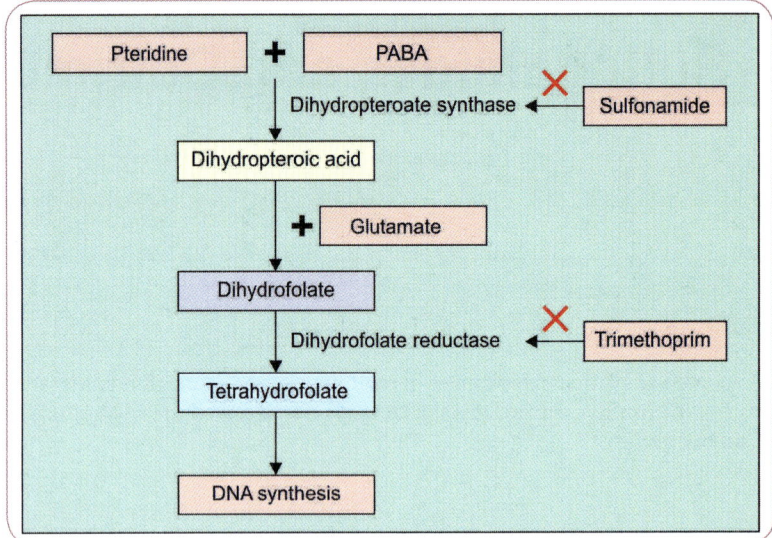

Figure 2: Bacterial folic acid synthesis and mechanism of action of sulfonamides

Resistance

Many bacteria that were initially sensitive have developed resistance to sulfonamides over the years. The mechanism of development of resistance include:

- Excess production of PABA
- Reduced affinity for the enzyme dihydropteroate synthase
- Development of an alternate metabolic pathway for folic acid synthesis
- Increase efflux of the drug

Pharmacokinetics

All sulfonamides (except those used for topical and local bowel effects) are well absorbed from the GIT. They are variably bound to plasma proteins, mainly albumin. Sulfonamides are distributed throughout the body tissues including CSF. They readily cross the placental barrier and reach the fetal circulation.

Sulfonamides are metabolized in the liver by acetylation. The metabolites are inactive but contribute to the adverse effects. Sulfonamides are excreted partly as unchanged drug and partly as metabolites, mainly in the urine.

In acidic urine, some of the older sulfonamides are insoluble and may precipitate leading to the formation of crystalline deposits. This can result in urinary obstruction.

Adverse Effects

Some of the key adverse effects of sulfonamides are mentioned in Figure 3.

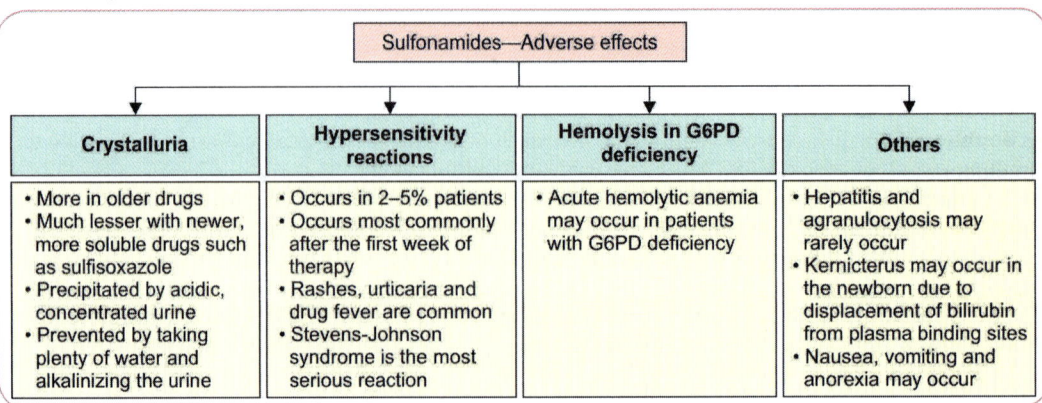

Figure 3: Adverse effects of sulfonamides

Drug Interactions

Sulfonamides potentiate the effects of oral anticoagulants, sulphonylureas, phenytoin and methotrexate by inhibiting their metabolism as well as displacing them from protein binding sites.

Clinical Uses

Sulfonamides are rarely used alone for systemic infections because of rapid development of resistance and availability of effective alternate antimicrobial agents. They are mostly used along with other drugs in these situations.

Some of the systemic and topical/local uses of sulfonamides are mentioned in Table 1.

TABLE 1	Clinical uses of sulfonamides
Toxoplasmosis	Sulfadiazine + pyrimethamine
Plasmodium falciparum malaria	Sulfadoxine + pyrimethamine
Pneumocystis jirovecii infection	Sulfamethoxazole + trimethoprim
Nocardiosis	Sulfamethoxazole + trimethoprim
Eye infections	Sulfacetamide (sodium salt) is preferred in ocular infections because of the following reasons: • High aqueous solubility • Neutral pH, hence nonirritating to the eye (other sulfonamides have alkaline pH and are highly irritating) • High penetration into ocular tissues • Less chances of hypersensitivity reactions
Preventing infection in burns	Silver sulfadiazine and mafenide are applied topically to prevent development of infection in burns • It is not used to treat an already established infection • Silver sulfadiazine slowly releases silver ions that are specifically toxic to the organisms
Inflammatory bowel disease (ulcerative colitis) and rheumatoid arthritis	Sulfasalazine is broken down by intestinal bacteria into sulfapyridine and mesalamine (5-aminosalicylic acid, 5-ASA) • 5-ASA is the effective agent in inflammatory bowel disease • Sulfapyridine is responsible for the adverse effects

COTRIMOXAZOLE

Cotrimoxazole is a fixed-dose combination (FDC) of sulfamethoxazole and trimethoprim in the ratio 5:1.

A **cotrimoxazole tablet** contains 400 mg of sulfamethoxazole + 80 mg of trimethoprim.

A **double strength cotrimoxazole tablet** is also available which contains 800 mg of sulfamethoxazole + 160 mg of trimethoprim.

Reason for Making the FDC of Sulfamethoxazole and Trimethoprim in the Ratio of 5:1

To achieve synergism, the ratio of concentrations of these 2 drugs in blood and tissues should be 20:1. This is possible if the ratio in the formulation is kept as 5:1 i.e. 20:4 (Figure 4).

Reason for making FDC (sulfamethoxazole and trimethoprim) ratio of 5:1

- For synergism, the ratio of concentration of these 2 drugs in blood and tissues should be 20:1. This ratio is equal to the ratio of the minimum inhibitory concentration (MIC) of these 2 drugs acting separately.
- As trimethoprim is more lipid-soluble than sulfamethoxazole, it has a larger volume of distribution and attains lower plasma concentration.
- Therefore, to achieve a ratio of 20:1 in blood and tissues, a higher concentration of trimethoprim is required in the FDC formulation.
- Hence, 5 parts of sulfamethoxazole is given along with 1 part of trimethoprim (as in the FDC).

Figure 4: Fixed-dose combination (sulfamethoxazole and trimethoprim) ratio of 5:1

Mechanism of Action

Cotrimoxazole produces a sequential block of folic acid synthesis (Figure 2). This means that the two components in cotrimoxazole, sulfamethoxazole and trimethoprim inhibit two subsequent steps in the same metabolic pathway. This results in synergistic effect.

In this case, sulfamethoxazole inhibits dihydropteroate synthase, while trimethoprim inhibits dihydrofolate reductase.

The pharmacokinetics of these 2 drugs are almost identical i.e. both have a half-life of around 10 hours. The advantages of combining sulfamethoxazole and trimethoprim are mentioned in Figure 5.

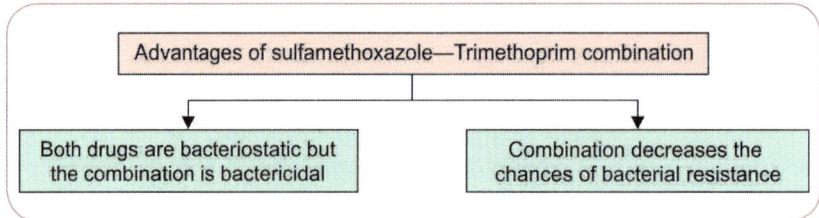

Figure 5: Sulfamethoxazole—Trimethoprim combination

Pharmacokinetics

Cotrimoxazole is well-absorbed orally. It is also available for parenteral use. It is distributed widely throughout the body tissues including the CSF and sputum. Trimethoprim (being a weak base) gets concentrated in prostatic and vaginal fluids which have an acidic environment than plasma. Hence, it is preferred in prostatic and vaginal infections.

The volume of distribution of trimethoprim is approximately 9 times than sulfamethoxazole. Cotrimoxazole is metabolized in the liver and excreted in the urine; therefore, dose reduction may be necessary in patients with renal impairment.

Adverse Effects

Cotrimoxazole is well tolerated. However, all the adverse effects caused by sulfonamides can be caused by cotrimoxazole as well.

The most common adverse effect includes skin reactions. The incidence of skin reactions is approximately 3 times higher with cotrimoxazole than with sulfamethoxazole. Rarely serious reactions such as exfoliative dermatitis, Stevens-Johnson syndrome or toxic epidermal necrolysis may occur.

The other adverse effects include GIT disturbances (nausea, vomiting, stomatitis etc.), megaloblastic anemia in folate deficient persons, bone marrow suppression and hepatitis.

Clinical Uses

Urinary Tract Infections (UTI)

Cotrimoxazole is effective in the treatment of acute uncomplicated UTI, chronic recurrent UTI in females and bacterial prostatitis (Figure 6).

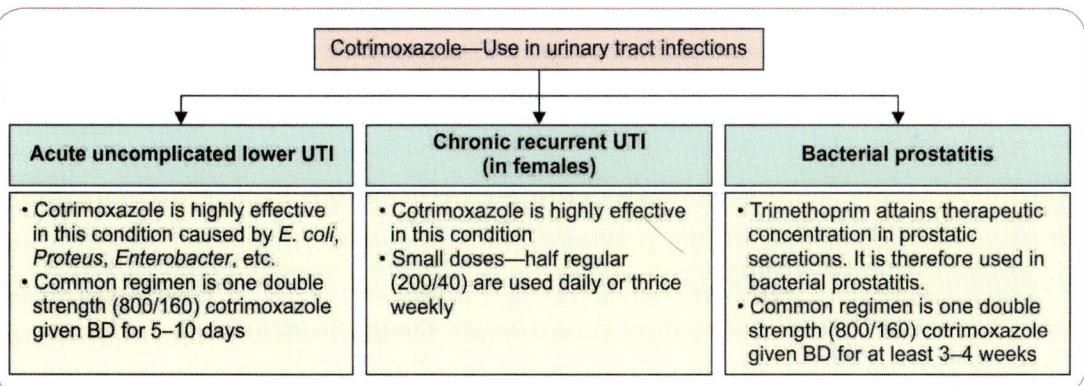

Figure 6: Cotrimoxazole use in urinary tract infections

Respiratory Tract Infections

Cotrimoxazole is effective in acute exacerbations of chronic bronchitis. One double strength (DS) cotrimoxazole twice a day is commonly used.

Cotrimoxazole is commonly used in acute otitis media in children and acute maxillary sinusitis in adults due to *Haemophilus influenzae* and *Streptococcus pneumococcus*.

Pneumocystis jirovecii Pneumonia

Cotrimoxazole is the drug of choice in *P. jirovecii* pneumonia in patients with neutropenia or AIDS. Cotrimoxazole is used both therapeutically as well as prophylactically. High doses are required.

Gastrointestinal Tract Infections

Cotrimoxazole is a second-choice drug in the following conditions:
- Typhoid fever—fluoroquinolones or ceftriaxone is the treatment of choice
- Shigellosis, traveller's diarrhea (due to *E. coli*), *Y. enterocolitica*—fluoroquinolones are the treatment of choice.

Nocardiosis

Cotrimoxazole is effective in the treatment of nocardiosis. However, it is used as an alternative to first line drugs such as doxycycline and aminoglycosides.

Chancroid

It is used as an alternative to ceftriaxone, azithromycin or fluoroquinolones in the treatment of chancroid caused by *Haemophilus ducreyi*.

ASSESS YOURSELF (Examination Questions of Various Universities)

1. What is cotrimoxazole? Give mechanism of action of cotrimoxazole and clinical uses of cotrimoxazole.

2. Adverse effects of sulfonamides

3. Rationale in the use of cotrimoxazole

MULTIPLE CHOICE QUESTIONS

1. Which among the following is the longest acting sulfonamide? *(Recent Question 2016)*
   a. Sulfisoxazole
   b. Sulfamethoxazole
   c. Sulfadiazine
   d. Sulfadoxine

2. All of the following are topically used sulfonamides except: *(Recent Question 2016)*
   a. Sulfacetamide   b. Sulfasalazine
   c. Silver sulfadiazine   d. Mafenide

3. Which of the following adverse effects is most likely to occur with sulfonamides?
   (Recent Question 2016)
   a. Neurologic effects including headache, dizziness, and lethargy
   b. Hematuria
   c. Fanconi anemia
   d. Skin reactions

4. The combination of trimethoprim and sulfamethoxazole is effective against which of the following opportunistic infections in the AIDS patient? *(Recent Question 2016)*
   a. Disseminated herpes simplex
   b. Cryptococcal meningitis
   c. Pneumocystis jirovecii
   d. Tuberculosis

5. Sulfonamide injection causes decrease in folic acid by: *(Recent Question 2016)*
   a. Competitive inhibition
   b. Noncompetitive inhibition
   c. Uncompetitive inhibition
   d. Allosteric inhibition

6. Composition of double strength septran:
   (Recent Question 2016)
   a. 80 mg trimethoprim + 400 mg
   b. Sulfamethoxazole
   c. 160 mg trimethoprim + 800 mg sulfamethoxazole
   d. 800 mg trimethoprim + 160 mg sulfamethoxazole

7. Mechanism of action of sulfonamides:
   (Recent Question 2016)
   a. Inhibition of cell wall synthesis
   b. Inhibition of formation of folic acid
   c. Inhibition of protein synthesis
   d. Altered DNA gyrase with reduced affinity

8. Which of the following is a side effect of sulfonamide? *(Recent Question 2016)*
   a. Constipation   b. Joint pain
   c. Crystalluria   d. Hyperkalemia

Ans.

1. (d)	2. (b)	3. (d)	4. (c)	5. (a)	6. (c)
7. (b)	8. (c)				

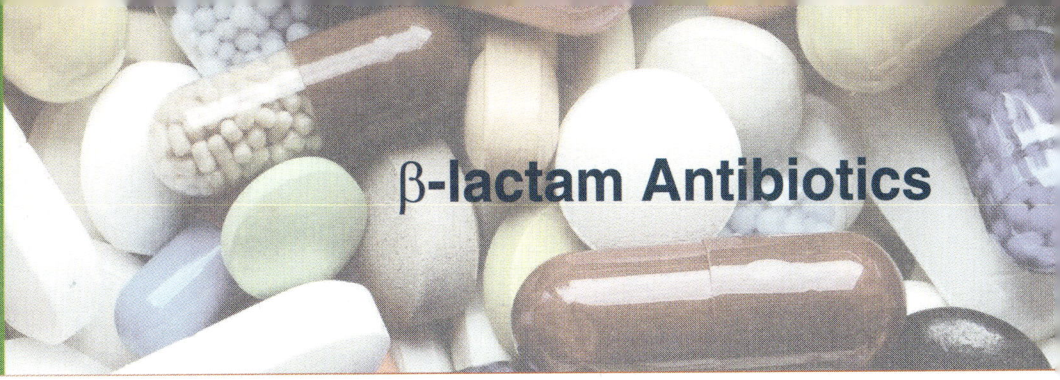

β-lactam Antibiotics

These antibiotics have a β lactam ring in their structure. β-lactam antibiotics include the following (Figure 1):
- Penicillins
- Cephalosporins
- Monobactams
- Carbapenems

β-lactam antibiotics			
Penicillins	**Cephalosporins**	**Monobactams**	**Carbapenems**
• Natural penicillins • Semisynthetic penicillins	• First generation • Second generation • Third generation • Fourth generation • Fifth generation	• Aztreonam	• Imipenem • Meropenem • Doripenem • Faropenem

Figure 1: β-lactam antibiotics

PENICILLIN

Penicillin was discovered by Alexander Fleming. It was initially obtained from the fungus *Penicillium notatum*. It is currently obtained from a mutant of *Penicillium chrysogenum*. Penicillin was the first antibiotic that was clinically used in the year 1941.

Structure

It is a beta lactam antibiotic and hence, has a β lactam ring in its structure. The three key elements in its structure are:
- Thiazolidine ring (contains sulfur)
- β-lactam ring
- Side chains attached to the above via amide linkage

Mechanism of Action

The bacterial cell wall is composed of peptidoglycan, which consists of cross-linked polymers of polysaccharides and polypeptides (Figure 2).

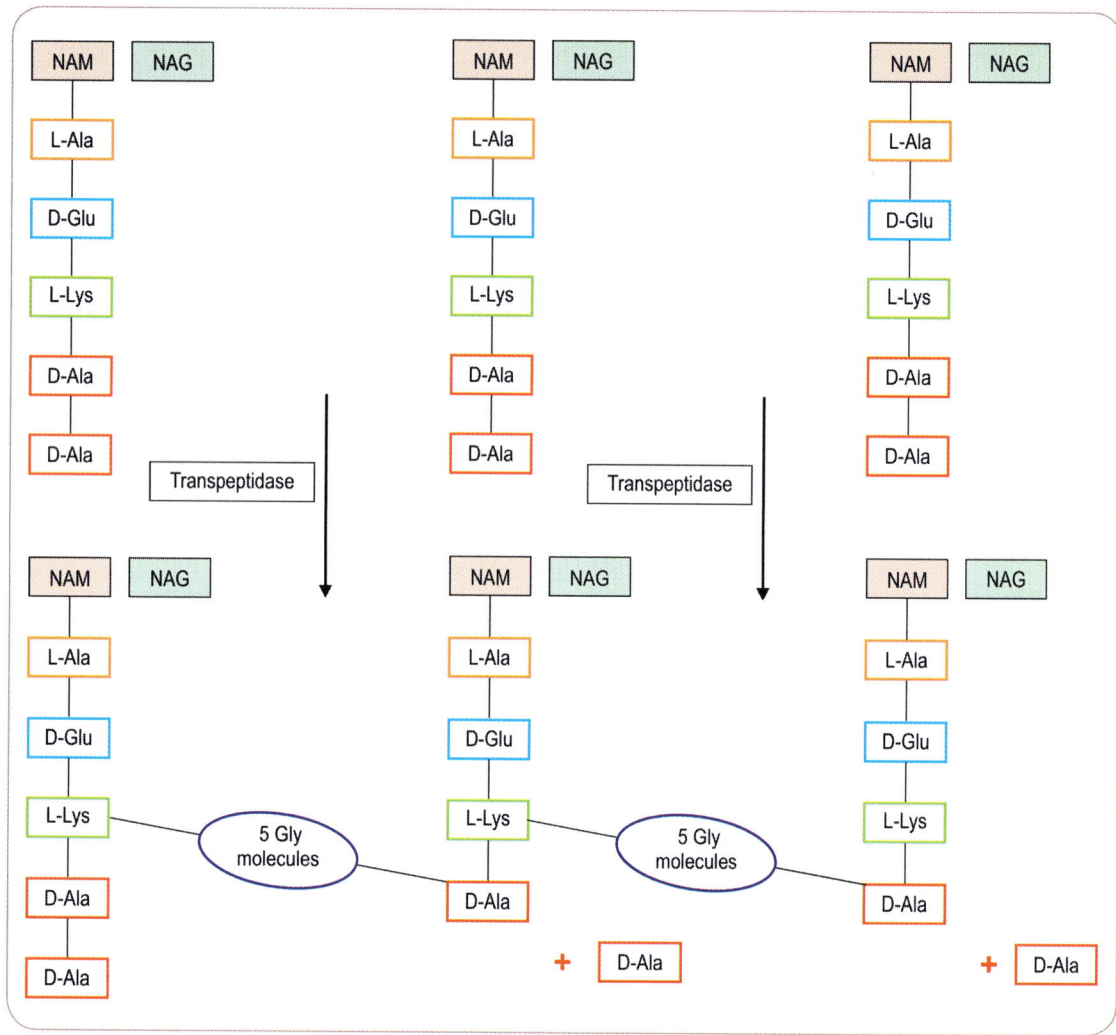

Figure 2: β-lactam antibiotics—mechanism of action

○ The polysaccharides involved are N-acetylmuramic acid (NAM) and N-acetylglucosamine (NAG).

○ The polypeptides involved are 5-amino-acid peptide (Ala-Glu-Lys-Ala-Ala) linked to the polysaccharide NAM. The transpeptidase enzyme cross links the adjacent polypeptides by removing a single amino acid alanine. This cross-linking provides structural integrity and strength to the bacterial cell wall.

β-lactam antibiotics inhibit the synthesis of bacterial (peptidoglycan) cell wall by blocking the transpeptidation reaction.

Therefore, cross-linking between the polypeptides do not take place.

When susceptible bacteria multiply in the presence of β-lactam antibiotics, cell wall synthesis becomes impaired. The interior of the bacteria being hyperosmotic, swell up and burst resulting in bacterial death.

Mechanism of Resistance

The bacteria develop resistance to penicillin in multiple ways as mentioned in Table 1.

TABLE 1	Bacterial resistance to penicillin	
Mechanism	Key action	Examples (some species)
Production of penicillinase (β-lactamase)	Penicillinase open the β-lactam ring of penicillin and hence inactivate the antibiotic	*S. aureus, E. coli, H. influenzae*
Modification of penicillin binding proteins (PBP)	Bacteria have a lower affinity to penicillin	Methicillin-resistant *S. aureus* (MRSA)
Reduced permeability of penicillin to reach PBP	A mutation of the porin channels prevents the penicillin from reaching the site of action	*Pseudomonas aeruginosa*

Classification of Penicillin

A classification of penicillin is mentioned in Table 2.

TABLE 2	Penicillin
Natural penicillins	• **Penicillin G** (Benzyl penicillin) • **Procaine penicillin G** • **Benzathine penicillin G**
Semisynthetic penicillins	• **Acid resistant** ▪ Phenoxymethylpenicillin (Penicillin V) • **Penicillinase resistant** ▪ Methicillin, oxacillin, cloxacillin, dicloxacillin • **Extended spectrum** ▪ Aminopenicillin—ampicillin, amoxicillin ▪ Carboxypenicillin—carbenicillin, ticarcillin ▪ Ureidopenicillin—mezlocillin, piperacillin

PENICILLIN G (BENZYL PENICILLIN)

It is a natural penicillin that has a narrow spectrum of antibacterial activity. It is mainly effective against gram-positive bacteria. Some gram-negative cocci are also sensitive to penicillin G.

Pharmacokinetics

Penicillin G is destroyed by the gastric acid (acid labile); hence, it is usually administered by the parenteral route.

It is excreted rapidly by the kidneys (mainly by tubular secretion); hence, elderly patients or those with impaired renal function will excrete penicillin slowly.

Administration of probenecid can prolong the action of penicillin G because probenecid blocks the tubular secretion of penicillin G.

Adverse Effects

Penicillin G is relatively safe in humans because the peptidoglycan cell wall does not exist in human cells. Some of the key adverse effects are mentioned in Table 3.

TABLE 3	Adverse effects of penicillin
Local and direct adverse effects	• Nausea → oral administration • Pain at injection site → IM administration • Thrombophlebitis → IV administration
Hypersensitivity reactions	**Clinical manifestations** • Skin rashes, dermatitis, bronchospasm, angioedema, urticaria, laryngeal edema, anaphylactic reaction including anaphylactic shock • Anaphylaxis including anaphylactic shock is usually a Type I (IgE mediated) immediate hypersensitivity reaction **Treatment** • It is a medical emergency • Drug therapy includes adrenaline, hydrocortisone, diphenhydramine • Supportive management including airway, breathing and circulation **Prevention** • Awareness of patient's history of prior administration or of allergic reactions • Partial cross reactivity has been observed with penicillin; hence, patients who have experienced hypersensitivity with one type of penicillin should not be administered any other type of penicillin • Sensitivity testing should be performed by an intradermal test • Emergency medications and resuscitation equipment such as adrenaline, hydrocortisone etc. should be kept ready to manage anaphylaxis • Patients having conditions such as asthma, hay fever etc. may be at an increased risk of penicillin hypersensitivity; hence, penicillin G should be avoided in such patients.
Jarisch-Herxheimer reaction	• Administration of penicillin G in a patient of syphilis may lead to sudden release of spirochetal lytic products that can result in shivering, fever, myalgia, exacerbation of lesions and vascular collapse. • The reaction usually lasts for 12–72 hours and does not require cessation of therapy. Aspirin and sedation can be used for the management.

Clinical Uses

The clinical use of penicillin G has decreased due to the risk of hypersensitivity reactions (including anaphylaxis) and the availability of better tolerated antimicrobial agents.

It is indicated for the treatment of infections caused by organisms that are sensitive to clinically administered doses of penicillin. Some of these uses are mentioned in Table 4.

TABLE 4	Clinical uses of penicillin G
Streptococcal infections • E.g. pharyngitis, rheumatic fever, otitis media	
Meningococcal meningitis	
Syphilis • Penicillin G is the drug of choice as *T. pallidum* is very sensitive	
Tetanus and gas gangrene • Antitoxins and supportive therapy is the main treatment • Penicillin G is used as an adjuvant drug	
Pneumococcal infections • Pneumonia, meningitis (only indicated if the organisms are sensitive)	
Gonorrhea • Not a preferred choice due to resistance	

Contd...

Diphtheria
- Antitoxin therapy is the main treatment
- Penicillin G can prevent the carrier state and is an adjuvant drug

Miscellaneous infections
- Anthrax, actinomycosis, trench mouth

Prophylactic therapy
- In patients of rheumatic fever (caused by Streptococci), bacterial endocarditis

SEMISYNTHETIC PENICILLINS

The natural penicillins have some limitations such as:
- Limited oral efficacy due to acid lability
- Narrow antimicrobial spectrum of action (mainly against gram-positive organisms)
- Susceptibility to penicillinase enzymes
- Risk of anaphylaxis—this risk has not been avoided in any preparation

Semisynthetic penicillins were developed in an attempt to overcome some of these limitations.

Acid Resistant—(Penicillin V) Phenoxymethylpenicillin

Phenoxymethylpenicillin is acid stable and hence, has a better oral absorption.

Penicillinase Resistant—Methicillin, Oxacillin, Cloxacillin, Dicloxacillin

These drugs have side chains that protect the β-lactam ring from being damaged by penicillinase produced by Staphylococci.

These drugs are indicated in infections that are caused by penicillinase producing Staphylococci.

Methicillin is administered parenterally (not acid resistant); whereas cloxacillin is acid resistant and hence can be administered orally and parenterally.

Extended Spectrum Aminopenicillin—Ampicillin, Amoxicillin

These drugs have amino substitution in the side chain. Apart from being effective against organisms that are sensitive to penicillin G, they are also effective against gram-negative bacilli such as *H. influenzae, Proteus, E. coli, Shigella* etc.

The key features of ampicillin and amoxicillin are mentioned in Table 5.

TABLE 5	Ampicillin and amoxicillin	
	Ampicillin	**Amoxicillin**
Classification	• Semisynthetic extended spectrum aminopenicillin	• Semisynthetic extended spectrum aminopenicillin
Pharmacokinetics	• Acid stable • Food interferes with absorption • Oral absorption is incomplete • Higher incidence of diarrhea	• Acid stable • Food does not interfere with absorption • Oral absorption is better • Lower incidence of diarrhea
Antimicrobial activity	• More effective against *Shigella*	• Less effective against *Shigella*

Clinical Uses

Bacterial resistance to aminopenicillin has increased; hence their clinical use is justified in scenarios where the bacteria are sensitive to their antimicrobial actions. The clinical uses of ampicillin are mentioned in Table 6.

TABLE 6	Clinical uses of ampicillin
• Urinary tract infections	
• Respiratory tract infections—including sinusitis, bronchitis, otitis media	
• Gonorrhea	
• Cholecystitis—Used because ampicillin achieves high concentration in the bile	
• Subacute bacterial endocarditis (SABE)	
• Meningitis	
• Septicemias and mixed infections	

Adverse Effects

Some of the key adverse effects of ampicillin include the following:
- Diarrhea is a frequent adverse effect
  - Occurs due to incomplete absorption of ampicillin from the GIT
  - It irritates the lower GIT and also causes alteration of the intestinal flora
- Rashes, particularly in patients of AIDS, EBV or leukemia
  - Co-administration of allopurinol increases the incidence of rashes
- Allergic reactions may develop
  - Patients with history of allergic reactions to penicillin may also develop allergic reactions to aminopenicillins
- Failure of oral contraceptives may occur
  - Occurs because ampicillin can inhibit intestinal flora and thereby interfere with deconjugation and enterohepatic cycling of oral contraceptives

Extended Spectrum: Carboxypenicillin—Carbenicillin, Ticarcillin

Carbenicillin

- Has activity against *Pseudomonas and Proteus*
- Inactive orally and hence used parenterally
- High doses may lead to bleeding as it interferes with platelet function
- Used in serious infections in patients of burns, septicemia, urinary tract infections due to susceptible organisms.

Ticarcillin

- More potent than carbenicillin against *Pseudomonas.*

Extended Spectrum: Ureidopenicillins—Mezlocillin, Piperacillin

Piperacillin

- Extended spectrum ureidopenicillins
- Has activity against *Pseudomonas, Klebsiella*
- Used in serious infections in patients of burns, neutropenia/immunocompromised states due to susceptible organisms.

■ BETA LACTAMASE INHIBITORS

β lactamases are enzymes produced by bacteria that open the β-lactam ring of the antibiotics. This leads to the inactivation of β-lactam antibiotics.

β-lactamase inhibitors have a structural resemblance to β-lactam drugs, but do not have any clinically significant antimicrobial action. β-lactamase inhibitors inactivate β lactamases by binding to them. This prevents the inactivation of the β-lactam drugs and increases their antimicrobial activity.

Clavulanic Acid

- Obtained from *Streptomyces clavuligerus*
- Exhibits progressive binding with β lactamase → initially the binding is reversible and later converts to an irreversible covalent binding. It is also called a suicide inhibitor as it gets inactivated after binding to the β lactamase enzymes.
- Pharmacokinetics (elimination $t_{1/2}$ and tissue distribution) is similar to amoxicillin. Therefore, it is used in combination with amoxicillin. The combination is known as "Co-amoxiclav".
- Clinically used along with amoxicillin in skin, soft tissue, respiratory and urinary tract infections.

Sulbactam

- Semisynthetic inhibitor
- Exhibits progressive binding with β-lactamase enzymes
- Combined with ampicillin and used for intra-abdominal and pelvic infections.

Tazobactam

- Pharmacokinetics similar to piperacillin; hence, used in combination with piperacillin
- Clinically used for severe infections due to gram-negative bacteria.

CEPHALOSPORINS

Cephalosporins are semisynthetic antibiotics.

Mechanism of Action

The mechanism of action of cephalosporin is similar to that of penicillin. They inhibit the bacterial cell wall synthesis. All cephalosporins are bactericidal.

Resistance to Cephalosporins

The mechanisms of development of resistance to cephalosporins is similar to that of penicillin.

First Generation Cephalosporins—e.g. Cefazolin, Cephalexin, Cefadroxil

- First generation cephalosporins were developed in 1960s
- High efficacy against gram-positive bacteria
- Low efficacy against gram-negative bacteria
- Cefazolin is highly susceptible to staphylococcal β-lactamase
- Clinical use includes surgical prophylaxis

Second Generation Cephalosporins—e.g. Cefuroxime, Cefaclor

- Second generation cephalosporins were introduced in 1970s
- High efficacy against gram-negative bacteria
- No activity against *Pseudomonas*
- Some drugs are active against anaerobes
- Cefuroxime is resistant to β lactamases produced by gram-negative bacteria
- Clinical uses include gonorrhea and respiratory tract infections.

Third Generation Cephalosporins—e.g. Cefotaxime, Ceftriaxone, Ceftazidime, Cefoperazone

- Third generation cephalosporins were introduced in 1980s
- High efficacy against gram-negative *Enterobacteriaceae*
- Less efficacy against gram-positive cocci and anaerobes
- Are resistant to β lactamases produced by gram-negative bacteria
- Antipseudomonas activity is observed with some drugs
- Cefotaxime is clinically used for meningitis due to gram-negative bacilli, infections in immunocompromised patients, septicemia, serious/life-threatening nosocomial infections

- Ceftriaxone has a longer duration of action and is clinically used in serious infections such as resistant typhoid fever, septicemia, complicated UTIs
- Ceftazidime is effective against *Pseudomonas* infections. Clinical uses include febrile neutropenia in patients with burns, hematological malignancies
- Cefoperazone has high activity against *Pseudomonas* infections.

Fourth Generation Cephalosporins—e.g. Cefepime, Cefpirome

Cefepime

- It was developed in 1990s
- Antimicrobial spectrum similar to third generation cephalosporins
- Resistance to β lactamases is high
- Clinically used in serious infections such as septicemia, nosocomial pneumonia, febrile neutropenia.

Cefpirome

- Clinically used in serious nosocomial infections such as septicemias.

Fifth Generation Cephalosporins - e.g. Ceftaroline, Ceftobiprole

Ceftaroline

- A broad-spectrum cephalosporin with activity against methicillin-resistant *Staphylococcus aureus*.
- Administered intravenously as a prodrug 'ceftaroline fosamil'.
- Apart from its activity against gram-positive bacteria, it also has broad-spectrum gram-negative activity similar to ceftriaxone.
- Currently indicated for the treatment of acute bacterial skin and soft tissue infections as well as community acquired bacterial pneumonia.

Ceftobiprole

- Is a newer cephalosporin currently approved in some countries in Europe.
- Is a broad-spectrum antibiotic effective against many gram-positive and gram-negative bacteria.
- Administered intravenously as a prodrug 'ceftobiprole medocaril'.
- Currently indicated for hospital-acquired bacterial pneumonia and community-acquired bacterial pneumonia.

Adverse Effects of Cephalosporins

Some of the key adverse effects with cephalosporins are mentioned below:

Hypersensitivity Reactions

- Incidence is lower than penicillin
- Some patients have cross reactivity with penicillin
- Manifestations include rashes, angioedema, anaphylaxis

Nephrotoxicity

- Cephaloridine has been withdrawn due to nephrotoxicity
- Cephalothin causes low grade nephrotoxicity

Bleeding

- Commonly seen with cefoperazone and ceftriaxone
- Due to hypoprothrombinemia and is common in patients with malignancies, renal failure or intra-abdominal infections

Disulfiram Like Reaction

○ Observed with cefoperazone

Neutropenia and Thrombocytopenia

○ Observed with ceftazidime

Others

○ Pain at the injection site
○ Diarrhea, vomiting

MONOBACTAMS—AZTREONAM

It is a β-lactam antibiotic. It is called a monobactam because it has one ring in its structure.

The antimicrobial spectrum is limited to aerobic gram-negative bacilli (such as *Pseudomonas, H. influenzae, Enterobacteriaceae* and *N. gonorrhoeae*).

It does not have any activity against gram-positive bacteria or anaerobes.

An advantage of aztreonam is that there is a lack of cross reactivity with other β-lactam antibiotics (except possibly ceftazidime); hence, it may be used in patients who are allergic to penicillin.

Clinical uses include nosocomial infections such as urinary tract and gastrointestinal tract infections.

CARBAPENEMS

Imipenem

It is a β-lactam antibiotic and the mechanism of action is to inhibit bacterial cell wall synthesis.

Imipenem has a broad spectrum of action and is effective against gram-positive cocci, gram-negative bacteria (e.g. *P. aeruginosa, Enterobacteriaceae*) and anaerobes (*C. difficile, B. fragilis*). It is resistant to most types of β lactamases.

Imipenem is administered along with cilastatin because cilastatin prevents the hydrolysis of imipenem by dehydropeptidase I enzyme and increases urinary concentration of imipenem Figure 3.

Combination of imipenem and cilastatin

- Imipenem is hydrolyzed by dehydropeptidase I enzyme in the renal tubules.
- Cilastatin is a reversible inhibitor of dehydropeptidase I enzyme. The pharmacokinetics of cilastatin is similar to imipenem (both have a $t_{1/2}$ of 1 hour).
- Hence, cilastatin and imipenem are combined to increase the urinary concentration of imipenem.

Figure 3: Combination of imipenem and cilastatin

The clinical uses of imipenem and cilastatin include serious nosocomial infections in patients with conditions such as malignancies and neutropenia.

Adverse effects include nausea, rashes, diarrhea and increased risk of seizures.

Meropenem

It is not hydrolyzed by dehydropeptidase I enzyme and hence cilastatin administration is not required.

Clinical uses include serious nosocomial infections such as septicemia, intra-abdominal and pelvic infections.

ASSESS YOURSELF (Examination Questions of Various Universities)

1. List Beta-lactam antibiotics. Write mechanism of action, adverse effects and uses of ampicillin
2. Enumerate beta lactam antibiotics. Describe in brief mechanism of action, adverse effect and clinical uses of Penicillin G.
3. Classify cephalosporins. Give mechanism of action, therapeutic uses and adverse effects of cephalosporins
4. Semi synthetic penicillins
5. Extended spectrum penicillins
6. Beta-lactamase inhibitors
7. Rationale of combining amoxicillin with clavulanic acid
8. Clavulanic acid
9. Why imipenem is administered with cilastatin

MULTIPLE CHOICE QUESTIONS

1. **All are true about cephalosporins, except:**
   (AIIMS May 2009)
   a. Ceftazidime is a 3rd generation cephalosporin
   b. Cefoperazone has got antipseudomonal effect
   c. Cefoxitin has got no activity against anaerobes
   d. Cephalosporins act by inhibiting cell wall synthesis

2. **Which of the following is most nephrotoxic cephalosporin?** *(Recent Question Dec 2016)*
   a. Cephaloridine
   b. Cephalothin
   c. Cefoperazone
   d. Ceftriaxone

3. **Which of the following is a fourth generation cephalosporin?** *(Recent Question 2016)*
   a. Ceftazidime
   b. Cefepime
   c. Cephaloridine
   d. Cefixime

4. **Drug of choice for syphilis in a pregnant lady is:**
   (Recent Question 2016)
   a. Penicillin
   b. Azithromycin
   c. Tetracycline
   d. Ceftriaxone

5. **Which of the following beta-lactam antibiotics can be safely used in a patient with a history of allergy to penicillins?** *(Recent Question 2016)*
   a. Aztreonam
   b. Monabactam
   c. Loracarbef
   d. Ceftriaxone

6. **All of the following antibacterial agents act by inhibiting cell wall synthesis except:**
   (Recent Question 2016)
   a. Carbapenems
   b. Monobactams
   c. Cephalosporins
   d. Nitrofurantoin

7. **Cilastatin is given along with:**
   (Recent Question 2016)
   a. Imipenem
   b. Amoxicillin
   c. Erythromycin
   d. Ampicillin

8. **Carbenicillin** *(Recent Question 2016)*
   a. Is effective in pseudomonas infection
   b. Has no effect in proteus infection
   c. Is a macrolide antibiotic
   d. Is administered orally

9. **A potent inhibitor of beta-lactamase is:**
   (Recent Question 2016)
   a. Carbenicillin
   b. Clavulanic acid
   c. Cefamandole
   d. Idoxuridine

10. **Jarisch-Herxheimer reaction is seen in syphilis with:** *(Recent Question 2016)*
    a. Tetracyclines
    b. Penicillins
    c. Co-trimoxazole
    d. Sulfonamides

11. **True about imipenem is:** *(Recent Question 2016)*
    a. It is a narrow spectrum antibiotic
    b. It is easily broke by β-lactam
    c. It can be used with cilastatin
    d. It is used with sulbactam

12. **All are third generation cephalosporin except:**
    (Recent Question 2016)
    a. Cefixime
    b. Ceftazidime
    c. Cefuroxime
    d. Cefoperazone

13. **Not a semi-synthetic penicillin:**
    (Recent Question 2016)
    a. Penicillin V
    b. Penicillin G
    c. Methicillin
    d. Amoxicillin

14. **True regarding aztreonam are all except:**
    (Recent Question 2016)
    a. Is a monobactam group
    b. Has activity against gram-positive bacteria
    c. Active against pseudomonas
    d. Can be given to a patient who develops sever hypersensitivity reaction to a penicillin

Ans.

1.	(c)	2.	(a)	3.	(b)	4.	(a)	5.	(a)	6.	(d)
7.	(a)	8.	(a)	9.	(b)	10.	(b)	11.	(c)	12.	(c)
13.	(b)	14.	(b)									

53

Quinolones and Fluoroquinolones

They are synthetic antibacterial drugs. The first quinolone was nalidixic acid that was effective against gram-negative bacteria. It was used in the treatment of urinary tract infections (UTI) and gastrointestinal tract infections.

Subsequently, fluoroquinolones which are fluorinated analogues of nalidixic acid were developed (Table 1).

TABLE 1	Quinolones and fluoroquinolones
Quinolones	Nalidixic acid
Fluoroquinolones	• **First generation** → Ciprofloxacin, norfloxacin, ofloxacin, pefloxacin • **Second generation** → Levofloxacin, lomefloxacin, sparfloxacin, moxifloxacin

QUINOLONES → NALIDIXIC ACID

Nalidixic acid is a quinolone that inhibits bacterial DNA gyrase and interferes with DNA replication. It has bactericidal effect.

Antimicrobial spectrum is mainly against gram-negative bacteria such as *E. coli, Klebsiella, Proteus* etc. It is not effective against *Pseudomonas.*

The adverse effects include rashes, CNS toxicity (headache, vertigo, convulsions) and GIT toxicity.

The clinical uses include urinary tract infections and diarrhea due to susceptible organisms.

FLUOROQUINOLONES

Fluoroquinolone antimicrobials are quinolones with fluorine substitutions.

Ciprofloxacin is a first-generation fluoroquinolone and is often considered a prototype drug.

Mechanism of Action

Fluoroquinolones are bactericidal drugs and they inhibit bacterial DNA synthesis (Figure 1).

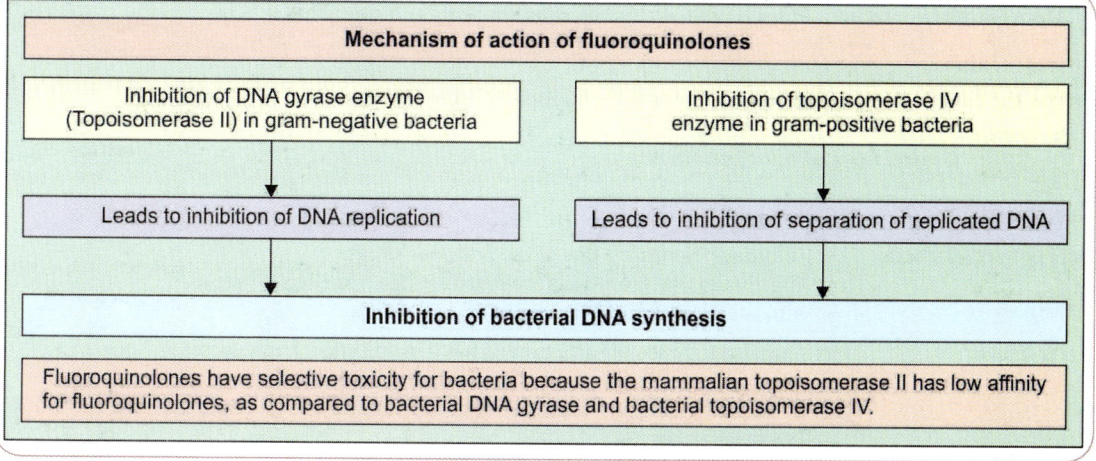

Figure 1: Mechanism of action of fluoroquinolones

Mechanism of Drug Resistance

The following mechanisms can lead to drug resistance to fluoroquinolones:
- Mutations in DNA gyrase or topoisomerase IV enzymes leading to decreased affinity to fluoroquinolones
- Reduced entry of drug in the bacteria or development of drug efflux mechanisms.

■ CIPROFLOXACIN

It is a first-generation fluoroquinolone and the antimicrobial spectrum includes the following:
- Gram-negative bacteria (e.g. *E. coli, K. pneumoniae, S. typhi, Proteus, N. meningitidis, N. gonorrhoeae, P. aeruginosa*)
- Gram-positive bacteria (e.g. *Bacillus anthracis, S. aureus, S. epidermidis*)
- *Mycobacterium tuberculosis*

Ciprofloxacin has high penetration in various tissues such as prostate, lungs, muscle, bones etc. Oral absorption is rapid, but is delayed by food. Excretion is mainly in the urine.

Adverse Effects

Some of the key adverse effects of ciprofloxacin are mentioned in Table 2.

TABLE 2	Adverse effects of fluoroquinolones
Gastrointestinal	• Nausea, vomiting, diarrhea
Musculoskeletal	• Tendonitis and tendon rupture • Cartilage damage has been observed in immature animals → fluoroquinolones should be avoided in young children
Skin and hypersensitivity	• Photosensitivity • Rashes, allergic reactions
Cardiotoxicity	• Arrhythmias, torsades de pointes, QT prolongation
Nervous system	• Dizziness, tremors, convulsions • Impairment of concentration
Fluoroquinolones should be avoided during pregnancy and in young children.	

Drug Interactions

The key drug interactions with ciprofloxacin are mentioned below:
- Ciprofloxacin inhibits the metabolism of theophylline and warfarin that can lead to an increase in plasma concentration of these drugs.
- CNS toxicity of fluoroquinolones can be enhanced by NSAIDs → convulsions can be precipitated
- Absorption of fluoroquinolones is reduced by iron salts, antacids and sucralfate.

Clinical Uses

Some of the clinical uses of fluoroquinolones are mentioned in Table 3.

TABLE 3	Clinical uses of fluoroquinolones	
Clinical uses	**Comments**	
Urinary tract infections	• Fluoroquinolones are one of the preferred drugs • Effective against gram-negative organisms such as *E. coli, Proteus* • Also useful in bacterial prostatitis	
Typhoid fever	• Ciprofloxacin is commonly used; it has a rapid action, has a decreased incidence of complications and relapse. Ciprofloxacin also prevents the carrier state as it is bactericidal, has good tissue penetration, and attains high concentrations in bile and intestinal mucosa. • Levofloxacin, pefloxacin and ofloxacin can also be used	

Contd...

Clinical uses	Comments
Gastroenteritis (bacterial)	• Effective in bacterial diarrhea caused by susceptible organisms such as *E. coli, Shigella, Salmonella*
Mycobacterial infections	• Used with other antimicrobials for multidrug resistant tuberculosis (MDR), Mycobacterium avium (MAC) infections in AIDS patients, atypical mycobacterial infections
Sexually transmitted infections	• Gonococcal infections—use has decreased due to resistance • Chancroid • Chlamydial infections
Soft tissues, wound and bone infection	• Used in combination therapy with other antimicrobials
Conjunctivitis	• Topical use
Anthrax	• Ciprofloxacin is used for treatment and prevention
Respiratory infections	• Levofloxacin and moxifloxacin are used for community acquired pneumonia, chronic bronchitis
Infections in neutropenic patients	• Used for prevention and treatment in susceptible patients

NORFLOXACIN

o First generation fluoroquinolone
o Mainly used for bacterial gastroenteritis, urinary and genital infections.

PEFLOXACIN

o First generation fluoroquinolone → methyl derivative of norfloxacin
o Preferred for meningeal infections as it has a high passage into the CSF
o Has high bioavailability (90–100%)
o Dose needs to be reduced in hepatic disease.

OFLOXACIN

o First generation fluoroquinolone
o Has a high bioavailability (85–95%)
o Clinical uses include patients with atypical pneumonia, tuberculosis and leprosy.

LEVOFLOXACIN

o Second generation fluoroquinolone
o Increased activity against some gram-positive bacteria (e.g. *S. pneumoniae)* and gram-negative bacteria
o Clinical uses include chronic bronchitis, pneumonia, sinusitis and pyelonephritis.

LOMEFLOXACIN

o Second generation fluoroquinolone
o Enhanced activity against chlamydia and some gram-negative bacteria.

SPARFLOXACIN

- Second generation fluoroquinolone
- Has higher activity against some gram-positive bacteria (e.g. *S. pneumoniae, Staphylococcus*), anaerobes and mycobacteria
- Clinical uses include chronic bronchitis, pneumonia, tuberculosis, leprosy and MAC infections in patients with AIDS
- Has a high incidence of phototoxicity; can also lead to prolongation of QTc interval.

MOXIFLOXACIN

- Second generation fluoroquinolone
- Has higher activity against some gram-positive bacteria (e.g. *S. pneumoniae)* and anaerobes
- Clinical uses include bronchitis, pneumonia and sinusitis
- Adverse effect profile is similar to other fluoroquinolones; can also lead to prolongation of QTc interval.

DRUGS USED FOR TYPHOID (ENTERIC) FEVER

The resistance to various antibiotics is increasing, especially in endemic areas; hence, susceptibility testing should be done to select the appropriate antibiotic.

In general, the antibiotics used for the management of typhoid fever include:

- Ceftriaxone
- Fluoroquinolones (e.g. ciprofloxacin, levofloxacin)
- Chloramphenicol
- Azithromycin
- Cotrimoxazole

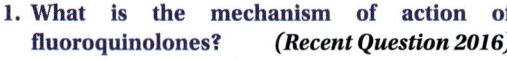

ASSESS YOURSELF (Examination Questions of Various Universities)

1. Fluoroquinolones and their therapeutic uses
2. Mechanism of action of fluoroquinolones
3. Ciprofloxacin
4. Nalidixic acid
5. Mention drugs used in treatment of enteric fever

MULTIPLE CHOICE QUESTIONS

1. What is the mechanism of action of fluoroquinolones? *(Recent Question 2016)*
   a. Block translocation of peptide chain from A to P site
   b. Inhibit peptidyl transferase
   c. Inhibit binding of aminoacyl-t-RNA to A site
   d. Inhibit DNA gyrase

2. Which of these is not used for the treatment of typhoid? *(Recent Question 2016)*
   a. Chloramphenicol
   b. Ciprofloxacin
   c. Ceftriaxone
   d. Cefixime

3. Maximum incidence of phototoxicity is associated with: *(Recent Question 2016)*
   a. Norfloxacin
   b. Sparfloxacin
   c. Lomefloxacin
   d. Cotrimoxazole

4. Gyrase inhibitors are: *(Recent Question 2016)*
   a. Fluoroquinolones
   b. Penicillins
   c. Aminoglycosides
   d. Azoles

5. Quinolone with highest CSF penetrating power: *(TN PG 2011)*
   a. Ciprofloxacin
   b. Ofloxacin
   c. Pefloxacin
   d. Levofloxacin

Ans.

| 1. | (d) | 2. | (d) | 3. | (b) | 4. | (a) | 5. | (c) |

TETRACYCLINES

These are broad-spectrum antibiotics and have four cyclic rings in their structure. The following drugs are included in the tetracycline group. They are mentioned in Figure 1.
- Tetracycline
- Oxytetracycline
- Demeclocycline
- Doxycycline
- Minocycline

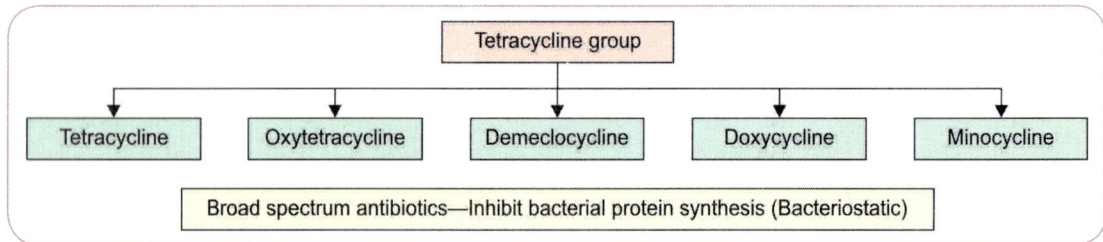

Figure 1: Tetracyclines

Mechanism of Action

The tetracyclines bind to 30S ribosomal unit of bacteria and prevent attachment of aminoacyl-t-RNA to the mRNA ribosome complex. This prevents the peptide chain from growing, thereby inhibiting bacterial protein synthesis.

Tetracyclines have selective toxicity for the microbes as compared to the human cells. This is because of the following reasons:
- Carrier involved in the active transport of tetracyclines is not present in the mammalian cells
- Reduced sensitivity of mammalian protein synthesizing apparatus to the effects of tetracyclines.

Antibacterial Spectrum

Tetracyclines were initially called broad-spectrum antibiotics as they were effective against multiple types of microbes. However, their efficacy has reduced due to development of drug resistance. The following organisms usually are sensitive to tetracyclines:
- *Rickettsia*
- *Chlamydia*
- *Mycoplasma*
- *Actinomyces*
- *Spirochetes*
- Gram-positive bacteria such as *Staphylococcus aureus, Bacillus anthracis*
- Gram-negative bacteria such as *Vibrio cholerae, Brucella*

Resistance

The mechanisms for the development of resistance to tetracyclines are mentioned in Figure 2.

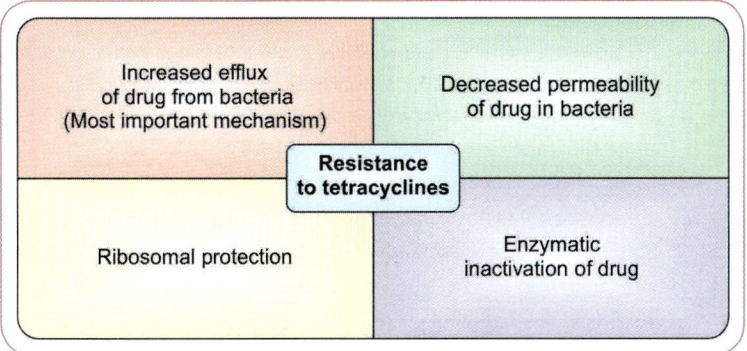

Figure 2: Resistance to tetracyclines

Pharmacokinetics

Tetracyclines are adequately absorbed following oral administration.

Tetracyclines have chelating properties and hence form unabsorbable and insoluble complexes with calcium, iron, magnesium and other metals.

Therefore, the absorption of tetracyclines is decreased if there is simultaneous administration of dairy products, antacids, iron and sucralfate (Figure 3).

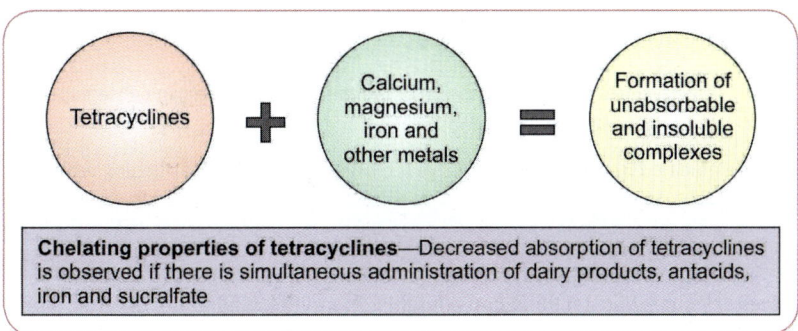

Figure 3: Chelating action of tetracycline

Tetracyclines are primarily excreted in the urine, except for doxycycline. Doxycycline is primarily excreted in the feces via bile. Doxycycline also undergoes enterohepatic circulation.

Adverse Effects

Some of the adverse effects observed with tetracyclines are mentioned in Table 1.

TABLE 1	Adverse effects of tetracyclines
Gastrointestinal	• Gastric pain, irritation, nausea, vomiting, diarrhea
Hepatotoxicity	• Fatty changes, hepatic necrosis • May lead to maternal hepatic toxicity (hepatic necrosis) if used during pregnancy. It can be fatal.
Renal toxicity	• Acute renal failure • Nephrogenic diabetes insipidus 　▪ Demeclocycline blocks the action of antidiuretic hormone (ADH) on renal tubules and may lead to nephrogenic diabetes insipidus

527

Contd...

	• Fanconi syndrome ▪ It is a disease characterized with dysfunction of the proximal renal tubule. It may manifest clinically as polyuria, polydipsia, electrolyte imbalance, acidosis. ▪ Exposure to expired tetracyclines products (epitetracyclines, anhydrotetracycline) is one of the causes of Fanconi syndrome.
Toxicity to teeth and bones	• Teeth ▪ Tetracyclines chelates in deciduous and permanent teeth. This may result in tooth discoloration, deformed teeth and increased susceptibility to caries. • Bones ▪ Tetracyclines may lead to suppression of bone growth • Tetracyclines should not be used during pregnancy or lactation.
Phototoxicity	• Phototoxicity (sunburn like reaction) may occur in some patients. • Increased incidence with doxycycline and demeclocycline.
Vestibular toxicity	• Vertigo, ataxia and nystagmus may occur • Observed with minocycline • Reversible on drug discontinuation
Antianabolic effect	• Reduce synthesis of proteins and have a catabolic effect
Pseudotumor cerebri	• Increased intracranial pressure is observed in some infants
Hypersensitivity	• Allergy, skin rashes, anaphylaxis
Superinfection	• Tetracyclines cause suppression of resident flora; hence can cause superinfections such as candida, pseudomembranous colitis.

Tetracyclines are contraindicated in children under 12 years, pregnancy and breastfeeding women.

Clinical Uses

Therapeutic use of tetracyclines has declined considerably due to the availability of other efficacious antibiotics. Some of the clinical uses of tetracyclines are mentioned below:
- **Rickettsial infections**
  - Rocky mountain spotted fever
  - Typhus
- **Atypical pneumonia** (*Mycoplasma pneumoniae*)
- **Venereal diseases**
  - Chlamydial urethritis
  - Lymphogranuloma venereum
  - Granuloma inguinale
- **Brucellosis**
- **Plague**
- **Relapsing fever**
- **Cholera**
- **Other uses of tetracyclines** include amoebiasis (along with other amoebicides), malaria (along with other antimalarial drugs for *P. falciparum* malaria), acne vulgaris (inhibition of *P. acnes* by tetracyclines)

Some of the differences between tetracycline and doxycycline are mentioned in Table 2.

TABLE 2	Tetracycline and doxycycline	
Criteria	Tetracycline	Doxycycline
Potency	Less potent	More potent
GIT absorption	Incomplete	Complete
Incidence of diarrhea	More	Less
Disturbance of intestinal flora	Significant	Less
Risk of nephrotoxicity	High	Low—because it is primarily excreted in bile and hence can be given in patients of renal disease

GLYCYLCYCLINES—TIGECYCLINE

Tigecycline is a minocycline analogue and binds to 30S ribosome with higher affinity. It is a broad-spectrum antibiotic and has a bacteriostatic action.

The main advantage with tigecycline is that it is active against many strains resistant to tetracyclines.

It is effective against methicillin-resistant *Staphylococcus aureus*, vancomycin-resistant *Enterococci* and multidrug-resistant *S. pneumoniae*.

The clinical uses include complicated skin, soft tissue and intra-abdominal infections.

The adverse effects include nausea and vomiting.

CHLORAMPHENICOL

Chloramphenicol was initially isolated from *Streptomyces venezuelae*. It is now produced synthetically.

It is a broad-spectrum antibiotic and has a bacteriostatic action.

It is active against a wide variety of aerobic and anaerobic gram-positive as well as gram-negative bacteria. It is effective against *Rickettsiae* but not against *Chlamydiae*.

Mechanism of Action

Chloramphenicol bind to 50S ribosomal unit of bacteria, and prevents the transfer of peptide chain to aminoacyl-t-RNA at the mRNA ribosome complex.

It prevents formation of peptide bonds, thereby inhibiting bacterial protein synthesis.

Chloramphenicol also acts on 70S ribosomes and inhibits mammalian protein synthesis.

Development of Resistance

The mechanisms for development of resistance to chloramphenicol include the following:
- Reduced permeability of the drug in the bacteria
- Production of enzyme acetyl transferase that inactivates chloramphenicol
- Ribosomal mutation that results in decreased affinity of chloramphenicol to the ribosomal binding site.

Pharmacokinetics

Chloramphenicol is well absorbed from the gastrointestinal tract. It can be administered either orally or intravenously. It readily crosses the blood-brain barrier.

It is metabolized in the liver through glucuronyl conjugation and excreted mainly via urine.

Adverse Effects

Some of the adverse effects reported with chloramphenicol are mentioned in Table 3.

TABLE 3	Adverse effects of chloramphenicol

Bone marrow depression	• Bone marrow depression is a very serious adverse effect
	• It can result in pancytopenia, agranulocytosis, thrombocytopenia, aplastic anemia
	• It can be of two types:
	  ▪ Dose dependent reversible bone marrow depression
	  ▪ Idiosyncratic non-dose dependent irreversible bone marrow depression—it can result in fatalities. Aplastic anemia is a common manifestation.

Gastrointestinal toxicity	• Nausea, vomiting, diarrhea
Hypersensitivity	• Rashes, fever, angioedema
Gray baby syndrome	• Administration of chloramphenicol in neonates, particularly in premature babies can lead to a dose dependent gray baby syndrome. • Mechanism is due to an inability of the neonates to adequately conjugate chloramphenicol. There is an inability to metabolize and excrete chloramphenicol. • Clinical manifestations include: cyanosis, abdominal distension, vomiting, inability to feed, hypothermia and cardiovascular collapse. It can be potentially fatal. • Chloramphenicol is to be avoided in neonates/premature babies.
Others	• Superinfections

Clinical Uses

The use of chloramphenicol has significantly reduced due to the risk of serious hematological toxicity. Some of the uses in susceptible organisms are as follows:

○ **Anaerobic infections including *B. fragilis***
○ **Typhoid fever**
  ❑ Fluoroquinolones and third generation cephalosporins are the preferred drugs
○ **Bacterial meningitis**
  ❑ Third generation cephalosporins are the preferred drugs for meningitis caused by *H. influenzae*
○ **Rickettsial infections**
  ❑ Tetracyclines are preferred drugs
○ **Eye and ear infections**
  ❑ Topical applications are done.

1. Clinical uses of tetracyclines
2. Adverse effects of tetracyclines
3. Differences between tetracycline and doxycycline
4. Chloramphenicol and grey baby syndrome

MULTIPLE CHOICE QUESTIONS

1. The following tetracycline has the potential to cause vestibular toxicity:
   (Recent Question 2016)
   a. Minocycline
   b. Demeclocycline
   c. Doxycycline
   d. Tetracycline

2. Which one of the following is primarily bacteriostatic? *(Recent Question 2016)*
   a. Ciprofloxacin
   b. Chloramphenicol
   c. Vancomycin
   d. Rifampicin

3. Tigecycline is a/an: *(Recent Question 2016)*
   a. Tetracyclines
   b. Erythromycin
   c. Penicillin
   d. Rifampicin

4. Drug used for prophylaxis of plague:
   (Recent Question 2016)
   a. Tetracycline
   b. Penicillin
   c. Erythromycin
   d. Cephalosporins

5. All the following can occur with tetracycline therapy during pregnancy except:
   (JIPMER 2011)
   a. Teeth discoloration
   b. Gingival hyperplasia
   c. Raised ICT
   d. Reduced bone growth

6. Gray color and yellow fluorescence in infant teeth is caused by: *(JIPMER 2010)*
   a. Phenytoin
   b. Porphyria
   c. Tetracycline
   d. Barbiturate

7. Gray baby syndrome is caused by:
   (TN PG 2010, 2005)
   a. Vancomycin
   b. Chloramphenicol
   c. Tetracyclines
   d. Sulfonamides

8. Tetracyclines are ineffective against:
   (TN PG 2007)
   a. Chlamydia
   b. Brucella
   c. Trichomonas
   d. Rickettsia

9. Which drug is primarily bacteriostatic?
   (TN PG 2001)
   a. Chloramphenicol
   b. Ceftriaxone
   c. Rifampicin
   d. Ciprofloxacin

Ans.

1.	(a)	2.	(b)	3.	(a)	4.	(a)	5.	(b)	6.	(c)
7.	(b)	8.	(c)	9.	(a)						

▌ AMINOGLYCOSIDES

Aminoglycoside antibiotics have a bactericidal action on the microbes.
They can be used systemically and topically (Figure 1).

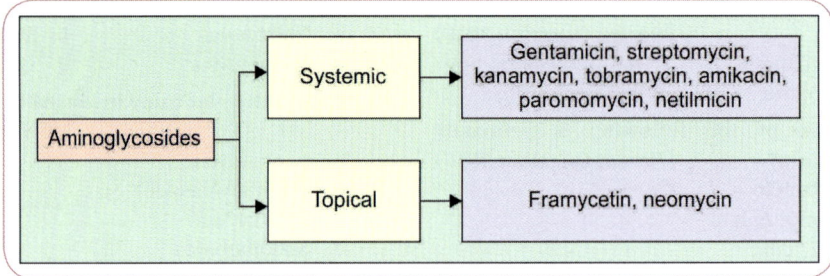

Figure 1: Classification of aminoglycosides

Mechanism of Action

Aminoglycosides bind to 30S ribosomes and inhibit protein synthesis in the bacteria (Figure 2). They have bactericidal activity.

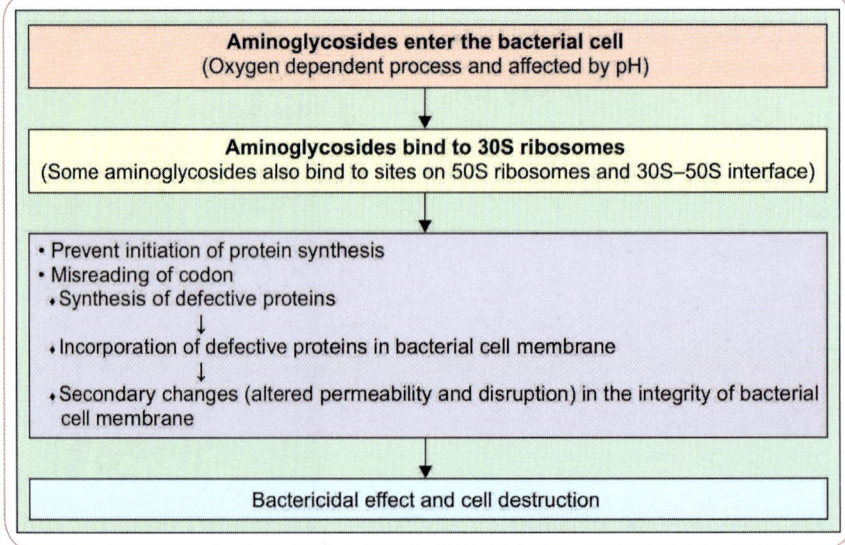

Figure 2: Mechanism of action of aminoglycosides

Anaerobes are resistant to aminoglycosides because the entry of aminoglycosides in the bacterial cell requires an oxygen dependent process.

Aminoglycosides are more active in alkaline pH because the entry of aminoglycosides in the bacterial cell is favored by high pH.

Aminoglycosides demonstrate concentration dependent bactericidal effect. This means that, an increase in the aminoglycoside concentration will lead to an increase in the bactericidal effect.

Aminoglycosides also demonstrate a postantibiotic effect. This means that the antibacterial action persists even when concentration of aminoglycoside decreases below the MIC (minimum inhibitory concentration). Hence, a once-daily dosage regimen can be effective despite the short half-life.

Resistance

Microbes develop resistance to aminoglycosides due to the following mechanisms:
- Inactivation of aminoglycosides by enzymes in the bacterial cell membrane
- Reduced entry of aminoglycosides in the bacterial cell
- Reduced affinity of ribosome to the aminoglycosides.

Adverse Effects

Aminoglycosides have a relatively narrow margin of safety and exhibit only partial cross resistance amongst them. Some of the key adverse effects reported with aminoglycosides include the following (Table 1):
- Ototoxicity
- Nephrotoxicity
- Neuromuscular blockade
- Others

TABLE 1	Adverse effects of aminoglycosides
Ototoxicity	• Manifests as cochlear and vestibular toxicity • Most important adverse effect that is related to dose and duration of treatment • Aminoglycoside ear drops are contraindicated in patients with perforated ear drum as they can cause ototoxicity • Refer to Figure 3
Nephrotoxicity	• Due to increased concentration of aminoglycosides in the renal cortex • Leads to tubular damage resulting in reduced urinary concentrating ability, reduced GFR, proteinuria, appearance of casts, retention of nitrogen • Can be reversible if drug is promptly discontinued • At risk groups include patients with underlying renal disease, elderly, or concomitant use of other nephrotoxic drugs such as amphotericin B, cisplatin, cyclosporine and vancomycin • Careful monitoring of the patient's renal function should be done
Neuromuscular blockade	• Aminoglycosides reduce the release of acetylcholine from the motor nerves • May result in apnea and respiratory paralysis in some patients; fatalities can occur • Should be used with caution in patients who have received muscle relaxants • Should be avoided in patients with myasthenia gravis due to enhanced susceptibility for neuromuscular blockade
Others	• Hypersensitivity reactions: Rashes, anaphylaxis • Pregnancy: Risk of fetal ototoxicity if aminoglycosides are used during pregnancy

Ototoxicity with aminoglycosides

- Accumulation of drug occurs in endolymph and perilymph of the inner ear
- Manifests as cochlear and vestibular toxicity due to damage to the VIIIth cranial nerve
- Progressive damage occurs to the vestibular and cochlear hair cells

Cochlear toxicity

- Damage to the cochlear hair cells and neurons
- Initial toxicity is asymptomatic (detected by audiometry). Patient can present with tinnitus and progressive hearing loss that can be irreversible

Vestibular toxicity

- Manifests as headache, nausea, vomiting, vertigo, ataxia, nystagmus
- Recovery can take 12–24 months and some residual damage may persist

Preventive measures

- Careful monitoring of the patient including renal, auditory and vestibular functions
- Shortest possible duration of therapy as per clinical judgement
- Identification of at risk groups → Elderly patients, patients with pre-existing auditory impairment, patients with impaired renal function, patients on therapy with other ototoxic drugs (e.g. loop diuretic (furosemide), minocycline) or nephrotoxic drugs (e.g. amphotericin B, cisplatin, cyclosporine, vancomycin)

Figure 3: Ototoxicity with aminoglycosides

Antimicrobial Spectrum and Clinical Uses

Aminoglycosides are mainly effective against gram-negative aerobic bacilli (e.g. *E. coli, Klebsiella, Proteus, Pseudomonas).* Gentamicin is a commonly used aminoglycoside.

Some of the clinical uses where these antibiotics can be considered for therapy against sensitive organisms are mentioned in Table 2.

TABLE 2 Clinical uses of aminoglycosides

- Urinary tract infections
- Tuberculosis (streptomycin, amikacin, kanamycin)
- Meningitis
- Plague (gentamicin, streptomycin)
- Pneumonia
- Tularemia (gentamicin, streptomycin)
- Peritonitis
- Brucellosis (gentamicin, streptomycin along with doxycycline)
- Sepsis
- Topical application for skin, ear and eye infections (gentamicin, neomycin, framycetin)
- Bacterial endocarditis

The adjustment of dose of aminoglycosides is done based on patient's bodyweight and renal function (creatinine clearance). Monitoring of serum concentrations of aminoglycosides may be required in specific instances.

INDIVIDUAL DRUGS

Streptomycin

It is used in combination therapy for tuberculosis. It can also be used for plague, brucellosis, tularemia. It has a low incidence of nephrotoxicity amongst aminoglycosides.

Gentamicin

Gentamicin is a commonly used aminoglycoside. It has a low therapeutic index and hence, is used is serious gram-negative aerobic bacilli infections.

Amikacin

It is semisynthetic derivative of kanamycin. It is resistant to aminoglycoside inactivating enzymes. Amongst the aminoglycosides, it has a broad spectrum of activity.

Paromomycin

The clinical uses of paromomycin include intestinal amoebiasis, giardiasis and vaginal trichomoniasis.

Neomycin

Neomycin is not used systemically as it is highly toxic (ototoxicity, nephrotoxicity). It is minimally absorbed from the gastrointestinal tract. Some of the clinical uses of neomycin are mentioned in Table 3.

TABLE 3	Clinical uses of neomycin
Topical use	• Skin and mucus membrane infections including infected wounds, ulcers, infected burns etc. • Eye and external ear infections • It is often used in combination with other drugs such as polymyxin, bacitracin
Oral use	Oral use is limited. It is used for local action on the GIT. • Used for preoperative preparation of the bowel. It may decrease postoperative infections. • Hepatic coma ▪ Neomycin reduces the intestinal bacterial flora. This results in decreased production of ammonia by the intestinal bacteria. A decrease in the blood ammonia levels is observed. However, lactulose is often preferred for this purpose due to lesser toxicity.

Framycetin

It is considered too toxic for systemic use. Hence, the clinical uses are limited to topical application in skin, ear and eye infections.

KEY FEATURES OF AMINOGLYCOSIDES

Some of the key features of aminoglycosides are mentioned in Table 4.

TABLE 4	Key features of aminoglycosides
• Aminoglycoside antibiotics have bactericidal action and are mainly effective against gram-negative aerobic bacilli (e.g. *E. coli, Klebsiella, Proteus, Pseudomonas*).	
• Not effective against anaerobes because the entry of aminoglycosides in the bacterial cell requires an oxygen dependent process.	
• Demonstrate concentration dependent bactericidal effect and a postantibiotic effect.	
• More active in alkaline pH because the entry of aminoglycosides in the bacterial cell is favored by high pH.	
• Have a narrow margin of safety. Key toxicities include ototoxicity, nephrotoxicity and neuromuscular blockade.	
• Adjustment of dose of aminoglycosides is done based on patient's bodyweight and renal function (creatinine clearance).	
• Mechanism of action is inhibition of protein synthesis in the bacteria.	
• Exhibit partial cross resistance amongst them.	
• Kinetics ▪ Highly polar compounds and have poor oral bioavailability. Predominantly distributed extracellularly. ▪ Poor penetration in the CSF. ▪ Not metabolized in body and excreted unchanged in the urine.	

ASSESS YOURSELF (Examination Questions of Various Universities)

1. Enumerate aminoglycosides. Describe common properties, shared toxicities and therapeutic uses of aminoglycosides

2. Gentamicin

3. Why neomycin is used in hepatic coma

4. Ototoxicity produced by aminoglycosides.

MULTIPLE CHOICE QUESTIONS

1. True about aminoglycosides is all except:
   (AIIMS May 2008)
   a. Are bacteriostatic
   b. Distributed only extracellularly
   c. Excreted unchanged in urine
   d. Teratogenic

2. Irreversible hearing loss caused by:
   (Recent Question 2016)
   a. Gentamycin
   b. Clarithromycin
   c. Both of the above
   d. None of the above

3. Which of the following drugs is most likely to cause loss of equilibrium and auditory damage? *(Recent Question 2016)*
   a. Amikacin   b. Ethambutol
   c. Isoniazid   d. Rifabutin

4. Bactericidal inhibitors of protein synthesis are:
   (Recent Question 2016)
   a. Tetracyclines   b. Aminoglycosides
   c. Macrolides   d. Lincosamides

5. Which of the following drugs is not excreted in bile: *(Recent Question 2016)*
   a. Erythromycin   b. Ampicillin
   c. Rifampicin   d. Gentamicin

6. All are aminoglycosides except:
   (Recent Question 2016)
   a. Netilmicin   b. Streptomycin
   c. Kanamycin   d. Azithromycin

7. The toxicity of depolarizing skeletal muscle relaxants are enhanced by:
   (Recent Question 2016)
   a. Daptomycin   b. Vancomycin
   c. Streptomycin   d. Azithromycin

8. Mechanism of action of streptomycin:
   (Recent Question 2016)
   a. Freezing of initiation
   b. Inhibits translocation
   c. Inhibits peptidyl transferase
   d. Inhibits cell wall synthesis

9. Aminoglycosides toxicity first affects:
   (Recent Question 2016)
   a. Outer hair cell and basal turn of cochlea
   b. Apex
   c. Cochlear nerve
   d. Vestibular nerve

10. Amikacin-mechanism of action:
    (Recent Question 2016)
    a. Protein synthesis inhibitors
    b. Inhibits DNA synthesis
    c. Inhibits cell wall synthesis
    d. Antimetabolite

11. Least nephrotoxic aminoglycoside is:
    (MH CET 2010)
    a. Amikacin   b. Gentamycin
    c. Streptomycin   d. Netilmicin

Ans.											
1.	(a)	**2.**	(a)	**3.**	(a)	**4.**	(b)	**5.**	(d)	**6.**	(d)
7.	(c)	**8.**	(a)	**9.**	(a)	**10.**	(a)	**11.**	(c)		

56

Macrolides and Other Miscellaneous Antibiotics

MACROLIDES

Macrolide antibiotics include erythromycin, roxithromycin, clarithromycin and azithromycin (Figure 1).

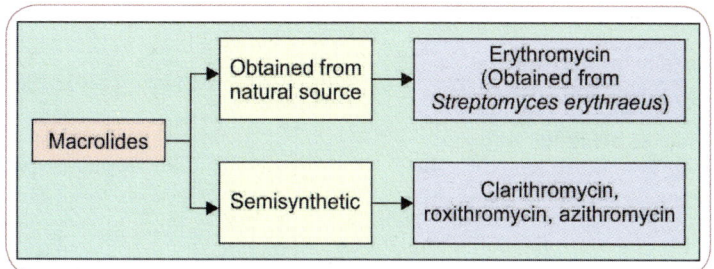

Figure 1: Macrolide antibiotics

Mechanism of Action

Macrolides inhibit microbial protein synthesis by binding to the 50S ribosomal subunit. The peptide chain is terminated prematurely. There is a specific inhibition of synthesis of larger proteins.

Macrolides are generally bacteriostatic, but can be bactericidal at high concentrations against certain organisms. The activity of macrolides is enhanced at alkaline pH.

Pharmacokinetics

Some of the salient points about the pharmacokinetics of erythromycin are mentioned below:
○ Erythromycin is acid labile. It requires enteric coating to prevent against destruction by gastric acid
○ Food can delay gastric emptying and interfere with the absorption of erythromycin
○ Erythromycin is partly metabolized by the liver and eliminated mainly via bile.

Adverse Effects and Drug Interactions (Table 1)

TABLE 1	Adverse effects and drug interactions to macrolides (Erythromycin)
Gastrointestinal	• Nausea, vomiting, diarrhea, epigastric pain • Erythromycin can stimulate the GI 'motilin' receptors. This may result in increased gastric emptying and intestinal motility.
Allergic reactions	• Hypersensitivity reactions, skin rashes
Hepatic	• Cholestatic hepatitis, jaundice, liver dysfunction, hepatotoxicity • Hepatitis occurs due to hypersensitivity to estolate ester • Incidence of hepatitis is higher in pregnancy
Hearing disorders	• Reversible hearing loss may be observed if high doses of erythromycin have been administered
Drug interactions	• Enzyme inhibition by erythromycin can result in increased blood levels of carbamazepine, ergotamine, sodium valproate, theophylline, warfarin • Inhibition of CYP3A4 enzymes by erythromycin or clarithromycin can lead to increased blood levels of terfenadine, astemizole, cisapride. This can result in serious arrhythmias such as QTc prolongation, torsades de pointes, ventricular arrhythmias. Fatalities can also occur.

Antimicrobial Spectrum and Clinical Uses

Macrolides have a narrow antimicrobial spectrum. They are mostly active against gram-positive bacteria, and also against some gram-negative bacteria.

They are usually effective against the following:

- Gram-positive bacteria → E.g. *Staphylococci, Streptococci, L. monocytogenes, C. diphtheriae*
- Gram-negative bacteria → E.g. *H. influenzae, N. meningitidis, N. gonorrhoeae, L. pneumophila*
- Other microbes → E.g. *M. pneumoniae, C. trachomatis*

Some of the clinical uses of macrolides are mentioned in Table 2.

TABLE 2	Clinical uses of macrolides
Preferred drugs for infections	
1.	Atypical pneumonia (due to *M. pneumoniae*)
2.	Whooping cough (due to *B. pertussis*)
3.	Chancroid (due to *H. ducreyi*)
Used as alternatives drugs to penicillin	
4.	Leptospirosis
5.	Tetanus
6.	Diphtheria
7.	Respiratory tract infections due to *pneumococci, H. influenzae*
8.	Streptococcal infections such as pharyngitis, tonsillitis, ear infections (otitis)
9.	Prophylactic therapy (patients allergic to penicillin) for rheumatic fever, bacterial endocarditis
Other infections	
10.	Legionnaires' pneumonia, chlamydial infections

INDIVIDUAL DRUGS

Erythromycin was the first macrolide antibiotic that was discovered in 1952. There are some limitations associated with erythromycin:

- Narrow antimicrobial spectrum
- Acid lability
- Gastrointestinal adverse effects
- Short duration of action
- Reduced oral bioavailability

Semisynthetic macrolides such as clarithromycin, roxithromycin and azithromycin were developed in an attempt to overcome some of the drawbacks of erythromycin.

Clarithromycin

- More acid stable as compared to erythromycin
- Similar adverse effect profile to erythromycin, but better GIT tolerance. Similar drug interactions profile to erythromycin.
- Similar antimicrobial spectrum to erythromycin, but additionally effective against *M. leprae, M. avium complex (MAC)* and some anaerobes
- Clinical uses are similar to erythromycin. Additional uses include:
  - Management of *H. pylori* infection (part of triple therapy regimen)
  - Management of MAC infection in AIDS patients (part of combination therapy regimen)

Roxithromycin

- Long acting drug that is acid stable
- Better gastric tolerability as compared to erythromycin

Azithromycin

- Expanded antimicrobial spectrum
- Long acting drug that is acid stable
- Better gastric tolerability as compared to erythromycin
- Can be administered as a once single dose (better compliance)

LINCOSAMIDES

Clindamycin

The mechanism of action is similar to erythromycin i.e. inhibits microbial protein synthesis by binding to 50S ribosomal subunit. It is mainly bacteriostatic.

The antimicrobial spectrum is similar to erythromycin, but clindamycin is additionally effective against anaerobic bacteria such as *B. fragilis*.

The adverse effects include the following:

- Rashes, urticaria, abnormal liver function, diarrhea, abdominal pain
- Pseudomembranous enterocolitis: It is a serious adverse effect and is due to superinfection with *C. difficile*. It occurs due to alteration of the usual intestinal flora while on therapy with antibiotics such as clindamycin. The management requires cessation of therapy with the offending antibiotic (clindamycin) and initiation of therapy with metronidazole or vancomycin.

The clinical uses include the following:

- Management of anaerobic infections in patients of pelvic, lung and abdominal abscesses
- Management of toxoplasmosis in AIDS patients (used along with pyrimethamine)
- Management of *P. jirovecii* pneumonia in AIDS patients (used along with primaquine)
- Acne vulgaris (topical application)

GLYCOPEPTIDE ANTIBIOTICS

Vancomycin

It is a glycopeptide antibiotic that acts by inhibition of bacterial cell wall synthesis.

Vancomycin is not absorbed orally. It is administered intravenously for the management of systemic infections.

Vancomycin has high toxicity and the adverse effects include the following:

- Allergic reactions such as rashes, anaphylactoid reactions, anaphylaxis
- Red man or red neck syndrome: Rapid intravenous administration of vancomycin may be associated with flushing, chills, urticarial reactions, tachycardia and severe hypotension. It is believed to be due to the vancomycin-induced release of histamine from mast cells.
- Nephrotoxicity
- Ototoxicity

Vancomycin is clinically used in the management of serious infections. The clinical uses include the following:

- Systemic administration (intravenous)
  - ❑ Serious infections due to methicillin-resistant *Staphylococcus aureus* (MRSA)
  - ❑ Enterococcal endocarditis in patients who are allergic to penicillin
  - ❑ Bacterial meningitis
- Oral administration
  - ❑ Pseudomembranous colitis due to *C. difficile*.

Teicoplanin

- ○ It is a glycopeptide antibiotic that acts by inhibition of bacterial cell wall synthesis.
- ○ Antimicrobial spectrum is similar to vancomycin.
- ○ It is administered parenterally (IM or IV).
- ○ Toxicity is lesser in comparison to vancomycin; adverse effects include rashes, hypersensitivity and ototoxicity.
- ○ Clinical uses include serious infections such as MRSA infections, enterococcal endocarditis and osteomyelitis.

OXAZOLIDINONE ANTIBIOTICS

Linezolid

- ○ It is a synthetic antibiotic.
- ○ It acts by inhibition of bacterial protein synthesis. It binds to the 23S fraction of the 50S ribosome.
- ○ Antimicrobial spectrum includes gram-positive aerobic bacteria and anaerobes.
- ○ Adverse effects include rashes, diarrhea, vomiting, headache and mild hematological toxicity (anemia, neutropenia, thrombocytopenia).
- ○ Linezolid is used in clinical conditions such as nosocomial and community acquired pneumonia, complicated skin and soft tissue infections and febrile neutropenia.

OTHER ANTIBIOTICS

The miscellaneous antibiotics are mentioned in Table 3.

TABLE 3	Miscellaneous antibiotics
Fusidic acid	• It is a narrow-spectrum antibiotic • It acts by inhibiting bacterial protein synthesis • Active against some gram-positive bacteria including *Staphylococcus* • Used topically for skin infections (e.g. boils, superficial folliculitis)
Bacitracin	• It is a polypeptide antibiotic • Acts by inhibiting bacterial cell wall synthesis • Antimicrobial spectrum includes gram-positive organisms • Parenteral administration can lead to severe toxicity (nephrotoxicity) → hence, it is used topically • Used topically for eye infections, infected ulcers, wound infections

Polymyxin B and colistin	• These are polypeptide antibiotics
	• Effective against gram-negative bacteria
	• Have bactericidal action
	• Mechanism of action is to interact with phospholipids and cause disruption of the bacterial cell membrane structure. This leads to the leakage of cellular contents (ions, amino acids etc.)
	• Adverse effects include nausea, vomiting, diarrhea upon oral administration
	• Clinical uses include
	  ▪ Topically: Infections of the skin, eye and ear caused by sensitive gram-negative bacteria
	  ▪ Orally: Diarrhea caused by sensitive gram-negative bacteria

URINARY ANTISEPTICS

Urinary antiseptics are antimicrobial drugs that upon oral administration attain antibacterial concentrations only in the urine. They have negligible systemic antibacterial action. These drugs are used to treat urinary tract infections (mainly lower UTIs).

Nitrofurantoin

It is a bacteriostatic drug. However, bactericidal effect may be observed in acidic urine.

The antimicrobial spectrum consists of sensitive gram-negative bacteria; mainly limited to *E. coli*.

The adverse effects include GI disturbances (epigastric pain, nausea, vomiting, diarrhea), hypersensitivity reactions, hemolytic anemia in G6PD deficiency, hepatotoxicity, acute pneumonitis, pulmonary infiltration, interstitial pulmonary fibrosis, neurological disorders and polyneuropathies.

Nitrofurantoin can result in brown discoloration of urine upon exposure to air.

Probenecid interferes with the antiseptic effect of nitrofurantoin by inhibiting the tubular secretion and lowering the urinary concentration of nitrofurantoin.

Nitrofurantoin is used in uncomplicated lower urinary tract infections.

Methenamine

Methenamine is a prodrug and is inactive. It is hydrolyzed in acidic urine to release ammonia and formaldehyde. Formaldehyde exerts an antibacterial effect.

Methenamine requires acidic urine (pH < 5.5) for its antibacterial effect. Hence, organic acids such as mandelic acid or ascorbic acid are administered to acidify the urine.

Methenamine is protected from decomposition in gastric acid by administering as enteric coated tablets.

The adverse effects include gastric irritation (due to formaldehyde release in the stomach), cystitis, bladder irritation and hematuria.

Contraindications include: hepatic dysfunction (detoxification of released ammonia is inhibited), renal failure (accumulation of mandelic acid can result in acidosis).

Methenamine can be used in patients with resistant, chronic urinary tract infection.

Phenazopyridine

- ○ It does not have antibacterial effect.
- ○ It is an orange dye that has analgesic effect in the urinary tract.
- ○ Adverse effects include epigastric pain, nausea, vomiting.
- ○ It is used for the symptomatic relief of pain, burning, frequency, urgency in patients with lower urinary tract infections.

DRUG THERAPY FOR URINARY TRACT INFECTIONS

The drug therapy for urinary tract infections is mentioned in Figure 2.

Drugs used in urinary tract infections (UTI)	
General factors to be considered for selection of the antibiotic(s) for UTI • Patient factors—underlying disorders, drug allergies • Local treatment protocol and patterns of drug resistance • Antibiotic availability and cost effectiveness • Lab reports of culture and sensitivity	
Acute cystitis (Lower UTI)	• Fluoroquinolones (e.g. ciprofloxacin, norfloxacin, ofloxacin) • Cotrimoxazole • Nitrofurantoin
Acute pyelonephritis (Upper UTI—involves the renal tissue)	• Fluoroquinolones (e.g. ciprofloxacin, norfloxacin, ofloxacin) • Cephalosporins (e.g. ceftriaxone, cefotaxime) • Ampicillin/gentamicin Hospitalization and parenteral therapy may be required. Duration of therapy is prolonged in patients of acute pyelonephritis as compared to acute cystitis.

Figure 2: Drug therapy for urinary tract infections

DRUG THERAPY FOR SEXUALLY TRANSMITTED INFECTIONS

The drug therapy for some of the sexually transmitted infections is mentioned in Table 4.

TABLE 4	Drugs used in the treatment of sexually transmitted infections	
Infection	**Organism**	**Drugs**
Chancroid	*Haemophilus ducreyi*	• Azithromycin or • Ceftriaxone or • Erythromycin or • Ciprofloxacin
Genital herpes	*Human herpesvirus*	• Acyclovir or • Famciclovir or • Valacyclovir
Gonorrhea	*Neisseria gonorrhoeae*	Dual therapy for gonococcal infections consists of: • Ceftriaxone + azithromycin or • Cefixime + azithromycin
Granuloma inguinale (Donovanosis)	*Klebsiella granulomatis*	• Doxycycline or • Azithromycin or • Erythromycin
Lymphogranuloma venereum	*Chlamydia trachomatis*	• Doxycycline or • Azithromycin or • Erythromycin
Syphilis	*Treponema pallidum*	• Benzathine penicillin or • Doxycycline or • Ceftriaxone
Trichomoniasis	*Trichomonas vaginalis*	• Metronidazole or • Tinidazole

PSEUDOMEMBRANOUS COLITIS

Some of the key features of pseudomembranous colitis are mentioned in Table 5.

TABLE 5	Pseudomembranous colitis (*Clostridium difficile* induced diarrhea)

- The leading cause of antibiotic associated colitis is *Clostridium difficile*
- Therapy with antibiotics can cause changes in the GI flora. It can result in intestinal overgrowth of *Clostridium difficile* and lead to pseudomembranous colitis
- Antibiotics with risk of causing pseudomembranous colitis include clindamycin, tetracyclines, ampicillin and aminoglycosides
- Treatment is with metronidazole or vancomycin

ASSESS YOURSELF (Examination Questions of Various Universities)

1. Enumerate macrolide antibiotics. Give therapeutic uses of erythromycin
2. Adverse effects of erythromycin
3. Clinical uses of clindamycin
4. Therapeutic status of vancomycin as an antibacterial agent
5. Linezolid
6. Drug therapy for urinary tract infections
7. Mention two drugs used in gonococcal infection

MULTIPLE CHOICE QUESTIONS

1. Erythromycin is given in intestinal hypomotility because: *(AIIMS Nov 2009)*
   a. It increases bacterial count
   b. It decreases bacterial count
   c. It binds to adenylyl cyclase
   d. It binds to motilin receptors

2. Bacitracin acts on: *(Recent Question 2016)*
   a. Cell wall
   b. Cell membrane
   c. Nucleic acid
   d. Ribosome

3. Red man syndrome occurs with: *(Recent Question 2016)*
   a. Clindamycin
   b. Teicoplanin
   c. Vancomycin
   d. Polymyxin

4. Pseudomembranous colitis false is: *(Recent Question 2016)*
   a. Treated by tetracycline
   b. Antibiotic associated with pseudomembranous colitis is clindamycin
   c. Life-threatening complication
   d. Presents with severe diarrhea, fever, and stools containing mucous membrane neutrophils

5. Linezolid is a: *(Recent Question 2016)*
   a. DNA gyrase inhibitors
   b. Bind to 30S unit
   c. Binds to 23S fraction of 50S ribosomes
   d. Bind to tetrahydrofolate reductase

6. In antibiotic associated colitis, organism involved is: *(PGI June 2006)*
   a. *Clostridium difficile*
   b. *Pseudomonas*
   c. *Staphylococcus*
   d. *Enterococcus*

7. Which of the following antibiotic is a glycopeptides? *(JIPMER 2012)*
   a. Clindamycin
   b. Vancomycin
   c. Azithromycin
   d. Linezolid

8. Which of the following prokinetic drugs acts on MOTILIN receptors? *(MH CET 2008)*
   a. Erythromycin
   b. Metoclopramide
   c. Loxiglumide
   d. Cisapride

9. Mode of action of vancomycin: *(WB PG 2011)*
   a. Cell wall inhibition
   b. Protein synthesis inhibition
   c. Direct DNA damage
   d. Peptidyl transferase inhibition

Ans.

1.	(d)	2.	(a)	3.	(c)	4.	(a)	5.	(c)	6.	(a)
7.	(b)	8.	(a)	9.	(a)						

57

Antimalarial Drugs

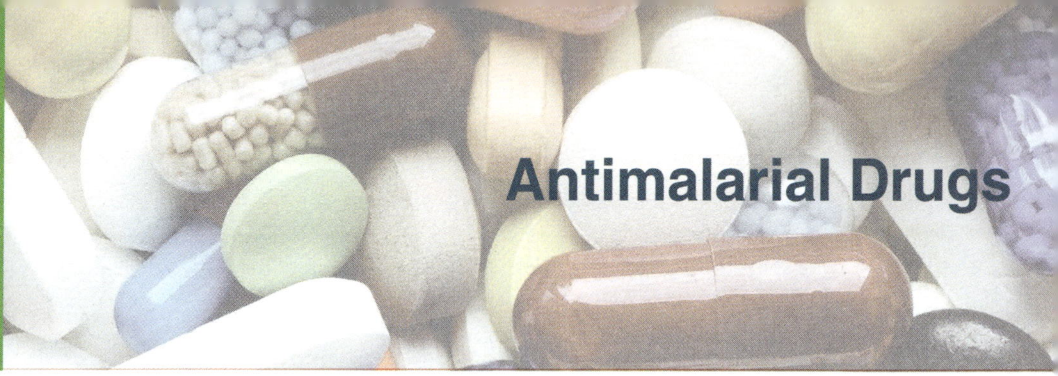

Malaria is caused by the *Plasmodium* parasite that includes the following species:
- *Plasmodium vivax* (common in India)
- *Plasmodium ovale*
- *Plasmodium falciparum* (common in India)
- *Plasmodium malariae*

The plasmodium infection is transmitted to the humans by the bite of infected female anopheles mosquito. The clinical features include fever (which may be periodic), chills, myalgia, headache, nausea and vomiting.

The lifecycle of the malarial parasite consists of the following:
- Sexual cycle (occurs in the female anopheles, mosquito)
- Asexual cycle (occurs in humans)

The key features of the malarial infection cycle are shown in Figure 1.

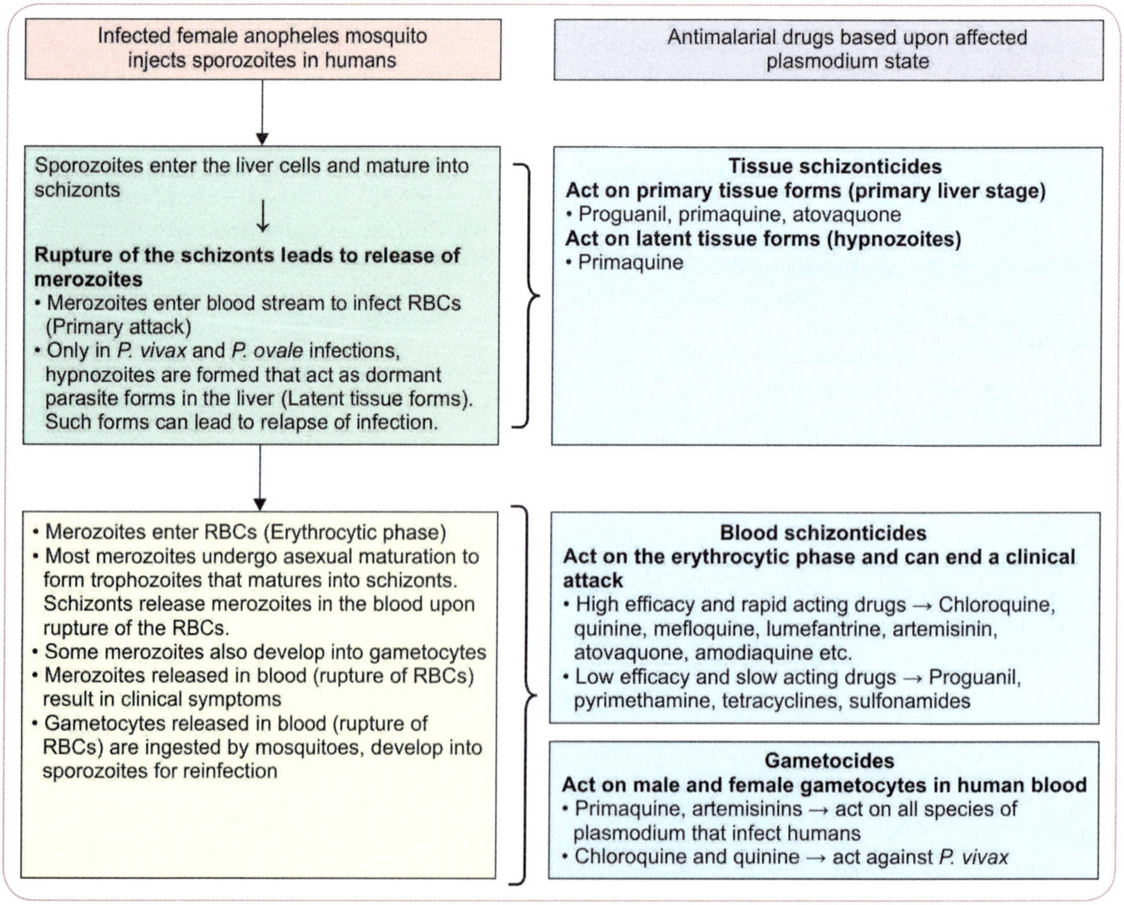

Infected female anopheles mosquito injects sporozoites in humans	Antimalarial drugs based upon affected plasmodium state
Sporozoites enter the liver cells and mature into schizonts ↓ **Rupture of the schizonts leads to release of merozoites** • Merozoites enter blood stream to infect RBCs (Primary attack) • Only in *P. vivax* and *P. ovale* infections, hypnozoites are formed that act as dormant parasite forms in the liver (Latent tissue forms). Such forms can lead to relapse of infection.	**Tissue schizonticides** **Act on primary tissue forms (primary liver stage)** • Proguanil, primaquine, atovaquone **Act on latent tissue forms (hypnozoites)** • Primaquine
• Merozoites enter RBCs (Erythrocytic phase) • Most merozoites undergo asexual maturation to form trophozoites that matures into schizonts. Schizonts release merozoites in the blood upon rupture of the RBCs. • Some merozoites also develop into gametocytes • Merozoites released in blood (rupture of RBCs) result in clinical symptoms • Gametocytes released in blood (rupture of RBCs) are ingested by mosquitoes, develop into sporozoites for reinfection	**Blood schizonticides** **Act on the erythrocytic phase and can end a clinical attack** • High efficacy and rapid acting drugs → Chloroquine, quinine, mefloquine, lumefantrine, artemisinin, atovaquone, amodiaquine etc. • Low efficacy and slow acting drugs → Proguanil, pyrimethamine, tetracyclines, sulfonamides
	Gametocides **Act on male and female gametocytes in human blood** • Primaquine, artemisinins → act on all species of plasmodium that infect humans • Chloroquine and quinine → act against *P. vivax*

Figure 1: Key features of the malarial infection cycle

CLASSIFICATION OF ANTIMALARIAL DRUGS

The classifications of antimalarial drugs are mentioned in Tables 1, 2 and 3.

TABLE 1	Classification of antimalarial drugs as per chemical structure
• 4-aminoquinoline	Chloroquine, amodiaquine, piperaquine
• Quinoline methanol	Mefloquine
• Biguanides	Proguanil, chlorproguanil
• Cinchona alkaloid	Quinine, quinidine
• Diaminopyrimidines	Pyrimethamine
• 8-aminoquinoline	Primaquine
• Sulfonamide and sulfone	Sulfadoxine, sulfamethoxypyrazine, dapsone
• Sesquiterpene lactone	Artesunate, artemether, arteether
• Amino alcohol	Halofantrine, lumefantrine
• Mannich base	Pyronaridine
• Naphthoquinone	Atovaquone
• Tetracycline	Tetracycline, doxycycline

TABLE 2	Classification of antimalarial drugs as per the type of therapy
Causal prophylaxis	• Drugs acting on the pre-erythrocytic phase (in the liver) ▪ Proguanil → mainly for *P. falciparum;* ▪ Primaquine → effective against all plasmodium species; not used commonly due to its toxicity
Suppressive prophylaxis	• Drugs suppress the erythrocytic phase and prevent the clinical attacks of malaria • These drugs are blood schizonticides and include: ▪ Chloroquine, primaquine, mefloquine, proguanil, doxycycline etc.
Clinical cure	• Drugs used to terminate an acute attack of malaria • These drugs are blood schizonticides and act on the erythrocytic phase and include: ▪ High efficacy and rapid acting drugs ➤ Chloroquine, quinine, mefloquine, lumefantrine, artemisinin, atovaquone, amodiaquine etc. ▪ Low efficacy and slow acting drugs ➤ Proguanil, pyrimethamine, tetracyclines, sulfonamides • High efficacy and rapid acting drugs are preferred especially in the management of *P. falciparum* malaria • Drugs used for clinical cure can also lead to radical cure of *P. falciparum* malaria. This is because *P. falciparum* infection does not lead to formation of hypnozoites (latent tissue forms) that causes relapse. • However, radical cure is needed for *P. vivax* and *P. ovale*, because in these infections, hypnozoites are formed that act as dormant forms of parasite in the liver (latent tissue forms) and can cause relapse.

Contd...

Radical cure	• Drugs attack the hypnozoites (latent tissue forms) of *P. vivax* and *P. ovale*—e.g. primaquine • Radical cure is needed in infections with *P. vivax* and *P. ovale*, because in these infections, hypnozoites are formed that act as dormant forms of parasite in the liver (latent tissue forms) and can cause relapse. • Radical cure is not needed for *P. falciparum* infection as it does not lead to formation of hypnozoites (latent tissue forms) that can cause relapse • Drugs used for radical cure of *P. vivax* and *P. ovale* are blood schizonticide (e.g. chloroquine) + primaquine
Gametocidal	• Drugs attack the male and female gametes of plasmodium in the blood of the patient • Artemisinin's and primaquine are gametocidal against all species of plasmodium that infect humans

TABLE 3	Classification of antimalarial drugs as per the affected plasmodium stage

Tissue schizonticides	• Drugs act on the primary tissue forms (primary liver stage)
	  ▪ Proguanil, primaquine, atovaquone
	• Drugs act on the latent tissue forms (hypnozoites)
	  ▪ Primaquine

Blood schizonticides	• Drugs act on the erythrocytic phase and can end a clinical attack
	  ▪ High efficacy and rapid acting drugs → Chloroquine, quinine, mefloquine, lumefantrine, artemisinin, atovaquone, amodiaquine etc.
	  ▪ Low efficacy and slow acting drugs → Proguanil, pyrimethamine, tetracyclines, sulfonamides etc.

Gametocides	• Drugs act on male and female gametocytes in human blood
	  ▪ Primaquine, artemisinin act on all species of plasmodium that infect humans
	  ▪ Chloroquine and quinine act against *P. vivax*
	• These drugs decrease the transmission to mosquitos

INDIVIDUAL ANTIMALARIAL DRUGS

■ CHLOROQUINE

Chloroquine is commonly used to treat all types of susceptible malarial infections.

Antimalarial Action

○ Rapidly acting blood schizonticide against *P. vivax, P. ovale, P. malariae* and chloroquine sensitive strains of *P. falciparum*
○ Gametocidal activity against *P. vivax,* but not against *P. falciparum*
○ No activity against liver stages of parasite (i.e. pre-erythrocytic and hypnozoites); hence, cannot prevent relapses in *P. vivax* and *P. ovale* infections.

Resistance to chloroquine is now quite common in *P. falciparum,* and has also been observed in *P. vivax* infections.

Mechanism of Action

The mechanism of action of chloroquine is not completely understood.

It is a basic drug that is actively taken up by the acidic food vacuoles of susceptible plasmodia. Once inside the parasite, chloroquine interferes with the conversion of toxic heme to nontoxic hemozoin. Accumulation of heme and the formation of chloroquine-heme complex are toxic to the plasmodia (Figure 2).

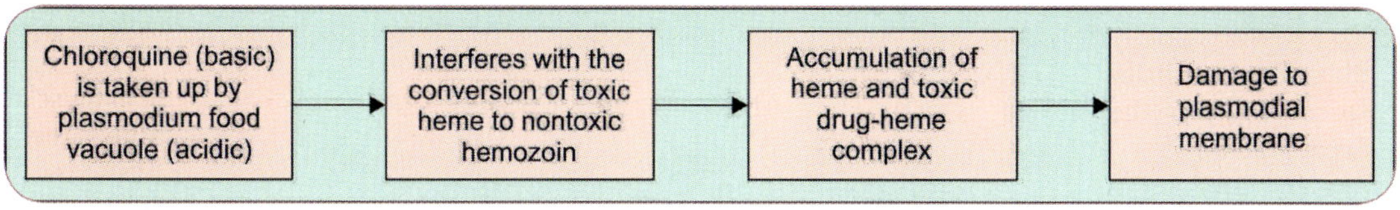

Figure 2: Mechanism of action of chloroquine

Pharmacokinetics

Chloroquine is well absorbed following oral and IM administration.

It gets concentrated mainly in liver, spleen, lung, kidney, skin and melanin-containing tissues. Accumulation in the retina can lead to ocular toxicity upon prolonged use.

It is mainly metabolized in liver and slowly excreted in urine. The initial half-life is 3–10 days and the terminal half-life is 1–2 months.

Adverse Effects

Chloroquine has low toxicity, but the adverse effects are frequent. It also has a narrow safety margin. Toxicity mainly relates to the CNS and CVS. Some of the adverse effects are mentioned in Table 4.

TABLE 4	Adverse effects of chloroquine
Usual antimalarial doses	Nausea, vomiting, abdominal pain, headache, itching, blurring of vision and rashes
Parenteral use (may lead to)	Hypotension, cardiac arrhythmias, cardiac arrest and CNS toxicity (e.g. convulsions)
Long term use (high dosage as in rheumatoid arthritis)	Retinopathy, peripheral neuropathy, myopathy and irreversible ototoxicity

Chloroquine can be used in pregnancy and in young children.

Precautions and Contraindications

Some of these include:
- Psoriasis
- Porphyria
- Epilepsy
- Myasthenia gravis
- Retinal/visual field abnormalities
- Liver, neurological or blood disorders

Mefloquine and chloroquine should not be given together due to risk of seizures. Patients on prolonged, high dose therapy should have ophthalmological and neurological examinations every 3–6 months.

Clinical Uses

The clinical uses of chloroquine include the following:

Malaria

- **Clinical cure of an acute attack of malaria** caused by *P. vivax, P. ovale, P. malariae* and chloroquine-sensitive strains of *P. falciparum.*
  - Fever generally resolves in 1–2 days and thick peripheral smears are usually negative by 2–3 days
  - In *P. vivax* and *P. ovale, chloroquine* does not eradicate the dormant forms (hypnozoites) in the liver; hence, primaquine must be added to achieve radical cure.
- **Suppressive prophylaxis of malaria** caused by *P. vivax, P. ovale, P. malariae* and chloroquine-sensitive strains of *P. falciparum.*

Other Uses

- Rheumatoid arthritis
- Discoid lupus erythematosus
- Lepra reactions
- Amoebic liver abscess
- Infectious mononucleosis

AMODIAQUINE

- It is a congener of chloroquine with properties similar as that of chloroquine.
- It is used (in combination with artesunate) for the treatment of uncomplicated *P. falciparum* malaria.
- It is not used for chemoprophylaxis of *P. falciparum* malaria due to toxicities (agranulocytosis and hepatotoxicity).

MEFLOQUINE

It is chemically related to quinine.

Mechanism of Action

- The mechanism of action is unclear, but is possibly similar to quinine and chloroquine.
- It is a blood schizonticide. It does not have any action on hepatic stages or gametocytes.

Pharmacokinetics

Mefloquine is administered orally because severe local irritation occurs with parenteral use. It has a prolonged terminal elimination half-life (about 20 days).

It is well-absorbed orally and is concentrated in many tissues such as liver, intestines and lung. It undergoes significant enterohepatic cycling.

Adverse Effects

The adverse effects of mefloquine include the following:
- Nausea, vomiting, dizziness, abdominal pain
- *Neurological and psychiatric toxicities* (e.g. balance abnormalities, hallucinations, seizures, ataxia, depression)
- Hematological, hepatic toxicity
- Concomitant administration of mefloquine with drugs such as quinine, quinidine, halofantrine) may lead to conduction abnormalities, QTc prolongation and cardiac arrest
- Contraindicated in patients with history of psychiatric disorders, epilepsy, arrhythmias and cardiac conduction abnormalities.

Clinical Uses

The clinical uses of mefloquine include the following:
- Chemoprophylaxis of malaria
- Treatment of uncomplicated falciparum malaria.
  - Used in combination with artesunate for uncomplicated falciparum malaria.

PRIMAQUINE

- It is the preferred drug for the prevention of relapses of *P. vivax* and *P. ovale* (by elimination of dormant liver forms i.e. hypnozoites).
- It is also used for chemoprophylaxis against all plasmodial species.

Antimalarial Action

- Active against hepatic stages (primary and latent tissue forms) of all human plasmodial species
  - Latent tissue forms exist only in *P. vivax* and *P. ovale*
  - It is the only drug available against the dormant hypnozoite stages of *P. vivax* and *P. ovale*
- Gametocidal against all human plasmodial species
- Not active against asexual blood stages of plasmodia.

Mechanism of Action

The exact mechanism of action is unknown. However, primaquine may be converted to electrophilic intermediates that may exert antimalarial effects by possibly generating reactive oxygen species.

Pharmacokinetics

Primaquine is well-absorbed orally and widely distributed in the body. It is metabolized in the liver and excreted in the urine with the half-life of 3–8 hours.

The metabolites have less antimalarial action but have an increased potential of inducing hemolysis.

Adverse Effects

The adverse effects of primaquine include the following:

- **Gastrointestinal intolerance:** Nausea, vomiting, epigastric pain, headache. These can be reduced by taking with food.
- **Hemolysis and hemolytic anaemia:** It is an important adverse effect and occurs in patients with G6PD deficiency.
- **Methemoglobinemia:** It can also occur with primaquine, particularly in patients with G6PD deficiency or with other hereditary metabolic defects.
- **Agranulocytosis, leukopenia**.

Precautions and Contraindications

- G6PD deficiency
  - G6PD deficiency should be ruled out prior to initiating primaquine
  - Primaquine should be avoided in pregnancy. This is because the fetus is relatively G6PD deficient and is at risk of hemolysis
- History of granulocytopenia or methemoglobinemia.

Clinical Uses

Malaria

- **Radical cure** of acute *P. vivax* and *P. ovale* malaria
  - For radical cure, since primaquine is effective only against the hepatic stages, it is given along with an erythrocytic schizonticide (usually chloroquine) to simultaneously eradicate the erythrocytic stages of plasmodia.
- **Terminal chemoprophylaxis** of *P. vivax* and *P. ovale* malaria
  - For terminal prophylaxis, primaquine should be initiated shortly before or immediately after a person leaves the malaria endemic area.

Other Uses

- *Pneumocystis jirovecii* infection
  - Primaquine + clindamycin is an alternative regimen for mild to moderate pneumocystosis as it is better tolerated than high dose cotrimoxazole or pentamidine.

QUININE

Quinine has been used in the treatment and prevention of malaria for a long time. It is an alkaloid that is derived from the bark of cinchona tree.

Mechanism of Action

The mechanism of action is unclear, but is similar to chloroquine. The antimalarial action is as follows:
- It is a blood schizonticide active against the four species of plasmodia.
- It also has gametocidal activity against *P. vivax*.
- Not active against the hepatic forms of plasmodia (primary liver stage or hypnozoites)

Other actions of quinine are:
- CVS → cardiac depressant, hypotension; rapid IV injection can lead to hypotension and cardiovascular collapse
- GIT → Increased gastric secretion
- Local irritant and anesthetic → can lead to nausea, vomiting and abdominal pain. It has a bitter taste. Injections can lead to muscle necrosis and venous thrombosis. Fibrosis can also be observed.
- Weak analgesic and antipyretic effect
- Can decrease skeletal muscle contraction.

Pharmacokinetics

Quinine is well-absorbed orally, primarily metabolized in the liver and excreted in the urine.

Adverse Effects

The key adverse effects of quinine are mentioned below. Quinine can lead to dose related toxicities.

Cinchonism

- Milder forms manifest as → deafness, tinnitus, vomiting, postural hypotension, headache, visual abnormalities (blurred vision, diplopia, night blindness etc.)
- Tinnitus can result from functional impairment of VIIIth cranial nerve
- Visual and hearing abnormalities possibly result from direct neurotoxicity along with constriction of auditory and retinal vessels
- GI manifestations include nausea, diarrhea, abdominal pain → due to the local irritant action of quinine
- Cutaneous manifestations include sweating, rashes, flushing and angioedema.

Hypoglycemia

- Quinine can cause hyperinsulinemia
- Can be life-threatening and requires prompt treatment with intravenous glucose.

Hypotension

- Uncommon, but serious complication
- Usually associated with rapid infusion of quinine.

Cardiac Toxicity

- Usually associated with high plasma concentrations
- Can include arrhythmias such as ventricular fibrillation and QTc prolongation. Can lead to fatal cardiac arrest.

Black Water Fever

- Rare type of hypersensitivity reaction to quinine
- Consists of massive hemolysis, hemoglobinemia, and hemoglobinuria that can result in anuria and renal failure. Fatalities can also occur.

Clinical Uses

The clinical uses of quinine include the following:
- Parenteral (IV) treatment of severe falciparum malaria (cerebral malaria)
- Oral treatment of uncomplicated resistant falciparum malaria
- Babesiosis—used along with clindamycin
- Treatment of nocturnal leg cramps

In pregnant women, quinine should only be used for infection that is life threatening. Monitoring of glucose levels is required due to the risk of hypoglycemia.

ARTEMISININ AND ITS DERIVATIVES

Artemisinin is the active component of a Chinese herbal medicine. It is obtained from a plant called *Artemisia annua*.

Pharmacokinetics

Artemisinin is not soluble in water or oil and can be used only orally.
The analogues of artemisinin have been developed to increase solubility and efficacy. The analogues are as follows:
- Artesunate
  - Water soluble
  - Used for oral, IM and IV administration
- Artemether
  - Lipid soluble
  - Used for oral & IM administration
- Dihydroartemisinin
  - Water soluble
  - Used for oral administration

Artesunate, artemisinin and artemether undergo rapid metabolism to the active metabolite dihydroartemisinin.

Mechanism of Action

Artemisinin and its analogs are highly effective blood schizonticides against all malarial plasmodial species. They are very rapid acting, highly potent and lead to faster cure and clearance of malarial parasite. They do not have any effect on the hepatic stages of the malarial parasite.

The antimalarial effect is believed to be due to the generation of free radicals from the cleavage of the endoperoxide bridge (iron-catalyzed) of the artemisinin compounds. The highly reactive free radicals cause lipid peroxidation, damage to the endoplasmic reticulum and inhibition of protein synthesis. The end result is the death of the parasite.

Adverse Effects

Artemisinin and its derivatives are usually well tolerated.

The adverse effects include nausea, vomiting, diarrhea, prolongation of QT interval, neutropenia, increased liver enzymes, allergic reactions etc.

Clinical Uses

Artemisinin based combination therapies (ACTs) are considered the standard of care in many endemic areas for the treatment of uncomplicated falciparum malaria.
The advantages of using artemisinin and its derivatives as combination therapies (ACTs) are:
- Increased efficacy of treatment leading to faster clinical cure with rapid clearance of malarial parasite
- Lower chances of drug resistance
- Prevention of recrudescence

The World Health Organization (WHO) has recommended the following 5 artemisinin based combinations for uncomplicated falciparum malaria:
- Artemether-lumefantrine
- Artesunate-amodiaquine
- Artesunate-mefloquine
- Dihydroartemisinin-piperaquine
- Artesunate-sulfadoxine-pyrimethamine

Artemisinins are also used in the treatment of complicated falciparum malaria. Artesunate (used intravenously) has the following advantages over quinine (used intravenously) in the treatment of complicated falciparum malaria:
- Faster parasite clearance time
- Better tolerability and safety profile

o   Better patient survival
o   Simpler dosing schedule.

ANTIFOLATES—PROGUANIL, PYRIMETHAMINE/SULFADOXINE

The mechanism of action of antifolates is mentioned in Figure 3.

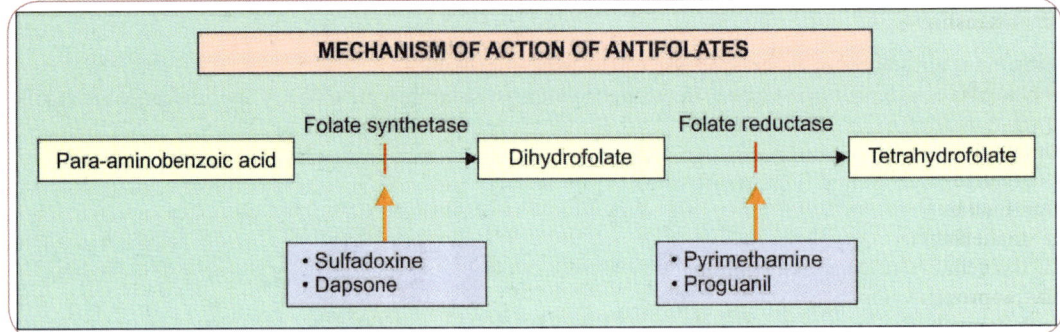

Figure 3: Mechanism of action of antifolates

PROGUANIL

Proguanil (a prodrug) is a slow acting erythrocytic schizonticide against all 4 plasmodia species. It is also effective against the primary hepatic stages of *P. falciparum*. It does not have any action against the hypnozoites. It also does not have any gametocidal action.

It is slowly but adequately absorbed from the GIT, with a terminal half-life of around 16 hours.

Proguanil is not used alone due to rapid development of resistance. Proguanil in combination with atovaquone is used for chemoprophylaxis and treatment of *P. falciparum* malaria.

Proguanil is generally well tolerated and the adverse effects include nausea, vomiting, diarrhea and abdominal pain. It is considered safe during pregnancy.

PYRIMETHAMINE

Pyrimethamine is a slow acting erythrocytic schizonticide against all 4 plasmodia species.

It is slowly but adequately absorbed from the GIT, with a terminal half-life of around 4 days.

Pyrimethamine is not used alone due to rapid development of resistance. Sulfadoxine-pyrimethamine in combination with artesunate is used for the treatment of *P. falciparum* malaria.

Pyrimethamine-sulfadiazine combination is also used in the treatment of toxoplasmosis in immunodeficient patients.

The adverse effects include skin rashes, megaloblastic anemia and nausea.

ATOVAQUONE

Atovaquone is used in combination with proguanil in a fixed-dose combination. Neither of these drugs are used alone due to the development of resistance. Atovaquone acts by disrupting the mitochondrial electron transport system.

It is administered only orally and has an erratic absorption. It has a half-life of around 2–3 days.

It acts as an erythrocytic schizonticide. It is also effective against the primary liver forms of *P. falciparum*. The clinical uses include the following:

o   Proguanil in combination with atovaquone is used for chemoprophylaxis and treatment of *P. falciparum* malaria.
o   *Pneumocystis jirovecii* infection

The adverse effects include nausea, vomiting, rash, headache and increase in liver enzymes.

LUMEFANTRINE

Lumefantrine is an aryl alcohol related to halofantrine that is an orally active erythrocytic schizonticide. It is only available as a fixed-dose combination with artemether for treatment of uncomplicated falciparum malaria. The absorption of lumefantrine is enhanced with meals. It is generally well tolerated; the adverse effects include headache, rashes, GIT disturbances and minor prolongation of the QT interval.

ANTIBIOTICS—TETRACYCLINE, DOXYCYCLINE, CLINDAMYCIN

These are modestly active antimalarial drugs and should not be used as single agents because their action is much slower than regular antimalarial drugs.

They act by inhibition of protein synthesis in malarial parasites and are active against erythrocytic schizonts. They are ineffective against hepatic stages of the malarial parasite.

Doxycycline is used in combination with quinine for treatment of falciparum malaria. Doxycycline is also used for chemoprophylaxis.

Clindamycin is used in patients in whom doxycycline cannot be used such as in children and pregnant women.

ANTIMALARIAL DRUG REGIMENS

There are multiple antimalarial regimens for the treatment and chemoprophylaxis of malaria. The regimens can change depending upon the local/regional applicability and resistance patterns. Some of these are mentioned in Figures 4 and 5.

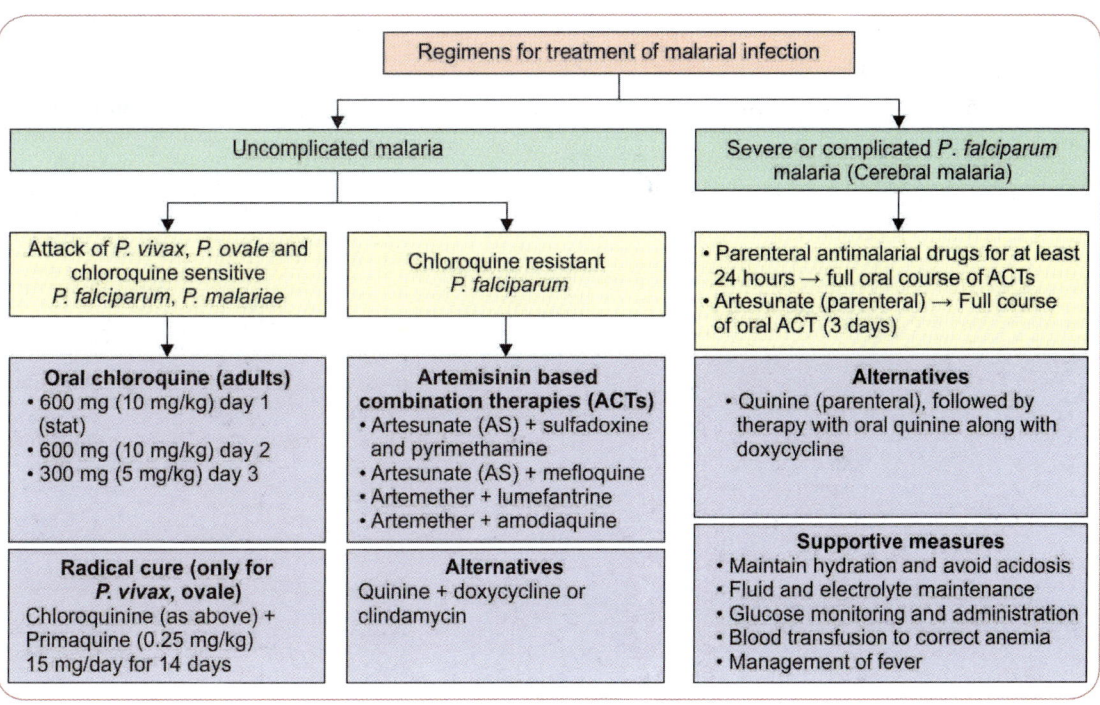

Figure 4: Regimens for treatment of malarial infection

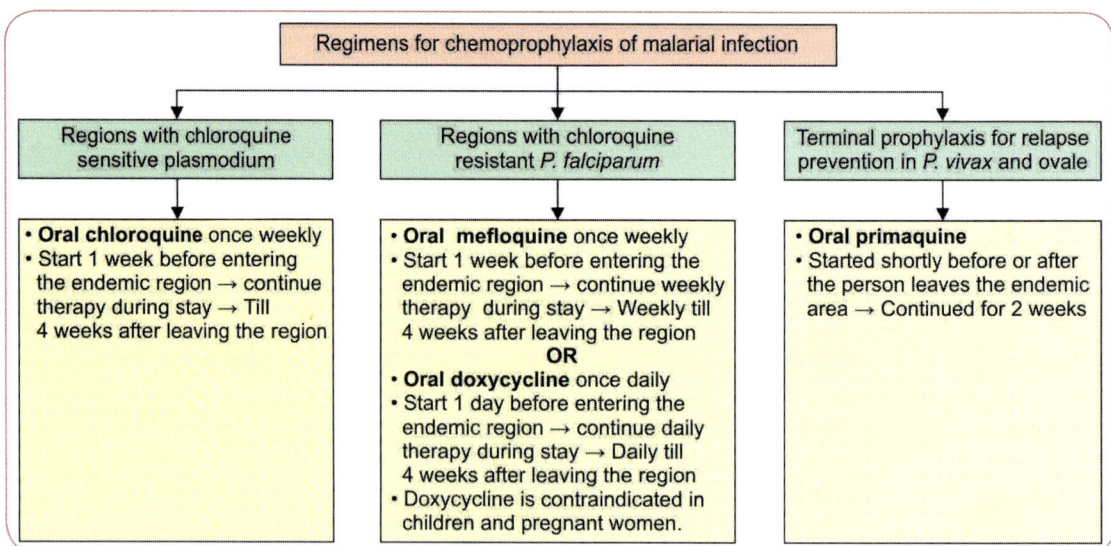

Figure 5: Regimens for chemoprophylaxis of malarial infection

ASSESS YOURSELF (Examination Questions of Various Universities)

1. Name drugs useful in malaria. Describe mechanism of action and therapeutic uses of chloroquine
2. Give mechanism of action, uses and adverse effects of artemisinin derivatives.
3. Artemisinin based combination therapy (ACT)
4. Define various terms used to describe antimalarial action of drugs in relation to life cycle of P. vivax
5. Classify anti-malarial drugs
6. Management of cerebral malaria
7. Mention non-malarial uses of chloroquine
8. Primaquine
9. Mefloquine
10. Radical cure in plasmodium vivax malaria
11. Chemoprophylaxis of malaria

MULTIPLE CHOICE QUESTIONS

1. Which of the following drugs can cause bull's eye retinopathy? *(Recent Question Dec 2016)*
   a. Chloroquine
   b. Amiodarone
   c. Ethambutol
   d. Vigabatrin

2. Most effective drug in severe falciparum malaria: *(AIIMS Nov 2014)*
   a. Quinine
   b. Chloroquine
   c. Artesunate
   d. Mefloquine

3. Drug causing megaloblastic anemia is: *(Recent Question 2016)*
   a. INH
   b. Chloramphenicol
   c. Pyrimethamine
   d. Methyldopa

4. Lumefantrine is an: *(Recent Question 2016)*
   a. Antimycobacterial
   b. Antifungal
   c. Antimalarial
   d. Antiamoebic

5. Which of the following antimalarial agents is most commonly associated with acute hemolytic reaction in patients with glucose-6-phosphate dehydrogenase deficiency? *(Recent Question 2016)*
   a. Chloroquine
   b. Clindamycin
   c. Mefloquine
   d. Primaquine

6. Drug deposited in retina: *(Recent Question 2016)*
   a. Isoniazid
   b. Chloroquine
   c. Rifampicin
   d. Pyrazinamide

7. Primaquine is the DOC for malaria in: *(TN PG 2003)*
   a. Radical cure
   b. Clinical cure
   c. Pregnancy
   d. Falciparum malaria

8. Which antimalarial drug is known to cause neuropsychiatric reaction as its adverse effect? *(MH CET 2010, 2007)*
   a. Artesunate
   b. Artimisinin
   c. Quinine
   d. Mefloquine

Ans.

1.	(a)	2.	(c)	3.	(c)	4.	(c)	5.	(d)	6.	(b)
7.	(a)	8.	(d)								

58

Antitubercular Drugs

TUBERCULOSIS

Tuberculosis (TB) is an infectious disease caused mainly by the bacterium *Mycobacterium tuberculosis*. It is one of the leading infectious causes of death across the world.

As per the WHO, India accounted for around 25% of the global burden of TB cases in 2012.

Characteristics of Mycobacteria

○ Mycobacteria are rod-shaped bacteria that multiply slowly (every 15–20 hours). The cell wall contains mycolic acid that gives an unusual, waxy coating on its surface. Due to the lipophilic cell walls, they resist staining with Gram's stain.

○ Acid-fast stains such as Ziehl-Neelsen are commonly used to identify *M. tuberculosis*. Once stained, the bacteria are not decolorized easily by various solvents; hence, the name 'acid-fast bacilli'.

○ *M. tuberculosis* is characterized by caseating granulomas in tissues (containing Langhans giant cells) which leads to tissue destruction.

Tuberculosis can occur in the form of pulmonary or extrapulmonary TB (Figure 1).

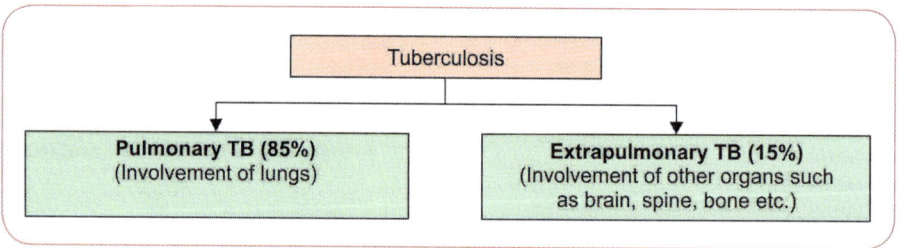

Figure 1: Tuberculosis

The infection most commonly occurs due to inhalation of infected droplet nuclei, which are generated by sneezing, coughing and spitting by patients with active TB.

When a person is infected with *M. tuberculosis*, there can be one of the following outcomes:

○ *Latent tuberculosis infection*
  ❑ In majority of cases, the infection is either cleared by the host immune system or subdued into an inactive form called latent tuberculosis infection (LTBI).
  ❑ These patients may develop active TB disease in future, which may then be called as 'TB reactivation'.
  ❑ The lifetime risk of reactivation of LTBI is estimated to be 5–10%. However, the chances are significantly higher in patients with risk factors (such as HIV infection, organ transplantation, silicosis, kidney dialysis, use of tumor necrosis factor-α blockers and close contact with an infectious patient).

○ *Active TB*
  ❑ Active disease
  ❑ Presence of symptoms including low-grade fever in the evening, night sweats, fatigue, weight loss and chronic cough with blood streaked sputum

The key differences between LTBI and active TB infection are mentioned in Figure 2.

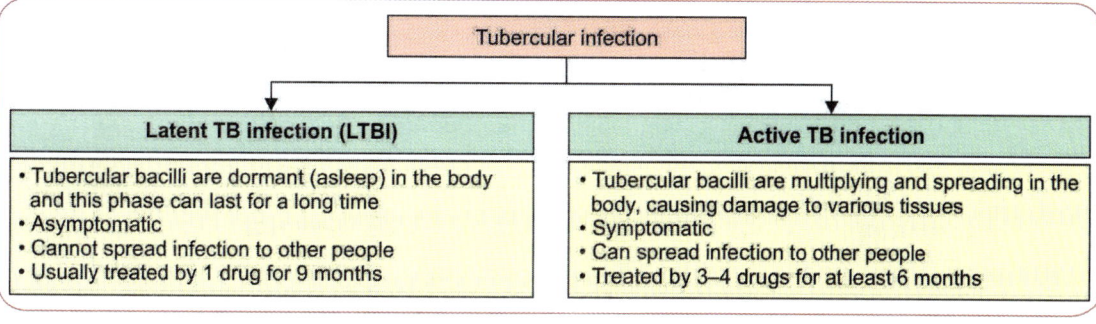

Figure 2: Difference between LTBI and active TB infection

Mycobacteria other than *M. tuberculosis* are known as 'atypical or nontubercular mycobacteria'. The atypical mycobacteria can cause disease similar to tuberculosis. Some atypical mycobacteria are mentioned in Table 1.

TABLE 1	Atypical (Nontubercular) mycobacteria
Pathogen	**Disease condition**
M. kansasii	Chronic pulmonary infection resembling pulmonary TB
M. marinum	Swimming pool granuloma
M. scrofulaceum	Cervical lymphadenitis
M. avium complex (comprises of *M. avium* + *M. intracellulare*)	Pulmonary and extrapulmonary disease in immunocompromised patients (most commonly AIDS)
M. leprae	Leprosy (Hansen's disease)

Important Considerations of Antitubercular Treatment

The mycobacteria are notorious due to the following challenges it poses during treatment:
- They have a lipid rich cell wall, which is impermeable to many antibiotics.
- They are mostly present inside the cells (intracellular) and reside inside the macrophages. The majority of antibiotics cannot penetrate inside the macrophages.
- They are well known for developing resistance to any single drug.

In order to overcome these challenges (specially to prevent resistance), the following measures are undertaken:
- Combine at least 2 or more antitubercular drugs.
- Drugs to be taken regularly (strict compliance).
- Continue treatment for months, as the response to therapy is slow.

CLASSIFICATION OF ANTITUBERCULAR DRUGS

The antitubercular drugs have traditionally been classified into 1st line drugs and 2nd line drugs (Figure 3).
- The 1st line drugs have higher efficacy and acceptable toxicity as compared to the 2nd line drugs.
- The 1st line drugs are to be used first for the treatment of any type of tuberculosis.
- The 2nd line drugs are to be used only when the 1st line drugs fail due to the development of resistance or if they are contraindicated for some reason.
- The WHO/Revised National Tuberculosis Control Program recommends the use of regimens comprising of 3–4 first-line drugs for a specified duration.

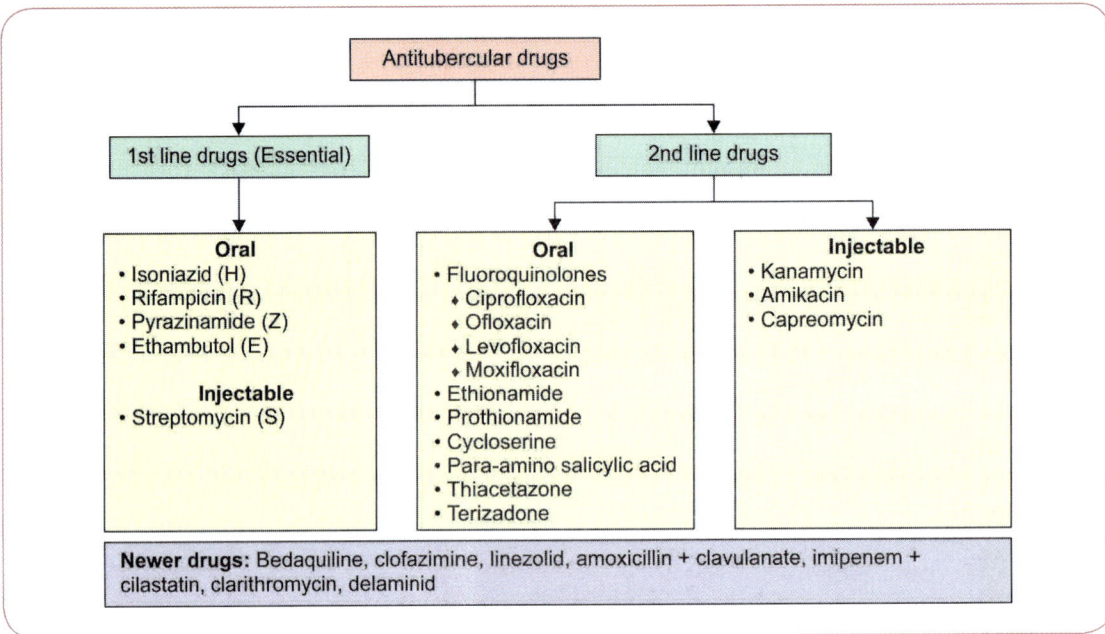

Figure 3: Classification of antitubercular drugs

FIRST LINE ANTITUBERCULAR DRUGS

The first line antitubercular drugs consist of isoniazid, rifampicin, pyrazinamide, ethambutol and streptomycin. The clinically employed daily doses of these drugs are mentioned in Figure 4.

Daily doses of first line antitubercular drugs				
Isoniazid (H)	**Rifampicin (R)**	**Pyrazinamide (Z)**	**Ethambutol (E)**	**Streptomycin (S)**
5 mg/kg Range 4–6 mg/kg Total dose—300 mg	**10 mg/kg** Range 8–12 mg/kg Total dose—600 mg	**25 mg/kg** Range 20–30 mg/kg Total dose—1500 mg	**15 mg/kg** Range 12–18 mg/kg Total dose—1000 mg	**15 mg/kg** Range 15–20 mg/kg Total dose—1000 mg

Figure 4: Daily doses of first line antitubercular drugs

ISONIAZID, ISONICOTINIC ACID HYDRAZIDE, INH (H)

Isoniazid is the most active, very potent and most widely used antitubercular drug.

Key Features of INH

- It is a prodrug that is converted to an active metabolite by mycobacterial enzyme, catalase peroxidase (KatG).
- It has structural similarity to pyridoxine.
- It is *bactericidal* for actively multiplying TB bacilli, and *bacteriostatic* for dormant TB bacilli.
- It is active against *both extracellular and intracellular bacteria* (within macrophages).
- It is highly active against *M. tuberculosis*, and to a lesser extent against *M. kansasii*.
- Most atypical (nontubercular) mycobacteria are resistant to INH.

Mechanism of Action

INH inhibits the synthesis of mycolic acid which is a unique and essential component of mycobacterial cell walls (Figure 5). No other microorganism contains mycolic acid in their cell walls; hence, INH is not effective against any other microorganism.

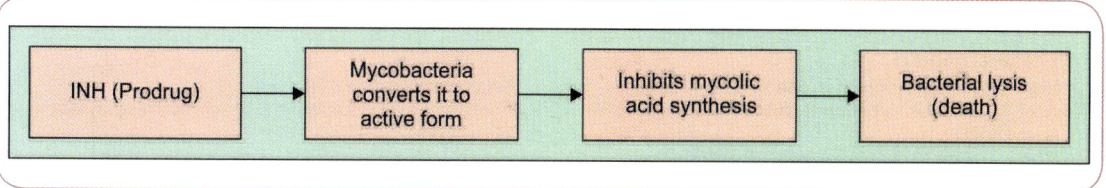

Figure 5: Isoniazid—mechanism of action

Mechanism of Resistance

The resistance in mycobacteria occurs due to chromosomal mutations. Some of the mutations are mentioned in Table 2.

TABLE 2	Isoniazid resistance—types of chromosomal mutations
Most common mutation	Mutation in the KatG gene (essential for conversion of INH prodrug to its active form)
Other mutation	Mutation in the InhA gene (essential for mycolic acid synthesis)

Pharmacokinetics

INH is well-absorbed orally. It readily diffuses in all body tissues, fluids and cavities (TB cavities, meninges, placenta and other body fluids).

INH is metabolized in the liver by acetylation. The rate of acetylation is under genetic control, so that there are slow and fast acetylators (Figure 6). The acetylated metabolites are excreted by the kidneys.

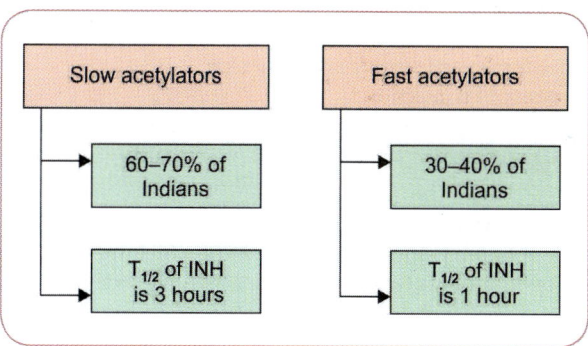

Figure 6: Isoniazid acetylation

Note:
- If INH is taken daily, the acetylator status does not affect the antitubercular response
- If INH is taken biweekly, the acetylator status affects the antitubercular response and may lead to decreased concentrations and response in a fast acetylator
- The acetylator status affects the INH toxicity profile

Adverse Effects

The key adverse effects of INH are mentioned in Figure 7.

Isoniazid—adverse effects	
Peripheral neuritis	**Hepatitis/Others**

Peripheral neuritis
• Dose dependent (occurs in doses >5 mg/kg/day)
• Acetylator status dependent (more common in slow acetylators)
• Risk is higher in chronic alcoholism, malnutrition, diabetes mellitus, AIDS etc.
• Common symptoms are paraesthesia, numbness etc.
• It is due to *relative pyridoxine (vitamin B₆) deficiency*, occurring because:
  ♦ INH interferes with pyridoxine utilization
  ♦ INH increases pyridoxine excretion in urine
• Concomitant pyridoxine use (10–40 mg/day) prevents the occurrence of peripheral neuritis
• Pyridoxine is also used for the treatment of peripheral neuritis, if it has already occurred
	Hepatitis
	• Major, serious adverse effect
	• Acetylator status dependent (more common in fast acetylators)
	• Risk is higher in elderly, chronic alcoholics and underlying liver disease
	• Reversible on INH discontinuation. Prompt discontinuation is required
	  However, if hepatitis remains unrecognized and INH is continued, it can lead to death
	Other adverse effects
	• Hypersensitivity reactions (fever, rash etc.)
	• GIT disturbance, hematological changes
	• Drug-induced SLE, psychosis, convulsions

Figure 7: Isoniazid—adverse effects

Drug Interactions

The key drug interactions of INH are:
- INH decreases the metabolism and increases the blood levels of warfarin, phenytoin and carbamazepine.
- Aluminum hydroxide (antacid) decreases INH absorption.

Clinical Uses

INH is used in the following clinical conditions:
- Treatment of active TB infection—used as combination therapy
- Treatment of latent TB infection—used as single drug therapy
- Prophylaxis for the prevention of TB infection

▮ RIFAMPICIN, RIFAMPIN (R)

Rifampicin is a widely used 1st line antitubercular drug.

It has a broader spectrum of antimicrobial action than INH, which means that apart from *M. tuberculosis*, it is also effective against many gram-positive and gram-negative bacteria such as *S. aureus, N. meningitides, H. influenzae, Klebsiella* etc.

Key Features of Rifampicin

- It is a derivative of rifamycin, which is an antibiotic produced by *Streptomyces mediterranei*.
- It is *bactericidal for both actively multiplying as well as dormant TB bacilli*. However, it acts best against slowly dividing bacilli (known as spurters).
- It is *active against both extracellular and intracellular bacteria* (within macrophages).
- It is known as a **sterilizing agent**. It is the only drug active against all subtypes of TB bacilli.
- It has good resistance preventing actions.
- It is also active against atypical (nontubercular) mycobacteria including *M. kansasii and MAC*.

Mechanism of Action

Rifampicin binds to and inhibits DNA dependent RNA polymerase in mycobacteria, and thereby inhibits RNA synthesis. Mammalian RNA polymerase does not bind rifampicin, therefore, there is no effect on human cells.

Pharmacokinetics

Rifampicin is well-absorbed orally. Food decreases its absorption; hence, it should be consumed on an empty stomach. It gets distributed widely throughout the organs and body fluids.

Rifampicin is metabolized in the liver and excreted in the bile. It undergoes enterohepatic recirculation. The metabolites are finally excreted in the feces with a small proportion excreted by the kidneys.

Rifampicin is a strong inducer of most CYP450 isoenzymes which increases the metabolism of many drugs. Rifampicin also undergoes autoinduction leading to its decreased plasma levels for the first few weeks.

Adverse Effects

Rifampicin is usually well tolerated. The key adverse effects of rifampicin are mentioned in Figure 8.

Rifampicin—Adverse effects			
GIT	**Hepatitis**	**Flu-like syndrome**	**Discoloration of body fluids***
• Nausea, vomiting • Abdominal distress • Commonly encountered adverse effects during rifampicin therapy	• Rare but an important adverse effect • Risk is higher in elderly, chronic alcoholics and in patients with pre-existing liver disease	• Symptoms include fever, chills, myalgia etc. • Occurs when rifampicin is given intermittently (i.e. less frequently than twice weekly)	• Causes a harmless orange-red discoloration of body fluids such as saliva, sweat, tears, urine, feces etc. • Contact lenses may become stained

*Patients should be counseled and forewarned regarding this harmless effect, so that drug compliance should not be impacted.

Figure 8: Rifampicin—adverse effects

Drug Interactions

Rifampicin is a strong inducer of most CYP450 isoenzymes (e.g. CYP1A2, CYP2C9, CYP3A4).

This leads to increased metabolism (and decreased blood levels) of other drugs given simultaneously such as oral contraceptives, oral anticoagulants, some anticonvulsants, HIV protease inhibitors and non-nucleoside reverse transcriptase inhibitors, ketoconazole, cyclosporine etc. Concurrent use may result in therapeutic failure of these drugs.

The patients should be warned of the possibility of oral contraceptive failure, when rifampicin is given along with oral contraceptives.

Clinical Uses

Tuberculosis

Rifampicin (along with INH and other antitubercular drugs) is used in the treatment of active TB infection. It is also used as chemoprophylaxis for the prevention of development of active TB infection.

Leprosy and Other Atypical Mycobacterial Infections

Rifampicin along with dapsone (with or without clofazimine) is used in multibacillary and paucibacillary leprosy. Rifampicin is also effective against some atypical mycobacterial infections.

Prophylaxis of H. influenzae and N. meningitides Meningitis

Rifampicin is useful in eradicating the nasopharyngeal carrier state of *H. influenzae* and *N. meningitides* infections. Hence, it is useful as a prophylactic drug to prevent the development of active infection. The usual doses employed are 600 mg twice a day for 2 days.

Staphylococcal Infections

Rifampicin may be used along with a beta lactam antibiotic or vancomycin in some cases of staphylococcal osteomyelitis, endocarditis etc.

PYRAZINAMIDE (Z)

Pyrazinamide is an analogue of nicotinamide. It is used orally only for the treatment of tuberculosis.

It is active only at acidic pH. It enters the macrophages and then exerts bactericidal action against tubercle bacilli residing in the acidic milieu of lysosomes.

Pyrazinamide is converted to the active form pyrazinoic acid (by mycobacterial enzyme) which then disturbs bacterial cell wall synthesis as well as membrane transport functions.

It is well-absorbed orally and is widely distributed throughout the body. It is metabolized in the liver and the metabolites are excreted by the kidneys. Hence, the dose must be reduced in patients with renal failure.

Adverse Effects

The key adverse effects of pyrazinamide are mentioned in Figure 9.

Pyrazinamide—Adverse effects		
Hepatotoxicity	**Hyperuricemia**	**GIT/Others**
• Most serious adverse effect • Elevation of transaminases is the earliest sign • Baseline hepatic function should be checked before start of therapy • Drug should be withdrawn in cases of apparent hepatic damage	• Inhibits uric acid excretion • Results in hyperuricemia in most patients • Acute attack of gout may rarely be precipitated in susceptible patients	• Nausea, vomiting, anorexia • Malaise, arthralgia • Drug fever • These adverse effects may occur with pyrazinamide use

Figure 9: Pyrazinamide—adverse effects

Clinical Uses

Pyrazinamide is effective against intracellular bacilli that may be responsible for causing relapses. Hence, it is also known as a sterilizing agent.

It is used along with INH, rifampicin and ethambutol in antitubercular regimens for treating active TB infection.

ETHAMBUTOL (E)

Ethambutol is a bacteriostatic drug. It inhibits arabinosyl transferases which are involved in the synthesis of mycobacterial cell wall.

Ethambutol is well-absorbed orally and is widely distributed throughout the body. It crosses the blood brain barrier only in situations when the meninges are inflamed. It is metabolized in the liver, but majority of the parent drug is excreted unchanged by the kidneys. Hence, the dose must be reduced in patients with renal failure.

Adverse Effects

Ethambutol is usually well tolerated by most patients. The key adverse effects of ethambutol are mentioned in Figure 10.

Ethambutol—Adverse effects	
Optic neuritis	**Hyperuricemia/others**

• Most important serious adverse effect
• Manifestations include:
  ♦ Reduced visual acuity
  ♦ Red-green color blindness
• Dose related effect (more chances with higher doses)
• Visual acuity and color discrimination testing must be done before start of therapy and then at periodic intervals
• Avoided in children as they are unable to permit visual examination
• Reversible if the drug is withdrawn early
	• Inhibits uric acid excretion
	• Results in hyperuricemia in ~50% of patients
	• Other adverse effects include:
	  ♦ Nausea, vomiting, abdominal pain
	  ♦ Rash, drug fever
	  ♦ Joint pain
	  ♦ Mental confusion
	  ♦ Disorientation

Figure 10: Ethambutol—adverse effects

Ethambutol is used along with INH, rifampicin and pyrazinamide in antitubercular regimens for treating active TB infection.

Ethambutol is a broad spectrum antitubercular drug i.e. apart from *M. tuberculosis*, it is also active against many atypical mycobacteria. However, apart from mycobacteria, it does not have activity against any other class of bacteria.

STREPTOMYCIN (S)

Streptomycin is a bactericidal drug. It is an aminoglycoside. It is not effective orally and is given by IM injection.

It penetrates poorly into the cells and is active primarily against extracellular bacilli. The adverse effects include ototoxicity and nephrotoxicity.

It is given along with INH, rifampicin and pyrazinamide in antitubercular regimens for treating active TB infection.

SECOND LINE ANTITUBERCULAR DRUGS

The 2nd line antitubercular drugs have a lower efficacy and higher toxicity than the 1st line drugs. Hence, they are the reserve drugs, and are to be used only when the 1st line drugs fail due to resistance or if there are some contraindications.

ETHIONAMIDE

Ethionamide is structurally similar to INH. It also inhibits mycolic acid synthesis. However, it has lesser efficacy than INH.

Ethionamide is a bacteriostatic drug. It is well-absorbed orally and is widely distributed throughout the body including the CSF. It is metabolized in the liver and excreted by the kidneys.

The common adverse effects include:

○ GIT disturbances–most common and includes nausea, vomiting, gastric irritation
○ Neurological toxicity–drowsiness, paraesthesia, depression
○ Others–hepatitis, rashes, acne, alopecia, gynecomastia

Pyridoxine (vitamin B_6) prevents/decreases the neurological toxicity, and it should be given concomitantly.

PARA-AMINO SALICYLIC ACID (PAS)

PAS is structurally similar to sulfonamides and *para*-aminobenzoic acid (PABA).

Like sulfonamides, it competitively inhibits the enzyme dihydropteroate synthase, and prevents the synthesis of folic acid, which is required for growth and multiplication of bacteria.

PAS is a bacteriostatic drug. It is well-absorbed orally and is widely distributed throughout the body except the CSF. It is metabolized in the liver and excreted by the kidneys.

The absorption from GIT is increased by the presence of food. Hence, PAS should be given after meals to increase the bioavailability as well as to decrease the GIT adverse effects.

It is acetylated in the liver, and the parent PAS as well as the acetylated metabolites are excreted by the kidneys. The adverse effects include:
- GIT disturbances–reduced by giving it along with food in divided doses
- Hypersensitivity reactions–fever, rashes, hepatitis, arthralgia, granulocytopenia etc.

PAS is a reserve drug being currently used in the treatment of multidrug resistant (MDR) TB.

CYCLOSERINE

Cycloserine is a structural analogue of d-alanine. It is an inhibitor of bacterial cell wall synthesis. It is a bacteriostatic drug.

It is well-absorbed orally and is widely distributed throughout the body including the CSF. Most of the drug is excreted unchanged by the kidneys.

The characteristic adverse effect includes *neuropsychiatric toxicity*. It may cause headache, convulsions, somnolence, psychosis, depression and suicidal ideation.

Cycloserine is a reserve drug being currently used in the treatment of MDR TB.

FLUOROQUINOLONES

Fluoroquinolones (FQ) are DNA gyrase inhibitors. They are bactericidal drugs.

Commonly used FQs in TB include ciprofloxacin, ofloxacin, levofloxacin, gatifloxacin and moxifloxacin.

They are currently used as 2nd line drugs for the treatment of MDR TB.

FQs are being increasingly included in the combination therapy for treating MDR TB and treatment of atypical mycobacteria because of the following reasons:
- Effectively kill intracellular bacilli
- Active against typical and atypical mycobacteria
- Orally effective
- Good tolerability
- Convenient dosing schedule

OTHER SECOND LINE ANTITUBERCULAR DRUGS

AMINOGLYCOSIDES (AMIKACIN AND KANAMYCIN)

Apart from streptomycin, amikacin and kanamycin are the other aminoglycosides used in the treatment of MDR TB. These are bactericidal drugs.

Both the drugs have significant ototoxicity and nephrotoxicity. They are therefore used as second-line drugs in MDR TB after streptomycin.

It has been observed that most MDR strains and those resistant to streptomycin are usually susceptible to amikacin. Amikacin is also effective against atypical mycobacteria.

CAPREOMYCIN

It is a peptide antibiotic. It is an injectable drug used in the treatment of MDR TB. The adverse effects are similar to that of aminoglycosides i.e. ototoxicity and nephrotoxicity. It also causes significant pain at the site of injection which may result in sterile abscesses. It is used in the treatment of MDR TB.

NEWER ANTITUBERCULAR DRUGS

BEDAQUILINE

Bedaquiline is the first drug with a novel mechanism of action. It inhibits the mycobacterial enzyme ATP synthase. This enzyme is necessary for the generation of energy in mycobacteria.

Inhibition of ATP synthase results in bactericidal effects on both replicating and nonreplicating mycobacteria. There is no cross-resistance between bedaquiline and other drugs used in tuberculosis.

It is well-absorbed orally and fatty meal increases its absorption. It is metabolized in the liver mainly by CYP3A4 isoenzyme. This may lead to numerous drug interactions.

The parent drug and the metabolites have a long terminal half-life of approximately 5.5 months.

The key adverse effects include hepatotoxicity and cardiac conduction toxicity (QT_c interval prolongation).

It is currently used in MDR TB, in combination with at least 3 other active anti-TB drugs for 24 weeks. The recommended dosing regimen is mentioned in Figure 11.

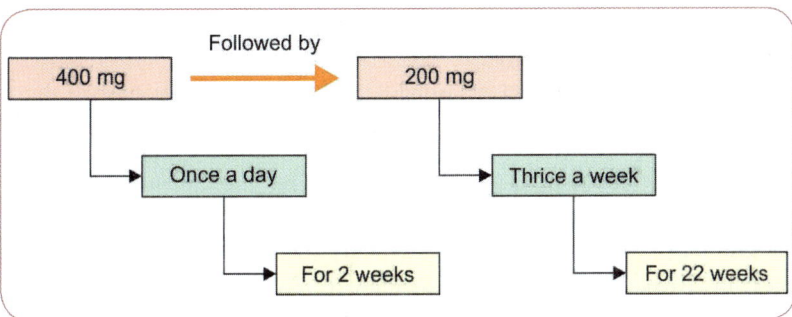

Figure 11: Dosing regimen of bedaquinile

RIFABUTIN

Rifabutin is an analogue of rifampicin. The similarities and differences with rifampicin are mentioned in Figure 12.

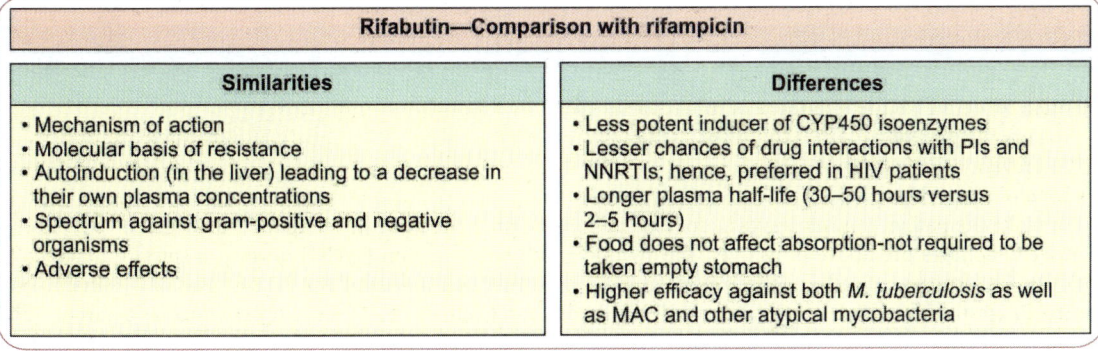

Rifabutin—Comparison with rifampicin	
Similarities	**Differences**
• Mechanism of action • Molecular basis of resistance • Autoinduction (in the liver) leading to a decrease in their own plasma concentrations • Spectrum against gram-positive and negative organisms • Adverse effects	• Less potent inducer of CYP450 isoenzymes • Lesser chances of drug interactions with PIs and NNRTIs; hence, preferred in HIV patients • Longer plasma half-life (30–50 hours versus 2–5 hours) • Food does not affect absorption-not required to be taken empty stomach • Higher efficacy against both *M. tuberculosis* as well as MAC and other atypical mycobacteria

Figure 12: Rifabutin and rifampicin

Rifabutin is used mainly in the following situations:

○ **Treatment of tuberculosis in HIV patients**—preferred due to its lesser propensity of inducing CYP450 isoenzymes. Therefore, the chances of drug interactions with PIs and NNRTIs (which are a part of HIV treatment) are much lesser.

o **Prevention and treatment of MAC infections in AIDS**—used along with clarithromycin/azithromycin, ethambutol and fluoroquinolones.

TERIZIDONE

It is a derivative of cycloserine. It is a bacteriostatic drug. The mechanism of action is similar to cycloserine.

It is active against both *M. tuberculosis* and *M. avium complex* and is used for the treatment of both pulmonary and extrapulmonary tuberculosis.

It is an important drug for the *treatment of urogenital tuberculosis*, because it achieves a much higher concentration in urine for a long duration of time.

The characteristic adverse effect (like cycloserine) includes *neuropsychiatric toxicity*. It may cause headache, convulsions, psychosis, depression and suicidal ideation.

DELAMINID

Delaminid is a new antimycobacterial drug indicated for use in pulmonary MDR TB, as a part of combination therapy in adults. It is a reserve drug for use when an effective treatment regimen cannot be provided. The drug is usually administered for a duration of 24 weeks.

The safety and efficacy in HIV-positive patients with MDR TB has not been established, due to limited clinical data.

MACROLIDES (AZITHROMYCIN, CLARITHROMYCIN)

Clarithromycin and azithromycin are used in the treatment and prophylaxis of atypical mycobacteria, most notably *mycobacterium avium complex* (MAC).

LINEZOLID

Linezolid has been found to be effective against intracellular bacilli and may be used in combination with other drugs for MDR TB.

The flip side is that the drug causes significant adverse effects (on prolonged use necessary for TB) including bone marrow suppression and irreversible optic and peripheral neuropathy.

Due to the magnitude of serious adverse effects, linezolid should be used only when the bacilli are resistant to numerous other first and second-line antitubercular drugs.

TREATMENT OF TUBERCULOSIS

The main objectives of the treatment of tuberculosis are:
o To cure the patient
o To prevent drug resistance
o To minimize relapses
o To make the patient noninfectious as soon as possible; hence, breaking the chain of transmission

In order to achieve the above objectives, the World Health Organization (WHO) devised a set of guidelines in 1995. The Government of India adopted these guidelines in 1997 and launched the Revised National Tuberculosis Control Program (RNTCP). Directly Observed Treatment Short Course (DOTS) was implemented as a part of WHO guideline/RNTCP.

The WHO released new guidelines in 2010, for the treatment of tuberculosis. The principles of the WHO guidelines have been adopted by the RNTCP in 2012. The aim of the new guidelines is to more effectively cure patients and prevent the development of MDR TB as well as more effective treatment of MDR TB.

DIRECTLY OBSERVED TREATMENT SHORT COURSE (DOTS)

The salient features of DOTS program are mentioned in Table 3.

TABLE 3	Directly observed treatment short course (DOTS)

- The anti-TB drugs are administered to the patient under direct supervision of a health worker or a trained person. This is done to make sure that the drugs are actually consumed.
- The thrice weekly dosing regimen is followed (in DOTS) only for Category 1 (i.e. new) patients.
- The aim is to ensure patient compliance and prevent the emergence of resistance.
- The patients are observed during the complete course of treatment. This is to make sure that the patient consumes correct drugs, at right doses, at right intervals, and for the appropriate duration.

The key features of RNTCP (which are based on WHO recommendations) are further mentioned in the following sections.

CLASSIFICATION OF PATIENTS BASED ON HISTORY OF TB TREATMENT

The distinction between patients based on the history of TB treatment is mentioned in Figure 13.

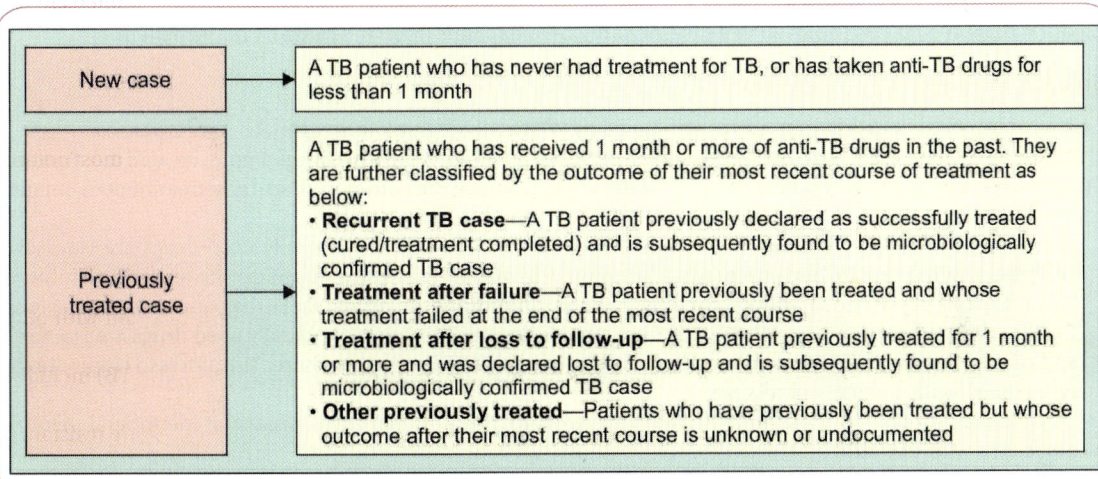

Figure 13: Classification of TB patients based on history of drug treatment

CLASSIFICATION OF PATIENTS BASED ON DRUG RESISTANCE

The distinction between patients based on the drug resistance is mentioned in Figure 14.

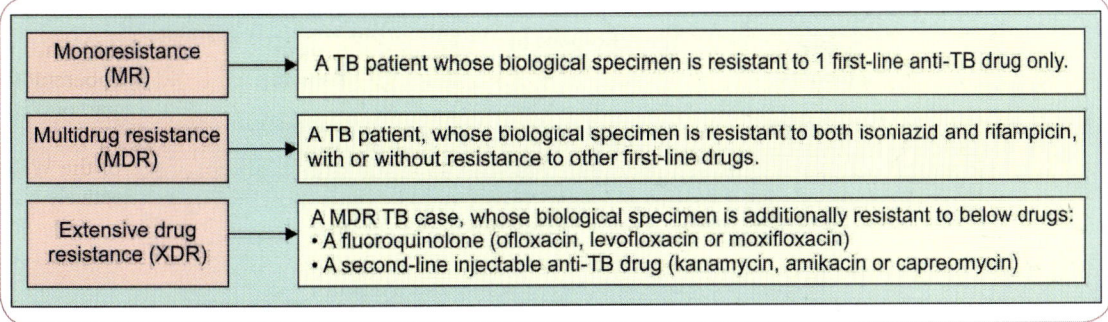

Figure 14: Classification of TB patients based on drug resistance

The WHO/RNTCP guidelines classify TB patients into Category I (new cases) or Category II (previously treated cases). The patients are also classified into MDR TB and XDR TB cases.

The anti-TB therapy is administered either as short-course regimens (for new cases and retreatment cases) or long-course regimens (MDR TB and XDR TB). Short-course regimens are given for 6–9 months while long-course regimens are given for 18–24 months.

In both short-course and long-course regimens, the drugs are administered in 2 phases: an intensive phase (IP) and a continuation phase (CP) (Figure 15).

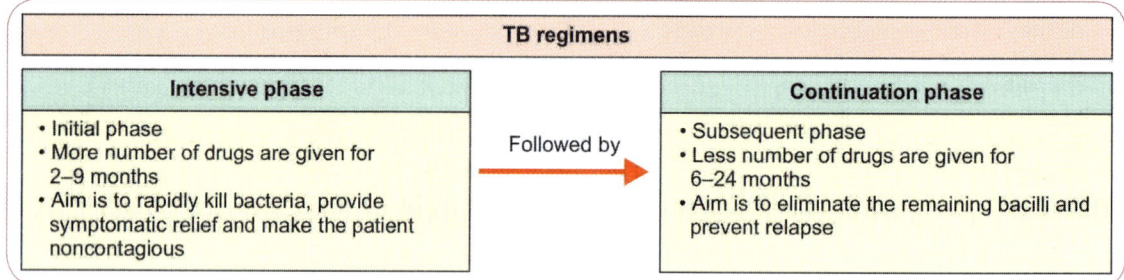

Figure 15: TB regimens—phases of treatment

The duration of IP and CP employed in a treatment regimen depends upon the category of the patient.

Short-term Treatment Regimen

The short-term treatment regimens were introduced by WHO. All the treatment regimens have 2 phases.

There are various short-term regimens being used. The treatment regimens, drugs employed, and the duration of treatment varies depending on the category of the patient. One of the common short-term treatment regimen is mentioned below:

- **Intensive phase for 2 months**—with 4 bactericidal drugs. The commonly orally used drugs are isoniazid, rifampicin, pyrazinamide and ethambutol. Streptomycin may be used intramuscularly instead of ethambutol. The aim of this phase is to rapidly kill bacteria, provide symptomatic relief and make the patient noncontagious.
- **Continuation phase for 4 months**—with 2 bactericidal drugs. The commonly orally used drugs are isoniazid and rifampicin. The RNTCP recommends the use of ethambutol also in this phase. The aim is to eliminate the remaining bacilli and prevent relapse.

Pyridoxine should be concomitantly administered to prevent the development of peripheral neuritis associated with isoniazid.

Category I (New Case)—Anti-TB Regimen

All new TB cases should be treated with an intensive phase of 2 months with HRZE daily followed by a continuation phase of 4 months of HRE daily (Figure 16).

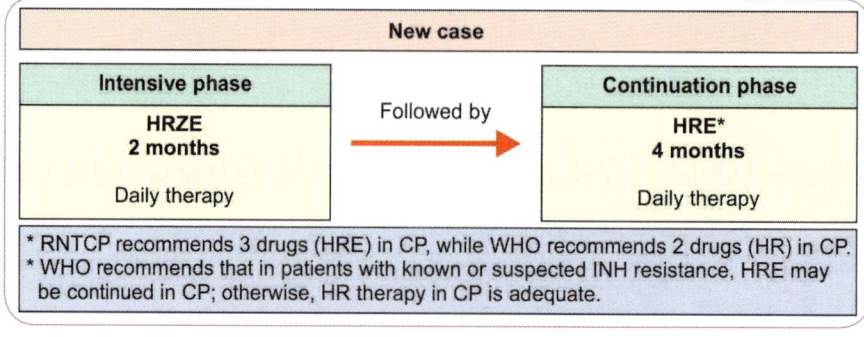

Figure 16: Category I (New Case)—anti-TB regimen

The WHO recommends that the optimal regimen is daily therapy in both IP and CP. Daily therapy should be followed, wherever possible. However, in situations, where daily therapy is not possible, the following approaches may be followed:

○ **Daily therapy in IP and thrice weekly therapy in CP**—thrice weekly therapy must be supervised (DOTS)
○ **Thrice weekly therapy in both IP and CP**—thrice weekly therapy must be supervised (DOTS) and the patient must not be living with HIV or in an HIV prevalent setting.

Category II (Previously Treated Case)—Anti-TB Regimen

The WHO recommends that all previously treated patients should have the specimens tested for culture and drug susceptibility testing (DST) at or prior to the start of therapy.

While awaiting the culture and DST results, two approaches can be followed:

○ When there is a low chance of patients having MDR TB (e.g. relapse/default patients), retreatment regimen with first-line drugs should be initiated.
○ When there is a high chance of patients having MDR TB (e.g. failure patients), a standard MDR regimen with second-line drugs should be initiated.

Once the results of DST are available, appropriate modifications in both the above approaches/regimens must be done.

The retreatment regimen for a previously treated case is mentioned in Figure 17. The MDR TB regimen is mentioned in the subsequent section.

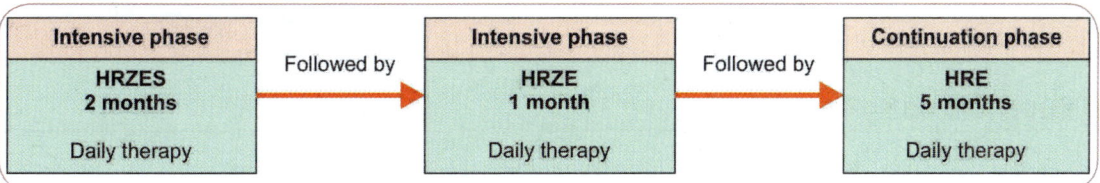

Figure 17: Previously treated case—retreatment regimen

Multidrug Resistant TB (MDR TB) Regimen

MDR TB means the patient is resistant to both INH and rifampicin with or without resistance to other first-line drugs.

It can be treated by standard MDR TB regimens; or by individual regimens in cases where DST results are available.

The WHO recommends that MDR TB should be treated with at least 4 drugs to which the bacilli are almost certainly susceptible. More than 4 drugs may be given if the bacilli susceptibility or the efficacy of the drugs is unknown.

The RNTCP regimen for the MDR TB is mentioned in Figure 18.

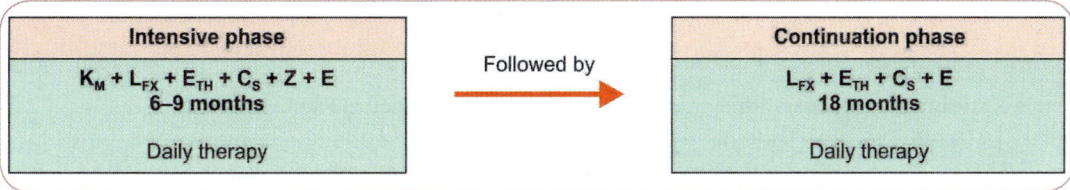

Figure 18: Multidrug resistant TB regimen

Abbreviations: K_M, kanamycin; L_{FX}, levofloxacin; E_{TH}, ethionamide; C_S, cycloserine; Z, pyrazinamide; E, ethambutol

Note: In case the patient is rifampicin resistant, but is either INH sensitive or INH unknown, INH should be added in both IP and CP.

The treatment for MDR TB should be initiated only where there are well established DOTS programs. The drugs used in MDR TB are administered daily under direct supervision.

For tackling MDR TB, WHO/RNTCP have implemented a DOTS plus strategy. DOTS Plus means the features of the DOTS program with additional measures for diagnosis, management and treatment of MDR TB.

Extensive Drug Resistant TB (XDR TB) Regimen

The drugs used in XDR TB are administered daily under direct supervision. The RNTCP regimen for the XDR TB is mentioned in Figure 19.

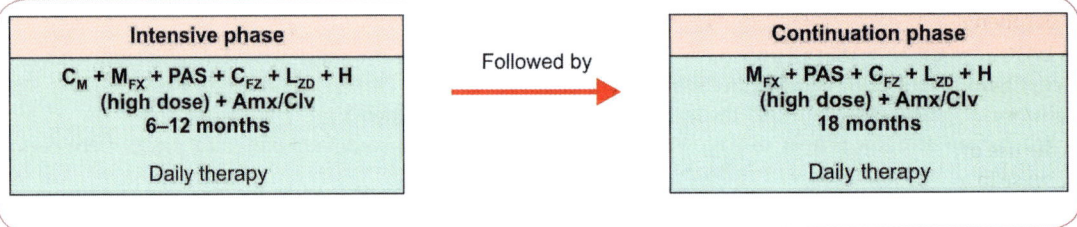

Figure 19: Extensive drug resistant TB regimen

Abbreviations: C_M, capreomycin; M_{FX}, moxifloxacin; PAS, para-amino salicylic acid; C_{FZ}, clofazimine; L_{ZD}, linezolid; H, isoniazid; Amx/Clv, amoxicillin/clavulinic acid

TREATMENT OF TB IN SPECIAL SITUATIONS

TUBERCULOSIS IN PREGNANCY

All the first-line drugs (H, R, Z, E) except for streptomycin, can be used during pregnancy. Streptomycin is contraindicated because it may cause ototoxicity in the fetus. Pyridoxine supplementation is necessary for pregnant patients consuming isoniazid.

The pregnant women should be counseled that successful TB treatment is critical for a successful pregnancy outcome.

TUBERCULOSIS IN HIV POSITIVE PATIENTS

The WHO recommends that HIV testing should be done in all patients presenting with tuberculosis.

The treatment of TB in HIV-positive patient is the same as that of HIV-negative patient. The patients are classified into 'new case' or 'previously treated case' and the regimens are accordingly employed.

The short-term chemotherapy is employed, and daily regimen is preferred in HIV patients. *The only difference is that rifabutin is preferred over rifampicin.* This is because rifabutin causes significantly less drug interactions with anti-HIV drugs (e.g. protease inhibitors and nonnucleoside reverse transcriptase inhibitors) as compared to rifampicin.

Cotrimoxazole Preventive Therapy

The role of cotrimoxazole preventive therapy in HIV patients is mentioned in Figure 20.

> **Cotrimoxazole preventive therapy in HIV-positive TB patients**
>
> • Cotrimoxazole preventive therapy should be initiated in all HIV-positive TB patients
> • It should be given throughout the duration of TB treatment
> • Advantage—It significantly reduces mortality in HIV-positive TB patients
> • It prevents *Pneumocystis jiroveci* and malaria infections and also impacts other bacterial infections

Figure 20: Cotrimoxazole preventive therapy

EXTRAPULMONARY TUBERCULOSIS

The extrapulmonary TB (EPTB) most commonly involves lymphatics and bone or joints. However, the most serious forms of EPTB occur with pericardial, meningeal or miliary (disseminated) TB.

EPTB (as for pulmonary TB) is treated with the same daily short-term regimens for a duration of 6-9 months. The following are some noteworthy points regarding EPTB:
- In tubercular meningitis, ethambutol should be replaced with streptomycin.
- In tubercular meningitis and pericarditis, corticosteroids' use as adjuvant therapy is recommended.

CHEMOPROPHYLAXIS

It is the use of antitubercular drugs, either to prevent the development of infection, or to prevent the development of disease in already infected individuals.
- The commonly used drug (for TB chemoprophylaxis) is isoniazid (INH) 300 mg (10 mg/kg/day in children) daily for 6 months.
- In some areas where INH resistance is prevalent, a combination of INH (5 mg/kg/day) and rifampicin (10 mg/kg/day) is given for 6 months.

The indications for TB chemoprophylaxis are mentioned in Table 4.

TABLE 4	Indications for TB chemoprophylaxis

- Close contacts of open (smear positive) cases
- Neonate of a mother with active tuberculosis
- Children (<6 years of age) with Mantoux positive skin test and having a TB positive family member
- Patients with Mantoux positive skin test + additional risk factors (e.g. AIDS, immunosuppression, diabetes, silicosis, malignancy etc.)

TREATMENT OF MYCOBACTERIUM AVIUM COMPLEX (MAC) INFECTIONS

MAC commonly causes disseminated disease in late stages of AIDS infection i.e. when the CD_4 cell counts are <50/μL.

MAC is not susceptible to the drugs employed for *M. tuberculosis*. The combination of drugs effective against MAC are mentioned in Table 5.

TABLE 5	Drugs employed against MAC
Treatment of MAC infections	Clarithromycin/azithromycin, ethambutol, rifabutin, ciprofloxacin, levofloxacin, moxifloxacin
Prophylaxis of MAC infections	Clarithromycin/azithromycin, rifabutin

ROLE OF CORTICOSTEROIDS IN TUBERCULOSIS

Although corticosteroids are generally not given in infections, and tuberculosis is a relative contraindication, they are used in the following situations (under effective cover of ant-TB drugs):
- In meningeal, pleural, pericardial tuberculosis—to prevent fibrosis, scar formation and its complications (e.g. constrictive pericarditis, pleural adhesions, focal neurological deficits etc.)
- To prevent and treat hypersensitivity reactions to anti-TB drugs

Corticosteroids should not be given in intestinal tuberculosis due to the risk of silent intestinal perforation.

Corticosteroids should be gradually withdrawn once the patient's condition improves, to avoid HPA-axis suppression.

ASSESS YOURSELF (Examination Questions of Various Universities)

1. Classify anti tubercular drugs. Discuss in detail the mechanism of action, side effects & uses of isoniazid

2. List anti tubercular drugs. Describe in detail about first line drugs

3. Describe the mechanism of action, pharmacokinetics, adverse effects and clinical uses of rifampicin

4. Explain why rifampin is not co-administered with oral contraceptives

5. Use of Bedaquiline in tuberculosis

6. Directly observed treatment short course (DOTS)

7. Drug therapy of multi drug resistant Tuberculosis (MDR-TB)

8. Second line antitubercular drugs

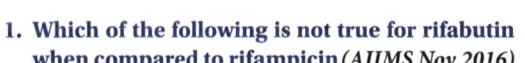

MULTIPLE CHOICE QUESTIONS

1. Which of the following is not true for rifabutin when compared to rifampicin *(AIIMS Nov 2016)*
   a. Rifabutin has a longer half-life than rifampicin
   b. Rifabutin is more effective for newly diagnosed TB
   c. Rifabutin has lesser incidence of drug interactions
   d. Rifampicin is more effective against MAC as compared to rifabutin

2. Anti TB drug associated with max ocular side effects is: *(Recent Question Dec 2016)*
   a. Rifampicin   b. Isonizad
   c. Ethambutol   d. Pyrazinamide

3. Which antitubercular drug causes hyperuricemia? *(Recent Question Dec 2016)*
   a. Isoniazid   b. Rifampicin
   c. Pyrazinamide   d. Ethambutol

4. Which of the following is a latest drug approved for MDR TB? *(AIIMS Nov 2015)*
   a. Bedaquilline   b. Tipranavir
   c. Levofloxacin   d. Linezolid

5. One of the antitubercular drugs is contraindicated in children below 6 years of age, because they may be unable to appreciate and report visual field defects or changes in vision, which is a known side effect of that drug. Which among the following is that drug?
   (Recent Question 2016)
   a. Ethambutol   b. INH
   c. Rifampicin   d. Pyrazinamide

6. Which of the following ATT is not hepatotoxic?
   (Recent Question 2016)
   a. Isoniazid   b. Rifampicin
   c. Pyrazinamide   d. Streptomycin

7. Arthralgia is commonly caused by which antituberculous drug? *(Recent Question 2016)*
   a. INH   b. Rifampicin
   c. Pyrazinamide   d. Ethambutol

8. Maximum sterilizing action is shown by which anti TB drug? *(Recent Question 2016)*
   a. Rifampicin   b. INH
   c. Pyrazinamide   d. Streptomycin

9. Flu like syptoms is side effect of which anti TB drug? *(Recent Question 2016)*
   a. INH   b. Rifampicin
   c. Pyrzinamide   d. Streptomycin

10. Bacteriostatic anti TB drug:
   (Recent Question 2016)
   a. INH   b. Rifampicin
   c. Ethambutol   d. Pyrazinamide

11. Pyridoxine should be given when treating with:
   (Recent Question 2016)
   a. Isoniazid   b. Rifampicin
   c. Pyrazinamide   d. Streptomycin

12. XDR TB is resistance to: *(Recent Question 2016)*
   a. Isoniazid
   b. Isoniazid + rifampicin
   c. Isoniazid + rifampicin + ethambutol
   d. Isoniazid + rifampicin + kanamycin

Ans.

| 1. | (d) | 2. | (c) | 3. | (c) | 4. | (a) | 5. | (a) | 6. | (d) |
| 7. | (c) | 8. | (a) | 9. | (b) | 10. | (c) | 11. | (a) | 12. | (d) |

13. **Hepatotoxic drug used in tuberculosis is:**
(Recent Question 2016)
   a. Isoniazid
   b. Streptomycin
   c. Kanamycin
   d. Ethambutol

14. **Ethambutol causes:** *(Recent Question 2016)*
   a. Retrobulbar neuritis
   b. Deafness
   c. Red urine
   d. Peripheral neuritis

15. **Slow acetylators of isoniazid are more prone to develop:** *(Recent Question 2016)*
   a. Failure of therapy
   b. Peripheral neuropathy
   c. Hepatotoxicity
   d. Allergic reactions

16. **The following is not a hepatotoxic antitubercular drug:** *(Recent Question 2016)*
   a. Ethambutol
   b. Isoniazid
   c. Ricampicin
   d. Pyrazinamide

17. **DNA dependent RNA synthesis is inhibited by:** *(Recent Question 2016)*
   a. Rifampicin
   b. Ethambutol
   c. Colchicine
   d. Chloromycetin

18. **Peripheral neuropathy is caused by:** *(Recent Question 2016)*
   a. Rifampicin
   b. Pyrazinamide
   c. INH
   d. Ethambutol

19. **Drug of choice for prophylaxis of TB is:** *(Recent Question 2016)*
   a. Rifampicin
   b. Isoniazid
   c. Pyrazinamide
   d. Streptomycin

20. **ATT drug causing contact lens staining:** *(Recent Question 2016)*
   a. INH
   b. Rifampicin
   c. Pyrazinamide
   d. Thioacetazone

21. **Side effects of isoniazid are all except:** *(Recent Question 2016)*
   a. Hepatitis
   b. Optic neuritis
   c. Peripheral neuropathy
   d. Thrombocytopenia

22. **Pregnant lady on ATT develops hearing abnormality and tinnitus. Causative drug is:** *(Recent Question 2016)*
   a. INH
   b. Rifampicin
   c. Ethambutol
   d. Streptomycin

23. **MDR-TB is defined as a strain resistant to:** *(Recent Question 2016)*
   a. Isoniazid and pyrazinamide
   b. Isoniazid and rifampicin
   c. Rifampicin and streptomycin
   d. Pyrazinamide and rifampicin

24. **XDR-TB is defined as:** *(Recent Question 2016)*
   a. Resistance isoniazid and rifampicin+ quinolone
   b. Resistance isoniazid + quinolone + injectable aminoglycoside
   c. Resistance isoniazid and rifampicin and quinolone + injectable aminoglycoside
   d. Resistance rifampicin + quinolone + injectable aminoglycoside anti-viral

25. **Antitubercular drug contraindicated in pregnancy:** *(TN PG 2015, 2013)*
   a. Isoniazid
   b. Rifampicin
   c. Ethambutol
   d. Streptomycin

26. **Drug not used in treating MDR-TB:** *(TN PG 2008)*
   a. Amikacin
   b. Kanamycin
   c. Capreomycin
   d. Isoniazid

27. **Isoniazid and pyridoxine are given together:** *(TN PG 2002)*
   a. To prevent peripheral neuritis
   b. To prevent INH resistance
   c. To increase drug absorption
   d. As liver supplement

28. **A known case of TB is now resistant to Rifampicin and Isoniazid. Which of the following would be most appropriate in treating this patient?** *(AIIMS Nov 2018)*
   a. 6 drugs for 4 months; 4 drugs for 12 months
   b. 6 drugs for 6 months; 4 drugs for 18 months
   c. 4 drugs for 4 months, 6 drugs for 12 months
   d. 5 drugs for 2 months; 4 drugs for 1 month; 3 drugs for 5 months

29. **Antitubercular drug causing ophthalmic toxicity is:** *(AIIMS Nov 2018)*
   a. Isoniazid
   b. Rifampicin
   c. Ethambutol
   d. None of above

Ans.

13.	(a)	14.	(a)	15.	(b)	16.	(a)	17.	(a)	18.	(c)
19.	(b)	20.	(b)	21.	(b)	22.	(d)	23.	(b)	24.	(c)
25.	(d)	26.	(d)	27.	(a)	28.	(b)	29.	(c)		

59

Antileprosy Drugs

INTRODUCTION

Leprosy (Hansen's disease) is a chronic granulomatous disease caused by *Mycobacterium leprae* which is an intracellular, obligatory parasite. It is a slow growing acid-fast bacillus.

The transmission of leprosy is through droplets, mainly via the respiratory tract. The incubation period for leprosy varies from a few weeks to up to 20 years with the average incubation period ranging from 5 to 7 years.

CLASSIFICATION OF ANTILEPROSY DRUGS

The classification of antileprosy drugs is shown in Table 1.

TABLE 1	Antileprosy drugs
Class	**Drug**
Sulfone	Dapsone
Phenazine derivative	Clofazimine
Antitubercular drug	Rifampicin
Miscellaneous antibiotics	• Fluoroquinolones—ofloxacin, pefloxacin • Macrolide—clarithromycin • Tetracycline—minocycline

TYPES OF LEPROSY AND TREATMENT REGIMENS

The two categories of leprosy along with the treatment regimens are mentioned in Table 2.

TABLE 2	Types of leprosy and treatment regimens	
Types of leprosy	**Paucibacillary (Tuberculoid)**	**Multibacillary (Lepromatous)**
Infectious	No	Yes
Hypoesthetic skin lesions	<5	>5
Peripheral nerve involvement	0–1 nerve	>1 nerve
Biopsy	Bacilli rarely found	Multiple bacilli found
Cell mediated immunity	Normal or partially deficient	Largely deficient
Lepromin test	Positive	Negative
Clinical course	Prolonged remissions with periodic exacerbations	Anesthesia of distal parts, ulcerations
Treatment regimen (Adult) (Doses are to be suitable adjusted in children)	• Rifampicin–600 mg monthly • Dapsone–100 mg daily Patient is released from treatment (end of treatment) upon completion of 6 monthly pulses	• Rifampicin–600 mg monthly • Dapsone–100 mg daily • Clofazimine–50 mg daily and 300 mg monthly Patient is released from treatment (end of treatment) upon completion of 12 monthly pulses

DAPSONE

Dapsone is closely related to sulfonamide and has a common mechanism of action i.e. inhibition of bacterial folate synthesis. It is the most widely used sulfonamide for long-term treatment of leprosy.

Resistance commonly develops if dapsone is used alone. Hence, it is used in combination with rifampicin and/or clofazimine.

Mechanism of Action

Dapsone is a leprostatic drug and inhibits the conversion of para-aminobenzoic acid into dihydrofolate by inhibiting the enzyme folate synthetase (Figure 1).

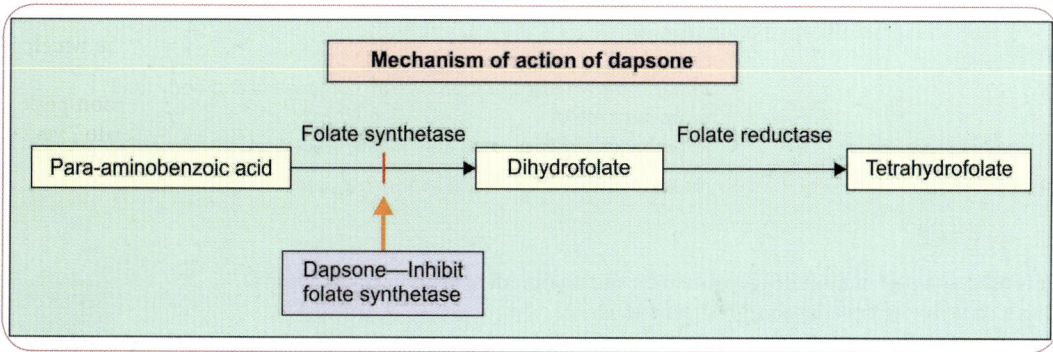

Figure 1: Mechanism of action of dapsone

Pharmacokinetics

Dapsone is well absorbed after oral administration, and is widely distributed in the body fluids and tissues. It tends to be concentrated in skin, liver, muscle and kidney. The skin heavily infected with *M. leprae* may contain a much higher concentration of the drug than normal skin.

It is acetylated in the liver, gets excreted in the bile, and undergoes enterohepatic circulation. The metabolites are ultimately excreted in the urine. It has a plasma half-life of 1–2 days.

Adverse Effects

Dapsone is mostly well tolerated in the usually employed doses of 100 mg/day.

Some of the key adverse effects are mentioned in Table 3.

TABLE 3	Adverse effects of dapsone
Hemolytic anemia	Dose related effect. It is particularly common in G6PD deficient patients. Methemoglobinemia may be observed.
Gastrointestinal	Anorexia, nausea, vomiting
Others	Fever, pruritus, rashes, dermatitis, headache, paraesthesia, hepatitis

Clinical Uses

- Leprosy—as a part of multidrug regimen for treatment of all forms of leprosy
- Malaria—treatment of chloroquine resistant malaria along with pyrimethamine
- *Pneumocystis jirovecii* pneumonia (in AIDS patients)—treatment and prophylaxis.

CLOFAZIMINE

- It is a phenazine dye with leprostatic activity.
- It has anti-inflammatory action. Hence, it is useful in the treatment of Type 2 Lepra reaction (erythema nodosum leprosum).

Mechanism of Action

Clofazimine binds to the DNA of *M. leprae* and inhibits its template function.

Pharmacokinetics

It is variably absorbed from the intestine and is mostly excreted in the feces. It is stored in the skin and reticuloendothelial tissues, from where it is slowly released. Hence, it has a long half-life of 70 days.

Adverse Effects

Some of the key adverse effects are mentioned in Table 4.

TABLE 4	Adverse effects of clofazimine
Skin	• Reddish-brown discoloration of skin, conjunctiva and body fluids is a prominent effect • Phototoxicity, skin dryness and itching
Gastrointestinal	• Nausea, vomiting, diarrhea, abdominal pain

Clinical Uses

- It is used as a part of multidrug regimen for the treatment of multibacillary leprosy.
- It is also active against dapsone-resistant *M. leprae*.
- Due to anti-inflammatory properties, it is used in Type 2 Lepra reactions (erythema nodosum leprosum).

◼ RIFAMPICIN AND OTHER ANTIBIOTICS

Rifampicin has bactericidal action against *M. leprae*. It is used as a part of multidrug therapy to decrease the incidence of resistance and improve the tolerability.

The other antibiotics are used as a part of alternative therapy regimens for leprosy (Table 5).

TABLE 5	Alternative regimens for leprosy
Patient unable to take rifampicin	• For first 6 months Clofazimine + any 2 of (minocycline, ofloxacin, clarithromycin) • For next 18 months Clofazimine + any 1 of (minocycline, ofloxacin)
Patient unable to take clofazimine	• For 12 months Dapsone + rifampicin + any 1 of (minocycline, ofloxacin)

◼ LEPRA REACTIONS

Some of the key features of Type 1 and Type 2 Lepra reactions are mentioned in Table 6.

TABLE 6	Lepra reactions	
Immunologically mediated reactions that occur during the course of the disease		
	Type 1 (Reversal reaction)	Type 2 (Erythema nodosum leprosum [ENL])
Occurrence	In both paucibacillary and multibacillary leprosy	Only in multibacillary leprosy
Cause	Delayed hypersensitivity (Type IV) to *M. leprae* antigen	Type III hypersensitivity reaction
Clinical features	Cutaneous ulceration and nerve	Red, painful, tender nodules; nerves may be affected
Treatment	Corticosteroids, analgesics	Corticosteroids, analgesics, clofazimine, thalidomide

ASSESS YOURSELF (Examination Questions of Various Universities)

1. Treatment of multibacillary leprosy and side effects of drugs used
2. Clofazimine in leprosy
3. Drug therapy of lepromatous leprosy
4. Therapeutic uses and adverse effects of dapsone
5. Management of lepra reaction

MULTIPLE CHOICE QUESTIONS

1. Which fluoroquinolone is highly active against mycobacterium leprae and is being used in alternative multidrug therapy regimens? *(Recent Question 2016)*
   a. Norfloxacin
   b. Ofloxacin
   c. Ciprofloxacin
   d. Lomefloxacin

2. The tetracycline with highest antileprotic activity is: *(Recent Question 2016)*
   a. Minocycline
   b. Doxycycline
   c. Demeclocycline
   d. Oxytetracycline

3. Which of the following anti leprosy drugs cause skin ichthyosis? *(Recent Question 2016)*
   a. Rifampicin
   b. Dapsone
   c. Clofazimine
   d. Ethionamide

4. A common side effect of dapsone is: *(Recent Question 2016)*
   a. Hemolytic anemia
   b. Thrombocytopenia
   c. Cyanosis
   d. Bone marrow depression

5. In leprosy, the best bactericidal agent is: *(Recent Question 2016)*
   a. Clofazimine
   b. Dapsone
   c. Rifampicin
   d. Ethionamide

6. Most common drug used in leprosy is: *(Recent Question 2016)*
   a. Dapsone
   b. Clofazimine
   c. Ethionamide
   d. Ofloxacin

7. Not a use of dapsone: *(Recent Question 2016)*
   a. Malaria
   b. G6PD deficiency
   c. Dermatitis herpetiformis
   d. Leprosy

8. Bactericidal drug active against lepra bacillus: *(TN PG 2010)*
   a. Rifampicin
   b. Clofazimine
   c. Dapsone
   d. Tetracycline

9. The drug used in lepra reaction is: *(TN PG 2005)*
   a. Dapsone
   b. Clofazimine
   c. Rifampicin
   d. Ofloxacin

Ans.

| 1. | (b) | 2. | (a) | 3. | (c) | 4. | (a) | 5. | (c) | 6. | (a) |
| 7. | (b) | 8. | (a) | 9. | (b) | | | | | | |

60

Antifungal Drugs

INTRODUCTION

The incidence of fungal infections has significantly increased in recent years. This is primarily because of an increase in HIV infection, advances in surgery and cancer treatment, prolonged use of immunosuppressing drugs, broad-spectrum antimicrobials etc.

The fungi (unlike bacteria) are eukaryotic, having cell wall made up of chitin (instead of peptidoglycans) and the cell membrane containing ergosterol (instead of cholesterol). Hence, their elimination requires different set of drugs than those used against bacteria.

The various type of fungal infections and their causative organisms are mentioned in Figure 1.

```
                              Fungal infections

         Superficial mycosis                      Deep/Systemic mycosis

    Dermatophytes          Yeast                   • Aspergillus
    • Epidermophyton       • Candida               • Blastomyces
    • Microsporum          • Malassezia furfur      • Candida
    • Trichophyton           (Pityrosporum orbiculare)  • Coccidioides
                           • Malassezia ovalis      • Cryptococcus
                             (Pityrosporum ovale)   • Histoplasma
                                                    • Mucormycosis
                                                    • Sporotrichosis
                                                      (subcutaneous inf.)
```

Figure 1: Types of fungal infections

CLASSIFICATION OF ANTIFUNGAL DRUGS

A classification based on the mechanism of action is mentioned in Figure 2.

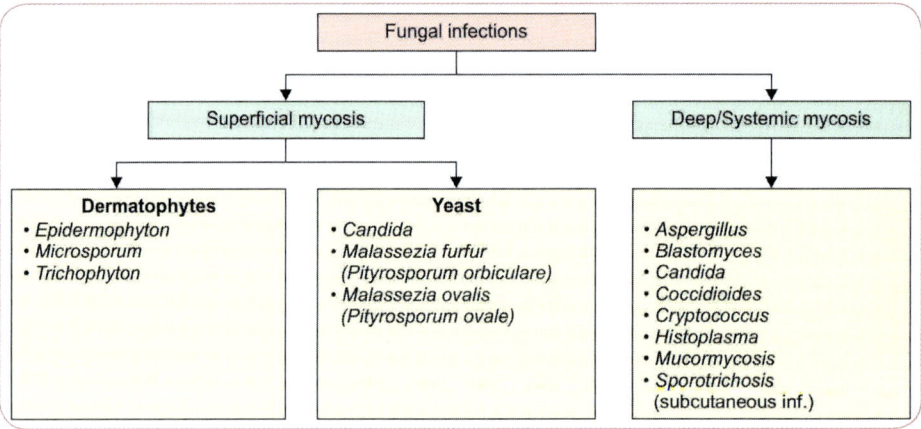

Antifungal drugs				
Inhibitors of cell wall synthesis	Inhibitors of cell membrane function	Inhibitors of ergosterol synthesis	Inhibitors of nucleic acid synthesis	Inhibitors of fungal mitosis
Echinocandins • Capsofungin • Micafungin • Anidulafungin	**Polyene antibiotics** • Amphotericin B • Nystatin • Hamycin	**Azoles** • Ketoconazole • Fluconazole • Itraconazole • Voriconazole • Posaconazole • Miconazole (topical) • Clotrimazole (topical) **Allylamines** • Terbinafine • Butenafine (topical)	**Antimetabolite** • Flucytosine	**Heterocyclic compound** • Griseofulvin

Figure 2: Classification based on mechanism of action

The antifungal drugs discussed further in this chapter are broadly divided into 3 categories:
- Systemic drugs (oral or parenteral) for systemic fungal infections
- Systemic drugs (oral) for superficial infections
- Topical drugs for superficial infections.

SYSTEMIC DRUGS (ORAL/PARENTERAL) FOR SYSTEMIC FUNGAL INFECTIONS

POLYENE ANTIBIOTICS

Amphotericin B

Amphotericin B (AMB) is a polyene antibiotic produced by *Streptomyces nodosus*. It has the broadest spectrum of action amongst the available antifungal drugs.

It is effective against deep systemic infections caused by fungus such as *Aspergillus, Blastomyces, Candida, Coccidioides, Cryptococcus, Histoplasma* and *Mucormycosis.*

Mechanism of Action

AMB binds to ergosterol present in the fungal cell membrane. It gets inserted into the membrane and leads to the formation of 'micropore'. This results in increased permeability, leakage of cell contents and fungal cell death (Figure 3).

Human cells contain cholesterol instead of ergosterol. AMB also binds to cholesterol but with a much lesser affinity. However, AMB is one of the most toxic antibiotics.

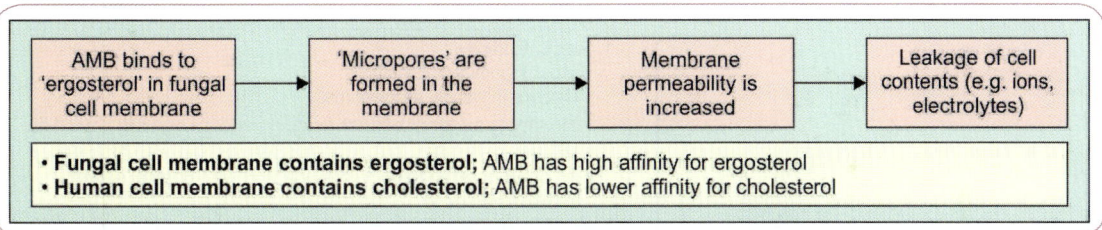

Figure 3: Mechanism of action of amphotericin B

Pharmacokinetics

AMB is not absorbed orally; therefore, it must be used parenterally (slow IV infusion) for systemic infections. It is widely distributed throughout the body, but poorly crosses the blood-brain barrier (BBB).

It binds to sterols in the tissues and gets released slowly (half-life 15 days); hence, it remains in the body for a longer duration of time. It is metabolized in the liver and excreted slowly by the kidneys.

Formulations

AMB is insoluble in water; hence, it is prepared by complexing it with sodium deoxycholate. This is called conventional amphotericin B (CAMB).

The CAMB has high toxicity potential, especially nephrotoxicity and infusion related toxicity. This led to the development of lipid formulations of AMB.

Four formulations of AMB are therefore available: 1 conventional formulation and 3 lipid-based formulations:
- Conventional amphotericin B (CAMB)
- Lipid formulations of amphotericin B
  - Amphotericin B colloidal dispersion (ABCD)
  - Amphotericin B lipid complex (ABLC)
  - Liposomal amphotericin B (LAMB)

The advantages and disadvantages of lipid formulations over CAMB are mentioned in Figure 4.

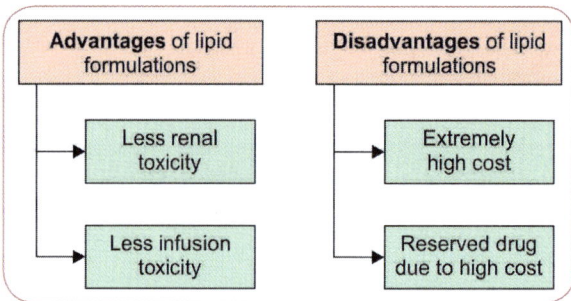

Figure 4: Lipid formulations: advantages and disadvantages

Adverse Effects

AMB is one of the most toxic antibiotics used. The adverse effects can be broadly categorized as immediately occurring effects and long-term effects (Figure 5).

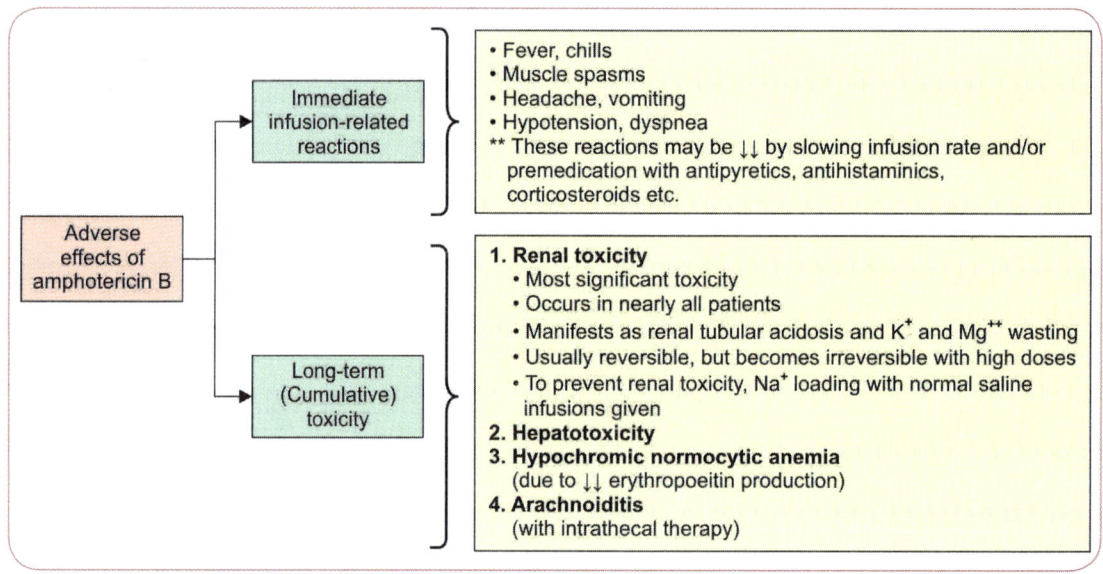

Figure 5: Adverse effects of amphotericin B

Drug Interactions

The key drug interactions of AMB are mentioned below:

○ **Flucytosine**—has synergistic action with AMB in cryptococcosis. AMB increases the penetration of flucytosine inside the fungal cell.

○ **Aminoglycosides, cyclosporine, vancomycin and other nephrotoxic drugs**—increase the renal toxicity caused by AMB.

Clinical Uses

AMB is a highly efficacious drug for systemic mycosis, but it has a high toxicity profile. Hence, it has been replaced by the azole group of drugs for the treatment of several systemic fungal infections.

Note:
- Azoles (fluconazole, itraconazole, posaconazole etc.) are much less toxic and can be easily administered as compared to AMB.

The clinical uses of AMB includes the following:

- Mucormycosis—AMB remains the drug of choice
- Histoplasmosis and blastomycosis
- Coccidioidomycosis, aspergillosis, sporotrichosis
- Candidiasis and cryptococcosis
- Leishmaniasis—used in resistant cases of Kala-azar and mucocutaneous leishmaniasis.

ANTIMETABOLITE

Flucytosine

Flucytosine is a synthetic antimetabolite that is mostly used in combination with AMB. It is a prodrug and is inactive as such. It is taken up by susceptible fungal cells and converted to an active metabolite.

Mechanism of Action

Flucytosine is taken up by the fungal cells and converted into 5-fluorouracil (5-FU). 5-FU is then further converted to other metabolites which inhibit the enzyme thymidylate synthase. This ultimately results in inhibition of fungal DNA synthesis (Figure 6).

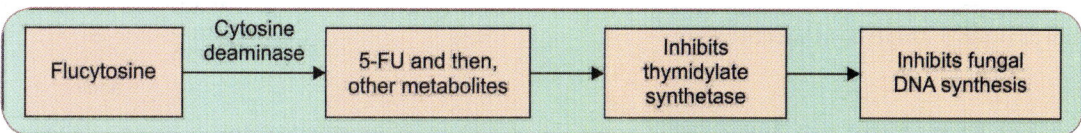

Figure 6: Mechanism of action of flucytosine

The human cells lack cytosine deaminase; hence, they cannot convert flucytosine to 5-FU. This explains the selective action of flucytosine on fungal cells.

Antifungal Spectrum

Flucytosine is a fungistatic drug. It has a narrow antifungal spectrum. It is effective against *Candida, Cryptococcus neoformans* and *Chromoblastomycosis.*

Pharmacokinetics

Flucytosine is available only in an oral formulation. It is well-absorbed orally, is poorly bound to plasma proteins and gets widely distributed in the body, including the CSF. It is mainly excreted unchanged by the kidneys.

Adverse Effects

The adverse effects mainly occur due to its conversion to antineoplastic drug 5-FU. The adverse effects include the following:

- **Bone marrow toxicity**—anemia, leukopenia, thrombocytopenia
- **Gastrointestinal toxicity**—nausea, vomiting, diarrhea, severe enterocolitis
- **Hepatotoxicity**—reversible elevation of liver enzymes.

Clinical Uses

Flucytosine is not used alone. It is used in combination with other drugs in the following fungal infections:

- Cryptococcosis and candidiasis (along with AMB)
- Chromoblastomycosis (along with itraconazole)

Note:
- Flucytosine has synergistic action with AMB. AMB increases the penetration of flucytosine inside the fungal cell. This also allows for a dose reduction of the more toxic AMB.

AZOLES

Azoles are synthetic drugs with a broad spectrum of action. The azoles are broadly divided into 2 main classes: imidazoles and triazoles (Figure 7).

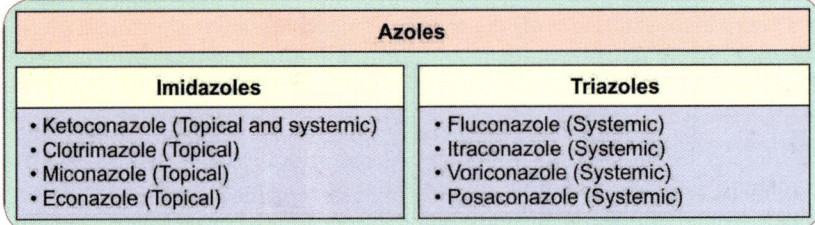

Figure 7: Classification of azoles

Both imidazoles and triazoles have similar mechanism and spectrum of action. As compared to imidazoles, triazoles have lesser adverse effects and drug interactions, and better oral absorption. Hence, triazoles have mostly replaced ketoconazole in the treatment of systemic mycosis.

Imidazoles (except ketoconazole) are mostly used topically and hence, are discussed in the section titled "Topical drugs for superficial infections".

Mechanism of Action

Azoles inhibit the fungal cytochrome 450 enzymes, lanosterol 14 α-demethylase. This leads to inhibition of ergosterol synthesis in the fungal cell membrane (Figure 8).

Azoles exhibit selective inhibition of fungal cytochrome 450 enzyme as compared to human enzyme. Therefore, they have selective toxicity for the fungus.

Imidazoles show lesser fungal selectivity than triazoles; hence, imidazoles have a higher incidence of adverse effects and drug interactions.

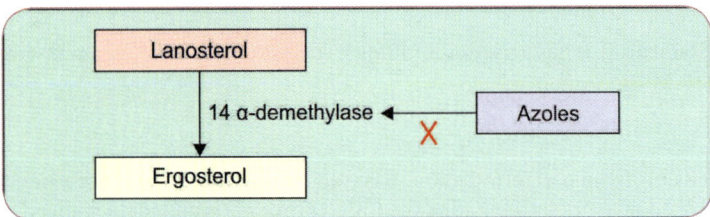

Figure 8: Mechanism of action of azoles

KETOCONAZOLE

Ketoconazole was the first orally effective azole used clinically. It has been used topically as well as orally, for the treatment of both superficial (dermatophytes, *Candida*) and deep (systemic) mycosis.

Due to the propensity of causing adverse effects and several drug interactions, ketoconazole is now mainly used topically for superficial mycosis. For the systemic mycosis, it has mostly been replaced by triazoles.

Pharmacokinetics

The oral absorption of ketoconazole is increased by gastric acidity. Therefore, drugs that increase gastric pH (e.g. H_2-receptor blockers, proton-pump blockers) decrease the oral absorption and bioavailability of ketoconazole.

It is metabolized extensively in the liver, well distributed throughout the body (except CSF) and metabolites are excreted in urine and feces.

Drug Interactions

As ketoconazole inhibits human cytochrome P450 3A4 isoenzyme, it can lead to many drug interactions. Some of the key drug interactions are mentioned in Figure 9.

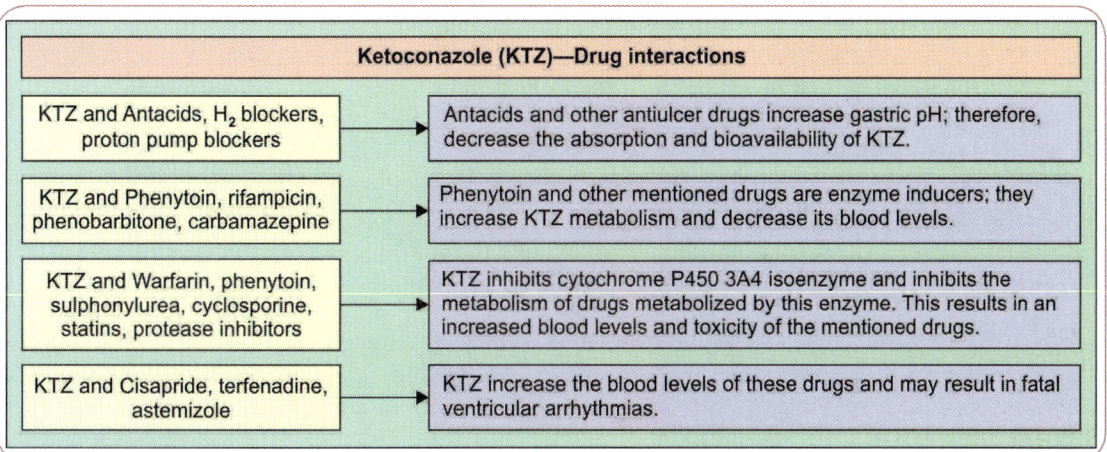

Figure 9: Drug interactions of ketoconazole

Adverse Effects

Ketoconazole is less toxic than AMB, but among azoles, it is the most toxic drug.

Some of the common adverse effects include GIT irritation i.e. nausea, vomiting and anorexia. This can be decreased by taking the drug with meals. It may also cause itching, rashes and reversible increase in liver enzymes. It inhibits the synthesis of testosterone, estrogen and androgen—this results in:

○ **Males:** Gynecomastia, decreased libido, oligozoospermia and impotence
○ **Females:** Menstrual abnormalities.

Clinical Uses

Ketoconazole is not used for systemic mycosis due to its toxicity and propensity for drug interactions. Therefore, for systemic mycosis, it has been replaced by triazoles.

It is still used in the following:

○ Superficial mycosis (dermatophytosis, candidiasis)—used as cream for *T. pedis, T. cruris, T. corporis*
○ Seborrheic dermatitis—used as a 2% shampoo
○ Other uses—Dermal leishmaniasis, Kala-azar and Cushing's syndrome.

FLUCONAZOLE

Fluconazole is a triazole with a broader antifungal spectrum than KTZ. It is effective in cryptococcal meningitis, coccidioidal meningitis and candidiasis (i.e. 3Cs).

It is available in oral and IV formulations.

Pharmacokinetics

It has high oral bioavailability (~94%). The oral absorption is not affected by food or gastric pH. The plasma protein binding is poor and is widely distributed throughout the body. It effectively penetrates the blood-brain barrier (unlike itraconazole).

It is mainly excreted unchanged in the urine. The drug interactions of fluconazole are like KTZ but to a much lesser extent.

Adverse Effects

Some of the common adverse effects include nausea, vomiting, abdominal pain, headache and skin rashes. It may also cause hepatotoxicity. It is not recommended in pregnancy due to teratogenic effect.

It does not inhibit the synthesis of testosterone, estrogen and androgen.

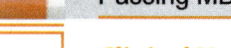

Clinical Uses

Fluconazole is used mainly in **C**ryptococcal meningitis, **C**occidioidal meningitis and **C**andidiasis (Figure 10).

Fluconazole—Clinical uses		
Cryptococcal meningitis	**Coccidioidal meningitis**	**Candidiasis**
• It is the drug of choice in treatment and prophylaxis of cryptococcal meningitis • It is used IV and is effective because it penetrates the BBB effectively	• It is the drug of choice in treatment of coccidioidal meningitis • It is used IV and is effective because it penetrates the BBB effectively • It provides an effective alternative to toxic AMB for this condition	• It is useful in the treatment of oropharyngeal, esophageal, cutaneous, vaginal and disseminated candidiasis

Figure 10: Clinical uses of fluconazole

ITRACONAZOLE

Itraconazole is a triazole with a broader antifungal spectrum than KTZ and fluconazole. It is effective in infection such as dermatophytosis, candidiasis, histoplasmosis, blastomycosis and sporotrichosis.

Pharmacokinetics

Itraconazole is available in oral and IV formulations. The oral absorption is variable and is increased by food and gastric acidity. It is highly plasma protein bound and is widely distributed throughout the body. It poorly penetrates the BBB (unlike fluconazole). It is metabolized in the liver and excreted in the feces.

Adverse Effects

The adverse effects include nausea, diarrhea, anorexia, headache, hypokalemia and hepatotoxicity.
It does not inhibit the synthesis of testosterone, estrogen and androgen.
It inhibits cytochrome isoenzymes and the drug interaction profile is similar to KTZ.

Clinical Uses

Itraconazole is commonly used in many of the systemic mycosis where meningitis is not associated. The clinical uses of itraconazole are mentioned in Figure 11.

Itraconazole—Clinical uses			
Histoplasmosis, blastomycosis and sporotrichosis	**Aspergillosis**	**Dermatophytosis and onychomycosis**	**Candidiasis**
• It is the drug of choice in these infections provided they are not associated with meningitis • This is because it poorly penetrates the BBB	• It is effective in the treatment of aspergillosis • However, voriconazole is the drug of choice	• It is extensively used in these conditions • It is effective against *T. capitis, T. corporis, T. unguium*, and *T. versicolor*	• It is useful in the treatment of oropharyngeal, esophageal, cutaneous, and vaginal candidiasis

Figure 11: Clinical uses of itraconazole

VORICONAZOLE

Voriconazole is a triazole with a broad antifungal spectrum like itraconazole. It is available in oral and IV formulations. It is metabolized by and inhibits cytochrome isoenzymes and the drug interaction profile is similar to itraconazole.

It is the drug of choice in invasive aspergillosis. It has excellent activity in invasive candidiasis.

The adverse effects include transient visual disturbances, prolongation of QT_C interval, hepatotoxicity and rashes.

POSACONAZOLE

It is a newer triazole used clinically. It has a broad antifungal spectrum with effect against *Candida, Aspergillus* and fungus causing mucormycosis. It has significant activity in mucormycosis.

It is metabolized in the liver by hepatic glucuronidation and not phase 1 oxidation. It however, inhibits the cytochrome CYP3A4 and hence, there is propensity for drug interactions.

The adverse effects include GIT disturbance (nausea, vomiting, diarrhea), headache and hepatotoxicity.

It is used in the following:
- **As a salvage therapy against invasive aspergillosis and candidiasis** in severe immunocompromised patients refractory to other drugs
- **As a salvage therapy against invasive mucormycosis and zygomycosis** that is refractory to AMB
- **Against oropharyngeal candidiasis**, but fluconazole is preferred due to low cost, better safety and long experience

A comparison of some of the key pharmacological features of various triazoles are mentioned in Figure 12.

Azoles—Comparison of key pharmacological features				
Properties	**Fluconazole**	**Itraconazole**	**Voriconazole**	**Posaconazole**
Bioavailability (%)	94	55	96	Variable
Effect of food/gastric pH on absorption	No effect	Increased	No effect	Increased
Plasma protein binding (%)	10–12	>99	56	>98
Blood-brain barrier penetration	Good	Poor	Good	Good
Route of elimination	Renal	Hepatic (Cytochrome)	Hepatic (Cytochrome)	Hepatic (Glucuronidation)
Antifungal spectrum	+ Cryptococcus Coccidioides Candida	++ Histoplasma Blastomyces Sporothrix Aspergillus Dermatophytes Candida	+++ (*) Aspergillus Candida	++++ (**) Aspergillus Candida Mucormycosis Zygomycosis

*Voriconazole is also active against fungus treated by itraconazole. However, it is mainly used against invasive aspergillosis and candidiasis.
**Posaconazole is also active against fungus treated by itraconazole. However, it is mainly used as a salvage therapy against invasive aspergillosis, candidiasis, mucormycosis and zygomycosis.

Figure 12: Comparison of key pharmacological features of various triazoles

ECHINOCANDINS

Caspofungin

Caspofungin is effective against *Candida* and *Aspergillus*. It is available only in IV formulations, as it is not active orally.

It inhibits the synthesis of (1,3) β-glucans in the fungal cell wall. This results in deficiency in cell wall structure, osmotic imbalance and fungal cell death.

Caspofungin is well tolerated. The adverse effects include phlebitis at the injection site, warmth, flushing and minor GIT effects.

It is used in the treatment of following infections:

o   Invasive candidiasis
o   Invasive aspergillosis—only as a salvage therapy, in case of failure of 1st line drugs such as AMB or voriconazole.

Micafungin

Micafungin has a similar mechanism of action as caspofungin, and is also available only in IV formulation.

It is used in the following infections:

o   Treatment of invasive candidiasis
o   Treatment of esophageal candidiasis
o   Prophylaxis of invasive candidiasis in patients undergoing hematopoietic stem cell transplantation.

SYSTEMIC DRUGS (ORAL) FOR SUPERFICIAL INFECTIONS

GRISEOFULVIN

Griseofulvin is a fungistatic drug. It is used orally only for the treatment of dermatophytosis. It is not active topically.

It is effective against most type of dermatophytes i.e. *Microsporum*, *Trichophyton* and *Epidermophyton*. It is not effective against any other fungi.

Mechanism of Action

Griseofulvin inhibits fungal mitosis by interfering with microtubule function. It attaches with polymerized microtubules and then disrupts them.

Pharmacokinetics

The GIT absorption is variable. The absorption is increased by the following:

o   Consuming it along with fatty meals
o   Using ultrafine or microfine preparation

It gets deposited in keratin precursor cells of skin, hair and nails. As it is fungistatic, it prevents the infection of new keratin cells by the fungus. It does not lead to killing (or eradication) of the fungus in already infected cells.

The fungus persists in the infected cells until the keratin cells are worn and shed off. Therefore, the duration of treatment is long and depends on the site of infection and the turnover rate of the keratin cells.

Griseofulvin is metabolized in the liver and excreted by the kidneys. It induces hepatic cytochrome isoenzymes; therefore, increases the metabolism and decreases the efficacy of warfarin and oral contraceptives.

Adverse Effects

Some of the key adverse effects of griseofulvin include the following:

o   Neurological: Headache, peripheral neuritis, fatigue, confusion, vertigo, blurred vision
o   Gastrointestinal: Nausea, vomiting, diarrhea, flatulence, stomatitis
o   Hematological: Leukopenia, neutropenia, basophilia
o   Hepatotoxicity

Clinical Uses

Griseofulvin is used only in the treatment of dermatophytosis due to *Microsporum*, *Trichophyton* or *Epidermophyton*.

The duration of therapy depends on the site of infection (i.e. turnover rate of the keratin cells). The duration of therapy is mentioned in Figure 13.

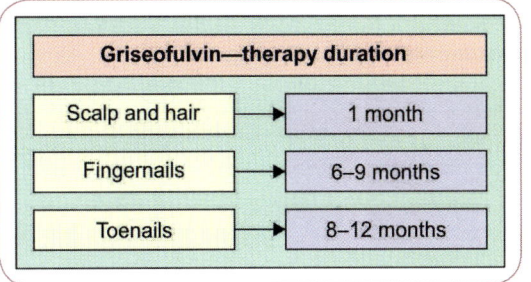

Figure 13: Griseofulvin—duration of therapy

The therapy should be continued until the fungal infected cells are completely replaced by normal skin, hair or nails from beneath.

Griseofulvin has mostly been replaced by itraconazole and terbinafine due to their better safety profile and efficacy.

TERBINAFINE

Terbinafine is a synthetic allylamine. It is available in topical and oral formulations.

It is effective against dermatophytes and *Candida*; however, it is often preferred for onychomycosis (i.e. dermatophyte infection of the nails).

Mechanism of Action

Terbinafine inhibits the fungal enzyme squalene epoxidase and leads to inhibition of ergosterol synthesis in the fungal cell membrane (Figure 14). The inhibition of this enzyme also results in accumulation of squalene, which is toxic to the fungus.

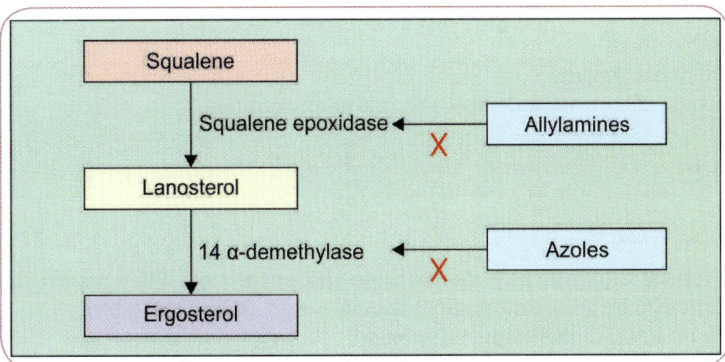

Figure 14: Mechanism of action of allylamines (Terbinafine, butenafine)

Pharmacokinetics

It is well absorbed but the bioavailability is only around 40% due to high first-pass metabolism in the liver. It is highly plasma protein bound, widely distributed and gets concentrated in the skin, nails and fat. It is metabolized in the liver and excreted in the urine and feces.

Adverse Effects

The adverse effects include GIT disturbance, headache, rash, and rarely skin reactions, neutropenia and hepatotoxicity.

Clinical Uses

Some of the clinical uses of terbinafine are mentioned in Figure 15.

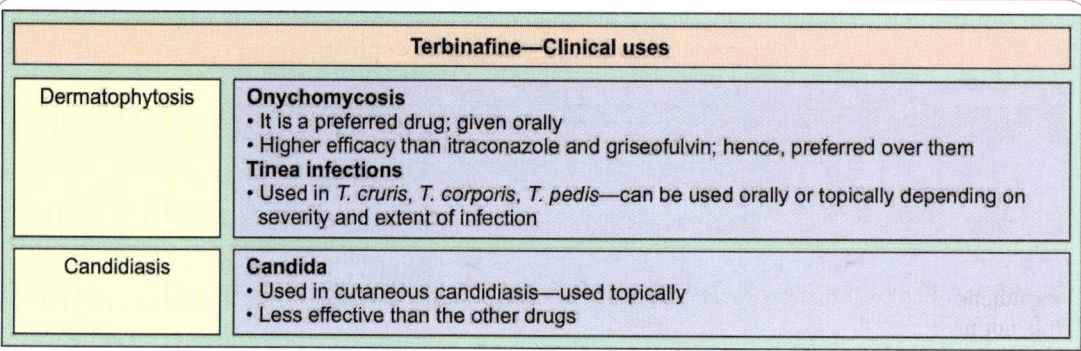

Figure 15: Clinical uses of terbinafine

TOPICAL DRUGS FOR SUPERFICIAL INFECTIONS

POLYENE ANTIBIOTICS

Nystatin

Nystatin has a similar mechanism of action and features as AMB, but has a much higher systemic toxicity. Therefore, it used only topically in superficial *Candida* infections. It is available as cream, ointment, suppository, powder, tablet etc.

It is poorly absorbed from the skin, mucous membranes and the GIT. It is used in the following infections:
○ Topical—candidiasis (cutaneous, oral, conjunctival, corneal etc.)
○ Oral—candidiasis (intestinal)
○ Suppository—candidiasis (vaginal)
The adverse effects include bitter taste and nausea on oral administration.

TOPICAL AZOLES

Clotrimazole, Miconazole

The commonly used topical azoles include clotrimazole and miconazole. They are available in the following formulations: cream, lotion, powder, solution, spray, vaginal cream and vaginal tablet.
These drugs are used topically in the following infections:
○ Dermatophytosis—used in *T. corporis, T. cruris, T. pedis, T. versicolor.* These drugs are applied twice a day for 3–6 weeks. The cure rate is 60–100%.
○ Candidiasis—used in cutaneous, oropharyngeal and vulvovaginal candidiasis. The cure rate is 80–100%.

TOPICAL ALLYLAMINES

Terbinafine, Butenafine

These are drugs used topically for the treatment of dermatophytosis (*T. corporis, T. cruris, T. pedis*). These are available as 1% cream or spray.

They are less effective against cutaneous candidiasis and *T. versicolor* but can also be used for these conditions.

MISCELLANEOUS DRUGS

CICLOPIROX OLAMINE

It is a synthetic drug used topically for the treatment of dermatophytosis, cutaneous candidiasis and *T. versicolor*. The drug penetrates the dermis and the hair follicles. High cure rates have been reported.

It may also be topically used (in high concentrations) for mild superficial onychomycosis. It may occasionally lead to hypersensitivity reactions.

TOLNAFTATE

It is a synthetic drug used topically for the treatment of dermatophytosis caused by *T. corporis* and *T. cruris*.

It is not used in *T. pedis*, *T. capitis*, onychomycosis and other hyperkeratinized lesions because it has poor penetrability. It is not effective in candidiasis and other superficial infections.

Relapses are common if it is used alone.

WHITFIELD'S OINTMENT

It is a combination of benzoic acid (6%) + salicylic acid (3%).

Benzoic acid has weak fungistatic action while salicylic acid has keratolytic action. Salicylic acid, due to keratolytic action, dissipates the infected tissue which helps benzoic acid to penetrate the fungal infected tissue.

It is mainly used in the treatment of *T. pedis* infection.

UNDECYLENIC ACID

It is a fungistatic drug. It is used in combination with zinc salt. It is used in *T. pedis*, *T. cruris*, diaper rash, and other minor fungal skin infections.

The cure rate (even with prolonged treatment) is around 50%, which is significantly lower than tolnaftate or topical azoles.

ASSESS YOURSELF (Examination Questions of Various Universities)

1. Classify the drugs used for the treatment of fungal infections. Explain the mechanism of action, adverse effects and therapeutic uses of griseofulvin
2. Liposomal amphotericin B
3. Ketoconazole
4. Azole antifungal agents
5. Fluconazole
6. Topical antifungal drugs

MULTIPLE CHOICE QUESTIONS

1. Drug whose absorption is increased in fatty meal: (*AIIMS Nov 2015*)
   a. Griseofulvin   b. Amphotericin-B
   c. Nimesulide   d. Azoles

2. Mucormycosis, drug of choice is:
                          (*AIIMS May 2013*)
   a. Amphotericin B   b. Itraconazole
   c. Voriconazole   d. Griseofulvin

3. The antimicrobial agent which inhibits the ergosterol biosynthesis:(*Recent Question 2016*)
   a. Ketoconazole   b. Amphotericin B
   c. 5-Flucytosine   d. Griseofulvin

4. A fungicidal drug that can be used orally for the treatment of onychomycosis:
                          (*Recent Question 2016*)
   a. Griseofulvin   b. Amphotericin B
   c. Clotrimazole   d. Terbinafine

5. Antifungal which can be used orally but not IV is: (*Recent Question 2016*)
   a. Voriconazole   b. Amphotericin B
   c. Terbinafine   d. None of the above

6. Amphotericin B causes deficiency of:
                          (*Recent Question 2016*)
   a. Sodium   b. Calcium
   c. Potassium   d. Chloride

7. Which of the following is not an antifungal drug?   (*Recent Question 2016*)
   a. Ketoconazole   b. Undecylenic acid
   c. Ciclopirox   d. Clofazimine

8. Topically used antifungal agent is:
                          (*Recent Question 2016*)
   a. Ketoconazole   b. Clotrimazole
   c. Amphotericin B   d. Voriconazole

9. Amphotericin B toxicity is monitored by:
                          (*Recent Question 2016*)
   a. Serum sodium measurement
   b. Serum potassium measurement
   c. Liver function test
   d. Blood sugar

10. Topical antifungal agent used for dermato-phytes: (*Recent Question 2016*)
    a. Hamycin   b. Natamycin
    c. Nystatin   d. Tolnaftate

11. The antifungal drug which is *not* an Azole:
                          (*NIMHANS 2013*)
    a. Ketoconazole   b. Mebendazole
    c. Miconazole   d. Voriconazole

12. Which of the following does not belong to Triazole?   (*NIMHANS 2013*)
    a. Posaconazole   b. Voriconazole
    c. Ketoconazole   d. Itraconazole

13. Which drugs causes gynecomastia?(*APPG 2008*)
    a. Ketoconazole   b. Fluconazole
    c. Itraconazole   d. Griseofulvin

14. Terbinafine hydrochloride is: (*MH CET 2012*)
    a. Antibacterial   b. Antifungal
    c. Antiviral   d. None

15. Which of the following drugs is/are used in treatment of mucormycosis: (*PGI May 2018*)
    a. Fluconazole   b. Amphotericin B
    c. Voriconazole   d. Posaconazole
    e. 5-flurocysteine

16. Which of the following is wrongly matched regarding mechanism of action of anti-fungal drugs?   (*AIIMS May 2018*)
    a. Azoles (fluconazole, itraconazole, micon-azole): Inhibit lanosterol alpha demethylase thereby preventing ergosterol synthesis
    b. Flucytosine: Inhibit microtubule synthesis thus preventing mitosis
    c. Echinocandins (Caspofungin): act by inhibiting beta 1,3 glucan synthesis
    d. Amphotericin B binds with ergosterol resulting in disruption of cell membrane causing micropores and leakage of ions and cell death

Ans.

1.	(a)	2.	(a)	3.	(a)	4.	(d)	5.	(c)	6.	(c)
7.	(d)	8.	(b)	9.	(b)	10.	(d)	11.	(b)	12.	(c)
13.	(a)	14.	(b)	15.	(b, d)	16.	(b)				

61

Antiprotozoal Drugs

The antiprotozoal drugs include the drug therapy for amoebiasis, giardiasis, leishmaniasis, trichomoniasis and trypanosomiasis.

ANTIAMOEBIC DRUGS

Amoebiasis is a protozoal infection caused by the organism *E. histolytica*. It is transmitted through the orofecal route. A classification of antiamoebic drugs is mentioned in Figure 1.

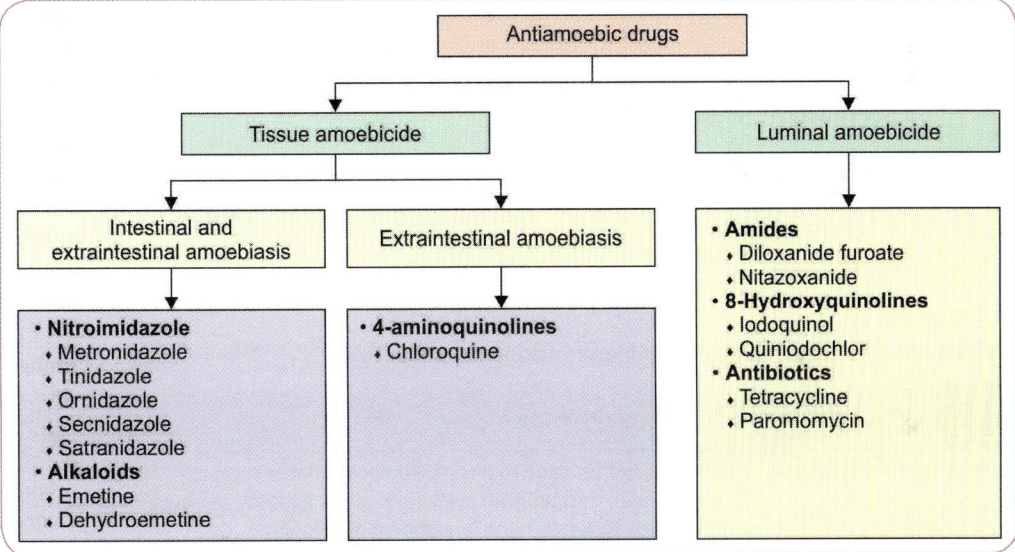

Figure 1: Classification of antiamoebic drugs

TISSUE AMOEBICIDE (USED FOR INTESTINAL AND EXTRAINTESTINAL AMOEBIASIS)

Metronidazole

- It is a nitroimidazole derivative.
- Metronidazole has broad spectrum activity against:
    - Protozoa (e.g. *Entamoeba histolytica, Giardia lamblia, Trichomonas vaginalis*)
    - Anaerobic bacteria (e.g. *Peptococcus, Bacteroides, Clostridium difficile*)
- It may also facilitate the extraction of adult guinea worm (*Dracunculus medinensis*).
- It is not effective against aerobic bacteria.

Mechanism of Action

Metronidazole is a prodrug that enters the cell and is reduced to a highly reactive nitro radical which has cytotoxic effect. Metronidazole has selective toxicity against anaerobic organisms. It is not active against aerobes because the presence of oxygen inhibits the reductive activation of metronidazole. The mechanism of action of metronidazole is mentioned in Figure 2.

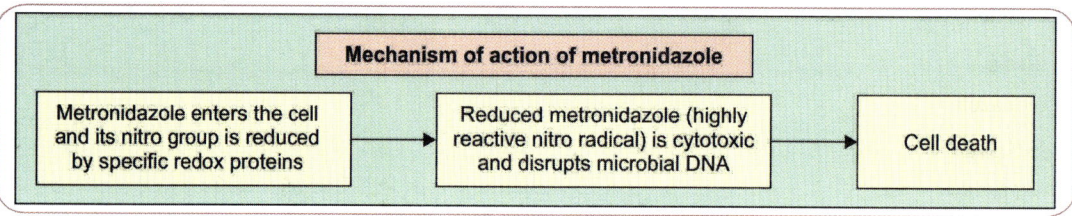

Figure 2: Mechanism of action of metronidazole

Pharmacokinetics

It is well-absorbed orally and is widely distributed in tissues and body fluids. Therapeutic levels are attained in saliva, semen, CSF and breast milk.

It is metabolized in the liver and the metabolites are excreted in the urine.

Adverse Effects

Some of the key adverse effects of metronidazole are mentioned in Table 1.

TABLE 1	Adverse effects of metronidazole
GIT	Nausea, metallic taste, anorexia, abdominal cramps, vomiting, diarrhea, headache
CNS	Dizziness, vertigo, irritability, seizures, ataxia, neuropathy, encephalopathy
Others	Allergic reactions, urticaria, flushing, itching, rashes

Drug Interactions

Some of the key drug interactions of metronidazole are mentioned in Table 2.

TABLE 2	Drug Interactions of metronidazole
Metronidazole and alcohol	Disulfiram—like reaction to alcohol can occur. Patients on metronidazole should be instructed to abstain from drinking alcohol. Patients can experience nausea, vomiting, headache, flushing, abdominal distress etc.
Metronidazole and cimetidine	Cimetidine can increase the level of metronidazole by inhibiting its metabolism.
Metronidazole and warfarin	Metronidazole can increase the action of warfarin by inhibiting its metabolism.
Metronidazole and lithium	Metronidazole can decrease the renal clearance of lithium and precipitate lithium toxicity.

Precautions and Contraindications

○ Neurological disease
○ Pregnancy (1st trimester)
○ Blood dyscrasias
○ Chronic alcoholism

Antimicrobial Spectrum and Clinical Uses

Amoebiasis

Metronidazole is the preferred drug for all forms of amoebic infections including intestinal and extraintestinal amoebiasis. It is also used for amoebic liver abscess.

A luminal amoebicide (e.g. diloxanide furoate) with tissue amoebicide (e.g. metronidazole, tinidazole) is required for eradication of *E. histolytica* from the colon and to prevent the development of the cyst passer or the carrier state.

Giardiasis

Metronidazole is highly effective in giardiasis.

Trichomonas Vaginitis

Metronidazole is highly effective in *Trichomonas vaginitis*. The male partner should also be treated in cases of recurrent infections.

Anaerobic Bacterial Infections

- Brain abscess, endocarditis and infections occurring after colorectal, pelvic and abdominal surgeries. Metronidazole is effective in the treatment and is generally used along with gentamicin or cephalosporins.
- Pseudomembranous colitis: It occurs due to *Clostridium difficile* infection. Metronidazole is an effective, safe and cost saving alternative to oral vancomycin.
- Helicobacter pylori gastritis/peptic ulcer: Metronidazole is given in combination with clarithromycin/amoxicillin and a proton pump inhibitor for treatment of *H. pylori* infection.
- Ulcerative gingivitis: Metronidazole is given in combination with tetracycline or amoxicillin for treatment of ulcerative gingivitis (as anaerobes are involved in this condition).
- Prophylactic agent for colorectal surgery.

Other Uses

- Guinea worm (Dracunculus medinensis): Metronidazole facilitates the extraction of the worm.
- Crohn's disease: Metronidazole may be useful in Crohn's disease. High doses for prolonged periods may be required, whereby neurotoxicity may limit its usefulness.

Some of the salient features of other nitroimidazoles are mentioned in Table 3.

TABLE 3	Other nitroimidazoles		
Tinidazole	Ornidazole	Secnidazole	Satranidazole
Longer duration of action and better tolerability as compared to metronidazole	Clinical use, tolerability is similar to tinidazole	Can be used as a single dose therapy; clinical use, tolerability is similar to metronidazole	Does not cause neurological toxicity and less likely to cause disulfiram like reaction with alcohol

Emetine and Dehydroemetine

Emetine is derived from *C. ipecacuanha* and dehydroemetine is semisynthetic derivative of emetine. They inhibit the synthesis of proteins in the amoebae. These drugs kill tissue trophozoites, but have no effect on the cysts.

Both the drugs are administered parenterally (IM) and not orally as they have an emetic effect (irritant, bitter and can cause nausea).

Their clinical uses are limited due to high toxicity and hence, have been replaced by metronidazole and its analogues. However, they can be used in situations where metronidazole cannot be used.

Adverse Effects

The adverse effects include:

- Cardiotoxicity—hypotension, cardiac arrhythmias, myocarditis. These drugs are administered in hospital setting with bed rest. Dehydroemetine is less cardiotoxic as compared to emetine
- Nausea and vomiting
- Muscle weakness, diarrhea, abdominal cramps
- Contraindications include patients with cardiac or renal disease, pregnancy.

TISSUE AMOEBICIDE (EXTRAINTESTINAL AMOEBIASIS)

Chloroquine gets concentrated in the liver and is effective against the trophozoites of *E. histolytica*.

It is used in the treatment of hepatic amoebiasis. It is not effective in intestinal amoebiasis because it does not attain sufficient concentration in the intestinal lumen and the wall.

LUMINAL AMOEBICIDE

Amides (Diloxanide Furoate)

Diloxanide furoate is a luminal amoebicide and kills trophozoites (responsible for formation of cysts) in the lumen of the gut. It has no action against tissue trophozoites.

It is used in mild intestinal amoebiasis and asymptomatic amoebiasis. It is given with a tissue amoebicide (e.g. metronidazole) in intestinal and extraintestinal amoebiasis for eradication of *E. histolytica* from the colon and to prevent the development of the cyst passer or the carrier state.

It is usually well tolerated; the adverse effect includes flatulence.

8-Hydroxyquinolines (Iodoquinol)

It is a luminal amoebicide and kills trophozoites (responsible for formation of cysts) in the lumen of the gut. It has no action against tissue trophozoites.

It is used in asymptomatic carriers. It is also used in giardiasis, local treatment of monilial and trichomonas vaginitis, bacterial and fungal skin infections.

Adverse Effects

The adverse effects include the following:
- Nausea, green colored stools
- Iodism can occur due to chronic iodine overload. It can present as furunculosis, mucous membrane inflammation.
- Subacute myelo-optic neuropathy (SMON) leading to visual impairment and blindness (especially in children). It may be due to repeated or prolonged use of the drug in high doses. It has been banned in many countries.

Antibiotics (Tetracycline, Paromomycin)

These drugs are luminal amoebicides. They are incompletely absorbed from the intestine and inhibit the bacterial flora in the colon which is needed for the amoeba to survive. Hence, they have an indirect action in decreasing the amoeba in the colon.

Some salient points regarding treatment of amoebiasis are mentioned in Table 4.

TABLE 4	Amoebiasis
Condition	**Treatment medications**
Asymptomatic carrier state (Cyst passers)	• Luminal amoebicide (e.g. diloxanide furoate, iodoquinol, paromomycin).
Intestinal amoebiasis (Amoebic dysentery or diarrhea)	• Metronidazole or tinidazole + luminal amoebicide (e.g. diloxanide furoate). • A luminal amoebicide (e.g. diloxanide furoate) is required with metronidazole or tinidazole for eradication of *E. histolytica* from the colon and to prevent the development of cyst passer or the carrier state. • Severe infection may require IV metronidazole along with supportive management to correct fluid and electrolyte balance.

Contd...

Severe amoebic dysentery and extraintestinal infection	<ul><li>Metronidazole or tinidazole + luminal amoebicide (e.g. diloxanide furoate).</li><li>May require IV metronidazole along with supportive management to correct fluid and electrolyte balance.</li><li>A luminal amoebicide (e.g. diloxanide furoate) is required with metronidazole or tinidazole for eradication of *E. histolytica* from the colon and to prevent the development of cyst passer or the carrier state.</li></ul>
Amoebic liver abscess	<ul><li>It is a serious condition—a complete eradication of trophozoites from the liver is required to prevent relapses.</li><li>Metronidazole or tinidazole + luminal amoebicide (e.g. diloxanide furoate).</li><li>Chloroquine may be required in some cases.</li><li>May require IV metronidazole and supportive management to correct fluid and electrolyte balance; may need surgical intervention.</li><li>A luminal amoebicide (e.g. diloxanide furoate) is required with metronidazole or tinidazole for eradication of *E. histolytica* from the colon and to prevent the development of cyst passer or the carrier state.</li></ul>

TREATMENT OF GIARDIASIS AND TRICHOMONIASIS

Some salient points regarding treatment of giardiasis and trichomoniasis is mentioned in Table 5.

TABLE 5	Giardiasis and trichomoniasis
Giardiasis	<ul><li>Pathogen is *Giardia lamblia*</li><li>Clinical features include diarrhea (can be watery); may lead to malabsorption</li><li>Treatment include:<ul><li>Metronidazole, tinidazole, secnidazole</li><li>Furazolidone → It is a nitrofuran compound; excreted in the urine and can turn it orange. Adverse effects include nausea, dizziness, headache</li><li>Nitazoxanide → It is a prodrug of tizoxanide which is a PFOR enzyme inhibitor</li></ul></li></ul>
Trichomoniasis	<ul><li>Pathogen is *Trichomonas vaginalis*</li><li>Can lead to vulvovaginitis</li><li>Treatment of the male partner may also be required to prevent cross infection</li><li>Treatment includes:<ul><li>Oral → Metronidazole, tinidazole, secnidazole</li><li>Intravaginal → Povidone iodine, clotrimazole, natamycin</li></ul></li></ul>

ANTILEISHMANIASIS DRUGS

Leishmaniasis is a parasitic disease caused by leishmania species.

SODIUM STIBOGLUCONATE

Sodium stibogluconate is a pentavalent antimonial compound.

The mechanism of action is not clear; however, it causes a rapid efflux of trypanothione and glutathione from the protozoal cells and also inhibits trypanothione reductase. This leads to a reduction in the levels of trypanothione and glutathione and causes a loss of thiol reduction potential in the cells.

Sodium stibogluconate is eliminated in 2 phases—a short initial half-life (~2 hours) and a long terminal half-life.

The adverse effects include pain at the injection site, gastrointestinal symptoms (nausea, vomiting), headache, myalgia, arthralgia, elevation of liver enzymes, ECG changes (T-wave changes and QT prolongation), myelosuppression and renal damage.

It is the preferred drug for treatment for cutaneous and visceral leishmaniasis except in some regions of the world (e.g. India) where the efficacy has significantly reduced due to extensive resistance.

MILTEFOSINE

It is the first orally effective drug recently introduced for visceral leishmaniasis. It is also effective against cutaneous leishmaniasis.

The adverse effects include nausea, vomiting, elevation of liver enzymes and serum creatinine.

The drug is teratogenic and contraindicated in pregnancy.

AMPHOTERICIN B (AMB)

It is an antifungal drug. It is also used in visceral leishmaniasis, especially in parts of India where there is a resistance to sodium stibogluconate. It can also be used in mucocutaneous leishmaniasis.

Both conventional AMB (AMB deoxycholate) and liposomal AMB may be used for visceral leishmaniasis.

Amphotericin B has high toxicity and can lead to acute reaction (infusion related) consisting of fever, chills, nausea, pain, dyspnea etc. Long-term toxicities include nephrotoxicity, hypokalemia, anemia, etc.

The characteristics of liposomal AMB (as compared to conventional AMB) are:

○ Better safety profile (milder acute reaction, lower nephrotoxicity, less anemia)
○ Higher cost

The liposomal preparation of amphotericin B can deliver the drug to the reticuloendothelial cells in the liver and spleen.

PAROMOMYCIN

It is an aminoglycoside antibiotic. It has also shown efficacy (as topical application) in cutaneous leishmaniasis. It can be used in the treatment of visceral leishmaniasis. The adverse effects include injection site pain, ototoxicity and elevation of liver enzymes.

Some salient points regarding treatment of leishmaniasis are mentioned in Table 6.

TABLE 6	Leishmaniasis

Visceral leishmaniasis (Kala-azar)	• Caused by *L. donovani* and is an infection of the reticuloendothelial system
	• Treatment medications include:
	  ▪ Amphotericin B liposomal
	  ▪ Miltefosine
	  ▪ Amphotericin B deoxycholate
	  ▪ Paromomycin
	  ▪ Sodium stibogluconate (in regions where parasite is sensitive)

Cutaneous leishmaniasis	• Caused by *L. tropica, L. major*
	• Treatment medications include:
	  ▪ Sodium stibogluconate
	  ▪ Paromomycin
	  ▪ Ketoconazole

Mucocutaneous leishmaniasis	• Caused by *L. braziliensis* • Treatment medications include: ▪ Sodium stibogluconate

TREATMENT OF TRYPANOSOMIASIS

The treatment of trypanosomiasis is mentioned in Table 7.

TABLE 7	Treatment of trypanosomiasis
African trypanosomiasis	**American trypanosomiasis**

• Caused by *T. brucei*
• Also known as African sleeping sickness
• Treatment includes:
  ▪ Pentamidine, eflornithine
  ▪ Suramin, melarsoprol
	• Caused by *T. cruzi*
	• Also known as chagas disease
	• Treatment includes:
	  ▪ Nifurtimox
	  ▪ Benznidazole

SECTION L ■ Antimicrobials

ASSESS YOURSELF (Examination Questions of Various Universities)

1. Classify anti amoebic drugs. Discuss the adverse effects, mechanism of action and other uses of metronidazole
2. Treatment of extra intestinal amoebiasis
3. Therapeutic status of chloroquine in hepatic amoebiasis
4. Diloxanide furoate
5. Treatment of trichomoniasis
6. Therapeutic status of liposomal amphotericin B in leishmaniasis
7. Stibogluconate sodium

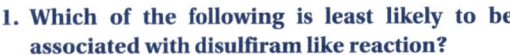

MULTIPLE CHOICE QUESTIONS

1. Which of the following is least likely to be associated with disulfiram like reaction?
   (Recent Question Dec 2016)
   a. Metronidazole   b. Tinidazole
   c. Satranidazole   d. Benznidazole

2. All of these are used in the treatment of visceral leishmaniasis except:
   (Recent Question 2016)
   a. Amphotericin
   b. Paromomycin
   c. Miltefosine
   d. Hydroxychloroquine

3. Choose the most effective drug for mild intestinal amoebiasis and asymptomatic cyst passers: *(Recent Question 2016)*
   a. Metronidazole
   b. Emetine
   c. Quiniodochlor
   d. Diloxanide furoate

4. The drug of choice for Kala-azar is:
   (Recent Question 2016)
   a. Pentamidine
   b. Suramin
   c. Sodium stibogluconate
   d. Ketoconazole

5. Which of the following drug is least effective luminal amoebicide?   *(Recent Question 2016)*
   a. Metronidazole
   b. Diloxanide furoate
   c. Iodoquinol
   d. Paromomycin

6. Metronidazole cause: *(PGI May 2011)*
   a. Disulfiram-like effect
   b. Antagonise warfarin
   c. It has metallic taste

7. Treatment of trichomoniasis infection of vagina: *(AP PG 2014)*
   a. Oral ciprofloxacin
   b. Oral metronidazole
   c. Oral doxycycline
   d. Topical Nystatin cream

8. Metronidazole is useful against all except:
   (TN PG 2000)
   a. Amoebiasis
   b. Trichomoniasis
   c. Giardiasis
   d. Kala-azar

Ans.

| 1. | (c) | 2. | (d) | 3. | (d) | 4. | (c) | 5. | (a) | 6. | (a, c) |
| 7. | (b) | 8. | (d) | | | | | | | | |

62

Antihelminthic Drugs

Helminths (also known as parasitic worms) infect human beings and cause a wide range of diseases. The various types of helminths along with the antihelminthic drugs are mentioned in Figure 1.

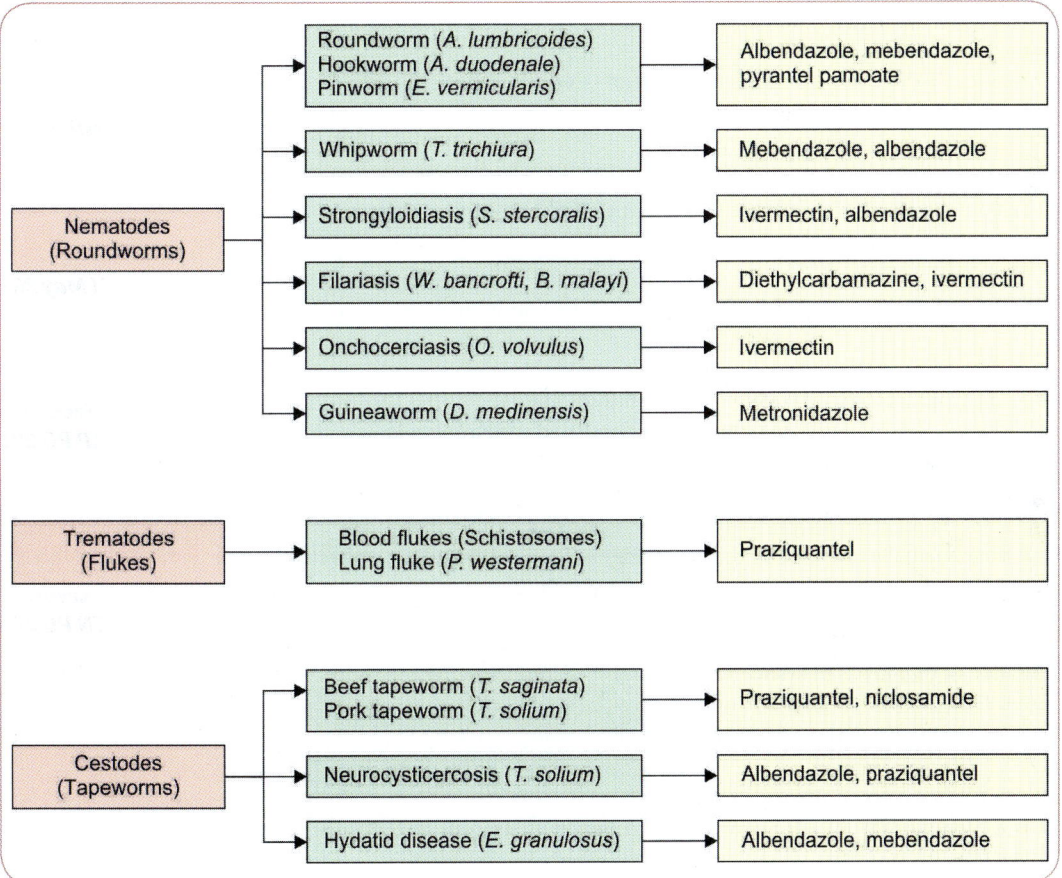

Figure 1: Antihelminthic drugs

MEBENDAZOLE

It is a benzimidazole with a broad-spectrum of antihelminthic activity.

Mechanism of Action

The possible mechanism of action of mebendazole is as follows:
○ Binds to β tubulin and inhibits microtubule polymerization
○ Blocks the uptake of glucose and depletion of glycogen stores in the parasite
○ The end result is immobilization and death of the parasite.

Pharmacokinetics

Mebendazole is poorly absorbed from the intestine. Following oral administration, most of the dose is excreted in the feces.

Adverse Effects

Mebendazole is usually tolerated well by the patients. Some of the adverse effects include:
- Abdominal discomfort, diarrhea, nausea and vomiting
- Allergic reactions, rashes, granulocytopenia
- Contraindicated in pregnant women
- It is not recommended in children aged less than 1 year.

Clinical Uses

- It is a broad spectrum antihelminthic and hence, is used in mixed infections (round worms, hookworms, pinworms, whipworms)
- It is more effective in trichuriasis than albendazole.

ALBENDAZOLE

It is a benzimidazole and has a broad-spectrum of antihelminthic activity.

Mechanism of Action

The possible mechanism of action of albendazole is similar to mebendazole.

Pharmacokinetics

The oral absorption of albendazole is variable; fatty food increases the absorption. It is metabolized in the liver and an active metabolite (albendazole sulfoxide) is produced which gets widely distributed in the body including brain and in hydatid cyst. Therefore, albendazole is preferred to mebendazole for the treatment of hydatid cyst.

Adverse Effects

Albendazole is usually tolerated well by the patients. Some of the adverse effects include:
- Abdominal discomfort, diarrhea, nausea and vomiting
- Allergic reactions, rashes, urticaria
- Hepatic dysfunction, leukopenia, thrombocytopenia, loss of hair may occur with higher doses/prolonged duration of therapy as in cysticercosis
- Contraindicated in pregnant women
- It is not recommended in children aged under 1 year.

Clinical Uses

- It is a broad-spectrum antihelminthic and hence, is used in mixed infections (round worms, hookworms, pinworms, whipworms)
- Hydatid disease
- Neurocysticercosis
  - Glucocorticoids are administered along with antihelminthics to decrease the inflammation resulting from dying parasites
  - Albendazole is preferred over praziquantel because of its shorter course, lower cost, increased concentration in the brain and CSF, better tolerability and increased drug levels (as compared to praziquantel)
  - It is contraindicated in ocular cysticercosis, as the host response can irreversibly harm the eye.
- Cutaneous larva migrans, trichinosis, lymphatic filariasis

PRAZIQUANTEL

It is effective in the treatment of *Schistosomiasis* and most other trematodes and cestodes. It is also effective in neurocysticercosis. It has no effect on nematodes.

Mechanism of Action

The mechanism of action believed to be responsible for antiparasitic action is mentioned below:
- Increased influx of calcium in the tegument leading to increase in muscular activity. This results in spastic paralysis and death of the parasite. This effect is observed at lowest effective concentration of the drug.
- At higher drug concentrations, tegumental damage occur leading to death of the parasite.

Pharmacokinetics

Praziquantel is rapidly absorbed following oral administration and undergoes extensive first pass metabolism in the liver. The metabolites are excreted mainly in urine. It crosses the blood brain barrier.

The bioavailability of praziquantel is reduced when taken along with phenytoin, carbamazepine and dexamethasone.

Adverse Effects

Some of the adverse effects of praziquantel include:
- Dizziness, sedation, headache
- Nausea, abdominal pain
- Urticaria, myalgia, joint pain, skin rashes

Precautions and Contraindications

- It is to be avoided in pregnancy
- It is contraindicated in ocular cysticercosis, as the host response can irreversibly harm the eye.

Clinical Uses

- Schistosomiasis: It is the drug of choice for all forms of schistosomiasis.
- Tapeworm infections
- Neurocysticercosis: Albendazole is the preferred drug; however, when it is not available or not appropriate, praziquantel can also be used.

NICLOSAMIDE

It is the second-choice drug for the treatment of most cestodes (tapeworm) infections.

Mechanism of Action

The adult worms are rapidly killed, but the ova are not affected. It presumably acts by inhibition of oxidative phosphorylation.

Adverse Effects

Some of the adverse effects of niclosamide include nausea, vomiting, diarrhea, headache, pruritus and malaise.

Clinical Uses

- Cestode (tapeworm) infections—*T. saginata*, *H. nana* and *D. latum* infections.

PYRANTEL PAMOATE

It is effective against *Ascaris lumbricoides* (roundworm), *Enterobius vermicularis* (pinworm) and *Ancylostoma duodenale* (hookworm) infections.

It is not active against *Trichuris* infections.

Mechanism of Action

It is a depolarizing neuromuscular blocker. It causes persistent activation of nicotinic acetylcholine receptors and inhibition of cholinesterase. This results in spastic paralysis of parasite followed by its expulsion.

Pharmacokinetics

It is poorly absorbed from the GIT. Most of the oral dose is excreted in the feces.

Adverse Effects

Some of the adverse effects of pyrantel pamoate include nausea, vomiting, diarrhea, abdominal cramps, headache, dizziness and skin rashes.

Clinical Uses

○ Nematode infections—*Ascaris lumbricoides* (roundworm), *Enterobius vermicularis* (pinworm) and *Ancylostoma duodenale/Necator americanus* (hookworm).

■ DIETHYLCARBAMAZINE CITRATE (DEC)

It is effective in the treatment of filariasis caused by *W. bancrofti* and *B. malayi*.

Mechanism of Action

DEC acts predominantly on microfilariae; adult worms are probably killed gradually upon prolonged therapy. DEC possibly causes an alteration of the membranes of microfilariae. This leads to their destruction by the host defense mechanisms. The mechanism of action of DEC against adult worms is unknown.

Pharmacokinetics

DEC is rapidly absorbed from the GIT. Metabolism occurs in the liver and is excreted in the urine. Faster excretion is observed in acidic urine.

Adverse Effects

Some of the adverse effects reported with the use of DEC are mentioned in Table 1.

TABLE 1	Adverse effects with diethylcarbamazine (DEC)
Direct toxic effects due to drug	• Nausea, vomiting, headache, anorexia, dizziness
Reactions due to dying parasite	• May lead to febrile reactions, swelling, lymphangitis, lymphoid abscess, rashes, hypotension • Can be mild (usually in bancroftian filariasis) or even severe reactions • Mazzotti reaction → Observed in patient with onchocerciasis. Develops soon after the first dose and presents as intense pruritus, rash, enlarged and tender lymph nodes, fever, headache, tachycardia, arthralgia. Can also lead to keratitis and uveitis. DEC is contraindicated in onchocerciasis. • Measures such as antihistaminics, corticosteroids and dosage reduction may be required.

Clinical Uses

The clinical uses of DEC include the following:
○ Filariasis caused by *W. bancrofti* and *B. malayi*
○ Tropical eosinophilia

IVERMECTIN

Ivermectin is the preferred drug for strongyloidiasis and onchocerciasis.

Mechanism of Action

The mechanism of action of ivermectin is as follows:
- It activates the glutamate gated chloride channels and increases GABAergic transmission in worms
- This leads to tonic paralysis of the worms resulting in death of the worms.

Pharmacokinetics

It is well absorbed following oral administration and has a wide distribution in the body.

Adverse Effects

Some of the adverse effects of ivermectin include:
- Fever, pruritus, nausea, vomiting, abdominal pain, myalgia, joint pains and transient ECG changes
- Reactions due to dying parasite may be observed and manifestations may include rashes, pruritus, joint paint, hypotension, tachycardia, edema etc. Severe reactions can be observed and may require treatment with corticosteroids. Mazzotti like reactions may be observed in patients with filarial infections.

Clinical Uses

The clinical uses of ivermectin include the following:
- Onchocerciasis
- Strongyloidiasis, ascariasis, cutaneous larva migrans
- Other uses—scabies, pediculosis.

Section L ■ Antimicrobials

1. Mebendazole
2. Albendazole
3. Therapeutic status of albendazole for neuro-cysticercosis
4. Diethylcarbamazine citrate
5. Write the mechanism of action and uses of ivermectin

MULTIPLE CHOICE QUESTIONS

1. Wrong statement about albendazole is:
   (Recent Question 2016)
   a. Poor CSF penetration
   b. Contraindicated in pregnancy
   c. Useful in neurocysticercosis
   d. Can cause hepatotoxicity

2. Drug of choice for schistosomiasis is:
   (Recent Question 2016)
   a. Albendazole
   b. Metronidazole
   c. Praziquantel
   d. Triclabendazole

3. What is true of ivermectin?
   (Recent Question 2016)
   a. It is the most effective drug for strongyloidiasis
   b. It is the drug of choice for onchocerciasis
   c. It can be used to treat scabies
   d. All of the above

4. An antihelminthic drug that is effective against blood fluke, liver fluke, lung fluke and cysticercosis is: *(Recent Question 2016)*
   a. Albendazole
   b. Praziquantel
   c. Ivermectin
   d. Thiabendazole

5. Drug of choice for treatment of infestation due to onchocerca volvulus is:
   (Recent Question 2016)
   a. Albendazole
   b. Ivermectin
   c. Praziquantel
   d. Suramin

6. Treatment of neurocysticercosis includes all of the following except: *(Recent Question 2016)*
   a. Albendazone
   b. Prednisolone
   c. Niclosamide
   d. Praziquantel

7. Ivermectin is indicated in all of the following except: *(JIPMER 2010)*
   a. Ascaris
   b. Filariasis
   c. Malaria
   d. Onchocerciasis

8. Effective drug for trematodes and many cestodes: *(TN PG 2001)*
   a. Niclosamide
   b. Praziquantel
   c. Pirenzepine
   d. Pyrantel pamoate

Ans.

| 1. | (a) | 2. | (c) | 3. | (d) | 4. | (b) | 5. | (b) | 6. | (c) |
| 7. | (c) | 8. | (b) | | | | | | | | |

63

Antiviral Drugs

Viruses survive only inside the host cells and their multiplication depends on cell's synthetic processes. Therefore, antiviral drugs, to become effective, must either block the entry or exit of virus from the host cells, or be active inside the host cells.

A classification of antiviral drugs is mentioned in Table 1.

TABLE 1	Antiviral drugs
Anti-herpesvirus drugs	
• Anti-herpesvirus drugs	Acyclovir, famciclovir, ganciclovir, valacyclovir, penciclovir, cidofovir, foscarnet, idoxuridine
Antiretroviral drugs	
• Nucleoside/nucleotide reverse transcriptase inhibitors (NRTIs)	Zidovudine, didanosine, stavudine, lamivudine, abacavir, emtricitabine, tenofovir
• Non-nucleoside reverse transcriptase inhibitors (NNRTIs)	Nevirapine, delavirdine, efavirenz, etravirine, rilpivirine
• Protease inhibitors (PI)	Indinavir, lopinavir/ritonavir, nelfinavir, saquinavir, atazanavir, darunavir, fosamprenavir, tipranavir
• Integrase inhibitors (Integrase strand transfer inhibitors [INSTIs])	Elvitegravir, raltegravir, dolutegravir
• Entry inhibitors	Enfuvirtide, maraviroc
Anti-influenza virus drugs	
• Oseltamivir, zanamivir	
• Amantadine, rimantadine	
Other antiviral drugs	
• Interferon alpha	
• Ribavirin	

ANTI-HERPESVIRUS DRUGS

Some of the types of herpesvirus with possible manifestations are mentioned in Table 2.

TABLE 2	Types of herpesviruses
Type of herpesviruses	**Manifestations include**
Human herpesvirus 1 (Herpes simplex virus type 1)	• Genital herpes, cutaneous herpes, encephalitis, herpes labialis, esophagitis
Human herpesvirus 2 (Herpes simplex virus type 2)	• Genital herpes

Contd...

Human herpesvirus 3 (Varicella-zoster virus [VZV])	• Chicken pox, herpes zoster
Human herpesvirus 4 (Epstein-Barr virus [EBV])	• Infectious mononucleosis, hepatitis, encephalitis
Human herpesvirus 5 (Cytomegalovirus [CMV])	• Retinitis, pneumonia, colitis

ACYCLOVIR

Acyclovir is a deoxyguanosine analogue drug having anti-herpesvirus activity.

Mechanism of Action

Acyclovir inhibits the synthesis of viral DNA and viral replication by the mechanism shown in Figure 1.

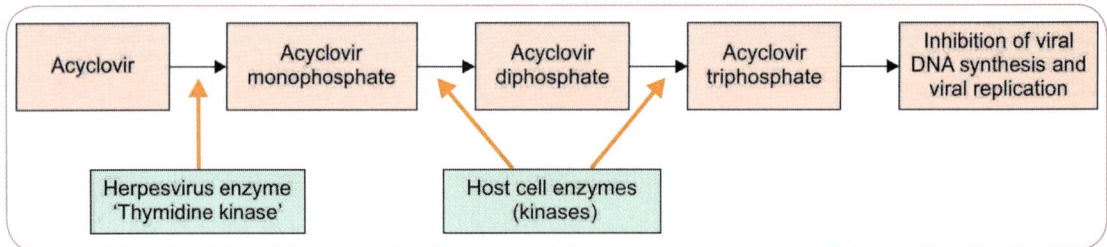

Figure 1: Mechanism of action of acyclovir

Pharmacokinetics

Acyclovir is available as oral, intravenous or topical formulation. It is widely distributed in the body and crosses the blood brain barrier.

It is excreted mainly unchanged by the kidneys with a half-life of 2–3 hours. Dose reduction is therefore required in renal impairment.

Adverse Effects

Acyclovir is generally well tolerated; however, nausea, malaise, vomiting and headache can occur.

High doses can lead to neurotoxicity (e.g. tremors, seizures, coma). Renal insufficiency can also occur. Irritation and burning sensation can occur after topical use.

Clinical Uses

Acyclovir is most effective against HSV type 1, followed by HSV type 2, VZV and EBV. The efficacy is similar for VZV and EBV.

Acyclovir is therapeutically not effective in CMV infections.

Some of the clinical uses of acyclovir are mentioned below:
- Genital herpes simplex
- Mucocutaneous herpes simplex
- Herpes simplex keratitis
- Herpes simplex encephalitis
- Chicken pox
- Herpes zoster

OTHER ANTI-HERPESVIRUS DRUGS

Some of the salient features of other anti-herpesvirus drugs are mentioned in Table 3.

TABLE 3	Other anti-herpesvirus drugs
Ganciclovir	• Analogue of acyclovir • Has activity against all herpesviruses • Adverse effects bone marrow depression, neutropenia, thrombocytopenia. CNS toxicity including convulsions, coma. It is reported to be carcinogenic, embryotoxic, and teratogenic in animals. • Used in patients of CMV retinitis and other severe CMV infections
Penciclovir	• Guanine nucleoside analogue • Inhibits viral DNA synthesis • Active against HSV and VZV
Famciclovir	• Prodrug of penciclovir • Effective orally • Adverse effects include nausea, diarrhea, headache, hallucinations, confusion • Clinical uses include genital or orolabial herpes and herpes zoster
Foscarnet	• Pyrophosphate analogue • Inhibits viral DNA polymerase and reverse transcriptase • Effective against herpes simplex, CMV and HIV • Poorly absorbed orally • Adverse effects include: nephrotoxicity, renal failure, anemia, hypocalcemia, hypomagnesemia, seizures, arrhythmias, electrolyte abnormalities • Clinical uses include CMV retinitis, other CMV infections and in acyclovir resistant HSV infections
Cidofovir	• Cytidine nucleotide analogue; inhibits viral DNA synthesis • Adverse effects include nephrotoxicity. It is contraindicated in patients on nephrotoxic drugs. Cidofovir is also mutagenic and teratogenic. • Oral probenecid and normal saline intravenous (IV) are administered with cidofovir to reduce the risk of nephrotoxicity • Clinical uses include CMV retinitis

ANTIRETROVIRAL DRUGS

Human immunodeficiency virus (HIV) is single stranded RNA retrovirus that attacks the body's immune system. Antiretroviral drugs are used against HIV. These drugs do not cure the infection but help in prolongation and improvement in quality of life. These drugs are also useful in postponing the complications of acquired immunodeficiency syndrome (AIDS) or AIDS related complex (ARC).

CLASSIFICATION OF ANTIRETROVIRAL DRUGS

A classification of antiretroviral drugs is mentioned in Table 4.

TABLE 4	Classification of antiretroviral drugs	
Class of drug	**Mechanism**	**Examples**
Nucleoside/Nucleotide reverse transcriptase inhibitors (NRTIs)	Inhibits HIV reverse transcriptase enzyme competitively	Zidovudine, didanosine, stavudine, lamivudine, abacavir, emtricitabine, tenofovir
Non-nucleoside reverse transcriptase inhibitors (NNRTIs)	Inhibits HIV reverse transcriptase enzyme noncompetitively	Nevirapine, delavirdine, efavirenz, etravirine, rilpivirine
Protease inhibitors (PIs)	Inhibits HIV protease enzyme competitively	Indinavir, nelfinavir, lopinavir/ritonavir, saquinavir, atazanavir, darunavir, fosamprenavir, tipranavir

Contd...

Integrase inhibitors (Integrase strand transfer inhibitors (INSTIs))	Binds to integrase enzyme and inhibits the insertion of proviral DNA into the genome of host cells	Elvitegravir, raltegravir, dolutegravir
Entry inhibitors	• Enfuvirtide is a fusion inhibitor that prevents the entry of HIV into the cell. It binds to the transmembrane glycoprotein gp 41 and prevents the conformational changes needed for the fusion of the virus with the cell membranes. • Maraviroc—blocks the CCR5 co-receptor that works along with gp 41 to facilitate entry of HIV in the host cells.	Enfuvirtide, maraviroc

NUCLEOSIDE/NUCLEOTIDE REVERSE TRANSCRIPTASE INHIBITORS (NRTIs)

These drugs are phosphorylated in the cytoplasm of host cells and are converted into the active triphosphate forms.

The active triphosphate forms then competitively inhibit the viral reverse transcriptase enzyme. This prevents the conversion of viral RNA into proviral DNA (Figure 2). The integration of proviral DNA with the host DNA is therefore prevented.

They are effective against both HIV-1 and HIV-2.

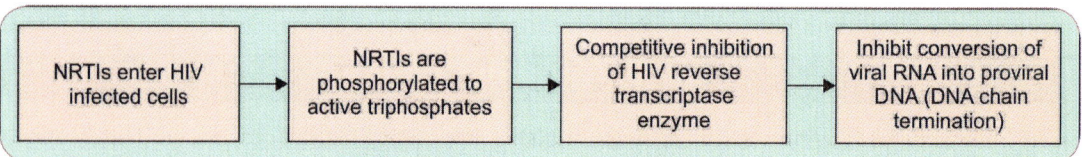

Figure 2: Mechanism of action of NRTIs

These drugs do not remove the virus that has already integrated into the host DNA, but they prevent infection of the new cells.

NRTIs are mostly used in combination with other classes of drugs such as NNRTI, PIs or integrase inhibitors.

Zidovudine (AZT)

- It is a prototype NRTI and is a thymidine analogue.
- AZT was the first antiretroviral drug approved for the treatment of AIDS.
- It is orally effective and is rapidly absorbed from the gastrointestinal tract (GIT). It crosses the blood brain barrier and placenta.
- It is metabolized in the liver by glucuronide conjugation and excreted by the kidney.

Adverse Effects

Some of the adverse effects of AZT include:
- Bone marrow suppression including macrocytic anemia and neutropenia are common adverse effects
- GIT intolerance, headache and insomnia tend to reduce gradually during therapy
- Other adverse effects include nail hyperpigmentation, skeletal muscle myopathy, hepatotoxicity, encephalopathy and lactic acidosis.

Drug Interactions

- Zidovudine and stavudine are not given together as they compete for intracellular phosphorylation – results in mutual antagonism.
- Zidovudine and paracetamol are not given together as both are metabolized by glucuronide conjugation. This may lead to increase in AZT levels and toxicity.
- Zidovudine can lead to bone marrow suppression. Hence, enhancement of bone marrow suppression may be observed if used with other drugs that suppress the bone marrow.

Clinical Uses

AZT is used in HIV patients in combination with other antiretroviral drugs. The clinical uses of AZT include the following:

- Treatment of HIV infection in adults and children
- Postexposure prophylaxis in HIV-exposed persons
- Prevention of mother to child transmission of HIV infection.

Some of the salient features of other NRTIs are mentioned in Table 5.

TABLE 5	Salient features of other NRTIs
Stavudine	• It is synthetic thymidine analogue • Peripheral neuropathy is a common adverse effect. Other adverse effects include lactic acidosis, hepatic steatosis and lipodystrophy • Stavudine should not be combined with didanosine due to increased risk of lactic acidosis, pancreatitis (can be fatal) and peripheral neuropathy • Stavudine should not be combined with zidovudine due to the occurrence of mutual antagonism
Lamivudine	• It is a cytidine analogue • It is usually well tolerated; mild adverse effects include headache, insomnia, dizziness, GI discomfort • In addition to HIV, it is also effective against HBV • One of the recommended drugs for use in pregnancy • Available in a fixed-dose combination with zidovudine and with abacavir
Didanosine	• It is a purine nucleoside analogue • Adverse effects include pancreatitis, peripheral neuropathy, hyperuricemia and optic neuritis • Didanosine should not be combined with stavudine due to increased risk of lactic acidosis, pancreatitis (can be fatal) and peripheral neuropathy
Abacavir	• It is a guanosine analogue • Adverse effects include a potentially fatal hypersensitivity syndrome usually within 6 weeks of therapy initiation • Concurrent use of alcohol may increase abacavir levels
Emtricitabine	• It is a cytidine analogue • Long intracellular half-life; hence, permits once-daily dosing • It has low toxicity amongst other antiretroviral drugs • Hyperpigmentation of skin may occur on prolonged use • In addition to HIV, it is also effective against HBV
Tenofovir	• It is a nucleotide analogue of adenosine • The mechanism of action is similar to nucleoside analogues • Generally, well tolerated; adverse effects include GIT complaints such as flatulence. Acute renal failure and Fanconi syndrome have been reported • In addition to HIV, it is also effective against HBV

NON-NUCLEOSIDE REVERSE TRANSCRIPTASE INHIBITORS (NNRTIs)

The non-nucleoside reverse transcriptase inhibitors (NNRTIs) are noncompetitive inhibitors of HIV-1 reverse transcriptase (RT). Unlike NRTIs, they do not require activation by intracellular phosphorylation (Figure 3). They are active against HIV-1 and have no activity against HIV-2.

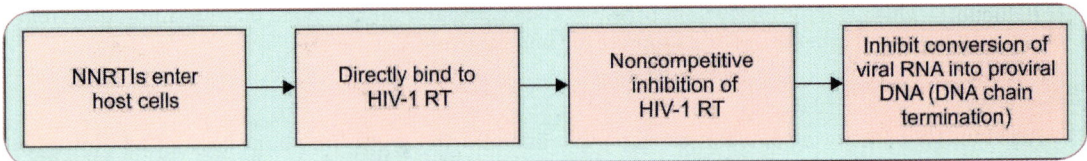

Figure 3: Mechanism of action of NNRTIs

Common Characteristics of NNRTIs

- Active against HIV-1 reverse transcriptase and not against HIV-2 reverse transcriptase
- Cross resistance can occur between NNRTIs but is not observed between NNRTIs and NRTIs or PIs
- Common adverse effects include skin rashes (including Stevens-Johnson syndrome) and gastrointestinal intolerance
- Metabolism by CYP450 system can result in many potential drug-drug interactions
- Used in combination regimens for the treatment of HIV infection.

Some of the salient features of NNRTIs are mentioned in Table 6.

TABLE 6	Salient features of NNRTIs
Nevirapine	• Well-absorbed orally, highly lipophilic and has a wide tissue distribution including CSF, breast milk and placenta • One of the recommended drugs for use in pregnancy; used to prevent HIV transmission from mother to newborn • Adverse effects include: 　▪ Skin rash (including Stevens-Johnson syndrome (SJS) and toxic epidermal necrolysis (TEN)—may be life-threatening) 　▪ Hepatic toxicity (may be fulminant and fatal) • Moderate inducer of CYP3A4 isoenzyme—can lead to drug interactions
Efavirenz	• Long duration of action; permits once-daily dosing • Should be taken empty stomach to reduce toxicity • Common adverse effects involve the CNS. May lead to dizziness, headache, insomnia, nightmares etc. Skin rashes have also been reported • To be avoided in pregnancy
Delavirdine	• Well-absorbed orally • Extensively metabolized by CYP isoenzymes; can lead to drug interactions • Adverse effects include skin rash, nausea and diarrhea • To be avoided in pregnancy
Etravirine	• Active against HIV strains that are resistant to 1st generation NNRTIs • Used for HIV treatment—experienced patients that have resistance to other NNRTIs • Common adverse effects include rash, diarrhea and nausea • It is a substrate and inducer of CYP3A4 and inhibitor of CYP2C9 and CYP2C19—multiple drug interactions can occur
Rilpivirine	• Used only in treatment-naïve patients with HIV RNA ≤100,000 copies/mL, and only in combination with at least 2 other antiretroviral drugs • Must be given with meals; oral bioavailability is significantly reduced in the presence of acid lowering drugs. Use with PPIs is contraindicated. • Common adverse effects include rash, depression, headache and insomnia

PROTEASE INHIBITORS (PIs)

Common Characteristics of Protease Inhibitors (PIs)

- Protease inhibitors competitively inhibit the HIV protease enzyme. The HIV protease enzyme is required for the cleavage of viral polyproteins into final structural proteins of HIV. Hence, protease inhibitors lead to the production of noninfectious, immature viral particles.
- Cross resistance is common amongst the PIs, but there is no cross resistance with NRTIs or NNRTIs. They are therefore, used in combination with NRTIs and NNRTIs.
- Adverse effects include nausea, diarrhea, dyslipidemia, fat redistribution, central obesity, cushingoid appearance, cardiac conduction abnormalities and hepatotoxicity. Hyperglycemia and insulin resistance can occur.
- Protease inhibitors undergo extensive metabolism by CYP3A4 → significant potential for drug-drug interactions.

Some of the salient features of some of the PIs are mentioned in Table 7.

TABLE 7	Salient features of protease inhibitors
Ritonavir	• It is a very potent inhibitor of CYP3A4; hence may result in large number of drug-drug interactions. However, this allows the use of ritonavir in low doses in combination with other protease inhibitors. • This 'booster therapy' has the following advantages: ▪ Increased bioavailability of other protease inhibitors leading to longer dosing intervals; decrease in the number/frequency of dosing ▪ Allows for better tolerability and increased efficacy • Nelfinavir is not combined with ritonavir • Adverse effects include GIT abnormalities and circumoral paraesthesia
Indinavir	• Common adverse effects include nephrolithiasis, crystalluria, hyperbilirubinemia and insulin resistance • Sufficient intake of fluids is recommended to decrease the incidence of nephrolithiasis/renal complications

INTEGRASE INHIBITORS (INTEGRASE STRAND TRANSFER INHIBITORS [INSTIs])

Integrase is an enzyme that is required for the replication of HIV-1 and HIV-2. Integrase inhibitors bind to integrase and inhibit the insertion of proviral DNA into the genome of host cells.

Integrase inhibitors are usually well tolerated and adverse effects include GIT disturbances, headache and neuropsychiatric effects. Rhabdomyolysis and hypersensitivity reactions can also occur.

Elvitegravir

- Available as a fixed-dose combination containing elvitegravir, cobicistat, emtricitabine, tenofovir
- Cobicistat is a pharmacokinetic enhancer or booster as it is a CYP3A inhibitor.

ENTRY INHIBITORS

Enfuvirtide

- Enfuvirtide is a fusion inhibitor that prevents the entry of HIV into the cell. It binds to the transmembrane glycoprotein gp41 and prevents the conformational changes needed for the fusion of the viral and host cell membranes.
- Requires subcutaneous injection for administration.
- Common adverse effects include injection site reactions (erythematous nodules), insomnia, headache and eosinophilia.

Maraviroc

- Blocks the CCR5 co-receptor that works along with gp41 to facilitate entry of HIV in the host cell
- Effective orally
- It is active against HIV that exclusively uses CCR5 co-receptor and is not active against HIV strains with CXCR4
- Adverse effects include cough, muscle pains, joint pains, hepatotoxicity, diarrhea, sleep disturbances and upper respiratory tract infections.

ANTIRETROVIRAL THERAPY (ART)

HIGHLY ACTIVE ANTIRETROVIRAL THERAPY (HAART)

There is a high incidence of resistance when HIV patients are treated with a single antiretroviral drug. Hence, HAART is used which is a combination of three or more drugs from two or more antiretroviral drug classes. The advantages of HAART therapy are:

- Decreases incidence of drug resistance
- Decreases morbidity and mortality rates in HIV infected patients
- Improves the quality of life

Management with ART is lifelong. Some of the key points about the antiretroviral therapy are mentioned in Table 8.

TABLE 8	Antiretroviral therapy (ART)
Criteria for initiation of ART in adults (>19 years of age)	Initiation of antiretroviral therapy should be done in all adults living with HIV, regardless of WHO clinical stage and CD4 cell count
First-line ART (adults)	• Two nucleoside reverse transcriptase inhibitors (NRTIs) PLUS a non-nucleoside reverse transcriptase inhibitor (NNRTI) or an integrase inhibitor (INSTI) ▪ TDF (tenofovir) + [(3TC (lamivudine) or (FTC (emtricitabine))] + EFV (efavirenz) ▪ Administered as a fixed-dose combination
Lab monitoring of ART	• Routine viral load monitoring
Second-line ART (adults)	• Two nucleoside reverse transcriptase inhibitors (NRTIs) PLUS a ritonavir boosted protease inhibitor (PI)
ART in pregnant women	• Two nucleoside reverse transcriptase inhibitors (NRTIs) PLUS a non-nucleoside reverse transcriptase inhibitor (NNRTI) or an integrase inhibitor (INSTI) **Drugs recommended during pregnancy** • **NRTIs** Recommended drugs—Lamivudine, zidovudine Alternate drugs—Abacavir, tenofovir, emtricitabine • **NNRTIs** Recommended drugs—Nevirapine **Protease inhibitors** Recommended drugs—Lopinavir/ritonavir Alternate drugs—Saquinavir, darunavir
ART for postexposure prophylaxis of HIV infection in adults	• ART regimen with two drugs is effective, but three drugs are preferred • TDF (tenofovir) + 3TC (or FTC) → two drugs • LPV/r (lopinavir/ritonavir) is the preferred third drug • 28 days prescription is given • Counseling is required

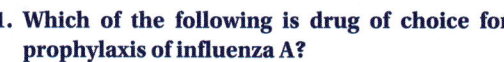

MULTIPLE CHOICE QUESTIONS

1. Which of the following is drug of choice for prophylaxis of influenza A?
   (Recent Question Dec 2016)
   a. Oseltamavir
   b. Zanamivir
   c. Amantidine
   d. Rimantidine

2. Drug of choice for bird flu: *(AIIMS Nov 2015)*
   a. Oseltamivir
   b. Ribavirin
   c. Entecavir
   d. Acyclovir

3. All are used in influenza B except
   (AIIMS Nov 2015)
   a. Oseltamivir
   b. Zanamivir
   c. Premavir
   d. Ribavirin

4. Which of the following is a protease inhibitor:
   (AIIMS May 2015)
   a. Abacavir
   b. Saquinavir
   c. Zidovudine
   d. Lamivudine

5. Nonnucleoside reverse transcriptase inhibitors (NNRTIs) include all of the following except:
   (AIIMS May 2014)
   a. Nevirapine
   b. Delavirdine
   c. Etavirine
   d. Lamivudine

6. Which of the following is an ocular side effect of HAART therapy? *(AIIMS Nov 2012)*
   a. Retinitis
   b. Uveitis
   c. Optic neuritis
   d. Scleritis

7. Efavirenz is used for treatment of HIV infections. It acts: *(AIIMS Nov 2011)*
   a. As protease inhibitor
   b. As reverse transcriptase inhibitor
   c. As integrase inhibitor
   d. By inhibiting the HIV entry into the cell

8. Which is the integrase inhibitor used in treatment of HIV? *(Recent Question 2016)*
   a. Raltegravir
   b. Indinavir
   c. Lopinavir
   d. Fosamprenavir

9. ART drug which is entry inhibitor:
   (Recent Question 2016)
   a. Enfuvirtide
   b. Abacavir
   c. Efavirez
   d. Amprenavir

10. Oseltamivir is: *(Recent Question 2016)*
    a. Neuraminidase inhibitor
    b. Neuraminidase activator
    c. Carboxylase inhibitor
    d. Carboxylase activator

11. HIV integrase inhibitor is:
    (Recent Question 2016)
    a. Elvitegravir
    b. Abacavir
    c. Maraviroc
    d. Tenofovir

12. Drug that is active against both HIV and hepatitis B virus: *(Recent Question 2016)*
    a. Lamivudine
    b. Indinavir
    c. Didanosine
    d. Efavirenz

13. Integrase inhibitor used in treatment of HIV:
    (Recent Question 2016)
    a. Raltegravir
    b. Indinavir
    c. Lopinavir
    d. Fosamprenavir

Ans.

1.	(a)	2.	(a)	3.	(d)	4.	(b)	5.	(d)	6.	(c)
7.	(b)	8.	(a)	9.	(a)	10.	(a)	11.	(a)	12.	(a)
13.	(a)										

14. **Nevirapine is:** *(Recent Question 2016)*
   a. Non-nucleoside reverse transcriptase inhibitor (NN-RTI)
   b. Nucleoside reverse transcriptase inhibitor (NRTI)
   c. Protease inhibitor
   d. Fusion inhibitor

15. **Zidovudine causes:** *(Recent Question 2016)*
   a. Neurotoxicity
   b. Nephrotoxicity
   c. Neutropenia
   d. Ototoxicity

16. **Enfuvirtide belongs to the class of:**
   (Recent Question 2016)
   a. Fusion inhibitors
   b. Protease inhibitors
   c. Gp 120 inhibitors
   d. Nucleotide reverse transcriptase inhibitors

17. **In antiretroviral therapy, zidovudine should not be combined with:** *(Recent Question 2016)*
   a. Lamivudine
   b. Nevirapine
   c. Didanosine
   d. Stavudine

18. **Reverse transcriptase inhibitor is:**
   (Recent Question 2016)
   a. Didanosine
   b. Acyclovir
   c. Enfuvirtide
   d. Maraviroc

19. **Reverse transcriptase inhibitor:**
   (Recent Question 2016)
   a. Ritonavir
   b. Saquinavir
   c. Amprenavir
   d. Tenofovir

20. **A patient is on indinavir, zidovudine, lamivudine and ketoconazole. He developed breast hypertrophy, nephrolithiasis, hyperlipidemia and central obesity; identify the drug causing these side effects amongst all:**
   (AIIMS Nov 2018)
   a. Lamivudine
   b. Indinavir
   c. Ketoconazole
   d. Zidovudine

Ans.

14.	(a)	15.	(c)	16.	(a)	17.	(d)	18.	(a)	19.	(d)
20.	(b)										

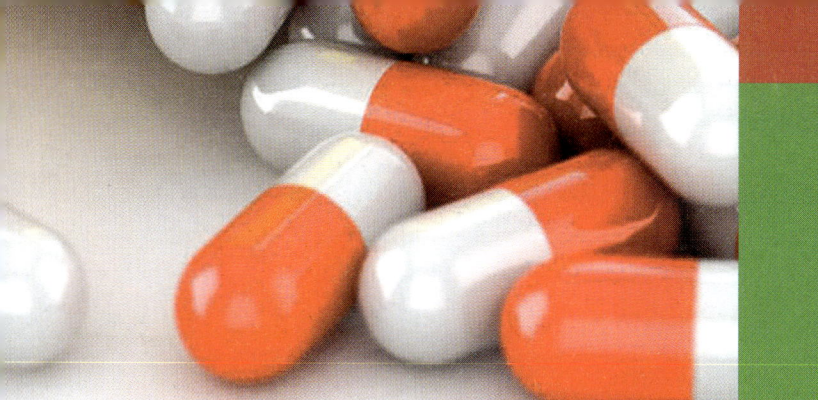

Anticancer Drugs

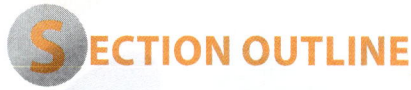

SECTION OUTLINE

- Anticancer Drugs

64

Anticancer Drugs

Anticancer drugs are used for various malignancies alone or in combinations. A combination of chemotherapy, surgery and radiotherapy may be the best approach in some malignancies.

CHEMOTHERAPY

- Primary chemotherapy → chemotherapy is administered as a primary treatment in patients with advanced malignancy for which an alternative therapy does not exist, e.g. patients with advanced metastatic malignancy.
- Neoadjuvant chemotherapy → used in patients with localized malignancy for which alternative local therapies do exist. However, these local therapies (e.g. surgery) are not completely effective. Neoadjuvant chemotherapy is administered to decrease the size of the primary tumor prior to surgery, e.g. cancer of the bladder, larynx.
- Adjuvant chemotherapy → administered after surgery or radiation to destroy residual cancer cells, e.g. colon cancer, gastric cancer.

Anticancer drugs can be either cell cycle specific or non-cell cycle specific (Figure 1).

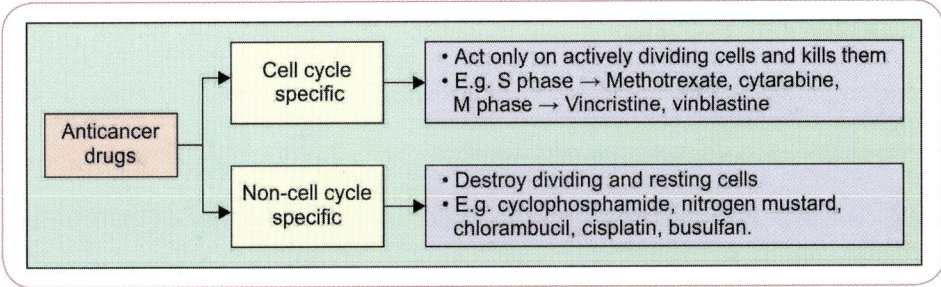

Figure 1: Anticancer drugs—cell cycle specific versus non-cell cycle specific

The phases of cell cycle and the examples of cell cycle specific drugs are mentioned in Figure 2 and Table 1.

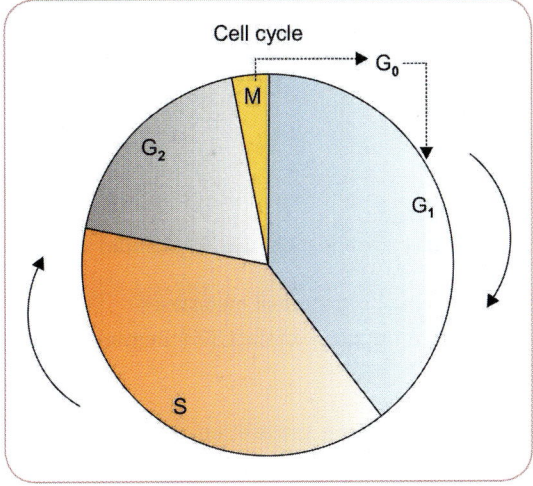

Figure 2: Cell cycle

TABLE 1	Phases of cell cycle and cell cycle specific anticancer drugs	
Phases of cell cycle	**Function**	**Examples of cell cycle specific drugs**
G_1 phase (Presynthesis)	Synthesis of cellular components (e.g. enzymes) required for DNA synthesis	Vinblastine
S phase (Synthesis)	DNA synthesis	Methotrexate, cytarabine, doxorubicin, 6-mercaptopurine, 5-fluorouracil
G_2 phase (Premitotic)	Synthesis of components for mitosis	Daunorubicin, etoposide, bleomycin, topotecan
M phase (Mitotic)	Mitosis	Vincristine, vinblastine, paclitaxel, docetaxel
G_0 phase (Resting)	Cells are not dividing (quiescent state)	

TOXICITY OF CYTOTOXIC (ANTICANCER) DRUGS

Anticancer drugs have significant effects on the rapidly growing cells. This is because nucleic acid and their precursors are an important target of anticancer drugs.

The tissues commonly affected by anticancer drugs include the bone marrow, GIT mucosa, hair and skin cells, reticuloendothelial system, gonads, fetus, etc.

Anticancer drugs are often administered in combination therapy to optimize the dose of each drug for maximum effectiveness and reduction in the incidence of toxicity.

BONE MARROW DEPRESSION

It can result in granulocytopenia, thrombocytopenia, aplastic anemia and agranulocytosis. Infections and bleeding are commonly observed in patients undergoing chemotherapy.

Therapeutic/preventive measures include the following:
- Recombinant erythropoietin therapy, packed RBC transfusions
- Platelet transfusions
- Granulocyte colony-stimulating factor (G-CSF) such as pegfilgrastim
- Bone marrow transplantation

IMMUNOSUPPRESSION

A reduction in the number and function of lymphocytes can lead to suppression of both cell-mediated and humoral immunity.

Patients also have damage to the epithelial surfaces and hence, are more prone to infections including opportunistic infections. Some of these infections can be *Candida, P. jirovecii*, cytomegalovirus, etc.

NAUSEA AND VOMITING

The causes of nausea and vomiting can include:
- Chemotherapy induced (e.g. cisplatin, cyclophosphamide, lomustine)
- Radiotherapy
- Other causes such as bowel obstruction or intracranial metastases

Nausea and vomiting can be due to direct stimulation of the CTZ (chemoreceptor trigger zone) by the drug or due to the emetogenic impulses generated from the GIT.

Drug therapy consists of the following:
- 5-hydroxytryptamine (5-HT$_3$) antagonists → e.g. granisetron, ondansetron
- Other drugs → e.g. dexamethasone, metoclopramide

GASTROINTESTINAL TRACT

Apart from nausea and vomiting, the following toxicities may be observed:
- Oral lesions such as stomatitis, ulcers, infections (e.g. candida), mucositis
- Diarrhea
- GI bleeding, hemorrhage

GONADS

- Males → oligospermia, impotence and infertility
- Females → amenorrhea, inhibition of ovulation and infertility

FETUS

Anticancer drugs can lead to abortion, fetal death or congenital anomalies.

SECONDARY MALIGNANCIES

Development of leukemias, lymphomas can occur in patients on therapy with anticancer drugs.

HYPERURICEMIA

Excessive cell destruction can lead to hyperuricemia. It can manifest as urate stones and gout.

Management (prevention) of hyperuricemia includes good hydration, allopurinol, corticosteroids etc. Allopurinol is an inhibitor of xanthine oxidase enzyme and reduces the synthesis of uric acid (Figure 3).

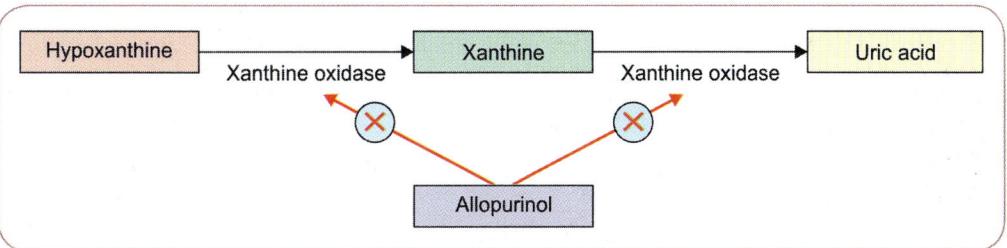

Figure 3: Mechanism of action of allopurinol

Allopurinol is a hypoxanthine analog that inhibits xanthine oxidase competitively, but it's major metabolite alloxanthine is a noncompetitive inhibitor of xanthine oxidase. Administration of allopurinol leads to a reduction in the levels of uric acid and an increase in the levels of hypoxanthine and xanthine which are more soluble and excreted in the urine. It can also cause some feedback inhibition of de novo purine synthesis.

HYPERCALCEMIA

It can result from some cancers (e.g. breast, prostate) or due to anticancer drugs. Therapy includes bisphosphonates (pamidronate, zoledronate, etc.), steroids and adequate hydration.

ALOPECIA AND DERMATITIS

A few examples of toxicities induced by specific anticancer drugs are mentioned in Table 2.

TABLE 2	Drug-induced toxicity
Anticancer drug(s)	**Specific toxicity**
Cyclophosphamide, ifosfamide	• Hemorrhagic cystitis • Therapy includes hydration, mesna (for systemic administration) and acetylcysteine (irrigation of bladder). • Both drugs contain thiol compounds that combine with and detoxify the toxic metabolites. Adequate hydration and frequent voiding of bladder is also helpful.
Methotrexate	• Megaloblastic anemia • Folinic acid is used for therapy. Folinic acid is also called citrovorum factor • Folic acid is not effective because it does not gets converted to the active coenzyme form (Figure 6)
Cisplatin	• Nephrotoxicity • Management includes mannitol and saline infusion
Doxorubicin, daunorubicin	• Cardiotoxicity
Busulfan, bleomycin	• Pulmonary fibrosis • Skin pigmentation

CLASSIFICATION OF ANTICANCER DRUGS

A classification of anticancer drugs is shown in Table 3.

TABLE 3	Classification of anticancer drugs
Alkylating agents	
Nitrogen mustards	• Mechlorethamine, cyclophosphamide, ifosfamide, chlorambucil, melphalan
Ethylenimine	• Thio-TEPA
Nitrosoureas	• Carmustine (BCNU), lomustine (CCNU)
Alkyl sulfonate	• Busulfan
Triazine	• Dacarbazine (DTIC)
Antimetabolites	
Folate antagonist	• Methotrexate (Mtx)
Purine antagonist	• 6-mercaptopurine (6-MP), azathioprine, fludarabine
Pyrimidine antagonist	• 5-fluorouracil (5-FU), cytarabine
Taxanes	
• Paclitaxel, docetaxel	
Vinca alkaloids	
• Vincristine, vinblastine	
Camptothecin analogues	
• Topotecan, irinotecan	
Epipodophyllotoxin	
• Etoposide	
Antibiotics	
• Actinomycin D (Dactinomycin), doxorubicin, daunorubicin, mitoxantrone, bleomycin	

Contd...

Tyrosine kinase inhibitors	
• Imatinib, dasatinib, erlotinib, sorafenib, sunitinib	
Miscellaneous	
• Cisplatin, carboplatin, hydroxyurea, procarbazine, L-asparaginase	
Hormones and drugs affecting the hormonal balance	
Glucocorticoids	Prednisolone
Estrogens	Fosfestrol
Selective estrogen receptor modulators (SERMs)	Tamoxifen, Toremifene
Selective estrogen receptor downregulators (SERDs)	Fulvestrant
Aromatase inhibitors	Anastrozole, letrozole
Androgens	Testosterone propionate
Antiandrogens	Flutamide, bicalutamide
5-α-reductase inhibitors	Finasteride, dutasteride
GnRH analogues	Buserelin, goserelin, nafarelin

ALKYLATING AGENTS

The alkylating agents have alkyl groups. They transfer the alkyl group to nucleophilic sites of the DNA by forming covalent bonds. This step is lethal to the DNA as it leads to abnormal base pairing/cross linking etc. (Figure 4).

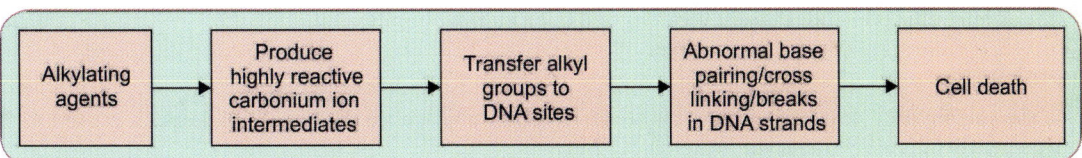

Figure 4: Mechanism of action of alkylating agents

Many of the alkylating agents are cell cycle nonspecific drugs, i.e. they act on resting as well as actively dividing cells. They also possess radiomimetic and cytotoxic activity.

Nitrogen Mustards

Cyclophosphamide

It is a prodrug. It is converted in the liver to an active metabolite aldophosphamide. Aldophosphamide undergoes nonenzymatic cleavage in tumor cells to produce phosphoramide mustard and a toxic metabolite acrolein (Figure 5).

Phosphoramide mustard produces cytotoxic effects and acrolein produces hemorrhagic cystitis.

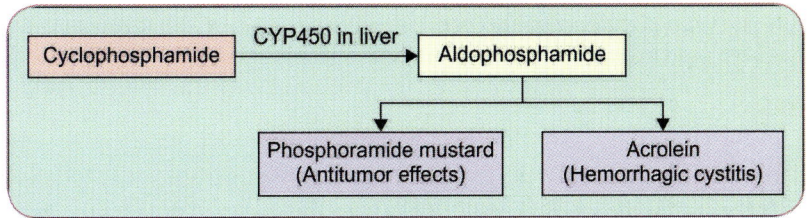

Figure 5: Cyclophosphamide and hemorrhagic cystitis

Cyclophosphamide is available as oral and IV formulations. The metabolites are primarily excreted in the urine.

Adverse Effects

The general adverse effects include nausea, vomiting, diarrhea, myelosuppression, alopecia, etc.

A unique toxicity of cyclophosphamide (and ifosfamide) is hemorrhagic cystitis, which is associated with hematuria and dysuria. The toxicity occurs due to the toxic metabolite acrolein. It can be reduced by:

○ Adequate hydration—which washes out the toxic metabolites including acrolein
○ IV injection of mesna (sodium 2-mercaptoethane sulfonate)—which neutralizes acrolein

Clinical Uses

It is a broad-spectrum antineoplastic drug. It also has strong immunosuppressive effect. It is used in the following conditions:

○ Neoplastic conditions—combination with other drugs for non-Hodgkin's lymphoma, other lymphoid cancers, breast and ovarian cancers, sarcoma, and other solid tumors in children.
○ Non-neoplastic conditions (immunosuppressive action)—rheumatoid arthritis, nephrotic syndrome, Wegener's granulomatosis.

Ifosfamide

Ifosfamide is a longer acting congener of cyclophosphamide. It also causes hemorrhagic cystitis. Mesna is given to reduce it.

The clinical uses include testicular cancer, breast cancer and sarcomas.

Mechlorethamine

It is highly reactive and causes severe local reactions. Hence, it can only be administered by intravenous route. It is rarely used currently and has been replaced by more stable nitrogen mustards. It was previously used as a part of MOPP regimen in Hodgkin's disease.

The adverse effects include nausea, vomiting and bone marrow suppression.

Chlorambucil

It is a slow acting drug. It is used orally. It is effective specifically against the lymphoid tissue. It is used in the management of chronic lymphocytic leukemia (CLL).

It can be given long-term as a maintenance therapy in CLL.

Melphalan

Melphalan is mainly used in the treatment of multiple myeloma. It is used in combination with other drugs such as dexamethasone or thalidomide.

It is mostly given IV as oral absorption is inconsistent. Bone marrow depression is a common adverse effect.

Nitrosoureas

Carmustine and Lomustine

Carmustine and lomustine are highly lipid soluble drugs that cross the blood-brain barrier. They are used in the treatment of brain tumors.

The adverse effects include profound but delayed bone marrow suppression. Adverse effects such as pulmonary fibrosis, renal failure and veno-occlusive disease (VOD) of the liver can occur with carmustine.

Carmustine has been used in malignant gliomas but is being replaced by temozolomide for this purpose.

Alkyl Sulphonate

Busulfan

It is effective specifically against the myeloid tissue. It has been the preferred drug for the treatment of chronic myeloid leukemia (CML).

The adverse effects include myelosuppression, pulmonary fibrosis, hyperuricemia, sterility, and veno-occlusive disease of the liver.

Triazene

Dacarbazine

It gets activated in the liver to an active metabolite. It kills cells in all cell cycle phases. It is used IV in the combination therapy for Hodgkin's disease. It is also used in malignant melanoma and adult sarcomas.

The adverse effects include nausea, vomiting, myelosuppression, flu-like syndrome, hepatotoxicity and alopecia.

Temozolomide

Temozolomide gets converted to an active metabolite. It kills cells in all phases of the cell cycle. It can be used orally or intravenously.

It is used in combination with radiotherapy for the treatment of malignant glioma and astrocytoma. It is also used in melanoma.

The adverse effects are similar to dacarbazine and include myelosuppression and hepatotoxicity.

Other Alkylating Drugs

Procarbazine

It is used mainly in the treatment of Hodgkin's lymphoma as a part of the combination chemotherapy.

It is gets converted to an active metabolite. The adverse effects include leucopenia, thrombocytopenia, vomiting, CNS depression, dermatitis and disulfiram like reactions.

ANTIMETABOLITES

The antimetabolites are structurally related to the normal components existing within the cell (e.g. DNA or enzymes involved in nucleic acid synthesis).

They competitively inhibit normal substrate utilization, or they are themselves incorporated forming dysfunctional molecules.

The 3 classes of antimetabolites are folate antagonists, purine antagonists and pyrimidine antagonists.

Folate Antagonist

Folic acid plays a key role in a variety of reactions that involve transfer of one-carbon units (methyl units) and is vital for cell replication. Methotrexate and pemetrexed are antifolate drugs.

Methotrexate is one of the commonly used and highly efficacious antineoplastic drug. It has antineoplastic, anti-inflammatory and immunosuppressant properties.

It acts during the 'S phase' of the cell cycle; therefore, it is most effective when the cells are dividing rapidly. Methotrexate mainly inhibits DNA synthesis, but it also has an effect on RNA and protein synthesis.

Mechanism of Action

Methotrexate is a folic acid analogue and competitively inhibits the enzyme, dihydrofolate reductase (DHFRase). This leads to inhibition of conversion from dihydrofolate (DHFA) to tetrahydrofolate (THFA). THFA is required for one-carbon transfer reactions involved in the *de novo* synthesis of thymidylate, purine nucleotides, and amino acids (serine and methionine). These, in turn, are required for the synthesis of DNA, RNA and important cellular proteins (Figure 6).

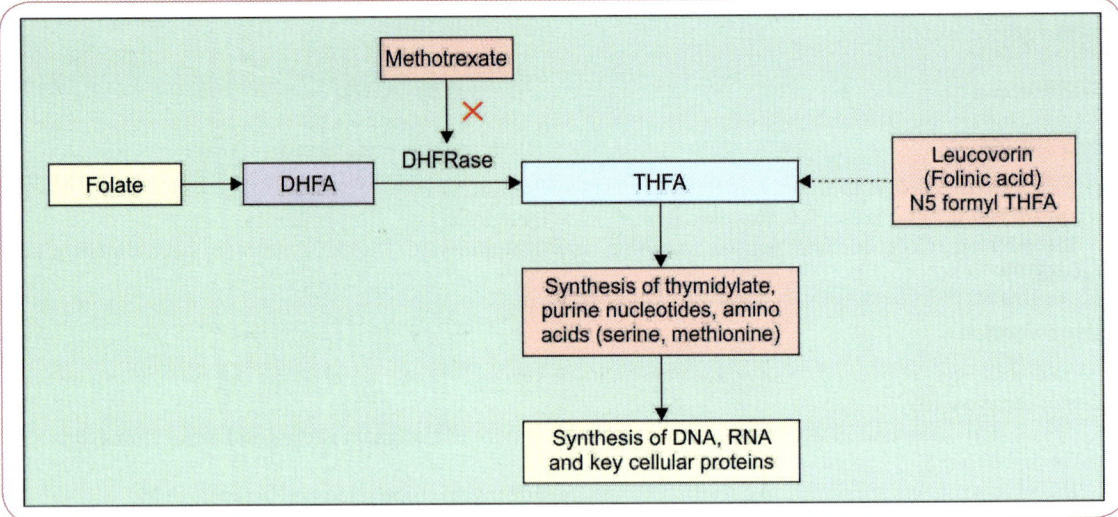

Figure 6: Methotrexate—Mechanism of action

Pharmacokinetics

Methotrexate is well-absorbed orally. It is also administered by parenteral routes (IV, IM).

Around 50% is bound to plasma proteins, and it is displaced from plasma albumin by several drugs such as salicylates, sulfonamides, phenytoin, tetracyclines, etc. This leads to increased methotrexate levels and toxicity.

The metabolism of methotrexate is minimal and it is largely excreted unchanged in the urine.

Folinic acid/Leucovorin/Citrovorum Factor Rescue

The toxicity of methotrexate on the normal cells can be reduced by administration of folinic acid (leucovorin). Folinic acid, which is an active coenzyme form (i.e. it does not need to be reduced by DHFRase) bypasses the methotrexate induced block and is able to quickly reverse the toxicity of methotrexate.

The use of folinic acid as a rescue medication has allowed the use of much higher doses of methotrexate for attaining better anticancer effect.

In contrast, folic acid is not effective as a rescue medication, because it does not gets converted to the active form THFA.

Adverse Effects

The adverse effects include nausea, diarrhea, stomatitis, myelosuppression, dermatitis, alopecia, megaloblastic anemia, pancytopenia, hepatotoxicity and nephrotoxicity.

Clinical Uses

Methotrexate is used in various malignant and nonmalignant conditions (Table 4).

TABLE 4	Methotrexate—clinical uses
Malignant conditions	• Choriocarcinoma • Acute lymphoblastic leukemia (ALL) in children • Burkitt's lymphoma/non-Hodgkin's lymphoma • Cancer of bladder, breast and head and neck
Nonmalignant conditions	• Rheumatoid arthritis • Severe psoriasis • Inflammatory bowel disease

Pemetrexed is an antifolate drug used in patients of non-small cell lung cancer.

Purine Antagonists

6-mercaptopurine (6-MP) and 6-thioguanine (6-TG) are converted in the body to their ribonucleotides, which inhibit purine biosynthesis and nucleotide interconversions (IMP to adenine and guanine nucleotides). Feedback inhibition of *de novo* purine synthesis also occurs. 6-MP also has immunosuppressant properties.

They act during the 'S phase' of the cell cycle; therefore, are most effective when the cells are dividing rapidly.

The absorption of 6-MP following oral administration is incomplete. The drug undergoes first-pass metabolism in the liver by the enzyme xanthine oxidase. The metabolites are then excreted in the urine.

If a xanthine oxidase inhibitor (allopurinol) is given along with 6-MP, the oral dose of 6-MP should be decreased by 75%. This results in reduced toxicity of 6-MP (Figure 7).

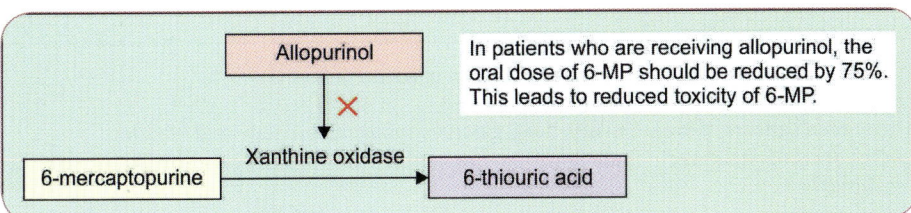

Figure 7: 6-mercaptopurine and allopurinol

The clinical uses of 6-MP include maintenance therapy of ALL. They are also used in choriocarcinoma and some solid tumors.

Bone marrow toxicity is the main adverse effect of 6-MP. The other adverse effects include GI toxicity (e.g. nausea, stomatitis, diarrhea) and hepatotoxicity.

Pyrimidine Antagonists

5-fluorouracil (5-FU) gets converted in the body to the nucleotide 5-fluoro-2-deoxyuridine monophosphate (FdUMP), which inhibits the enzyme thymidylate synthase resulting in an inhibition of DNA synthesis (Figure 8).

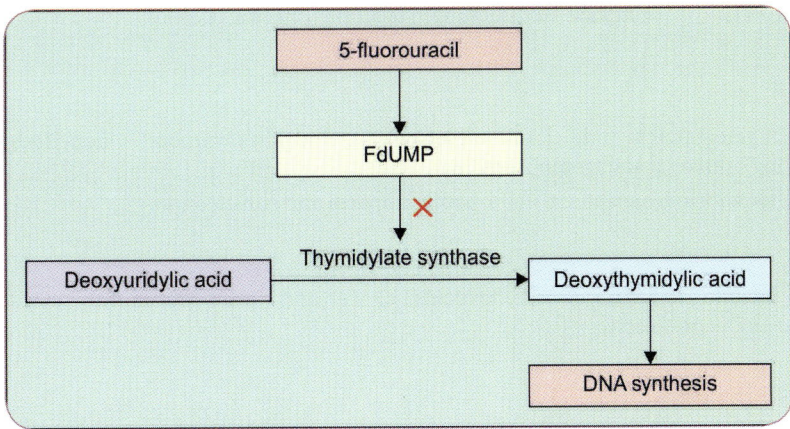

Figure 8: Mechanism of action of 5-fluorouracil

5-FU is used in solid tumors such as colorectal, breast and liver cancers. 5-FU is also used topically in basal cell cancer of the skin.

TAXANES

Paclitaxel is a taxane that was isolated from the bark of Western yew tree. Docetaxel is a recent more potent congener of paclitaxel.

Paclitaxel has a unique mechanism of action (which is opposite to that of vinca alkaloids and colchicine) in that it binds to β-tubulin and enhances its polymerization. The microtubules are stabilized and their depolymerization does not occur. This leads to inhibition of mitosis (Figure 9).

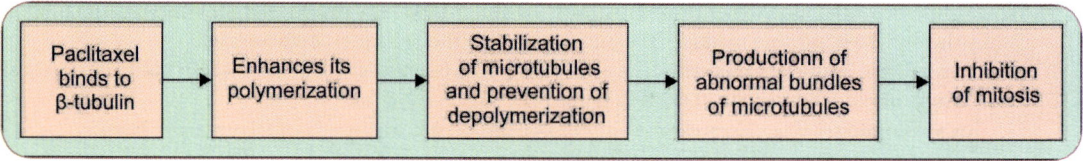

Figure 9: Mechanism of action of taxanes

It is used in advanced cancers of breast, ovary, lung, gastroesophageal, prostate and bladder.

The adverse effects of paclitaxel include bone marrow suppression, peripheral neuropathy, arthralgia, myalgia and hypersensitivity.

VINCA ALKALOIDS

Vinca alkaloids are mitotic inhibitors. Their mechanism of action is shown in Figure 10.

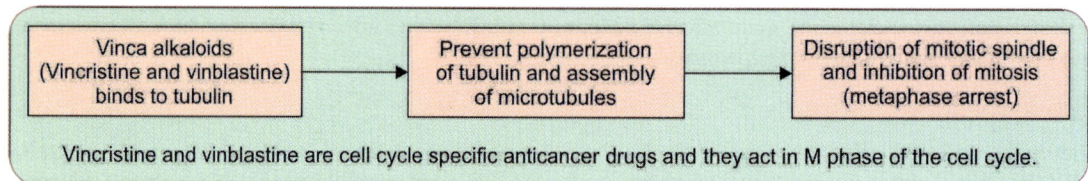

Figure 10: Mechanism of action—vinca alkaloids

Vincristine (Oncovin)

The clinical uses of vincristine include childhood leukemias, Hodgkin's lymphoma, non-Hodgkin's lymphoma, Wilms' tumor, Ewing's sarcoma and lymphosarcoma.

The adverse effects include peripheral neuropathy, alopecia and constipation.

Vinblastine

The clinical uses include Hodgkin's disease, testicular cancer and breast cancer. The adverse effects include myelosuppression and neurotoxicity.

CAMPTOTHECIN ANALOGUES

Both topotecan and irinotecan cause inhibition of DNA topoisomerase-I. This results in damage to the DNA leading to cell death.

Topotecan

The clinical uses of topotecan include advanced ovarian cancer and small cell lung cancer.
The adverse effects include myelosuppression and GIT toxicity (vomiting, diarrhea).

Irinotecan

Irinotecan is a prodrug and clinical uses include metastatic colorectal cancer, lung cancer and ovarian cancer. The adverse effects include myelosuppression, GIT toxicity (vomiting, diarrhea).

Irinotecan inhibits acetylcholinesterase activity and can lead to cholinergic effects (e.g. diarrhea, lacrimation, diaphoresis, hypersalivation, etc.).

EPIPODOPHYLLOTOXIN

Etoposide is a semisynthetic derivative of podophyllotoxin. Etoposide inhibits the DNA topoisomerase II enzyme leading to cell death.

Etoposide inhibits the cell cycle in S and G_2 phase.

The clinical uses of etoposide include lung cancer, testicular tumors, bladder cancer and Hodgkin's lymphoma. The adverse effects include myelosuppression, alopecia and GIT toxicity (such as nausea, vomiting).

ANTIBIOTICS USED FOR MALIGNANCIES

Many of these antibiotics interfere with template function of the DNA. They intercalate between specific bases of the DNA, block DNA synthesis and interfere with replication of the cell. Some of the key features of the anticancer antibiotics are mentioned in Table 5.

TABLE 5	Anticancer antibiotics
Actinomycin D (Dactinomycin)	• Used in Wilms' tumor, rhabdomyosarcoma • Adverse effects include GIT toxicities (nausea, vomiting, diarrhea, stomatitis), myelosuppression, alopecia
Doxorubicin	• Mechanism includes inhibition of topoisomerase II and generation of free radicals that bind to DNA and cause DNA damage, intercalation into DNA • Used in breast cancer, Hodgkin's and non-Hodgkin's lymphoma, ovarian cancer, Wilms' tumor • Is potentially mutagenic and carcinogenic • Adverse effects include cardiotoxicity (ECG changes, arrhythmias, cardiomyopathy, CHF), myelosuppression, GIT toxicities (nausea, vomiting, diarrhea), alopecia
Daunorubicin	• Mechanism includes inhibition of topoisomerase II and generation of free radicals that bind to DNA and cause DNA damage, intercalation into DNA • Used in acute myelogenous leukemia (AML) and acute lymphoblastic leukemia (ALL) • Is potentially mutagenic and carcinogenic • Adverse effects include cardiotoxicity (ECG changes, arrhythmias, cardiomyopathy, CHF), myelosuppression, GIT toxicities (nausea, vomiting, diarrhea), alopecia
Mitoxantrone	• Analogue of doxorubicin • Used in metastatic breast cancer, non-Hodgkin's lymphoma, advanced prostate cancer • Reported to have a lower incidence of cardiotoxicity • Adverse effects include nausea and vomiting, myelosuppression, cardiotoxicity
Bleomycin	• Mechanism includes generation of free radicals that lead to DNA breaks • Used in testicular tumors, Hodgkin's lymphoma, squamous cell malignancies of head and neck, skin, oral cavity • Adverse effects include pulmonary toxicity (pulmonary fibrosis) and skin hyperpigmentation. It causes little myelosuppression.

TYROSINE KINASE INHIBITORS

Tyrosine kinases are a group of enzymes that are involved in multiple important cellular processes such as cell division and signal transduction.

Imatinib

It is a tyrosine kinase inhibitor and is clinically used in patients of chronic myeloid leukemia (CML).

Adverse effects include GI toxicity (nausea, vomiting), myelosuppression, hepatotoxicity, fluid retention and congestive cardiac failure.

Erlotinib

It is an inhibitor of epidermal growth factor receptor tyrosine kinase. Clinical uses include non-small cell lung cancer and pancreatic cancer. The adverse effects include diarrhea, skin rashes and interstitial lung disease (may be fatal).

Sorafenib

It is a tyrosine kinase inhibitor and clinical uses include renal cell carcinoma and hepatocellular carcinoma. Adverse effects include nausea, hypertension, rashes and bleeding.

HORMONES AND DRUGS AFFECTING THE HORMONAL BALANCE

Glucocorticoids

Glucocorticoids can have various applications in oncology. Some of these are mentioned in Table 6.

TABLE 6	Glucocorticoids in oncology
<ul><li>Glucocorticoids have lympholytic effects and are used in the treatment of acute leukemias in children and malignant lymphomas in adult and children.</li><li>They are also used as a part of combination therapy in Hodgkin's and non-Hodgkin's lymphoma, multiple myeloma and chronic lymphocytic leukemia (CLL).</li></ul>	
<ul><li>They can be used along with radiotherapy to decrease edema associated with tumors of brain, spinal cord and superior mediastinum.</li><li>They can be used for complications such as hypercalcemia, bleeding (due to thrombocytopenia) and hemolysis.</li></ul>	
<ul><li>They can be used as antiemetic prophylaxis and as antipyretic agents.</li><li>They can produce mood elevation or feeling of wellbeing.</li></ul>	

Some of other drugs affecting the hormonal balance with applications in oncology are mentioned in Table 7.

TABLE 7	Drugs affecting hormonal balance
1.	**Estrogens** <ul><li>Provide symptomatic relief in prostate cancer as it is an androgen dependent malignancy; estrogens are physiological antagonists of androgens.</li><li>Fosfestrol has been used in prostate cancer.</li></ul>
2.	**Selective estrogen receptor modulators (SERMs)** <ul><li>E.g. tamoxifen has antiestrogen activity and is used in carcinoma breast.</li></ul>
3.	**Selective estrogen receptor downregulators (SERDs)** <ul><li>These are also known as 'pure antiestrogens'.</li><li>E.g. fulvestrant is a competitive estrogen receptor antagonist and is used in postmenopausal women with carcinoma breast.</li></ul>

Contd...

4.	**Aromatase inhibitors**
	• E.g. anastrozole, letrozole → used in postmenopausal women with carcinoma breast.
5.	**Antiandrogens**
	• E.g. flutamide, bicalutamide → used in patients with prostate cancer.
6.	**GnRH agonists (Buserelin, goserelin, nafarelin)**
	• Inhibit the secretion of estrogen/androgens by suppressing the release of FSH and LH from pituitary gland. They cause suppression of gonadal function.
	• Used in prostate and breast cancer.

PLATINUM-CONTAINING COMPOUNDS

These drugs have broad spectrum antineoplastic activity and are used in ovarian, bladder, esophageal, colon, lung and head and neck cancers. These drugs are mutagenic, teratogenic and carcinogenic.

Cisplatin

It is non-cell cycle specific drug, and acts both on resting and dividing cells. It enters the cells where it forms highly reactive platinum complexes. These react with the nucleophilic sites of the DNA leading to DNA damage (Figure 11).

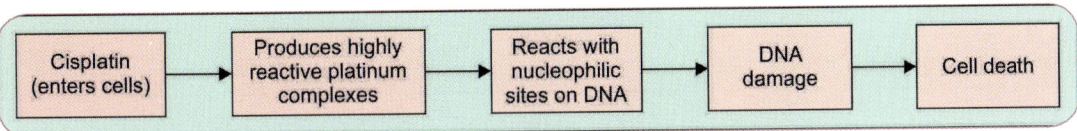

Figure 11: Mechanism of action of cisplatin

It is highly bound to plasma proteins and is slowly excreted by the kidneys. It gets concentrated in liver, kidney, intestine and testes. It has poor penetration into the central nervous system.

Adverse Effects

Cisplatin is a highly emetogenic drug and can produce nausea and vomiting. Antiemetic drugs (e.g. ondansetron) are commonly used to control nausea and vomiting.

Some of the other important toxicities include:
- Nephrotoxicity—can be reduced by adequate hydration and chloride diuresis
- Ototoxicity—manifests as tinnitus and high-frequency hearing loss. It is more frequent with repeated doses and in children. It is unaffected by diuresis.
- Neurotoxicity—can lead to progressive peripheral motor or sensory neuropathy
- Electrolyte disturbances—hypokalemia, hypocalcemia, hypomagnesemia and hypophosphatemia
- Others—bone marrow suppression

Clinical Uses

Cisplatin is highly effective in testicular and ovarian cancer. It is also used in bladder, lung, head and neck and gastroesophageal cancers.

Carboplatin/Oxaliplatin

The mechanism of action of carboplatin and oxaliplatin is similar to cisplatin. Some of the key points regarding these drugs are mentioned below.

Carboplatin

- Differs from cisplatin in chemical, pharmacokinetic and toxicological properties.
- It is relatively better tolerated and causes lesser nausea/vomiting, nephrotoxicity, ototoxicity and neurotoxicity than cisplatin. However, the dose limiting toxicity is bone marrow suppression, mainly thrombocytopenia.

- It is rapidly excreted by the kidneys due to lesser plasma protein binding.
- It is mainly used in ovarian cancer and lung cancer. In other cancers (e.g. esophageal, head and neck), it may be less effective than cisplatin.
- It is an effective alternative in patients (with responsive tumors) who are unable to tolerate cisplatin due to toxicities.

Oxaliplatin

- It is mainly used in gastric and colorectal cancers.
- Peripheral neuropathy is the main dose limiting toxicity. Acute allergic reactions may occur.

ENZYME-L-ASPARAGINASE

L-asparaginase is an enzyme that is sometimes used in the treatment of childhood acute lymphoblastic leukemia (ALL).

Normal cells are able to synthesize asparagine. However, cancer cells in ALL are unable to synthesize asparagine because they lack asparagine synthetase and need to obtain asparagine from plasma.

L-asparaginase breaks down asparagine to aspartic acid and ammonia. Therefore, the cancer cells are deprived of asparagine leading to cell death.

The adverse effects of L-asparaginase include hypersensitivity reactions including anaphylaxis that can be fatal, hemorrhage, hyperglycemia (due to insulin deficiency), hypertriglyceridemia and pancreatitis.

HYDROXYUREA

Hydroxyurea interferes with the synthesis of DNA by inhibiting the enzyme ribonucleoside diphosphate reductase. This blocks the conversion of ribonucleotides to deoxyribonucleotides.

The clinical uses of hydroxyurea include chronic myeloid leukemia, polycythemia vera and some solid tumors.

The main toxicity of hydroxyurea is myelosuppression (leukopenia, thrombocytopenia, anemia). Other toxicities include GI disturbances, stomatitis and neurological manifestations.

CHEMOTHERAPY REGIMENS

The management of malignancy requires considerable skill in utilizing chemotherapy and considering other treatment measures such as surgery and radiotherapy.

The benefits and risks along with the applicability of different treatment measures for a particular malignancy along with the patient's characteristics should be taken into consideration.

Some of the factors that are considered in utilizing drugs for combination chemotherapy are as follows:

- Utilization of drugs that are known to be effective when used alone for a specific cancer.
- Drugs having different mechanisms of action and different mechanisms for the development of drug resistance.
- The toxicity of the drug is not similar to toxicities with other drugs in the combination.
- Understanding mechanisms of drug interactions (e.g. biochemical, molecular, pharmacokinetic) of the medications used in the combination.
- Activity of a drug in specific phase(s) of cell cycle.
- Utilization of optimum dosage of the drugs.

Some of the combination chemotherapy regimens are mentioned in Table 8.

TABLE 8	Combination chemotherapy	
1.	**CHOP regimen** used in non-Hodgkin's lymphoma	• Cyclophosphamide, doxorubicin, vincristine, prednisolone
2.	**MOPP regimen** used in Hodgkin's disease	• Mechlorethamine, vincristine, procarbazine, prednisolone
3.	**ABVD regimen** used in Hodgkin's disease	• Doxorubicin, bleomycin, vinblastine, dacarbazine

ASSESS YOURSELF (Examination Questions of Various Universities)

1. Classify alkylating anticancer drugs with examples. Explain the mechanism of action. Enumerate therapeutic uses of any one. Enlist commonly encountered adverse effects with anticancer drugs.
2. Classification of anti-cancer drugs
3. Aromatase inhibitors
4. Cisplatin
5. Citrovorum factor rescue
6. Paclitaxel
7. Role of Vinca alkaloids and taxanes in cancer

MULTIPLE CHOICE QUESTIONS

1. Hemorrhagic cystitis is caused by:
   (AIIMS Nov 2010, Recent Question 2016)
   a. Cyclophosphamide
   b. 6 mercaptopurine
   c. 5 fluorouracil
   d. Busulfan

2. Most emetogenic anticancer drug is:
   (AIIMS May 2009)
   a. Cisplatin
   b. Carboplatin
   c. High dose cyclophosphamide
   d. High dose methotrexate

3. Ifosfamide belongs to which group of anticancer drugs?
   (AIIMS Nov 2008; AI 2009; 2008)
   a. Alkylating agents
   b. Antimetabolites
   c. Mitotic inhibitors
   d. Topoisomerase inhibitors

4. Which of the following drugs is associated with untoward side effect of renal tubular damage?
   (AIIMS May 2006)
   a. Cisplatin
   b. Streptozocin
   c. Methysergide
   d. Cyclophosphamide

5. A 35-year-old patient is having carcinoma lung with a past history of lung disease. Which of the following drugs should not be given?
   (Recent Question 2016)
   a. Vinblastine   b. Bleomycin
   c. Mithramycin   d. Adriamycin

6. Alkylating agents are all except:
   (Recent Question 2016)
   a. Buslfan   b. Carmustine
   c. Dacarbazine   d. Etoposide

7. Nitrosoureas used in the treatment of cancer are: *(Recent Question 2016)*
   a. Carmustine   b. 5 FU
   c. Methotrexate   d. Cisplatin

8. Which antineoplastic drug has a very high cardiac toxicity?   *(Recent Question 2016)*
   a. Bleomycin   b. Actinomycin-D
   c. Doxorubicin   d. Mitomycin-C

9. Cyclophosphamide is? *(Recent Question 2016)*
   a. Alkylating agent
   b. Antitumor antibiotic
   c. Monoclonal antibody
   d. Antimet abolites

10. True about cyclophosphamide:
    (Recent Question 2016)
    a. Antimetabolites
    b. Alkylating agent
    c. Platinum compound
    d. Topoisomerase inhibitors

11. Pulmonary fibrosis is a complication of:
    (Recent Question 2016)
    a. Methotrexate   b. Doxorubicin
    c. Cisplatin   d. Busulfan

12. Anticancer drug causing nephrotoxicity:
    (Recent Question 2016)
    a. Imitanib   b. Irinotecan
    c. Fosfestrol   d. Cisplatin

Ans.

1.	(a)	2.	(a)	3.	(a)	4.	(a)	5.	(b)	6.	(d)
7.	(a)	8.	(c)	9.	(a)	10.	(b)	11.	(d)	12.	(d)

13. **All of the following are G2 phase inhibitors except:** *(AIIMS May 2016)*
   a. Paclitaxel
   b. Etoposide
   c. Topotecan
   d. Daunorubicin

14. **Methotrexate is used for the management of all of these conditions except:** *(AIIMS May 2011)*
   a. Rheumatoid arthritis
   b. Psoriasis
   c. Sickle cell anemia
   d. Organ transplantation

15. **Which of the following is an anti-metabolite?** *(AIIMS May, 2007)*
   a. Methotrexate
   b. Cyclosporine
   c. Etoposide
   d. Vinblastine

16. **Which antineoplastic is cell cycle S phase inhibitor:** *(Recent Question Dec 2016)*
   a. Vincristine
   b. 5 FU
   c. Paclitaxel
   d. Cyclophosphamide

17. **Antidote for methotrexate poisoning is:** *(Recent Question Dec 2016)*
   a. Folic acid
   b. Folinic acid
   c. Pyridoxine
   d. Vitamin B-12

18. **Hydroxyurea: mechanism of action in cancer is by inhibiting the enzyme:** *(Recent Question 2016)*
   a. Ribonucleoside diphosphate reductase
   b. Ribonucleotide oxidase
   c. DNA lyase
   d. DNA synthetase

19. **Microtubule formation is inhibited by:** *(Recent Question 2016)*
   a. Paclitaxel
   b. Vincristine
   c. Etoposide
   d. Irinotectan

20. **Mechanism of action of 5-FU is:** *(Recent Question 2016)*
   a. Antimetabolite
   b. Direct DNA chelating agent
   c. Anti-mitotic
   d. Topoisomerase inhibitor

21. **Drug used to counteract methotrexate toxicity:** *(Recent Question 2016)*
   a. Folinic acid
   b. Folic acid
   c. VitBu
   d. Mesna

22. **Methotrexate mechanism of action:** *(Recent Question 2016)*
   a. Inhibit dihydrofolate reductase
   b. Stimulate dihydrofolate reductase
   c. Inhibit tetrahydrofolate reductse
   d. Stimulate tetrahydrofolate reductse

23. **The drug imatinib acts by the inhibition of:** *(AIIMS May 2006)*
   a. Tyrosine kinase
   b. Glutathione reductase
   c. Thymidylate synthetase
   d. Protein kinase

24. **Nephrotoxicity is a side effect of:** *(AP PG 2010)*
   a. Cisplatin
   b. Buslphan
   c. Methotrexate
   d. Adriamycin

25. **Mechanism of action of TAXANES is:** *(WB PG 2009)*
   a. Depolymerization of microtubules
   b. Increase polymerization of microtubules
   c. Inhibitor of topoisomerase I
   d. Inhibitor of topoisomerase II

26. **Leucovorin rescue is related to:** *(WB PG 2006)*
   a. MTX toxicity
   b. Cyclophosphamide toxicity
   c. Oncovin toxicity
   d. Cisplatin toxicity

Ans.

13.	(a)	14.	(c)	15.	(a)	16.	(b)	17.	(b)	18.	(a)
19.	(b)	20.	(a)	21.	(a)	22.	(a)	23.	(a)	24.	(a)
25.	(b)	26.	(a)										

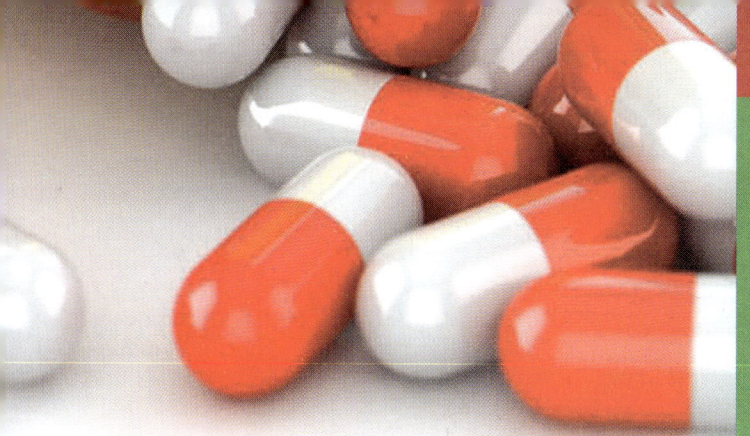

Miscellaneous Drugs

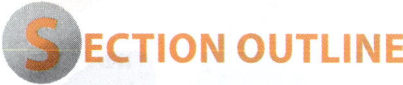

SECTION OUTLINE

- ○ Chelating Agents
- ○ Immunosuppressant Drugs

65

Chelating Agents

Chelating agents form ring like structures after combining with metallic ions. These structures are stable, nontoxic, water soluble and are rapidly excreted from the body. Chelating agents are used in poisoning with heavy metals (Figure 1 and Table 1).

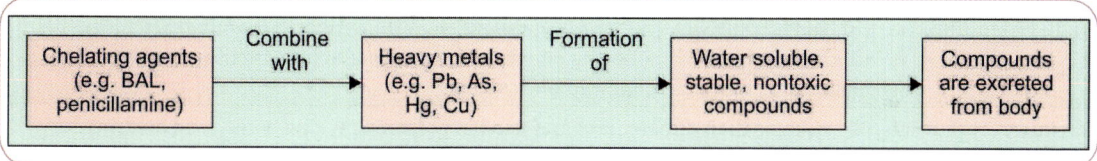

Figure 1: Chelating agents

TABLE 1	Chelating agents—clinical uses
Chelating agent	**Clinical uses**
Dimercaprol (BAL)	• Acute poisoning by heavy metals such as arsenic, mercury, gold, bismuth, antimony, copper • Used (as an adjuvant therapy) with penicillamine in Wilson's disease, copper toxicity • Used (as an adjuvant therapy) with calcium disodium edetate in lead poisoning
Disodium edetate	• Anticoagulant (*in vitro*) • Emergency management of hypercalcemia • Not clinically used for lead toxicity
Calcium disodium edetate	• Poisoning with lead, zinc, copper, iron, manganese
D-penicillamine	• Acute poisoning with copper, zinc, mercury and lead • Wilsons's disease (hepatolenticular degeneration) • Cystinuria and prevention of cystine stones • Severe, active rheumatoid arthritis • Scleroderma

Desferrioxamine	• Acute iron poisoning—It is the drug of choice and is administered parenterally
	• Chronic iron overload
	  ▪ Transfusion hemosiderosis (e.g. thalassemia patients)
	  ▪ Hemochromatosis
	• Aluminum overload—in patients with end stage renal failure on dialysis

Deferiprone	• Transfusion hemosiderosis (e.g. thalassemia patients) • Acute iron poisoning

DIMERCAPROL (BAL)

BAL also stands for British anti-lewisite. It was developed during World War II as an antidote to arsenic containing gases.

Dimercaprol contains two SH (sulfhydryl) groups that combine with heavy metals to form a chelating complex. The clinical uses and adverse effects of dimercaprol are mentioned in Table 2.

TABLE 2	Dimercaprol (BAL)
Clinical uses	• Acute poisoning by heavy metals such as arsenic, mercury, gold, bismuth, antimony, copper. • Used (as an adjuvant therapy) with penicillamine in Wilson's disease and copper toxicity. • Used (as an adjuvant therapy) with calcium sodium edetate in lead poisoning.
Adverse effects	• Headache, tingling of hands, anxiety, hemolysis, hypertension, tachycardia, hepatotoxicity and renal impairment. • It should be used with caution in hypertensives or those with impaired renal function. • It is contraindicated in poisoning due to iron and cadmium because the complexes (iron-dimercaprol, cadmium-dimercaprol) are toxic.

Succimer: It is considered less toxic than dimercaprol and used in poisoning with arsenic, lead and mercury.

DISODIUM EDETATE

It chelates calcium and can cause tetany on IV injection. Therefore, it is not clinically used for lead toxicity.

It is used as an anticoagulant (*in vitro*) and in the emergency management of hypercalcemia.

CALCIUM DISODIUM EDETATE

It does not reduce the calcium levels. It is used in poisoning with lead, zinc, copper, iron and manganese.

The adverse effects include nephrotoxicity (proximal tubular necrosis), febrile reactions including chills, rigor etc.

D-PENICILLAMINE

The D-isomer of penicillamine is clinically used because the L-isomer is more toxic and can cause optic neuritis.

Penicillamine is obtained as a degradation product of penicillin and hence, there is a risk of cross reactivity with penicillins.

Penicillamine chelates copper, zinc, mercury and lead.

Clinical Uses

○ Acute poisoning with copper, zinc, mercury and lead
○ Wilsons's disease (hepatolenticular degeneration)
  ❑ Autosomal recessive disease of copper metabolism wherein there is a deficiency of ceruloplasmin (that binds and removes copper).
  ❑ This results in increased levels of copper in the body and deposition of copper in sites such as liver, basal ganglia etc.
  ❑ Penicillamine is a copper chelating agent that leads to excretion of copper from the body. This results in reduced levels of copper.
  ❑ Usually lifelong therapy with penicillamine may be required.
○ Cystinuria and prevention of cystine stones
  ❑ Penicillamine enhances the excretion of cystine. It also prevents the precipitation of cystine in the urinary tract.
○ Severe, active rheumatoid arthritis
○ Scleroderma

A summary of clinical uses and adverse effects of D-penicillamine is mentioned in Table 3.

TABLE 3	D-penicillamine
Clinical uses	• Acute poisoning with copper, zinc, mercury and lead • Wilsons's disease (hepatolenticular degeneration) • Cystinuria and prevention of cystine stones • Severe, active rheumatoid arthritis • Scleroderma
Adverse effects	• Hematological → Thrombocytopenia and proteinuria • Skin → Rashes, pruritus, Stevens Johnson syndrome, pemphigus • Renal → Proteinuria • Allergic reaction, pyrexia

DESFERRIOXAMINE

It is a chelating agent for iron and aluminum.

It chelates iron from ferritin, hemosiderin as well as loosely bound iron. It does not remove iron from hemoglobin or cytochrome.

Clinical Uses

○ Acute iron poisoning—It is the drug of choice and is administered parenterally
○ Chronic iron overload
  ❑ Transfusion hemosiderosis (e.g. thalassemia patients)
  ❑ Hemochromatosis
○ Aluminum overload—in patients with end stage renal failure on dialysis

Adverse Effects

○ Allergic reactions such as rashes, hypotension, urticaria, anaphylactic reactions
○ Injection site reactions such as pain, swelling
○ Nephrotoxicity, hearing and visual impairment

DEFERIPRONE

It is an iron chelating agent that is orally effective.

The clinical uses include transfusion hemosiderosis (e.g. thalassemia patients) and acute iron poisoning.

The adverse effects include nausea, vomiting, abdominal pain and agranulocytosis.

ASSESS YOURSELF (Examination Questions of Various Universities)

1. List and elaborate briefly on various chelating agents used in clinical practice
2. Iron chelating agents
3. Dimercaprol (BAL)
4. Penicillamine

MULTIPLE CHOICE QUESTIONS

1. Select the correctly matched pair of heavy metal and their chelating agent:
   (Recent Question 2017)
   a. Mercury – Calcium disodium edetate
   b. Copper – d-Penicillamine
   c. Iron – BAL (British antilewisite)
   d. Arsenic - Desferrioxamine

2. Which of the following drug contains disulphide group: *(Recent Question 2017)*
   a. EDTA
   b. BAL
   c. Penicillamine
   d. Penicillin

3. Iron poisoning in a 4-year old child is treated by: *(Recent Question 2017)*
   a. X-ray abdomen
   b. Blood transfusion
   c. Desferrioxamine IV 100 mg
   d. Stomach lavage

4. Which of the following chelating agent is a penicillin-derived compound:
   (Recent Question 2017)
   a. EDTA
   b. Penicillamine
   c. Dimercaprol
   d. Desferrioxamine

Ans.

| 1. | (b) | 2. | (b) | 3. | (c) | 4. | (b) |

66

Immunosuppressant Drugs

Immunosuppressants suppress cellular or humoral immune responses, or both. The clinical indications of immunosuppressants include:

o Organ transplantation (e.g. liver, kidney, cardiac, bone marrow)
o Autoimmune diseases (e.g. rheumatoid arthritis, SLE)

The classification of immunosuppressants is mentioned in Table 1.

TABLE 1	Immunosuppressant drugs
Calcineurin inhibitors	• Cyclosporine • Tacrolimus
Cytotoxic (Antiproliferative) drugs	• Azathioprine, mycophenolate mofetil, methotrexate, cyclophosphamide, chlorambucil
Glucocorticoids	• Prednisolone
Biologics	• Antibodies → Antithymocyte globulin (ATG), Muromonab CD3 • IL-1 inhibitors → Anakinra • TNF-α inhibitors → Infliximab, etanercept, adalimumab
Proliferation signal inhibitors (PSI)	• Sirolimus (rapamycin) • Everolimus

CALCINEURIN INHIBITORS

Cyclosporine

It is a calcineurin inhibitor that is extracted from the soil fungus *Beauveria nivea*.

It preferentially inhibits cell-mediated immunity. It does not have toxic effects on the bone marrow and the reticuloendothelial system. It does not inhibit hemopoiesis (Figure 1).

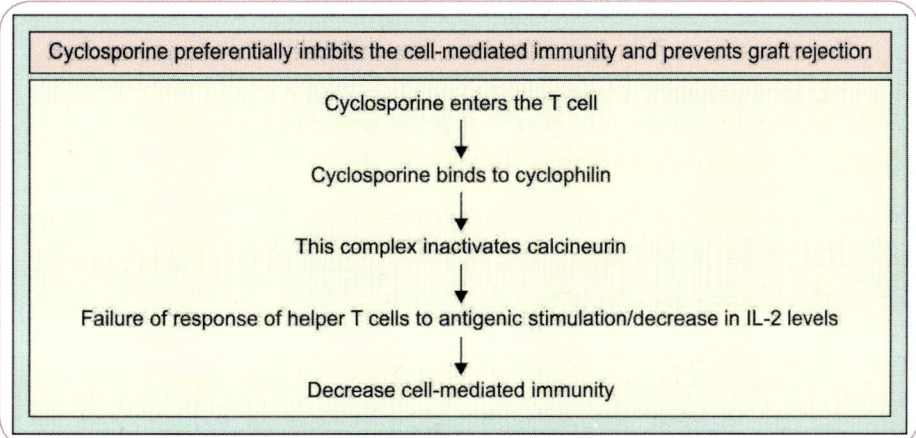

Figure 1: Mechanism of action of cyclosporine

Clinical Uses

○ Organ transplantation
  ❑ Prevention and treatment of graft rejection in organ transplantation (e.g. liver, kidneys, heart, bone marrow)
○ Nontransplant indications
  ❑ Rheumatoid arthritis
  ❑ Psoriasis
  ❑ Atopic dermatitis
  ❑ Dermatomyositis

Adverse Effects

○ Nephrotoxicity (the major toxicity)
○ Hepatotoxicity
○ Hypertension, hyperlipidemia, hyperglycemia
○ Hirsutism
○ Increased risk of infections
○ Increased risk of lymphomas and other malignancies

Drug Interactions

○ Avoid nephrotoxic drugs (e.g. aminoglycosides, amphotericin B, vancomycin, NSAIDs).
○ Drugs that induce CYP3A4 and/or P-glycoprotein can decrease cyclosporine levels. Such drugs include phenytoin, barbiturates, carbamazepine and rifampicin. A reduced level of cyclosporine can lead to rejection of the transplant.
○ Drugs that inhibit CYP3A4 and/or P-glycoprotein can increase cyclosporine levels and cause toxicity. Such drugs include erythromycin, ketoconazole and metoclopramide.
○ Use of potassium sparing diuretics can result in hyperkalemia.

A summary of key features of cyclosporine is mentioned in Table 2.

TABLE 2	Cyclosporine
Mechanism of action	• Inactivation of calcineurin leads to failure of response of helper T cells to antigenic stimulation/decrease in IL-2 levels • Preferentially inhibits the cell-mediated immunity and prevents graft rejection
Clinical uses	• Prevention and treatment of graft rejection in organ transplantation (e.g. liver, kidneys, heart, bone marrow) • Rheumatoid arthritis, psoriasis, atopic dermatitis, dermatomyositis
Adverse effects	• Nephrotoxicity, hepatotoxicity • Hypertension, hyperlipidemia, hyperglycemia, hirsutism • Increased risk of infections • Increased risk of lymphomas and other malignancies

Tacrolimus (FK-506)

Tacrolimus is a macrolide antibiotic. It is more potent than cyclosporine.
The mechanism of action, clinical uses and adverse effect profile are similar to cyclosporine.

CYTOTOXIC (ANTIPROLIFERATIVE) DRUGS

These drugs predominantly inhibit the clonal expansion of B and T lymphocytes and exert significant immunosuppressant effects. Some cytotoxic drugs are mentioned in Table 3.

TABLE 3	Cytotoxic (Antiproliferative) drugs
Azathioprine	• Purine antagonist • Used to prevent graft rejection in organ transplant patients • Also used in patients of severe rheumatoid arthritis, systemic lupus erythematosus • Adverse effects include infections, neoplasms (benign and malignant), bone marrow depression, hepatotoxicity

Contd...

Methotrexate	• Folate antagonist
	• It has antineoplastic, anti-inflammatory and immunosuppressant activities
	• It is used in conditions such as rheumatoid arthritis, severe psoriasis, Crohn's disease
	• Adverse effects include stomatitis, myelosuppression, rash, alopecia, megaloblastic anemia, pancytopenia and hepatotoxicity
Mycophenolate mofetil	• It is a prodrug
	• It inhibits inosine monophosphate dehydrogenase → inhibition of lymphocyte proliferation, decreased production of antibodies, reduction of humoral and cell mediated immunity
	• It is used along with cyclosporine and corticosteroids for the prophylaxis of acute transplant rejection in organ transplant patients (renal, hepatic, cardiac)
	• The adverse effects include: ▪ Increased risk of developing lymphomas and other malignancies ▪ Increased risk of opportunistic infections ▪ GIT ulceration, hemorrhage ▪ Teratogenicity ▪ Bone marrow suppression

BIOLOGICS

Some of the key biologics are mentioned in Table 4.

TABLE 4	Biologics
Antibodies	
Antithymocyte globulin (ATG)	• ATG are polyclonal antibodies
	• They bind to the surface of T lymphocytes. Destruction of T lymphocytes occurs resulting in immunosuppression.
	• Used in the management of renal transplant rejection episodes
	• Adverse effects include infections, allergic reactions, anaphylaxis, pyrexia and serum sickness
Muromonab CD3 (OKT3)	• Murine monoclonal antibody
	• It acts against the CD3 antigen of the T cells
IL-1 inhibitors	
Anakinra	• Used in rheumatoid arthritis
	• Adverse effects include injection site reactions, serious infections
TNF-α inhibitors	
Infliximab, etanercept, adalimumab	• Used in patients of rheumatoid arthritis, psoriasis
	• Adverse effects include risk of infections, risk of malignancies and anaphylactic reactions

PROLIFERATION SIGNAL INHIBITORS (PSI)

Sirolimus (Rapamycin)

It is a macrolide immunosuppressant.

Sirolimus inhibits the activation of mTOR (mammalian target of rapamycin). This inhibits multiple signal transduction pathways leading to suppression of lymphocyte activation. The end result is immunosuppression.

Sirolimus is used for the prophylaxis of organ rejection in adult renal transplant patients.

The adverse effects include hypersensitivity reactions, hyperlipidemia, hypertension, thrombocytopenia, anemia, malignancies and infections.

ASSESS YOURSELF (Examination Questions of Various Universities)

1. Name immunosuppressants, their therapeutic indications along with adverse effects
2. Azathioprine
3. Mycophenolate mofetil
4. Sirolimus

MULTIPLE CHOICE QUESTIONS

1. Which of the following is a calcineurin inhibitor? *(AIIMS Nov 2015)*
   a. Cyclosporine
   b. Basiliximab
   c. Azathioprine
   d. Sirolimus

2. All of the following drugs are used as immunosuppressants except: *(AIIMS Nov 2008)*
   a. Glucocorticoids
   b. Cyclosporine
   c. Cephalosporin
   d. Azathioprine

3. Mechanism of action of tacrolimus is: *(Recent Question 2016)*
   a. Inhibition of calcineurin
   b. Antimetabolite
   c. mTOR inhibitor
   d. Inhibition of DNA synthesis

4. TNF-α inhibitors are: *(PGI June 2014, Nov 2012)*
   a. Bevacizumab
   b. Ranibizumab
   c. Adalimumab
   d. Infliximab
   e. Etanercept

Ans.

| 1. | (a) | 2. | (c) | 3. | (a) | 4. | (c, d, e) |

The "wow" factor of the book is the brief explanation of each section and innumerable diagrams for quick revision. Overall the book is very good, the content is precise. Recent questions given chapterwise are enough for practice. Book covers all the important point according to latest exam pattern. Overall layout and presentation is outstanding.

Vidhya Bhat
Gulbarga Inst. of Medical Sciences, Kalaburgi

The pictorial and lucid presentation is the WOW Factor here.
Anatomy isn't brought or confusing anymore,
with such extra ordinary color and pictures the book is gripping,
the charts are so Good!!
Rajkumar Patel, AMCMET Medical College, Ahmedabad

Synopsis is amongst the best. Putting the entire anatomy, Embryology and histology so concisely shows the knowledge, endeavour and talent of the authors
Shivam Sabharval Dr SN Medical College, Jodhpur

Extensive coverage of contents, colored images, to the point text, high yield facts makes the book interesting. The clinical aspects helps us to correlate and reading is much Easy. Anatomy reading is very hard but the hard work of the authors have made our job much easier.
Mainak Mandal, KIMS, Bhubaneshwar

A must buy to ease your anatomy preparation. I have always found reading anatomy difficult, in 1st mbbs and even for preparing for pg exams but when I studies this book it made my FRICTION of DIFFICULTY into CLEAR AND SMOOTH knowledge of easiness. It is so easy to read and understand that you will LOVE anatomy as a subject after giving it a look. Nicely and crisply penned down by one of the best subject experts.
I will love to consult it to my juniors for preparing for pg entrance exams and even for 1st mbbs students to get their thoughts clear.
Syed A.

Needed information for PGMEE are given in well arranged. Easy to read format. If anyone want to read and revise the only book I will advise to buy this CBS Anatomy book. All the regional Anatomy is given superb with Images,clinical boxes and remember boxes
Sandeep P S, Tagore Medical College, Chennai

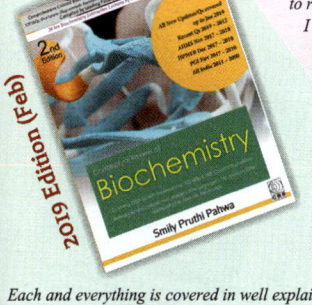

The book focuses on "to know everything about something & something about everything" by giving a comprehensive approach to Anatomy which is a strategy to clear exams like NEET, AIIMS, PGI, JIPMER. The book contains simplified, fully colored diagrams with meticulous labeling along with authentic content
Alish R Mehta
SBH Govt. Medical College, Dhule

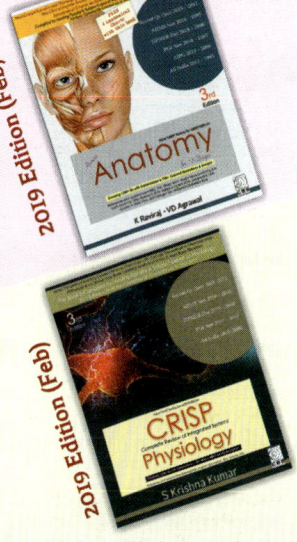

Each and everything is covered in well explained manner, colorful book, Interesting to read, hard topics covered in very easy manner, Recent questions updated, overall the best book of biochemistry so far.
Prabal Singh, SGRD Medical College, Amritsar

The colourful pages of the book doesn't make a reader sleep with a subject like biochemistry. I feel someone cannot get a simpler version of biochemistry than this book. The author has excellently simplified every topic.
P Harish
Kaminei Inst. Of Medical Sciences, Hyderabad

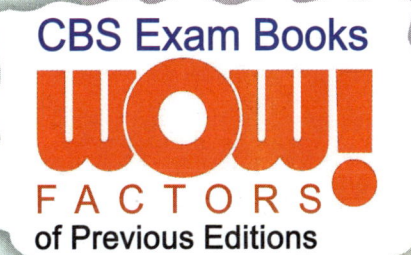
CBS Exam Books
WOW!
FACTORS
of Previous Editions

Its concept making skills can be illustrated from 1st chapter itself. She doesn't just state a fact but gives a reason behind it as well. Each line and sentence is through provoking and also contains one liner, and post each concept a small diagram for easy review is present. Reading text is sufficient to answer any question. Synopsis as a whole is sufficient for attempting all the questions and the question and answers are good for concept building and should be attempted after synopsis.
Saranya Mohan, Lady Hardinge Medical College, Delhi

Book contains the entire Biochemistry in the most concise and conceptual ways. The division of the syllabus in the various understandable units and chapter is quite adorable. The various high yielding boxes like additional edge, fundamental box, etc. is a major boost. In synopsis, the division of syllabus into the various different heading is done exceptionally well. It appears to be the most applauding feature. The number of questions and their explanation appears suitable and exact
Shivam Sabharwal, SN Medical College, Jodhpur

It's a good book as it is concise, biochemistry is a nightmare for everyone the point based manner of the book makes it easy to study and remember the overall layout is good and everything is covered. Practice questions are up to date and many are there so its very useful.
Apeksha, ESI Medical College, Bengaluru

Difficult topics are supplemented by Diagrams. Easy to understand. Awesome creation of High Return box, fundamental Box & MCQ are clearly explained. This book is enough for PGMEE
Theeran R, GMC, Villupuram

The best thing is INTEGRATED APROACH to all systems. Like how well he has covered Endocrinology, just wow. If you read a system from his book before reading the same system in medicine it saves you a hell lot of time. He is covered all physiology plus associated pathology and pharmacology wherever needed plus many syndromes.
Aditya Gudheniya, Lokmanya Tilak Municipal Medical College, Mumbai

Really the wow factor is its appearance, colourful, high quality smooth colour papers, clinical importance tables are high yielding as well as conceptual. Nice layouts and presentations for diagrams. Two column concept is excellent. Concise Content and concept oriented. Lots of new question patterns added
Prithvi Raj, Govt Thiruvarur Medical College, Thiruvarur

Well presented in student friendly manner, CRISP content with integration from all subjects with detailed explanations with proper references, good page quality. IBQ'S and well-illustrated graphs are the strong features of the book
Rachit Singhania, North Bengal Medical College, Darjeeling

Well this no doubt the best book in the market in physiology. Integration of different systems as the name suggests is the key part of the book. And what's more interesting is the integrated view sir possess which includes mentioning about the subjects like medicine, pathology, pharmacology.
Vatsal Sampat, PDU, Rajkot

Remember & high yield points in between the chapters thus helping students understand what is focus on. Clubbing of pharmacology with physiology that's the best thing done. I don't think author has left any topic untouched with make it unique and apt to clear any exams physiology questions.
Alish R Mehta, SBH Govt Medical College, Dhule

The clinical correlation of every subject in this book is the best thing that makes every student to read this book. I never read such a book in my past, the final hard work of author is truly visible. Everything- the explanation, clinical correlation, IBQs synopsis all are better. No book will beat this book in the future.
Sandeep PS, Tagore Medical College, Chennai

Scan the QR Code to View Sample Pages of the Books

It is very presentable than any other review books on this subject, Conceptual box makes learning of pharmacology a pleasant experience, The brilliant use of colors and explanation of concept makes this book a Go-to-reference for all the doubts that went unasked.

Balasaranya S
Coimbatore Medical College, Coimbatore

Excellent book, concept oriented, presentation is good with lot of flow charts that add to the beauty. Only review of pharma with maximum image based questions and numerical in general pharma. BIGGEST ADVANTAGE "ALL LATEST DRUGS COVERED". Practice questions in this book are much much better. I really appreciate the quality of MCQs (as well as IBQs)

Ch Idrees Rashid, GMC, Srinagar

The book is concise version of so vast PATHOLOGY which makes it best book for PG preparation. Since I am a final year student this book really needed to revise through pathology with recent updates which form base of medicine. The best feature of book is to the point info in tables. This really aids the learning. The concept maps to images are really good which are easy to understand. Everything is good but the synopsis is really best. The theory is aided with question answer and every MCQ is explained which has enhanced the learning level.

Shubha Singh
Malda Medical College, Malda

Wow factor is concept explanation, Orientation; I think quality of MCQs and image based questions is best. Also the best thing of book is all latest drugs are covered. Mechanism of action is explained in easy way with this book, we can also write theory exams also well. Pharmacology is very difficult to remember, but this book has made it easy by giving mnemonics. This is the best book for those who are preparing for PG entrance exams.

Bhuvana N
ESIC Medical College, Gulbarga

The overall presentation of the context put the book far ahead of other competitors. Makes the concepts clear and understandable Covers the entire pharmacology. Numerous "Small- small" things that other book lack; make one to love this book and say "WOW". Synopsis covers the entire syllabus in the text. All the major points of the subjects are covered in the form of table; boxes; prose; etc. Practice Questions are at par with AIIMS and NEET level.

Shivam Sabharwal
SN Medical College, Jodhpur

The 'wow' factor of the book is the question coverage. There are so many questions that brushes up every aspect of concept. The book has included all the contents required efficiently. Other best part is the conceptual box and mnemonics box. It is colourful and really interesting presentation. The explanation is really relevant and given in a simple manner which makes it easy to grasp. The questions are really very good – from simple ones to hard ones.

Shivani Singh
Kathmandu School of Medical Sciences, Nepal

A carol of Pathology books, a concise review of the entire pathology, A great collection of MCQs and image based questions, Apt diagram, illustrations and flow chart, Annexures in the initial pages are the major boost; provide a through, quick and concise review. Synopsis in the book is concise, conceptual and an excellent guide to Pathology, the number of MCQ's covering the previous year's questions, practice questions, etc. are apt. their explanation doubtfully correct.

Shivam Sabharwal
SN Medical College, Jodhpur

Image based questions are covered just after the end of chapter review which cover a good portion of papers. Only Recent years questions are included as we know the pattern of paper is quite variable so it's useless to practice old paper questions. Though every author provides very good explanation of mcq answers but in this book , the relevant information is also mentioned in box. The pages of book are coloured and of good quality. Overall representation of chapter review content is awesome with tables, graph .

Rashi

Annexures are superb....Key points & Key recent updates & high field facts are nice...Table content of explanations for many major topics...Flow charts that helps to understand easily. The flow charts & Table contents are made difficult topics into easy.

Theeran R
GMC, Villupuram

"Everything is WOW" let it be Annexures, high yield boxes, recent update sections or authentic images in a lucid language. Layout and presentation, makes the reader truly hooked up to the book. Absolute Book for Pathology.

Rajkumar Patel
AMCMET Medical College, Ahmedabad

Covered and included all the recent updates req for the ongoing and upcoming next meet. Better explainations for the difficult portions of Park text. Given all recent MCQs. Minimum no. Of very old questions. Considering present NEET pattern new questions are framed.

Abhijeet Hiremath

PSM is a boring subject in MBBS, but Mukhmohit singh sir explained the subject very interestingly in the book. High Yielding points are reader friendly, boxes are very useful. All recent questions are covered in this book. The pages are of good quality and nice presentation.

Siva Subramanian
Madurai Medical College, Madurai

This is one of the best books of Pathology in the market. The concepts are dilating with proper & logical thinking and are to the point. The tables in the book are high-yielding. The "high –yielding facts" are very much helpful and are an extra- edge to the book. The updates from robins 10th edition are really of great help too. The answers to the questions are well-dealt in most of the questions and are well explained. The IBQs also according to latest NEET exam pattern and are really explained.

Sayan Banerjee
Malda Medical College, Malda

All the latest updates are covered till date. The national programs and policies are given topic wise in each chapter instead of keeping all the programs at one place which is a good thing by the way. Best thing about this book is that all the chapters are given equal justice. The chapter of immunization and vaccine is one to mention here. Well the epidemiology section was literally amazing, all the tables , the diagrams ,charts made everything so easy. One of the nightmares is biostatistics for many students, well guys this book has covered that too in a proper way I must say. Lastly the 'good to remember', 'must remember' and 'high yield points' makes us differentiate the importance of the data in a way what to remember first. Must must buy book. This book is best for the subject instead of memorizing the data from the same old updated edition of the named book which was the only option until now.

Vatsal Sampat, PDU, Rajkot

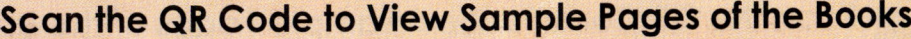

Vast and concise coverage of all important topics for proff exams as well a pg entrance exams. Presentation of topics are so arranged that are easy to remember via help of flowcharts and colourful diagrams. Detailed description of difficult questions helps to understand the concept. Topic wise practice questions helps to establish grip over the chapter topic by topic. IBQs are like cherry over the cake because IBQs are increasing in recent exam trends

Ankit Tiwari
Bundelkhand Medical College, Sagar

SURGERY SIXER very nice book for PG preparation it contains all important points in all standard books like Sabiston ,Bailey ,Schwartz etc. Surgery Sixer book is very easy to prepare during last preparation & during last time revision best book is surgery sixer ,high yield one liners in all chapters was very nice clear image in all chapters with brief explanations ,this book is apt for all exam preparations ,image based questions was nice

Karthick Raja, GMC, Vilupuram

Excellent book written by one of the top faculty of Medicine. Fully – colored layouts and it is reader – friendly. Synopsis is given in the form of bullet points which help in easy revision. MCQs are explained in a way to eliminate the options and opt for the best choice.

Liyakat Ahmed
Navodaya Medical College, Raichur

Surgery Sixer book's One line creation is awesome to revise easily in last time. Recent advances, Bailey's update is correctly mentioned in this book... Image based questions with explanations are excellent. Surgery Sixer book is simplified book of Bailey & Love... The synopsis of this book are easily understood than any other book... It's easy to prepare

Theeran R, GMC, Villupuram

Surgery Sixer for NBE by R Rajamahendran is the most reffered MCQ book for surgery and so I got a copy of it. The book gives us a 15 day plan to complete it plus 5 days for revision just before the exam. The PGI section is sorted separately towards the end and the students not aspiring for that can skip that part. It also has MCQs on Instruments and image based questions which is the recent pattern in the entrance exams. Quick tables for last minute revision are also there making revision even more easy!!

Shivani Desai
(Feedback on CBS Exam Books FB Page)

Absolutely Stunning Book ..!! Surgery Presented in Easiest Way Possible. Colorful Presentations , High Quality Paper, Seperate Boxes for Controversies, Bailey 27e Updates ..! Everything is Top Notch . No Second Thoughts . Go For it !!
Prithivi Raj
(Feedback on CBS Exam Books FB Page)

Concise matter that plays a vital role during revision. Centre of attraction in this book is separate column of bailley updates. Controversy desk as a column is a nice concept. I like it diagrammatic representation is best part of this book, practice questions by author are best selected questions from surgery. Helps in proff exams too. Hence, Undoubtedly best book for surgery in market. separate theory part is better for learning in comparison to other available surgery books in market.GIT in this book is so well presented that it made me fall for it. Correlated images favours it as best book of surgery. Instrument images and controversy desk leaves no stone unturned.
Shubham Jain, NSCB, Jabalpur

Question bank available for practice is good n enough comparing other books. Crisp concepts and brief explanations are given for quick revision to topics while solving questions. The volume of the book is tried to be kept as its minimum without compromising the quality. Language is student friendly even for hindi medium students and proper use of highlighting fonts n colours.
Naman Tiwari, GMC, Kota

WOW factor for me is Dr Deepak Marwah Sir. A must have book for every medical student due to its excellent content which is covered in a beautiful layout and presentation of colourful pages (best quality), soothing to eyes and conceptual boxes. Excellent presentation of theory part, way too many MCQs with logical references, not too much length to make it difficult to revise
Syed Aijaz Ahmad, GMC, Srinagar

Wow factors are point wise description of content, uses of tables and diagrams, all updates included, conceptual diagnostic algorithm.
Rashi Jain
JLN Medical College, Ajmer

Tables, Harrison updates and practice questions are the best part of the book. The number of practice questions are plenty for better preparation
P Harish
Kamineni Inst. Of Medical Sciences, Hyderabad

2019 Edition (Feb)

Medicine
Deepak Marwah

Wow is its concise appearance, colorful, high quality smooth colour papers, Reading monotonous papers are really tiring. Nice layout and presentation. Two column concept is excellent. Concise content. IBQs are given sufficiently. Clear Radiology images. Above All, CRYSTAL CLEAR CONCEPTS.
Prithvi Raj, GMC, Thiruvarur

CBS Exam Books
WOW!
FACTORS
of Previous Editions

Surgery Sixer
R Rajamahendran
2019 Edition (Feb)

2019 Edition (Feb)
Radiology

Excellent Explanation of basic radiology. Almost everything covered in contents. Overall, what I liked most in that book is interactive at many places (in many concept boxes). I liked the images of the book, which I don't think any other review has, and also the way these images has been explained with arrows, that makes concept more clear.
Ishtiyaq Ahmad Ganaie, ACOMS Jammu

The wow factor of the book is the content and the detailed explanation of the physics involved in each including the explanation of electromagnetic spectrum. Image based MCQs are amazing. All that is required for PG NEET is present in the book. Students need not refer to any additional source. The layout is presented well.
Apeksha, ESI Medical College, Bangaluru

I should say whole book itself is a wow factor. The book is one of its kind so well explained, this is concise and adequate for undergraduates to prepare for entrance as well as for practical knowledge. I liked every bit of it the X Ray, CT Scan, USG all are so well explained in starting and here by disease wise. I think this is the best book for Radiology I have ever seen.
Shubhda Singh, Malda Medical College, Malda

The book by Dr MAK is the best book in the subject for PG Aspirants. It covers many radiological images which have made understanding easy not only radiology but also related subjects. Extensive content and topic wise distribution of chapters have given the book an extra edge with such a great presentation. Radiology learning will be fun and interesting in SIR's way. The text in each chapter is very helpful to know the subject and then solving the practice questions is very helpful.
Mainak Mandal
KIMS, Bhubaneshwar

Scan the QR Code to View Sample Pages of the Books

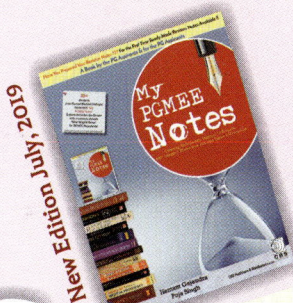

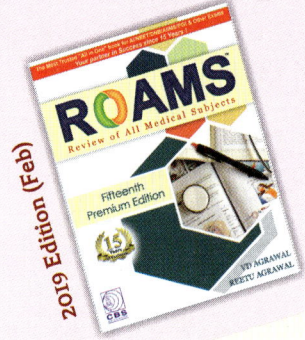
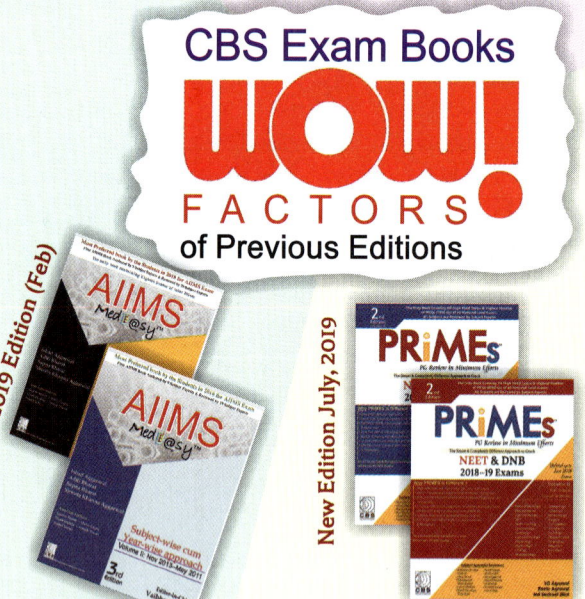

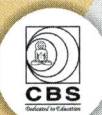
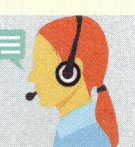

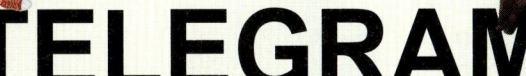

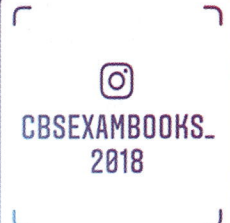

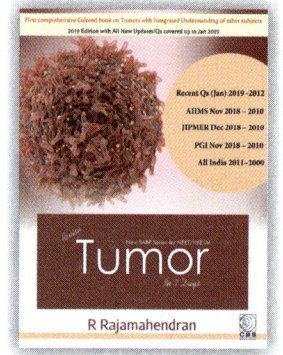
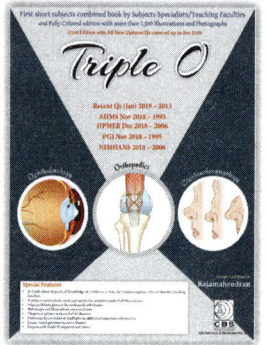
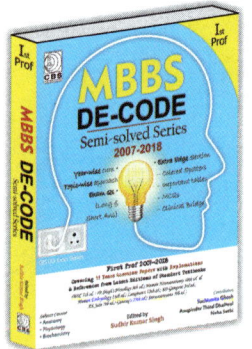
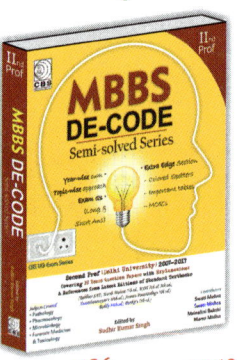
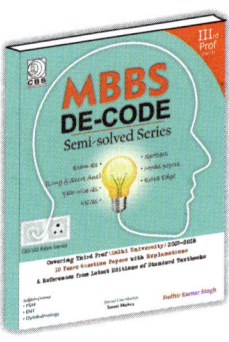
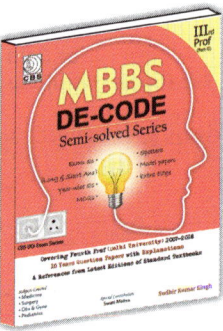
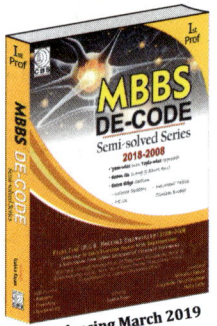
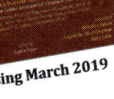
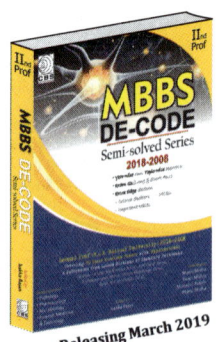
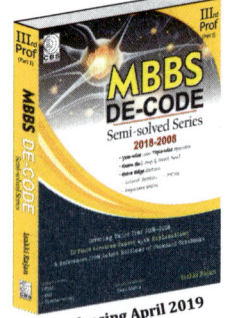
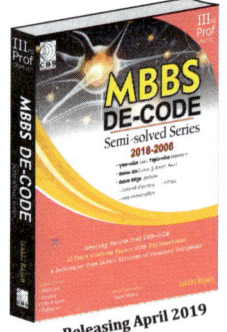